**TEXTBOOK OF SURGERY**

This publication is dedicated to you by

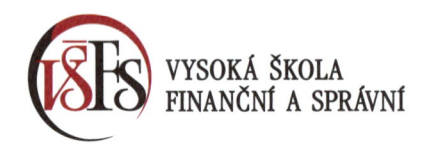

**VYSOKÁ ŠKOLA FINANČNÍ A SPRÁVNÍ**

GENERAL SPONSOR

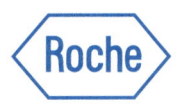

Roche

Coloplast

# TEXTBOOK OF SURGERY

## Current Surgical Diagnosis and Treatment

### Jiří Hoch
MD, PhD
Professor of Surgery
Head, Department of Surgery, 2nd Faculty of Medicine
Charles University, Prague

### Jan Leffler
MD, PhD
Associate Professor of Surgery
Department of Surgery, 2nd Faculty of Medicine
Charles University, Prague

**maxdorf** publishing

## Authors

- **Prof. Jiří Hoch, MD, PhD**
  Dept. of Surgery, 2nd Faculty of Medicine, University Hospital Motol, Charles University, Prague

- **Assoc. Prof. Jan Leffler, MD, PhD**
  Dept. of Surgery, 2nd Faculty of Medicine, University Hospital Motol, Charles University, Prague

All rights reserved.

No part of this publication may be reproduced, stored in a retrieval system or transmitted in any form or by any means electronic, mechanical, photocopying, recording or otherwise, without the prior written permission of the publisher.

Jiří Hoch, Jan Leffler et al.
TEXTBOOK OF SURGERY, Current Surgical Diagnosis and Treatment

Translated from Czech original J. Hoch, J. Leffler a kol. Speciální chirurgie, 3rd edition, Maxdorf Jessenius 2011

Copyright © Jiří Hoch, Jan Leffler 2013
Copyright © Maxdorf 2013
Illustrations © Maxdorf 2013
Cover Layout © Jan Hugo 2013
Cover Photo © iStockphoto/Khonji

**Maxdorf Publishing**, Na Šejdru 247/6a, CZ, 142 00 Prague 4
info@maxdorf.cz, www.maxdorf.cz.

Copy Editor: **Mgr. Jan Lany**
Cover Layout: **Jan Hugo**, Maxdorf Publishing
Typesetting: **Blanka Filounková**, Maxdorf Publishing
Drawings: **Ing. Jaroslav Nachtigall, PhD**, Maxdorf Publishing
Printed in the Czech Republic by **Books print s.r.o.**

ISBN 978-80-7345-375-6

# Co-Authors

- **Petr Bavor, MD**
  Dept. of Surgery, 2nd Faculty of Medicine, University Hospital Motol, Charles University, Prague
- **Prof. Karel Cvachovec, MD, PhD, MBA**
  Dept. of Anaesthesiology and Resuscitation, 2nd Faculty of Medicine, University Hospital Motol, Charles University, Prague
- **Prof. Petr Goetz, MD, PhD**
  Institute of Biology and Medical Genetics, 2nd Faculty of Medicine, University Hospital Motol, Charles University, Prague
- **Ivana Hochová, MD**
  Dept. of Clinical Hematology, University Hospital Motol, Prague
- **Zbyněk Jech, MD**
  Dept. of Surgery, 2nd Faculty of Medicine, University Hospital Motol, Charles University, Prague
- **Prof. Roman Kodet, MD, PhD**
  Institute of Pathology and Molecular Medicine, 2nd Faculty of Medicine, University Hospital Motol, Charles University, Prague
- **Tomáš Krejčí, MD**
  Dept. of Surgery, 2nd Faculty of Medicine, University Hospital Motol, Charles University, Prague
- **Jiří Lisý, MD, PhD**
  Dept. of Imaging Methods, 2nd Faculty of Medicine, Charles University, Prague
- **Jan Neumann, MD, PhD**
  Dept. of Surgery, 2nd Faculty of Medicine, University Hospital Motol, Charles University, Prague
- **Otakar Nyč, MD, PhD**
  Institute of Medical Microbiology, 2nd Faculty of Medicine, University Hospital Motol, Charles University, Prague
- **Filip Pazdírek, MD**
  Dept. of Surgery, 2nd Faculty of Medicine, University Hospital Motol, Charles University, Prague
- **Ronald Pospíšil, MD**
  Dept. of Surgery, Regional Hospital, Kladno
- **Assoc. Prof. Jana Prausová, MD, PhD, MBA**
  Radiotherapeutic-Oncological Dept., University Hospital Motol, Prague
- **Assoc. Prof. Miloslav Roček, MD, PhD, FCIRSE, EBIR**
  Dept. of Imaging Methods, 2nd Faculty of Medicine, University Hospital Motol, Charles University, Prague
- **Jan Schwarz, MD**
  Dept. of Surgery, 2nd Faculty of Medicine, University Hospital Motol, Charles University, Prague
- **Jiří Svoboda, MD**
  Dept. of Surgery, Regional Hospital, Příbram
- **Assoc. Prof. Marek Šetina, MD, PhD**
  Complex Cardiovascular Center, General University Hospital, Prague
- **Assoc. Prof. Jaromír Šimša, MD, PhD**
  Dept. of Surgery, 1st Faculty of Medicine and Thomayer Hospital, Charles University, Prague
- **Jaroslav Špatenka, MD, PhD**
  Center of Transplantation, University Hospital Motol, Prague
- **Assoc. Prof. Michal Tichý, MD, PhD**
  Dept. of Neurosurgery, 2nd Faculty of Medicine, University Hospital Motol, Charles University, Prague
- **Martin Wald, MD, PhD**
  Dept. of Surgery, 2nd Faculty of Medicine, University Hospital Motol, Charles University, Prague

# PREFACE

The idea for this book grew from two earlier efforts (2001, 2003) published in Czech language. In these two editions we tried to develop a treatment of the art of surgery based on understanding the structure and functions of human body and its defects.

During the past ten years, since the last publication of Special Surgery, we got convinced that our effort to present this textbook as an attempt to provide a comprehensive integrated study of human surgery corresponds to the requirements of both undergraduate and postgraduate students is correct. The second edition quickly disappeared from booksellers' shelves and found its readers not only at the 2nd Medical Faculty of Charles University, but, to the delight of its authors and publisher, also among the wide range of medical professionals.

Surgery is a large subject. We have tried to make it more digestible by organizing the text into clearly demarcated sections, using statement headings to define what the reader can find in each section, and identifying important new terms by bold typeface.

This third revised and extended edition has a completely new form. Besides translating the book into English for the benefit of English speaking students, the texts have been updated, illustrations have been re-designed and new chapters have been added. A significant change is the addition of the chapters Cardiovascular Surgery, and Neurosurgery. Newly included in this edition of surgery textbook are brief chapters on anesthesiology, oncology, hematology, microbiology, pathology, genetics, and imaging methods, i.e. the fields related to surgery, without which current surgery might not exist. The themes and extent of these chapters generally correspond to the advancement of respective specializations in the field of surgery.

A new section of the textbook is the picture appendix. We expect that, similarly to the drawings, it will help students to remember at least some surgical findings and will remind them of practices and devices mentioned in the book.

The texts have been prepared in cooperation with a number of professionals from the Clinic of Surgery and other clinics, departments and institutes of the 2nd Medical Faculty of Charles University in Prague-Motol. Despite the fact that the diction of individual authors and their focus on details are different, all of them tried hard to prepare readable, comprehensible and concise texts. Currently, the pace of research in the field of surgery (e.g. transplantations) is extremely rapid, and new information and insights are pouring out of the surgical rooms and laboratories at an almost unimaginable rate. To cope with this flood, students need two tools: a good framework of principles, established by this book, and the ability to use modern informatics.

We owe thanks to Ms. Jana Valterová for her diligent and thorough assistance during the preparation of the textbook. We are indeed grateful for the proof reading of the texts provided by Jan Lány.

Revolutionary times are nothing if not exciting. We have tried to convey the feel of fast-moving research, while providing a description in some depth of the techniques and data that are helping us to understand the evolution, nature and function of human body. This book will have succeeded if readers finish it sharing our excitement and enthusiasm for the continuing voyage of discovery. The journey is far from finished.

We hope that this textbook will be a good aid during the surgery studies, and the basis of surgical knowledge in the medical practice of the students and all other readers.

*Jiří Hoch and Jan Leffler*

# CONTENTS

PREFACE . . . . . . . . . . . . . . . . . . . . . . . . . . . . . . . . . . . . . . . . . . . . . . . . . . . . . . . . . . 6
ABBREVIATIONS . . . . . . . . . . . . . . . . . . . . . . . . . . . . . . . . . . . . . . . . . . . . . . . . . . 15

| | | |
|---|---|---|
| **1** | **NECK SURGERY**  *(Petr Bavor)* . . . . . . . . . . . . . . . . . . . . . . . . . . . . . . . . . . | 19 |
| 1.1 | Neck Cysts, Lymph Nodes . . . . . . . . . . . . . . . . . . . . . . . . . . . . . . . . . . . | 19 |
| 1.2 | Inflammations, Tumors . . . . . . . . . . . . . . . . . . . . . . . . . . . . . . . . . . . . . | 20 |
| 1.3 | Thyroid Gland . . . . . . . . . . . . . . . . . . . . . . . . . . . . . . . . . . . . . . . . . . . . | 21 |
| 1.4 | Parathyroid Glands . . . . . . . . . . . . . . . . . . . . . . . . . . . . . . . . . . . . . . . . | 31 |
| 1.5 | Compressive Neck Syndromes . . . . . . . . . . . . . . . . . . . . . . . . . . . . . . . | 34 |
| | | |
| **2** | **THORACIC SURGERY**  *(Ronald Pospíšil)* . . . . . . . . . . . . . . . . . . . . . . . . . | 35 |
| 2.1 | Thoracic Wall. . . . . . . . . . . . . . . . . . . . . . . . . . . . . . . . . . . . . . . . . . . . . | 35 |
| 2.2 | Pleura. . . . . . . . . . . . . . . . . . . . . . . . . . . . . . . . . . . . . . . . . . . . . . . . . . . | 39 |
| 2.3 | Lungs. . . . . . . . . . . . . . . . . . . . . . . . . . . . . . . . . . . . . . . . . . . . . . . . . . . | 47 |
| 2.4 | Mediastinum . . . . . . . . . . . . . . . . . . . . . . . . . . . . . . . . . . . . . . . . . . . . . | 54 |
| 2.5 | Thoracic Trauma . . . . . . . . . . . . . . . . . . . . . . . . . . . . . . . . . . . . . . . . . . | 57 |
| 2.6 | GI Surgery Using a Thoracic Approach . . . . . . . . . . . . . . . . . . . . . . . . . | 61 |
| | | |
| **3** | **MAMMARY GLAND SURGERY**  *(Martin Wald)* . . . . . . . . . . . . . . . . . . . . | 63 |
| 3.1 | Introduction . . . . . . . . . . . . . . . . . . . . . . . . . . . . . . . . . . . . . . . . . . . . . . | 63 |
| 3.2 | Classification of Breast Diseases. . . . . . . . . . . . . . . . . . . . . . . . . . . . . . | 63 |
| 3.3 | Diagnosis of Breast Diseases . . . . . . . . . . . . . . . . . . . . . . . . . . . . . . . . | 65 |
| 3.4 | TNM Classification of Breast Cancer . . . . . . . . . . . . . . . . . . . . . . . . . . | 70 |
| 3.5 | Breast Cancer Therapy . . . . . . . . . . . . . . . . . . . . . . . . . . . . . . . . . . . . . | 71 |
| 3.6 | Prognosis of Patients with Breast Cancer . . . . . . . . . . . . . . . . . . . . . . | 74 |
| 3.7 | Complications of Surgical Treatment . . . . . . . . . . . . . . . . . . . . . . . . . | 74 |
| 3.8 | Medical Surveillance after Breast Cancer Therapy . . . . . . . . . . . . . . . | 76 |
| 3.9 | Breast Reconstruction after Mastectomy. . . . . . . . . . . . . . . . . . . . . . . | 77 |
| | | |
| **4** | **SOFT TISSUE TUMORS IN ADULTS**  *(Jan Leffler)* . . . . . . . . . . . . . . . . . . | 78 |
| 4.1 | General Characteristics . . . . . . . . . . . . . . . . . . . . . . . . . . . . . . . . . . . . . | 78 |
| 4.2 | Incidence and Localization of Soft Tissue Sarcomas . . . . . . . . . . . . . . | 79 |
| 4.3 | Symptoms of Soft Tissue Sarcomas . . . . . . . . . . . . . . . . . . . . . . . . . . | 79 |
| 4.4 | Diagnostics and Surgical Treatment . . . . . . . . . . . . . . . . . . . . . . . . . . | 79 |
| 4.5 | Conclusions for Clinical Practice . . . . . . . . . . . . . . . . . . . . . . . . . . . . . | 82 |
| | | |
| **5** | **MALIGNANT MELANOMA**  *(Tomáš Krejčí)*. . . . . . . . . . . . . . . . . . . . . . . | 83 |
| 5.1 | Introduction . . . . . . . . . . . . . . . . . . . . . . . . . . . . . . . . . . . . . . . . . . . . . . | 83 |
| 5.2 | Classification, TNM Classification and Staging . . . . . . . . . . . . . . . . . . | 83 |
| 5.3 | Risk Factors, Causes . . . . . . . . . . . . . . . . . . . . . . . . . . . . . . . . . . . . . . . | 85 |
| 5.4 | Diagnostics . . . . . . . . . . . . . . . . . . . . . . . . . . . . . . . . . . . . . . . . . . . . . . | 86 |
| 5.5 | Therapy . . . . . . . . . . . . . . . . . . . . . . . . . . . . . . . . . . . . . . . . . . . . . . . . . | 87 |
| 5.6 | Prognosis . . . . . . . . . . . . . . . . . . . . . . . . . . . . . . . . . . . . . . . . . . . . . . . . | 88 |

# CONTENTS

**6 ABDOMINAL WALL AND HERNIAS** *(Filip Pazdírek)* ........................89
6.1 Hernias..........................................................................89
6.2 Inflammations and Tumors ...........................................94
6.3 Developmental Defects ................................................95

**7 ESOPHAGUS AND DIAPHRAGM SURGERY** *(Ronald Pospíšil)* ..............96
7.1 Esophagus ....................................................................96
7.2 Diaphragmatic Hernias ...............................................105

**8 GASTRIC AND DUODENAL SURGERY** *(Jan Schwarz)* .....................107
8.1 Introduction – Anatomical and Physiological Comments ........107
8.2 Symptomatology of Gastroduodenal Diseases ......108
8.3 Examinations of the Gastroduodenum .....................109
8.4 Gastric and Duodenal Diseases .................................109
8.5 Gastroduodenal Surgical Procedures........................116

**9 SURGERY OF THE SMALL AND LARGE INTESTINES, RECTUM AND ANUS** *(Jiří Hoch)* ..............................................................124
9.1 Anatomical and Functional Notes..............................124
9.2 Symptoms of Intestinal Diseases................................127
9.3 Diagnostic Notes .........................................................128
9.4 Small Intestine.............................................................130
9.5 Large Intestine.............................................................140
9.6 Rectum and Anus.........................................................150

**10 LIVER SURGERY** *(Jan Leffler)* ........................................163
10.1 Symptomatology of Liver Diseases............................163
10.2 Clinical Findings .........................................................164
10.3 Paraclinical Assessments............................................165
10.4 Benign Focal Liver Diseases .......................................166
10.5 Malignant Liver Diseases ...........................................169

**11 GALLBLADDER AND EXTRAHEPATIC BILE DUCTS** *(Jan Leffler)* ............171
11.1 Symptomatology of Gallbladder and Bile Duct Diseases...............172
11.2 Clinical Findings .........................................................173
11.3 Paraclinical Assessments............................................173
11.4 Treatment of Gallbladder and Bile Duct Diseases ...175
11.5 Basic Surgical Procedures in Gallbladder and Bile Ducts ............177
11.6 Prognosis of Patients with Gallbladder and Bile Duct Diseases........179

**12 PORTAL HYPERTENSION** *(Jan Leffler)*................................181
12.1 Types of Portal Hypertension ....................................181
12.2 Pathophysiology of Portal Hypertension..................182
12.3 Symptoms of Portal Hypertension.............................182
12.4 Clinical Findings and Complications of Portal Hypertension...........182
12.5 Diagnostics of Portal Hypertension Complications.....................183
12.6 Bleeding from Esophageal Varices ............................183
12.7 Ascites – Possible Ways of Conservative and Surgical Treatment .......186

# TEXTBOOK OF SURGERY

**13  PANCREAS** *(Jan Leffler)* .......................................... 187
13.1  Symptoms of Pancreatic Diseases ............................... 188
13.2  Clinical Findings in Pancreatic Diseases ........................ 188
13.3  Laboratory Assessments ....................................... 189
13.4  Imaging Methods ............................................. 189
13.5  Acute Pancreatitis ........................................... 191
13.6  Chronic Pancreatitis ......................................... 195
13.7  Cystic Processes of the Pancreas .............................. 199
13.8  Pancreatic Tumors ........................................... 200

**14  SPLEEN SURGERY** *(Jiří Hoch)* ..................................... 205
14.1  Anatomy .................................................... 205
14.2  Function and Physiology of the Spleen ......................... 205
14.3  Splenic Malformations ....................................... 206
14.4  Spleen Surgery .............................................. 206
14.5  Splenomegaly ............................................... 209

**15  ACUTE ABDOMEN IN GENERAL, BASIC DIAGNOSTICS** *(Martin Wald)* ....... 210
15.1  Introduction and Definition .................................. 210
15.2  Classification of Acute Abdomen .............................. 211
15.3  Diagnostics ................................................. 212
15.4  Differential Diagnostics ..................................... 218

**16  ILEUS – INTESTINAL OBSTRUCTION** *(Zbyněk Jech)* .................. 220
16.1  Definition .................................................. 220
16.2  Ileus Classification Based on Its Causes ..................... 220
16.3  Pathophysiology of the Ileus and Ileus Disease Development .... 222
16.4  Symptoms of Ileus ........................................... 223
16.5  Ileus Diagnostics ........................................... 224
16.6  Therapy ..................................................... 227
16.7  Prognosis ................................................... 230

**17  PERITONITIS** *(Jan Leffler)* ..................................... 231
17.1  Definition .................................................. 231
17.2  Pathophysiology of Peritonitis and Sepsis ..................... 232
17.3  Peritonitis Classification ................................... 233
17.4  Clinical Symptoms ........................................... 234
17.5  Paraclinical Diagnostics .................................... 236
17.6  Indications for Surgical Treatment ........................... 237
17.7  Peritonitis Therapy ......................................... 238
17.8  Prognosis in Patients with Peritonitis ....................... 241

**18  ABDOMINAL TRAUMA** *(Jiří Hoch)* .................................. 242
18.1  Introduction ................................................ 242
18.2  Liver Injuries .............................................. 245
18.3  Splenic Injuries ............................................ 248

**19  GIT HEMORRHAGE** *(Jan Schwarz)* .................................. 249
19.1  Upper GIT Hemorrhage ........................................ 251
19.2  Lower GIT Hemorrhage ........................................ 254

| | | |
|---|---|---|
| **20** | **MINI-INVASIVE SURGERY** *(Jiří Svoboda)* | 255 |
| 20.1 | Laparoscopic Cholecystectomy | 258 |
| 20.2 | Laparoscopic Appendectomy | 260 |
| 20.3 | Laparoscopic Inguinal Hernioplasty | 261 |
| 20.4 | Gastroesophageal Reflux Disease and Hiatal Hernias | 262 |
| 20.5 | Laparoscopic Colorectal Procedures | 262 |
| 20.6 | Diagnostic and Therapeutic Thoracoscopy | 263 |
| 20.7 | The Future of Minimally Invasive Therapy | 264 |
| | | |
| **21** | **VASCULAR SURGERY** *(Marek Šetina)* | 265 |
| 21.1 | Introduction | 265 |
| 21.2 | History of the Discipline | 265 |
| 21.3 | Vascular Replacement and Sutures | 266 |
| 21.4 | Acute Arterial Closures (Outline) | 271 |
| 21.5 | Chronic Arterial Closures | 274 |
| 21.6 | Large Vessel Injuries | 275 |
| 21.7 | Individual Large Vessel Affections | 277 |
| 21.8 | Vascular Approaches for Hemodialysis | 296 |
| | | |
| **22** | **CARDIAC SURGERY** *(Marek Šetina)* | 298 |
| 22.1 | Introduction | 298 |
| 22.2 | Cardiac Surgery in History and Present Days | 298 |
| 22.3 | Principle of Extracorporeal Circulation | 300 |
| 22.4 | Preoperative Examinations | 301 |
| 22.5 | Surgical Approaches in Cardiac Surgery | 302 |
| 22.6 | Coronary Artery Disease | 302 |
| 22.7 | Valvular Defects | 308 |
| 22.8 | Aneurysm of the Thoracic Aorta | 317 |
| 22.9 | Aortic Dissection | 318 |
| 22.10 | Cardiac Tumors | 319 |
| 22.11 | Surgical Treatment of Arrhythmias | 319 |
| 22.12 | Mini-invasive Procedures in Cardiac Surgery | 320 |
| 22.13 | Heart Transplantation, Mechanical Cardiac Supports | 321 |
| 22.14 | Heart Injuries | 321 |
| 22.15 | Congenital Cardiac Defects | 323 |
| | | |
| **23** | **NEUROSURGERY** *(Michal Tichý)* | 328 |
| 23.1 | Craniocerebral Injuries | 328 |
| 23.2 | Spine and Spinal Cord Injuries | 333 |
| 23.3 | Peripheral Nerve Injuries | 334 |
| 23.4 | Degenerative Spinal Disorders | 335 |
| 23.5 | Constriction Syndromes | 338 |
| 23.6 | CNS Congenital Anomalies and Hydrocephalus | 338 |
| 23.7 | Infectious Diseases of the CNS | 342 |
| 23.8 | Vascular Brain Diseases | 344 |
| 23.9 | Brain Tumors | 347 |
| 23.10 | Surgical Treatment of Epilepsy | 356 |

| | | |
|---|---|---|
| 24 | **MODERN TECHNIQUES OF CUTTING, DISSECTION, COAGULATION, HEMOSTASIS, SUTURE AND TISSUE ADHESION, VISCEROSYNTHESIS** *(Jiří Hoch)* | 358 |
| 25 | **ORGAN TRANSPLANTATION** *(Jaroslav Špatenka)* | 361 |
| 25.1 | Introduction | 361 |
| 25.2 | Issues of Organ Donation – Multi Organ Harvesting | 365 |
| 25.3 | Kidney Transplantation | 371 |
| 25.4 | Liver Transplantation | 373 |
| 25.5 | Heart Transplantation | 375 |
| 25.6 | Lung Transplantation | 380 |
| 25.7 | Pancreas Transplantation | 382 |
| 25.8 | Intestinal Transplantation and Multi Organ Transplantation | 384 |
| 25.9 | Immunosuppression and Complications of Organ Transplantations | 384 |
| 25.10 | Future of Organ Transplantation | 386 |
| 26 | **SENTINEL LYMPH NODES** *(Jaromír Šimša)* | 388 |
| 26.1 | Introduction | 388 |
| 26.2 | Possibilities of Detection of Sentinel Lymph Nodes | 389 |
| 26.3 | Importance of the Method in Particular Tumors | 389 |
| 26.4 | In Vitro Examination | 390 |
| 27 | **BARIATRIC SURGERY** *(Jiří Hoch)* | 391 |
| 27.1 | Definition of Obesity | 391 |
| 27.2 | Treatment of Obesity | 392 |
| 28 | **INTENSIVE CARE IN SURGERY** *(Jan Neumann)* | 395 |
| 28.1 | Postoperative Monitoring | 396 |
| 28.2 | Monitoring the Cardiovascular System | 397 |
| 28.3 | Monitoring the Respiratory System | 397 |
| 28.4 | Examination of Blood Gases and Acid-Base Homeostasis | 399 |
| 28.5 | Consciousness | 399 |
| 29 | **PERIOPERATIVE NUTRITION** *(Jan Neumann)* | 400 |
| 29.1 | Enteral Nutrition | 400 |
| 29.2 | Parenteral Nutrition | 402 |
| 30 | **INFECTION IN SURGERY, ANTIBIOTIC THERAPY AND PROPHYLAXIS** *(Otakar Nyč)* | 405 |
| 30.1 | Surgical Site Infection | 405 |
| 30.2 | Classification of SSI | 406 |
| 30.3 | Microbiology of SSI | 406 |
| 30.4 | Classification of Operative Wounds According to the Risk of SSI | 406 |
| 30.5 | Risk Factors for the Development of SSI | 407 |
| 30.6 | Microbiological Diagnostics of SSI | 407 |
| 30.7 | Antibiotic Use in the Treatment of SSI | 408 |
| 30.8 | Principles of Antibiotic Prophylaxis during Surgical Procedures | 411 |

## CONTENTS

| | | |
|---|---|---|
| **31** | **HEMATOLOGICAL ISSUES IN SURGERY** *(Ivana Hochová)* | 413 |
| 31.1 | Antithrombotic Prophylaxis in Surgery | 413 |
| 31.2 | Operation on Patients Receiving Chronic Anticoagulant and Antiaggregant Therapy | 414 |
| 31.3 | Surgical Treatment in Patients with Neutropenia and Thrombocytopenia | 416 |
| 31.4 | Significant Acquired Bleeding Disorders in Surgical Patients | 417 |
| 31.5 | Splenectomy and its Management | 419 |
| **32** | **ANESTHESIOLOGY AND RESUSCITATION IN SURGERY** *(Karel Cvachovec)* | 420 |
| 32.1 | Terminology Used | 421 |
| 32.2 | Anesthesiological Techniques | 421 |
| 32.3 | The Most Widely Used Pharmaceuticals | 423 |
| 32.4 | Providing for Anesthesiological Care | 424 |
| 32.5 | Collective Cooperation with the Anesthesiologist | 429 |
| **33** | **MULTIMODAL ONCOLOGICAL TREATMENT** *(Jana Prausová)* | 431 |
| 33.1 | Surgical Treatment | 432 |
| 33.2 | Chemotherapy | 433 |
| 33.3 | Radiotherapy | 434 |
| 33.4 | Hormonal Therapy | 435 |
| 33.5 | Biological Targeted Therapy | 436 |
| **34** | **TUMOR GENETICS** *(Petr Goetz)* | 437 |
| 34.1 | Hereditary Non-Polyposis Colorectal Cancer (HNPCC, Lynch Syndrome) | 439 |
| 34.2 | Familial Adenomatous Polyposis (FAP) | 440 |
| 34.3 | Hereditary Breast and Ovarian Cancer Syndrome | 441 |
| 34.4 | Multiple Endocrine Neoplasia Type 1 (MEN 1 Syndrome) | 442 |
| 34.5 | Multiple Endocrine Neoplasia Type 2 (MEN 2 Syndrome) | 443 |
| 34.6 | Medullary Thyroid Carcinoma (MTC) and MEN 2 Syndromes | 443 |
| **35** | **PATHOLOGY** *(Roman Kodet)* | 445 |
| 35.1 | The Discipline of Pathology in Surgery | 445 |
| 35.2 | Autopsy | 445 |
| 35.3 | Bioptic Pathology | 446 |
| 35.4 | Generalization of Optimum Practice in Clinical Pathology | 455 |
| **36** | **IMAGING METHODS IN SURGERY** *(Miloslav Roček, Jiří Lisý)* | 457 |
| 36.1 | Radiodiagnostics | 457 |
| 36.2 | Interventional Radiology | 469 |
| **IMAGING METHODS IN SURGERY – GALLERY** | | 473 |
| **COLOR IMAGE GALLERY** | | 505 |
| **AUTHORS** | | 567 |
| **INDEX** | | 577 |

# ABBREVIATIONS

AA .................................. acute abdomen
ABCDE rule ..................... Asymmetry, Border, Color, Diameter, Enlarging
ACB ................................. aortocoronary bypass
ACD ................................. right coronary artery
ACS ................................. left coronary artery; acute coronary syndrome
AF ................................... atrial fibrillation
ANC ................................ absolute neutrophil count
AP ................................... acute pancreatitis
APC ................................. argon-plasma coagulation
APE ................................. appendectomy
AR ................................... radial artery
ARDS ............................... acute respiratory distress syndrome
ARU ................................ Anesthesiology and Resuscitation Unit
ASA ................................. American Society of Anesthesiologists
AV ................................... atrioventricular
AVM ................................ arteriovenous malformation
BMI ................................. body mass index
BP ................................... blood pressure
CAD ................................ coronary artery disease
CFA ................................. common femoral artery
CKTCH ............................. Centrum kardiovaskulární a transplantační chirurgie
CNS ................................. central nervous system
COMECON ...................... Council for Mutual Economic Assistance
CPAP ............................... continuous positive airway pressure
CRC ................................. colorectal cancer
CRP ................................. C-reactive protein
CT ................................... computed tomography
CTS ................................. carpal tunnel syndrome
CVA ................................ cerebrovascular accident
CVP ................................. central venous pressure
ČTS ................................. Česká transplantační společnost
DCC ................................ deleted in colorectal carcinoma
DGHAL ............................ Doppler-guided hemorrhoidal artery ligation
DIC ................................. disseminated intravascular coagulopathy
DNET ............................... dysembryoplastic neuroepithelial tumor
DSA ................................ digital subtraction angiography
EC ................................... extracorporeal circulation
ECG ................................ electrocardiography
EEA ................................. entero-enteroanastomosis
EF ................................... ejection fraction
EGFR and VEGF ................ growth factor receptors
ECHO .............................. echocardiography
EMG ................................ electromyography
EO ................................... endocrine orbitopathy
EPT ................................. endoscopic papillotomy
ERCP ............................... endoscopic retrograde cholangiopancreatography
ES ................................... esophageal sphincter

| | |
|---|---|
| EUS | endosonography |
| FAP | familial adenomatous polyposis |
| FBSS | back surgery syndrome |
| FMTC | familial MTC |
| FNAB | fine needle aspiration biopsy |
| FNH | focal nodular hyperplasia |
| FOBT | fecal occult blood |
| fT3 | triiodothyronine |
| fT4 | thyroxine |
| FW | Fahraeus-Westergren (test) |
| GCS | Glasgow coma scale |
| GEA | gastroenteroanastomoses |
| GER | gastroesophageal reflux |
| GERD | gastroesophageal reflux disease |
| GIST | gastrointestinal stromal tumors |
| GIT | gastrointestinal tract |
| GM | glioblastoma multiforme |
| GSV | great saphenous vein |
| HBD | heart-beating donors |
| HCC | hepatocellular carcinoma |
| HNPCC | hereditary nonpolyposis colorectal cancer |
| HR | heart rate |
| ICU | Intensive Care Unit |
| IE | infectious endocarditis |
| ICH | intracerebral hematoma |
| IKEM | Institute of Clinical and Experimental Medicine (Prague) |
| IMA | internal mammary artery |
| IPAA | ileal-pouch anal anastomosis |
| IPC | idiopathic proctocolitis |
| ITA | internal thoracic artery |
| KST | Coordinating Transplant Centre (Koordinační středisko tansplantací) |
| LA | left atrium |
| LMWH | low-molecular-weight heparin |
| LT | total lobectomy |
| MALT | mucosa associated lymphoid tissue |
| MAP | MYH associated polyposis |
| MAP | mean arterial pressure |
| MEN | multiple endocrine neoplasia |
| MI | myocardial infarction |
| MIBI | methoxyisobutylisonitrile |
| MIDCAB | minimally invasive direct coronary artery bypass |
| MIU | international units |
| MODS | multiple organ dysfunction syndrome |
| MOF | multiple organ failure |
| MOH | multi organ (multiple organ) harvesting |
| MRCP | magnetic resonance cholangiopancreatography |
| MRI | magnetic resonance imaging |
| MRM | magnetic resonance mammography |
| MRSA | methicillin resistant Staphylococcus aureus |
| MTC | medullary thyroid carcinoma |
| NG | nasogastric |
| NHBD | non-heart-beating donors |

# ABBREVIATIONS

| | |
|---|---|
| NMM | nodular melanoma |
| NMR | nuclear magnetic resonance |
| NOTES | natural orifice transluminal endoscopic surgery |
| NRL | laryngeal recurrent nerve |
| NSAID | non-steroid antirheumatics |
| OCHG | optochiasmatic-hypothalamic gliomas |
| OPSI | overwhelming post splenectomy infection |
| PCA | patient controlled analgesia |
| PEEP | positive end expiratory pressure |
| PEG | percutaneous endoscopic gastrostomy |
| PET | positron emission tomography |
| PMPS | postmastectomy pain syndrome |
| PNO | pneumothorax |
| PTA | percutaneous transluminar angioplasty |
| PTC | percutaneous transhepatic cholangiography |
| PTD | percutaneous transhepatic drainage |
| RC | ramus circumflexus |
| RES | reticuloendothelial system |
| RET | rearranged during transfection |
| RFA | radiofrequency ablation |
| RIA | ramus interventricularis anterior |
| RIND | reversible ischemic neurological deficit |
| SAH | subarachnoid hemorrhage |
| SILS | single incision laparoscopic surgery |
| SIRS | surrounding fatty tissue, inducing generalized inflammatory response |
| SLN | sentinel lymph node |
| SND | sentinel lymph node dissection |
| SPECT | single photon emission computed tomography |
| SSI | surgical site infection |
| SSM | superficial spreading melanoma |
| STE | subtotal resection of the thyroid gland |
| TAPP | transabdominal preperitoneal plasty |
| TBC | tuberculosis |
| TEM | total mesorectal excision |
| TEP | total extraperitoneal plasty |
| TgAK | antibodies against thyroglobulin |
| TIA | transitory ischemic attack |
| TIPS | transjugular intrahepatic portosystemic shunt |
| TIPSS | transjugular Intrahepatic portosystemic stent shunt |
| TNF | tumor necrosis factor |
| TOS | thoracic outlet syndrome |
| TRAK | antibodies against a TSH-receptor |
| TRAM | transverse rectus abdominus myocutaneous |
| TSH | thyroidea stimulating hormone |
| TTE | total thyroidectomy |
| US | ultrasound |
| USS | ulnar sulcus syndrome |
| VAC | vacuum assisted closure |
| VAS | visual analog scale |
| VATS | video-assisted thoracoscopy |
| VTE | venous thromboembolism |
| WL | waiting lists |

# 1  NECK SURGERY

> 1.1  Neck Cysts, Lymph Nodes
> 1.2  Inflammations, Tumors
> 1.3  Thyroid Gland
> 1.4  Parathyroid Glands
> 1.5  Compressive Neck Syndromes

## 1.1  Neck Cysts, Lymph Nodes

In terms of neck organ diseases, surgical treatment in this region pertains to neck cysts, thyroid diseases, inflammations and lymphadenopathies.

**Medial neck cysts** are formed from the thyroglossal duct, the embryonic route of the descending thyroid gland, whose base develops in the area of the foramen cecum of the tongue. The thyroglossal duct is commonly obliterated to form a fibrous band, or it persists less commonly as a cranial projection from the thyroid gland isthmus as the pyramidal lobe. When the cranial part fails to close, an inner fistula develops, i.e. an opening at the tongue root. Retention of its content leads to the formation of a cystic structure under the skin on the hyoid bone level. The cyst may perforate and appear outside due to secondary infection or trauma, thus leading to formation of a complete medial fistula. As for differential diagnostics, medial cysts may be represented by a dermoid cyst or, more rarely, an ectopic thyroid gland, which may be the single tissue of the thyroid gland. Unless the tumor exhibits clear cystic characteristics, scintigraphy focused on the thyroid gland should be performed before surgical treatment. Medial cysts are excised together with the medium part of the hyoid bone, while ligating the inner mouth. A relapse may occur upon incomplete removal.

**Lateral neck cysts** are formed from the persisting thymopharyngeal duct. They have two mouths: The inner mouth is found on the arch of the soft palate, and cysts run along the inner carotid artery, while the outer mouth is found in the sternoclavicular fossa, at the medial edge of the sternocleidomastoid muscle. More commonly, lateral fistulas are incomplete. Radical excision should be performed in lateral neck fistulas during the first year of life, before the cyst becomes infected.

**Cystic hygroma colli** are polycystic structures filled with thin liquid, formed from the rudiment of the embryonic lymph sac. They are usually located on the lateral side of the neck below the mandible. Cranially, they may reach from the floor of the mouth up to the tongue, and caudally up to the axilla. Hygroma symptoms depend on the size and localization. A hygroma becomes hazardous in cases where it spreads on the tongue and in the mediastinum, which is manifested by dyspnoea. The treatment is based on extirpation as soon as possible after birth.

**Lymphadenopathy** – a neck lymph node disorder – is affected by primary and secondary (metastases) tumors or manifestation of a system disease. It may be benign or malignant.

Lymphadenities, as a response to acute inflammations in the surrounding areas, are the main benign cause of neck lymph node enlargement. The main malignant cause of neck lymphadenopathy consists in cancer metastases that stem from tumors of the pharynx, larynx, trachea, esophagus, bronchi, digestive tract (Virchow's node – in the supraclavicular region on the left) and the thyroid gland. Malignant involvement of neck lymph nodes usually occurs with a lymphoma – Hodgkin's lymphogranulomatosis.

Surgical removal of the node for histological assessment is essential in differential diagnostics of neck lymphadenopathies.

## 1.2 Inflammations, Tumors

**Carbuncle** (carbunculus nuchae) is a typical inflammatory manifestation in the neck area. Most often, it develops in diabetics through the fusion of several furuncles, reaching deep down to the solid fascia. It tends to be highly painful; the solid fibrous subcutis and fascia prevent the inflammation and edema from spreading in the area. It is treated by wide excision of the inflammatory tissue up to the fascia. The defect is left to heal **per secundam**. A less radical method consists in a wide cross incision, always in connection with antibiotic treatment.

Deep **phlegmones** occur rarely, and they may originate from oral cavity diseases, a penetrating injury of the pharynx, esophagus, trachea or an advanced purulent inflammation of neck lymph nodes. These inflammations put the patient at risk of a septic condition or involvement of important neck structures (blood vessels, trachea, etc.), particularly upon late diagnosis. The condition is treated surgically by opening the lesion, draining it and administrating antibiotics.

As for benign tumors, fibromas and lipomas, felt as palpable resistances, predominate; often they are asymptomatic. Surgical extirpation is used to manage the condition. Histological assessment is always needed.

**Primary malignant tumors** affecting the area of the neck include particularly **thyroid and larynx cancers** and they are discussed in respective chapters. **Secondary tumors** affect the entire lymphatic system.

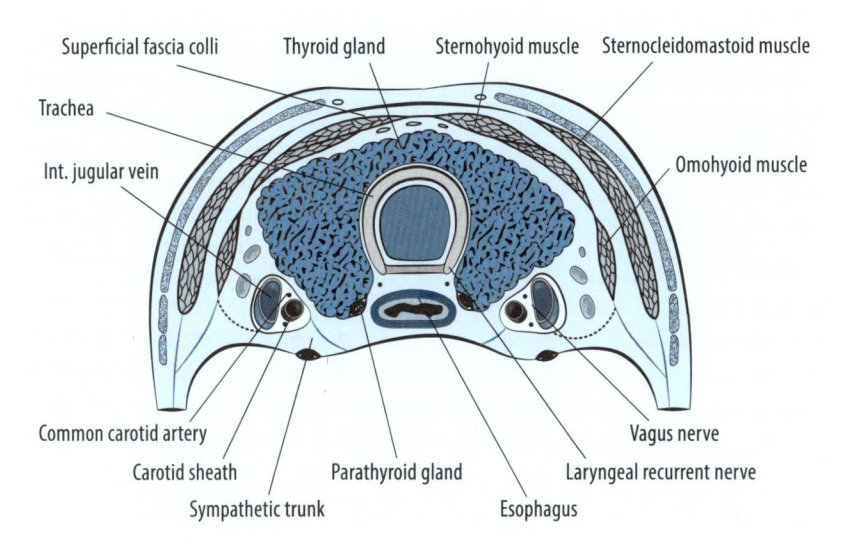

Fig. 1.1 *Cross-section of the neck at the height of the thyroid gland*

## 1.3 Thyroid Gland

The thyroid gland is butterfly-shaped and consists of two lobes connected with an isthmus of varied width. The thyroid gland is located ventrally and laterally from the trachea and the larynx. The isthmus is found on the level of the 2nd and 3rd annular cartilages. The non-constant pyramidal lobe runs cranially from the isthmus and is an embryonic residue of the thyroglossal duct. Nutrition for the thyroid gland is ensured by superior thyroid arteries (the first branch of the external carotid artery) and inferior thyroid arteries (originating in the thyrocervical trunk). Venous outflow is directed to the internal jugular vein. Lymph drainage reaches the pre- and paratracheal nodes first (the central group), then nodes along the internal jugular vein (lateral group) and the upper mediastinum. Parathyroid glands are found in the immediate vicinity of the thyroid gland, ventromedially, and recurrent nerves run dorsolaterally in the tracheoesophageal sulcus. Anatomical conditions and relationships are illustrated in Figs. 1.1, 1.2, and 1.3.

### 1.3.1 Symptoms

The symptoms of thyroid disorders are **local** – conditioned by anatomical changes of the gland, associated with pressure exerted on the surrounding structures (neck "enlargement", a feeling of pressure, difficult swallowing, respiration disorders, pain, and voice disorders) – and **general**, caused by a functional disorder of the gland. Functional disorders of the thyroid gland are manifested as hypo-

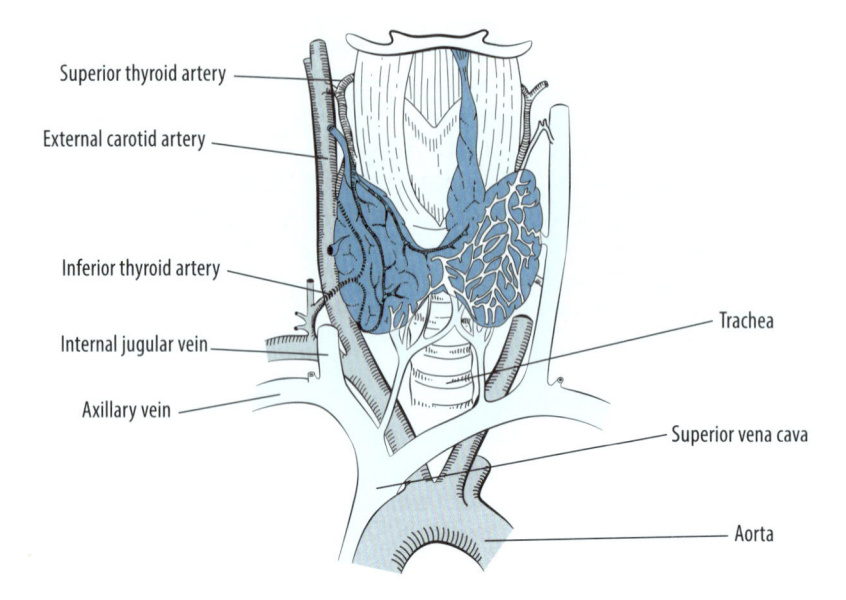

**Fig. 1.2** *Anatomical situation of the thyroid gland – vascular supply*

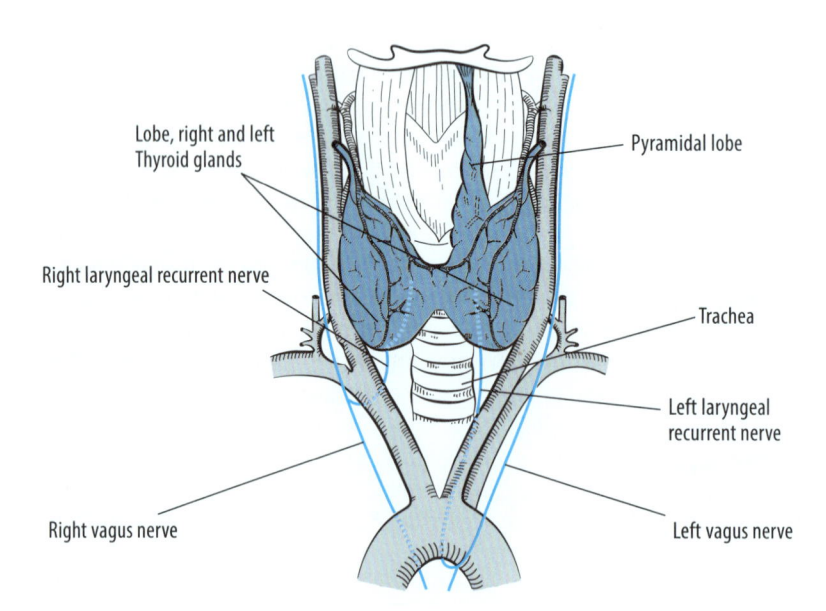

**Fig. 1.3** *Anatomical situation of the thyroid gland – course of recurrent nerve*

thyroidism or hyperthyroidism. Typical symptoms of **hyperthyroidism** include intermittent heart pounding (palpitations), rhythm disorders, heat flushes, unrest, nervousness, emotional lability, heat intolerance, increased sweating, weight loss with preserved appetite, fatigue, insomnia, eye problems, and crural swelling. Typical symptoms of **hypothyroidism** include cold intolerance, feeling tired, and sleeppiness often. In addition, slowness can be observed (up to lethargy), weight gain, constipation, and development of dry, scaly, doughy skin (pretibial myxedema).

### 1.3.2 Assessment

The following factors are assessed during physical examination: The size, movability, concurrent movement with swallowing, pain, elasticity of the tissue and its consistency, presence of nodules and any possible enlargement of lymph nodes in the surrounding areas. The stages (Tab. 1.1) are assessed based on the goiter size during physical examination.

**Sonography** can be used to determine the size or volume of the thyroid gland, its boundaries and relationship to the surrounding structures. This method is most valuable to determine any nodules, which may be benign adenomas with normal or impaired function or regressive changes, focal inflammations or malignancies. Blood flow through the gland can be assessed using sonography, which is important for more detailed assessment of hyperfunctional goiters. Compared to assessments using palpation, sonography provides higher sensitivity when examining nodules in the middle and lateral compartments.

**Scintigraphy** is a method used to determine functional topography of the thyroid gland. Today, the increasing quality of sonographic examination has pushed scintigraphy aside; in practice, this method is now used only where a gland rebuilt in terms of hyperfunction and nodules is examined. Scintigraphy is of crucial importance when it comes to determining residual tissue of the thyroid gland after surgery due to cancer before administration of a therapeutic dose of radioiodine.

**CT examination** of the thyroid gland is indicated in cases where a retrosternal goiter is suspected. This method makes it possible to assess the relationship of the gland to mediastinal organs, given that the mediastinum is not accessible for

Table 1.1 Goiter size stages (WHO)

| Stage | Characteristics |
| --- | --- |
| 0 | No goiter (i.e. not palpable, invisible) |
| I | Palpable small goiter, visible only with the head bent backward |
| II | Clearly visible and palpable goiter – without the head bent backward |
| III | Clearly visible goiter also from a distance (including retrosternal propagation) |

sonography. It is also important in the preoperative consideration of the possible need of a thyroidectomy or a sternotomy.

**SPECT/CT** – Computer-processed recording of an isotope examination combined with conventional computed tomography. This imaging technique, used from 2005, provides a combination of the advantages of both afore-mentioned examinations. It is important particularly for reoperations of a thyroid gland.

**Fine Needle Aspiration Biopsy – FNAB** is used to verify the biological nature of the nodules in the thyroid gland, e.g. whether the changes are benign, regressive, inflammatory or clearly malignant or whether malignancy is only suspected based on any cell atypia found.

**As for laboratory parameters** used to assess thyroid function from peripheral blood, examination of basal **TSH** – thyroidea stimulating hormone in the serum – is the most important. A normal TSH value corresponds to normal function of the thyroid gland. Hyperthyroidism is associated with decreased TSH values, while increased TSH values are indicative of hypothyroidism. Determination of free **thyroxine (fT4) and triiodothyronine (fT3)** serum levels is used for accurate determination of peripheral function. A reduced T4 level is indicative of hypothyroidism, while T3 elevation is used to determine hyperthyroidism (including the grade).

**Indirect laryngoscopy** used to assess vocal cord function in order to demonstrate proper recurrent nerve innervation is a typical examination before any surgery. Any changes of the voice and in the vocal cords cannot be accurately assessed based on clinical examination (auscultation).

Determination of **calcium** serum levels is used to assess the function of parathyroid glands.

A radiographic scan of the upper thoracic aperture, used often in the past, is not necessary given that more detailed information on the finding is provided by sonography.

### 1.3.3 Eufunctional Goiter

Diffuse or nodular enlargement of the thyroid gland with no change in its function is denoted as an eufunctional goiter. It does not include inflammation or malignancy, and in most cases it is caused by a lack in iodine – an endemic goiter. Women are affected approximately 7 times more often than men. Diffuse eufunctional goiters are not encountered very often in the Czech Republic. In children and young adults, the reduction of the size of the gland may be achieved by administration of a therapeutic dose of iodine and thyroid hormones. Usually no surgery is required.

A large goiter, i.e. grade II and higher (see Tab. 1.1), often multi-nodular, is an indication for surgery. The indication is supported by symptoms – feeling of pressure and tension in the neck, worsened respiration, and unresponsiveness of the goiter to suppressive treatment. Pressure exerted on the trachea leads to its narrowing, stenosis associated with respiratory problems; pressure exerted on the esophagus is the cause of dysphagias; and pressure exerted on large blood vessels makes venous return more difficult and may become the cause of superior vena cava syndrome. The so-called **mechanical syndrome** is associated predominantly with retrosternal goiters.

Diagnostic explanation of the nature of a solitary node is of primary importance. Such nodules may be solid adenomas (colloid nodules, follicular neoplasia, and autonomous adenomas), regressive changes or cysts, and also malignant tumors. More malignant tumors are found in childhood age and in adolescents, therefore indications for surgery are more numerous in these populations, even if no clear confirmation of a malignant tumor can be obtained based on preoperative examination. The suspicion of malignancy rises with the following constellation of findings – hypoechogenity based on sonography and a cold nodule based on scintigraphy.

### 1.3.4 Hyperthyroidism

**Two terms are distinguished:**
- **Hyperthyroidism** – elevated production of thyroid hormones determined from peripheral blood
- **Thyrotoxicosis** – harmful effect of elevated hormonal levels on peripheral organs

Elevated function of the thyroid gland is characterized by a pathologically increased effect of hormones in the periphery. Women are affected 5–8 times more often and all age categories show the same incidence. Any deviation in the size, structure and biological nature of the thyroid gland may be associated with hyperthyroidism. In clinical practice, patients are symptomatic, i.e. patients with thyrotoxicosis, in virtually all cases.

Thyrotoxicosis is classified as follows:
- **Autonomous,** more frequent in endemic regions
- **Autoimmune,** in other than endemic regions, thus also **in the Czech Republic**

#### IMMUNOGENIC THYROTOXICOSIS

Immunogenic thyrotoxicosis (Graves-Basedow disease) is a genetically conditioned disease and various factors are involved in its clinical manifestation, e.g., smoking, stress and other influences of the environment. Antibodies (IgG) against individual components of the thyroid gland are formed. Antibodies against the TSH-receptor, thyrocyte, usually have a stimulating, less often attenuating effect on the growth of the gland and on hormonal production. Upon stimulation, a **diffuse goiter and hyperfunction** develop sooner or later. Antibodies against a TSH-receptor (TRAK), against microsomal thyroidal antigens (antibodies against peroxidases TPO/MAK), and against thyroglobulin (TgAK) are most commonly determined. The clinical image includes concurrent findings of **endocrine orbitopathy (EO)** and **circumscriptive myxedema**, in addition to general manifestations of thyrotoxicosis (tachycardia, palpitations, etc., see above). The same antibodies (TRAK, TPO, and TgAK) seem to participate in formation of the goiter as well as in goiter development. EO may develop before, concurrently with or even later than a goiter with thyrotoxicosis.

Initially, immunogenic thyrotoxicosis is **treated conservatively**. Administration of **thyrostatics** suppresses the manifestations of hyperfunction. It has no effect on antibody levels or on the components of the gland and orbital inflammation. Remission may occur in the course of 6 to 12 months. Sometimes, antibody levels also drop temporarily after thyrostatic therapy. More often – in about 60–80% of cases – a relapse should be expected. Therefore definitive, ablative therapy is preferred for long-term success – **surgery or radioiodine application**.

### AUTONOMOUS THYROTOXICOSIS

Thyroidal autonomy usually occurs in 3 forms:
- **Unifocal** (autonomous, independent – toxic – adenoma)
- **Multifocal**, often associated with a polynodous goiter
- **Diffuse toxicosis** with diffuse involvement of the whole gland where its differentiation from immunogenic hyperthyroidism is difficult

The signs of thyrotoxicosis may be missing until hormonal production in thyroidal autonomy does not exceed the needs of the body. Every increase in iodine intake (food, medications, and contrast agents) increases the risk of thyrotoxicosis manifestation. Although thyrotoxicosis may be removed temporarily by conservative therapy in thyroidal autonomy, the effect is never long-term. Reducing or ablative therapy is the definitive measure. If no contraindications are known, **surgery** should be preferred to **radioiodine therapy** for its fast and reliable effect.

The scope of the surgical procedures include: Lobectomy for a solitary toxic adenoma, total thyroidectomy for diffuse involvement, i.e. bilateral complete removal of the parenchyma.

Before surgery on any type of toxic goiter, the symptoms of elevated thyroid function must be removed using medicamentous therapy. Thyrostatics are usually used, often with an addition of beta-blockers for effect on the periphery. High iodine doses in the form of Lugol's solution are now used only sporadically as part of preoperative preparation.

**Thyrotoxic crisis** is a life threatening condition caused by the escalation of thyrotoxicosis symptoms. Formerly, it appeared in connection with insufficient preparation of the patient for surgery due to thyrotoxicosis, occasionally after a narcosis, in connection with an overlooked disease of the thyroid gland, often after iodine contamination, for example, during contrast radiography. Alarming symptoms include **tachycardia** with threatening cardiac failure, high **fever**, adynamia, confusion and **somnolence or even coma**. Therapy consists in administration of high doses of thyrostatics, sedatives, liquids, antipyretics and beta-blockers. Today, thyrotoxic crisis very rarely occurs.

## 1.3.5 Malignant Tumors of the Thyroid Gland

Malignant tumors of the thyroid gland represent 1% of all malignancies. According to histological findings, they are highly varied and differ considerably in terms of therapy success and prognosis. Each stage is described based on the TNM system.

As to frequency, **differentiated cancer**, mostly papillary, predominates **in 70–80%** of cases. **Papillary carcinoma** affects particularly younger age categories, and is not rare even in children and adolescents. It tends to development as early **metastases in regional neck lymph nodes** – lymphogenic metastases, spreading to the periphery in the hematogenic mode only at a significantly later stage. The prognosis is favorable when treated in early stages, with long survival even with metastases present. Incidences of papillary cancer have been rising in the population.

**Follicular carcinoma** is typical for middle age patients. It exhibits hematogenic formation of metastases, particularly in the **lungs and bones**. The prognosis is worse than that of papillary carcinoma.

**Anaplastic carcinoma** is a non-differentiated structure cancer that grows rapidly and invasively, fails to respect organ boundaries, grows through the trachea, larynx, esophagus or large neck blood vessels, forming metastases quickly. The chance for healing is very small. This type of cancer leads to death in the course of several months, similarly to rare **sarcomas** of the thyroid gland.

**Medullar carcinoma** is a special kind of tumor that stems from C-cells (i.e. parafollicular cells) of the thyroid gland. It produces calcitonin that can be determined as a marker in the serum. Medullar cancer is sporadic and hereditary. Prognosis of a hereditary tumor is more favorable than in a sporadic one; however, generally worse than in differentiated types of thyroid cancer. All tend to develop lymphogenic metastases. Missing or present metastases at the beginning of therapy are decisive for therapeutic prospects and survival.

**Total thyroidectomy** is the basic therapeutic principle for differentiated thyroid tumors. This procedure is the only one to reach radicality in tumors that may be multicentric. Elimination of all tissue of the thyroid gland makes it possible to administer further therapy – radioiodine in radiosensitive papillary and follicular carcinoma. Neck lymph nodes affected by metastases are removed using radical **en bloc resection of the lymph nodes** in various modifications. Malignant tumors of the thyroid gland are not sensitive to chemotherapy. Highly lethal anaplastic carcinoma is usually radically inoperable at the time of diagnosis; therefore palliative external actinotherapy is used.

## 1.3.6 Thyroid Inflammations

**Acute thyroiditis** – suppurative inflammation of the thyroid gland – is formed in a hematogenic mode or through the spreading of inflammation from the surrounding area, and most often is caused by staphylococci or streptococci. It is manifested by fever, local swelling, reddening, dysphagia and pain; an abscess may develop in exceptional cases. The therapy is conservative, symptomatic, with administration of antibiotics and antiflogistics. Incision and drainage is necessary when an abscess (fluctuation) is present.

**De Quervain subacute thyroiditis** is a rare disease that develops as a consequence of viral infection, injury or external irradiation. The symptoms are local – pain, a feeling of pressure in the anterior part of the neck, shooting up to the angle of the lower jaw, and in the ears, and **general** – subfebrile, weakness, fatigue, pain in the joints and signs of **thyroid function disorder** – starting with hyperfunctional symptoms, followed by a period of eufunction and ending with hypofunction. The therapy is **conservative**, and symptomatic, e.g., antipyretics, antiflogistics, and beta-blockers when hyperfunction is present.

**Hashimoto's chronic thyroiditis** is an autoimmune disease with a lymphoplasmocytic infiltrate of the gland. Except in endemic regions, this is the most frequently occurring type of thyropathy. Antibodies are present, particularly against thyroidal peroxidasis. It may occur in the hypertrophic form (Hashimoto's goiter); however, the atrophic form is more common. Temporarily, the disease may manifest with signs of hyperthyroidism at the beginning, while hypothyroidism is associated with atrophy. The diagnosis is specified through a fine needle puncture and through the proof of antibodies in the serum. Hashimoto's thyroiditis may be associated with orbitopathy. Given the replacement of the thyroid tissue itself with fibrous tissue, the thyroid gland is often very solid and even a slightly enlarged gland may be associated with mechanical syndrome and indicates the need for a total thyroidectomy.

**Riedel's fibrotizing** (chronic) **thyroiditis** is very rare. The cause of this development is not known. The disease leads to the formation of a fibrous scarred change of the thyroid gland, occasionally with the consequence of tracheal compression and paresis of the recurrent nerve. **Conservative** therapy is usually applied; or surgical treatment, only if tracheal compression occurs, aimed at removing mechanical syndrome.

## 1.3.7 Surgical Treatment of Thyroid Diseases

Surgical treatment of thyroid diseases is indicated in:
- Malignant tumors
- Nodular goiters (single- or multinodular), which seem to grow even in spite of suppressive (medicamentous) therapy, especially with the compression of the trachea, esophagus or blood vessels present

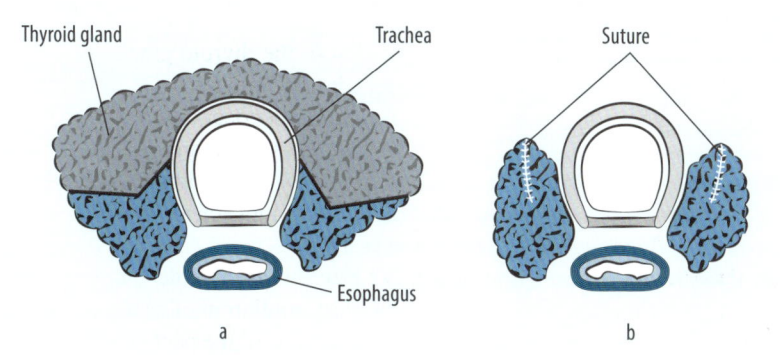

**Fig. 1.4** *Thyroid gland surgery – subtotal thyroidectomy bilateral (STE); a) Extent of resection; b) Condition after STE*

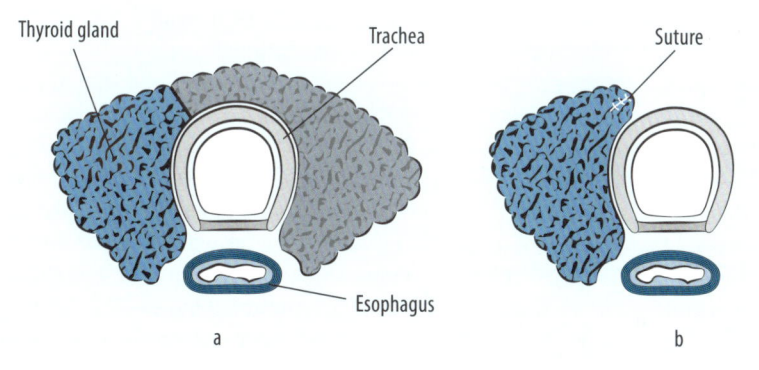

**Fig. 1.5** *Thyroid gland surgery – total lobectomy (LT); a) Extent of resection; b) Condition after STE*

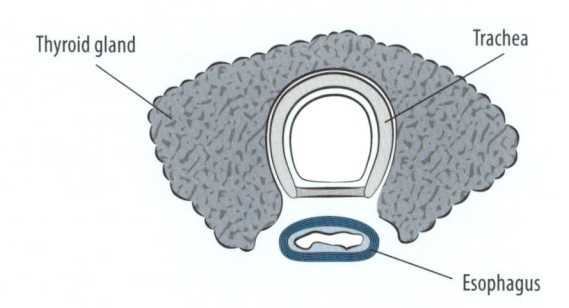

**Fig. 1.6** *Thyroid gland surgery – total thyroidectomy (TTE)*

- Toxic (hyperfunctional) disorders where medicamentous therapy is unsuccessful, achieving eufunction is not successful, or relapses of the toxicosis occur
- Autoimmune diseases (Hashimoto's thyroiditis or Graves-Basedow thyrotoxicosis) where endocrine orbitopathy is shown
- Inflammations with abscess formation (rare)

**Partial procedures,** such as nodular extirpation, partial resection or enucleation – removal of a pathological lesion while leaving healthy tissue, are all procedures that are rarely performed today. Disease relapses used to occur frequently after such procedures, as well as bleeding from non-removed parenchyma. A lower incidence of complications compared to radical procedures was not proven. A certain exception can be seen in the solitary nodule in the area of the isthmus where isthmus resection can be performed while leaving both healthy lobes of the thyroid gland.

**Subtotal resection of the thyroid gland (STE)**: The aim of this operation is to reduce the hormone-producing tissue so that it is preserved in a scope sufficient for the production of physiological amounts of thyroid hormones (Fig. 1.4). Today, this procedure is applied only in exceptional cases.

**Thyroidectomia fere totalis** – almost total thyroidectomy – removal of nearly the entire thyroid gland while leaving only a minimum residue of the tissue near the recurrent nerve, to prevent injury.

**Total lobectomy (TL)**: Complete removal of the whole lobe of the thyroid gland together with the isthmus. This procedure is used in one-sided nodules (both normo- and hyperfunctional) that fail to respond to conservative therapy (Fig. 1.5).

**Total thyroidectomy (TTE)**: The most radical procedure used in malignant tumors, autoimmune diseases (Hashimoto's thyroiditis, Graves-Basedow toxicosis, etc.) and in relapsing goiters. This entails complete removal of the thyroid tissue including the pyramidal lobe and split-off adenoma, found in low numbers, next to the thyroid gland (Fig. 1.6).

**Surgical procedure** – a dermal incision (Kocher or collateral incision) is made 2–3 cm above the jugular fossa. After lifting the cranial lobe formed by the skin, subcutis and platysma muscle, infrahyoid muscles are split longitudinally along the middle line, thereby obtaining access to the thyroid gland. The lateral part is mobilized at first; the branches of the upper thyroid artery are ligated subsequently immediately at the surface of the gland so that any injury to upper parathyroid glands is prevented. Ligation of branches of the lower thyroid artery and vein loosens the lower pole of the gland. The lobe is then prepared along the laterodorsal edge, upon prior identification of the recurrent nerve. The lobectomy is finished by loosening the lobe from the trachea. In a total thyroidectomy, the procedure is identical also in the contralateral lobe. When the gland has been removed, any presence of bleeding is checked in the bed using the Valsalva overpressure maneuver, which reveals bleeding from untreated collapsed veins.

A Redon drain is inserted in the bed after perfect hemostasis, and the procedure is finished by continued suture of the wound in layers.

### 1.3.8 Complications of Thyroid Surgeries

**Specific complications** of thyroid procedures include injuries to the vocal cord nerve – **paresis of the laryngeal recurrent nerve (NLR), function disorder of the parathyroid glands** associated with postoperative hypoparathyrosis and **postoperative bleeding**.

**Hoarseness or possibly aphonia** is the manifestation of a one-sided function disorder of the laryngeal recurrent nerve, **stridor** in the case of a bilateral lesion, and **respiration** disorders due to the paramedial position of paralyzed vocal cords, with narrowing of the respiratory crevice. NLR transient – temporary paresis, which subsides within 6 months or usually earlier with adjustment of the function **ad integrum**, and permanent paresis are distinguished. A permanent lesion of the recurrent nerve on one-side is usually sufficiently compensated by the function of the other vocal cord. A bilateral NLR lesion indicates the need for a tracheostomy to prevent suffocation. The incidence of permanent NLR paresis has been reported in an interval of 0.5–10%.

When the parathyroid glands have been impaired, the **signs of tetany** occur within 24–48 hours, which requires an immediate substitution of calcium. Vitamin D precursors are added in severe forms of hypocalcemia. Hypocalcemia is transient in most cases as well. Long-term tetany due to right parathyroprive hypocalcemia is registered in less than 1% of persons treated; transient hypocalcemia occurs in 3–15% of patients operated on after a total thyroidectomy.

**Postoperative bleeding** with formation of a hematoma in the wound is a serious complication. This condition poses a threat to the patient not due to blood loss but due to compression of the trachea and the larynx. This condition must be resolved by urgent revision of the surgical wound with evacuation of the hematoma and treating the source of the bleeding.

## 1.4 Parathyroid Glands

The number and localization of the parathyroid glands are not constant. Four glands are developed in most cases, but a lower or higher number is not a rare phenomenon. **Upper parathyroid glands** develop from the 4$^{th}$ brachial arch. They are found beyond the upper pole of the thyroid gland, most often near the entry of the laryngeal recurrent nerve in the cricothyroidal membrane. **Lower parathyroid glands** develop from the 3$^{rd}$ brachial arch and surpass the upper parathyroid glands during embryogenesis. They are found beyond the lower parts of the thyroid gland, most often near the lower pole of the thyroid gland or in the fibrous tissue structure between the lower pole and the thymus, in the so called thyrothymic ligament. The variability of the position of lower glands is higher than in upper ones, and they may also be located above the upper pole of the thyroid gland or in the mediastinum. The weight of a normal parathyroid gland is 30–70 mg; it is 3 to 5 mm long, 2 to 4 mm wide and about 1–3 mm thick. The vascular supply of the parathyroid glands is derived from the thyroid artery branches.

The function of the parathyroid glands consists in **parathormone** production, which is responsible for calcium homeostasis. Parathormones act on three organs:
- The skeleton
- The distal tubule of the kidneys
- The intestines

In bones, parathormones cause a rise in osteocyte and osteoclast osteolysis. When parathormones predominate, bones are degraded. In kidneys, parathormones attenuate reverse phosphate resorption in the distal tubule and lead to phosphaturia. Contrary to phosphorus excretion, calcium excretion is reduced. In the intestines, parathormones increase intestinal absorption of calcium.

These effects of parathormones maintain extracellular calcium levels in the normal range.

### 1.4.1 Hyperparathyrosis

The term "hyperparathyrosis" should be understood as an **elevated secretion of parathormones** caused by an adenoma, hyperplasia or carcinoma of the parathyroid glands. This chronic hypersecretion may be caused by the glands themselves (**primary hyperparathyrosis**) or it may be a response to a pathological condition that stimulates elevated secretion (**secondary hyperparathyrosis**).

#### ■ PRIMARY HYPERPARATHYROSIS

Pathophysiology: In primary hyperparathyrosis, parathormone secretion is higher than what the body needs. The regulatory feedback mechanism of the parathyroid glands is probably impaired, which stops parathormone secretion, with normal peripheral calcium levels.

The incidence of primary hyperparathyrosis is found in 20–33 patients per 100,000 inhabitants. The disease affects women more often. In about 80–90% of patients, primary hyperparathyrosis is caused by a **solitary adenoma** of one parathyroid gland. **Hyperplasia**, where all four glands are affected in most cases, occurs in 10–20% of patients. **Multiple adenomas** have been reported in 5–8% of cases. Parathyroid carcinoma is the cause in less than 1% of patients.

**Nephrolithiasis** as a consequence of hypercalcemia is the most frequent manifestation of hyperparathyrosis. Also, symptoms such as reduced performance, fatigue, polyuria and polydipsia, depressive mood, nausea or functional abdominal problems, the so-called **hypercalcemic syndrome,** are commonly seen.

With early detection of hypercalcemia, about 10–30% of patients have no symptoms. "Biochemical hyperparathyroidism" is sometimes mentioned, i.e. laboratory signs of primary hyperparathyrosis are present but clinical symptoms are missing. Today, involvement of the skeleton as part of the primary hyperparathyrosis is understood as a sign of late diagnosis.

The diagnosis differentiates between examinations of the metabolism on the one hand, e.g. differential diagnostic determination of whether the problems are caused by a parathyroid disorder, and localization diagnosis on the other, used to determine which of the glands is involved. Serum calcium, phosphorus and parathormone levels are assessed. The primary sign is represented by **hypercalcemia higher than 2.7 mmol/L**. The determination of serum phosphates is important, while the determination of calciuria is not obligatory. **Alkaline phosphatase is elevated** when bones have been affected. Elevated phosphatase levels precede **radiographic changes in the bones**, therefore no bone changes need to be sought with the help of radiography, with normal levels of alkaline phosphatase. Sonography examination of kidneys may indicate nephrolithiasis or nephrocalcinosis.

**Localization diagnosis**: Numerous methods can be used to localize the parathyroid glands – US, CT, NMR. These methods provide a sensitivity of 60–80%. The experience of specialized centers indicates a 90–95% sensitivity in surgical exploration. Among localization preoperative methods, the combination of US and isotope examination using MIBI is considered as the "gold standard". Technetium-marked methoxyisobutyl isonitrile selectively accumulates only in the hyperfunctional tissue of the parathyroid glands.

The treatment of primary hyperparathyrosis consists in the removal of excessively functioning parathyroid tissue. If more than one gland is enlarged, the condition indicates hyperplasia. In this case, 3 glands have to be removed and the 4th gland is removed only partially. When a parathyroid carcinoma is present, it is recommended to remove the adjacent lobe of the thyroid gland and associated fatty tissues together with central neck lymph nodes on the side of the tumor.

After successful treatment of primary hyperparathyrosis, serum calcium levels become normalized no later than 48 hours after the surgery, provided that the renal function is normal. Serum calcium levels may decrease below the normal values, particularly if bones have been affected, leading to the symptoms of "hungry bones", or hypocalcemia – paresthesia.

## SECONDARY HYPERPARATHYROSIS

Secondary hyperparathyrosis occurs predominantly in patients who must undergo hemodialysis due to chronic renal insufficiency, and/or in patients with terminal insufficiency before or after renal transplantation. Very rarely, chronic intestinal diseases (Crohn's disease, sprue) that cause an impairment of calcium absorption may lead to secondary hyperparathyrosis.

The diagnosis of secondary hyperparathyrosis stems from the same parameters as primary hyperparathyrosis, i.e. serum calcium, phosphorus and parathormone levels assessment.

The therapy of secondary hyperparathyrosis is conservative – administration of calcium and vitamin D metabolites. Standard surgery consists in total parathyroidectomy with autotransplantation of 20 fragments of parathyroid glands in the volume of 1 mm³ in the forearm musculature.

Tertiary hyperparathyroidism is a condition where compensatory secondary hyperparathyroidism is transposed to autonomy.

## 1.5 Compressive Neck Syndromes

**Thoracic outlet syndrome** (TOS) includes difficulties caused by compression of the neurovascular bundle of the upper limbs. This condition is caused by neck rib syndrome or scalene syndrome.

**Cervical ribs.** The supernumerary cervical rib departs from the transversal projection of the 7th cervical vertebra. Its external edge may be loose or ventrally connected to the end of the first rib, and it is more common in women. Hypoperfusion of the limb is manifested by the feeling of cold in the hand, cyanosis of the fingers, weakening or even vanishing of a pulse in the radial artery. Compression of the brachial plexus produces neuralgic pain in the forearm after any head movement, sensation disorders from the arm joint up to the fingers, and paresthesias of the fourth and fifth fingers. A late manifestation consists in motor disorders and atrophy of the small muscles of the hand. The diagnosis is supported by radiographic examination of the cervical spine. Therapy consists in resection of the cervical rib.

**Scalene syndrome** is caused by compression of the neurovascular bundle between hypertrophic scalene muscles. Its clinical image is similar to cervical rib syndrome. The resection of scalene muscles applied in the past has been replaced with resection of the first rib to which the scalenes are attached.

# 2 THORACIC SURGERY

- 2.1 Thoracic Wall
- 2.2 Pleura
- 2.3 Lungs
- 2.4 Mediastinum
- 2.5 Thoracic Injuries
- 2.6 GIT Surgeries Using a Thoracic Approach

## 2.1 Thoracic Wall

### 2.1.1 Anatomical Notes

The thoracic wall is formed by three layers. The surface layer is composed of the skin and subcutis, the middle layer is formed by the anterior, lateral and posterior groups of muscles with nerve and vascular supply. The deep layer consists of the bone skeleton of the chest, intercostal areas with muscles and intrathoracic fascia. Proximally, the entry point in the chest is opened by the superior thoracic aperture, while distally it is the $12^{th}$ rib together with the $12^{th}$ thoracic vertebra, both of which circumscribe the inferior thoracic aperture covered with the diaphragm.

The mechanical function of the thoracic wall in respiration is its main role and is effectuated by enlarging the thoracic volume through elevation of the ribs and declining of the diaphragm. Protection of vital organs is the second function of the thoracic wall.

### 2.1.2 Thoracic Wall Diseases

#### SUPERIOR THORACIC APERTURE SYNDROME

The superior thoracic aperture syndrome (thoracic outlet syndrome) is the compression of the subclavian artery and brachial plexus in the costoclavicular area, resulting in neurological and vascular problems of the upper limbs.

**Etiology** – Superfluous cervical rib, extended transverse process of the $7^{th}$ cervical vertebra, fibrous band between the $7^{th}$ vertebra and the $1^{st}$ rib, hypertrophic scalene muscles, clavicle fracture or the fracture of the $1^{st}$ rib healed in a poor position. The anatomical reasons cannot be exactly defined in some cases.

**Symptomatology** – Symptoms of brachial plexus disorder predominate in the clinical image: pain in the upper limb shooting toward the shoulder blade and to the lateral side of the neck, upper limb paresthesia, Raynaud's symptom. As for vascular symptoms, claudication pain of the upper limb upon physical exertion is present.

**Diagnostics** – The cervical rib can be felt locally. Essential assessments include radiography of the thoracic skeleton, 3D CT with thoracic wall reconstruction, complete neurological assessment, vascular assessment, and angiography if any signs of vascular involvement are present.

**Therapy** – Initially, conservative therapy is applied: vasodilatants, sympatolytics, rehabilitation exercise of the cervical spine and upper limbs. If no organic source of the syndrome is found based on the assessments, this therapy is usually successful, as it is in cases where organic involvement is not fully expressed (hypertrophy of scalene muscles). Surgical treatment is indicated upon the failure of conservative therapy, in cases where marked problems are present, and if the syndrome has occurred based on the cervical rib. Surgery consists in the removal of the 1st rib; if the cervical rib or an artificial fibrous band is present, they are resected as well.

**Complications** - An injury of the subclavian artery or brachial plexus may occur during the surgery. Both injuries must be treated immediately. There is a risk of the disease relapsing if the resection of the 1st rib is not sufficient.

## THORACIC WALL INFECTIONS

An infection of the thoracic wall may cause isolated involvement of soft tissues of the thoracic wall, the bony skeleton or the whole complex of the thoracic wall.

### Thoracic Wall Phlegmona

Phlegmona of the thoracic wall is most often caused by a mixed staphylococcal, streptococcal or colibacillary infection, rarely by an anaerobic infection. Its source may be infected lymph nodes in the axilla, infections in the thoracotomy wound, a canal after puncture or drainage of an inflammatory intrathoracic lesion or suppurative pericarditis, complications of pacemaker implantation, or spreading of an inflammation of the mammary gland in rare cases. If the inflammatory lesion becomes circumscribed and coliquated, a **subpectoral** or **subscapular abscess** is formed, based on the localization.

**Symptomatology** – Signs of an inflammation are apparent locally, and the general response of the body is present when the finding is more advanced.

**Diagnostics** – The finding is usually apparent from physical examination. Laboratory assessment shows an increase in inflammatory markers. When an abscess is suspected, sonography will contribute to the diagnosis, possibly with targeted puncture or drainage of the lesion.

**Therapy** is surgical and consists in opening the lesion by making a sufficient incision and in subsequently draining the lesion. Contraincision is performed in case of more advanced findings. It is always necessary to remove the necrotic tissue and send the contents for bacteriological assessment. The wound should be redressed regularly until completely healed.

Antibiotics are indicated according to sensitivity, for extensive phlegmonas with a general response.

**Complications** – In exceptional cases, the infection may be transferred to the pleural cavity upon insufficient treatment, causing emphysema of the chest.

The prognosis is favorable provided that properly managed therapy is initiated in time, and complete healing is achieved.

## Osteomyelitis of the Ribs and Sternum

Osteomyelitis of the ribs and sternum is usually a complication of a thoracotomy or sternotomy.

Staphylococci and *E. coli* are the most common infectious agents. Osteomyelitis may also develop as a secondary disease due to hematogenic spread of general infectious diseases, particularly in children.

**Symptomatology** – The course may be acute with septic fever, tachycardia, considerable pain in chest, particularly upon movement and cough; or subacute with most of the changes being local (edema, inflammatory infiltrate). A chronic form may also occur, associated with development of abscesses, non-healing fistulas and sequesters.

**Diagnosis** is most often determined on the basis of clinical symptoms, frequently upon complicated healing of a surgical wound. Radiography is not beneficial before development of chronic inflammation, at least 4 weeks from occurrence, when osteolysis and formation of sequesters become apparent.

**Therapy** – In the acute stage: parenteral application of broad spectrum antibiotics, and incision and drainage if an abscess has formed. In the subacute and chronic stage: resection of the involved part with subsequent drainage or lavage. Therapy in these stages is long-term and difficult, usually leaving cosmetic defects in the thoracic wall.

## THORACIC WALL TUMORS

Tumors occur in both benign and malignant variants and may originate in all layers of the thoracic wall. Metastases of intrathoracic tumors, breast carcinoma, kidney carcinoma, etc. are found relatively often in the thoracic wall.

1. **Benign tumors of soft tissues** include lipomas, fibromas, neurofibromas, lymphangiomas and hemangiomas. They are usually asymptomatic and are manifested through local resistance. The diagnosis stems from finding such resistance during physical examination, from sonography examination and radiography of the chest. (Radiography is negative in benign lesions except cavernous hemangioma which destructs the bone.) **Therapy** consists in extirpation, and also resection of adjacent bone for cavernous hemangioma. The prognosis is excellent.

TEXTBOOK OF SURGERY

2. **Malignant tumors of soft tissues** in this localization include particularly sarcomas whose current classification is based on immunohistochemical, cytogenetic and molecular-genetic techniques. Most commonly, these include fibrosarcoma, liposarcoma, and primitive neuroectodermal tumors.
   Etiological factors mentioned in the literature include:
   - Exposure to organic chemicals such as dioxin, chlorophenols, etc.
   - External radiation
   - Infectious agent (HIV, human herpes virus 8)
   - Some immunodeficiency syndromes
   - Genetic factors (Gardner syndrome, neurofibromatosis type I)
   - Chronic inflammation and repeated trauma
     – Symptomatology - Initially, the tumors are asymptomatic, their first symptom being non-painful resistance in the thoracic wall. At the time of diagnosis, distant metastases are already established in up to 30% of cases.
     – Diagnostics - Besides standard radiography, assessments performed include CT or nuclear magnetic resonance (NMR), sonography; and as part of staging, also skeletal scintigraphy and liver sonography. An open biopsy is needed for exact classification of the tumor, with the subsequent definitive surgical procedure as soon as possible.
     – Therapy consists in radical en-bloc resection of the thoracic wall and its replacement with an allotransplant or musculocutaneous flap. Oncological therapy follows. Symptomatic therapy is usually applied in case of generalization.
     – Complications - A serious complication of the post-operative period is early infection, which may even require removing the allotransplant. A large akinetic zone is formed upon extensive resection of the thoracic wall and its replacement with foreign material, which may exert a negative effect on respiration.
     – Prognosis of these tumors is not good; 5-year survival does not exceed 30% even after a radical operation.
3. **Benign skeletal tumors of the thoracic wall** include chondromas, osteochondromas, myxochondromas, and fibrous dysplasias. They are normally localized in the parasternal region, causing no pain, and they are manifested through palpable resistance only. Usually, they are discovered through a non-targeted radiography finding. The therapy consists in local excision, associated with good prognosis after the removal.
4. **Malignant primary skeletal tumors of the thoracic wall** most often include chondrosarcomas (approx. 40%), osteosarcomas and Ewing's sarcomas. Their etiology, symptomatology and diagnostics are similar to soft tissue tumors. Surgical treatment consists in radical en bloc resection of the thoracic wall and its replacement. Complex oncological treatment follows after the surgery. Prognosis is very poor, and 5-year survival is rare.

5. **Malignant secondary skeletal tumors of the thoracic wall** most often include metastases of epithelial tumors – of bronchogenic carcinoma, renal carcinoma and mammary gland carcinoma. Ribs are involved in most cases, while metastases in the sternum are relatively rare. In case of isolated metastases offering technical respectability, surgical removal of the affected part of the skeleton should be opted for, with potential replacement of the thoracic wall to ensure that respiratory mechanics is not affected. If multiple metastatic involvement of the chest skeleton is present, surgical treatment is not indicated and palliative oncological treatment can be considered (analgesic irradiation of the thoracic wall, pharmacotherapy – Bonefos and biological treatment).

### 2.1.3 Thoracic Wall Surgeries

Surgical access to the thoracic cavity can be provided by the following procedures:
- Longitudinal complete sternotomy
- Longitudinal partial sternotomy
- Posterolateral thoracotomy
- Anterolateral thoracotomy
- Dorsal thoracotomy
- Bilateral anterior thoracotomy with transverse sternotomy

Sternotomies are used to provide access to the anterior and central mediastinum, for cardiac surgeries, and to large blood vessels in the superior mediastinum. Both thoracic cavities can also be explored at the same time by means of sternotomy, and surgery can be performed in the lungs in one session. Longitudinal partial sternotomies are designated for resolving tumors of the superior mediastinum, for treating stenoses in the middle part of the trachea, and for resolving tracheobronchial fistulas in this localization. As for thoracotomies, posterolateral access to the thoracic cavity is used most often for surgeries of the lungs, esophagus and to access the posterior mediastinum.

An intrathoracic drain must be inserted before closing the thoracotomy; based on the type of procedure, in the cavity the drain is connected to active suction (pulmonary resection) or inactive suction such as Bülau drainage below the liquid level (pneumonectomy, surgery with no disruption of pulmonary parenchyma).

## 2.2 Pleura

### 2.2.1 Anatomical Notes

The pleural sac is formed by two sheets. The visceral pleura covers the surface of the lung and cannot be separated from the lungs. It is seamlessly bound with parietal pleura in the area of the pulmonary hilum and mediastino-pulmonary ligament. The parietal pleura has four parts: costal pleura, diaphragmatic, mediastinal and cervical pleurae. The space between both sheets forms the pleural cavity, which is filled with a small amount of serous liquid and enables the movement of the lungs. Under normal conditions, negative pressure is present in the pleural cavity; it ranges from -9 mmHg (-1.2 kPa) in the inspirium to -3 mmHg (-0.4 kPa) in the expirium. Besides the hilar part, the visceral pleura is not sensitive; however, the parietal pleura is innervated from intercostal nerves, the brachial plexus and from the phrenic nerve, and it is very sensitive. Pathological affections in this area are manifested by severe pain.

### 2.2.2 Pneumothorax

Pneumothorax means accumulation of air in the pleural cavity. It is not a separate disease but rather a symptom of another basic disease.

Based on **etiology**, pneumothorax is classified as:
- Spontaneous
- Traumatic
- Iatrogenic

Based on **pathophysiology**, it is classified as follows:
- Closed – usually a single entry of air in the pleural cavity and relatively stable volume
- Open – the pleural cavity communicates directly with the outside atmosphere and the volume of air varies with respiratory excursions
- Tension – a higher amount of air enters the pleural cavity, more than the amount that can escape, thus the pressure in the pleural cavity keeps rising

In terms of **pathological anatomy** and **based on the extent**, pneumothorax can be:
- Sheath – in this case, loose air forms about 15–20% of the thoracic cavity volume. Subjective problems are minimal and the clinical finding is poor
- Partial – the volume of loose air reaches 50–60%. This type usually occurs in the presence of pleural adhesion
- Complete – the volume of air is higher than 60%. This type is usually symptomatic.

#### ▪ SPONTANEOUS PNEUMOTHORAX

Spontaneous pneumothorax (primary spontaneous pneumothorax) is a disease of younger persons with typical prevalence between 20 and 30 years of age, occurring more commonly in men whose numbers predominate over women at the ratio of 9:1, and in asthenic individuals. Etiology is not completely known; currently, the enzyme-based theory of pathological disproportion between pulmonary elastases and proteases predominates. Small subpleural bullae can be found macroscopically in approximately 70% of individuals, while pneumothorax is caused by their rupture. It shows a tendency to relapse.

## SECONDARY PNEUMOTHORAX

Secondary pneumothorax is one of the symptoms of another disease. Most commonly, it is a chronic obstructive pulmonary disease, bronchial asthma, cystic fibrosis, various interstitial pulmonary processes and lung infections. As for other than lung diseases, it is commonly associated with endometriosis and Marfan syndrome.

## IATROGENIC PNEUMOTHORAX

Iatrogenic pneumothorax is usually a complication of invasive diagnostic and therapeutic methods. For example: cannulation of the central venous stream, artificial pulmonary ventilation, pleural exudate puncture. Therapeutic pneumothorax is no longer used.

With an **open pneumothorax**, air is sucked into the thoracic cavity rapidly during inspirium, leading to the paradoxical mediastinal movement to the healthy side, while the movement is opposite during expirium and the mediastinum is deviated to the affected side. This effect is called **mediastinal flutter** and is greatly involved in the development of respiratory insufficiency, particularly in old patients with associated cardiorespiratory diseases. With **tension pneumothorax**, additional air enters the pleural cavity with every inspiration through the valve mechanism, while the air has nowhere to escape. The mediastinum thus moves to the healthy side, causing myocardial compression, deteriorated venous return, until the condition results in circulatory and respiratory failure.

**Symptomatology** – The clinical image of all types of pneumothorax is similar. The symptoms depend on its size, the speed of its development, and the underlying condition of the cardiorespiratory apparatus. The symptoms may vary from an asymptomatic course up to global respiratory insufficiency. Pain in the affected side of the chest, below the scapula, initially sharp and later dull, is a typical symptom. Sudden onset dyspnea and dry irritating cough are usual. Hemoptysis and cyanosis may be present in rare cases. Subcutaneous emphysema may be present in the case of open pneumothorax, at the place of the injury.

Symptoms of tension pneumothorax are dramatic. The patient is restless, anxious, sweating, and central cyanosis commonly occurs. Tachycardia, tachypnea and later hypotension are present. The affected side of the chest is more voluminous than the healthy one.

**Diagnostics** – Medical history data are important (any trauma, young patient, respiratory disease diagnosis). Hypersonor percussion different on both sides and weakened up to non-audible respiration found during physical examination. The anteroposterior scan of the lungs is the predominant diagnostic method, where lung markings are missing on the pneumothorax side and the mediastinum position is changed.

**Therapy** is surgical, establishing thoracic drainage with subsequent active suction. A small sheath pneumothorax is an exception; no drainage is applied in this case and the patient is only observed.

### Drainage Procedure

Under aseptic conditions under local anesthesia, an incision is performed in the middle or posterior axillary line, in the 4$^{th}$ or 5$^{th}$ intercostal space. A thoracic drain of 20–24 Ch is inserted using a trocar after pulling apart the soft tissues, and it is placed near the upper edge of the lower rib. The drain is fixed to the skin and connected to active suction – 10 cmH$_2$O (0.98 kPa). Radiography is performed after drainage to check the condition. The drain is left connected to active suction until the lung has fully reexpanded. Subsequently, the drain is closed for 24 hours, and after a radiographic check-up, when the lung is well expanded, the drainage is removed (Fig. 2.1).

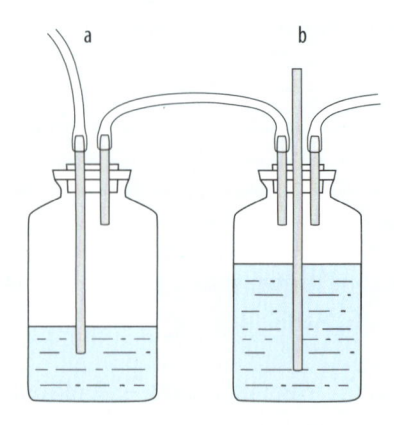

*Fig. 2.1 Thoracic drainage system: a) Drain from the patient; b) Active suction –15 to –20 mmHg*

Indications for surgical treatment, performed exclusively through thoracoscopy today, include:
- Pneumothorax persisting during drainage (5 to 7 days)
- Massive air escape that prevents the lung from reexpanding
- Relapsing pneumothorax (already the first relapse is a clear indication for thoracoscopic treatment)
- Bilateral pneumothorax
- Radiographic finding of large cysts
- The first attack in patients of special professions (pilots, divers)
- Pneumothorax complications (hemothorax, empyema)

Revision of thoracic cavity is performed during thoracoscopy. If a pathological finding is proven – pulmonary bullae in most cases – the affected part of the lung is resected. The procedure is finished with mechanical abrasion of the pleural cavity or partial pleurectomy. If the affected place cannot be found, the procedure is performed in the pleura and a small lung biopsy is taken from the apical segment. The surgery is ended with thoracic drainage.

**Acute treatment of open pneumothorax** as part of first aid consists in provisional closure of the entry wound from 3 sides, using the one-way valve principle. For the **tension pneumothorax**, an urgent procedure of the pleural cavity puncture using a wide cannula is performed, thus converting the problem to open pneumothorax.

**Complications** – An untreated or insufficiently treated pneumothorax may result in respiratory insufficiency and fibrous changes of the visceral pleura, or in pyothorax. Tension pneumothorax, unless treated in time, results in cardiorespiratory failure and exitus of the patient. Bleeding (from the lungs, thoracic wall) or development of an infection and empyema in the chest may appear as a rare complication of drainage or thoracoscopy.

**Prognosis** is excellent for spontaneous pneumothorax after adequate treatment; its healing brings no further limitations. The prognosis of traumatic and iatrogenic pneumothorax depends on the trauma or underlying disease.

### 2.2.3  Pleural Effusion – Fluidothorax

Pleural effusion – fluidothorax – means the presence of loose liquid in the pleural cavity. It is classified as follows, based on the liquid type:
- Hydrothorax (serous liquid)
- Pyothorax (thoracic empyema)
- Hemothorax
- Chylothorax

#### ■ HYDROTHORAX

Based on the serous exudate characteristics, hydrothorax is divided into transudate – specific weight lower than 1.015 g/L, protein content lower than 30 g/L; and exudate – specific weight higher than 1.015 g/L, protein content over 30 g/L.

**Etiology** – The most frequent causes of transudate include: cardiac failure, liver cirrhosis, nephrotic syndrome, hypoproteinemia, and sarcoidosis. Exudate has the following causes: lung and pleura tumors, viral and mycotic pneumonias, system diseases, pulmonary infarction, post-irradiation syndrome and some gastrointestinal tract diseases (pancreatitis, subphrenic and liver abscesses).

**Symptomatology** – Pleural pain is the most common symptom of inflammatory diseases, increasing with deep inspirium. The pain subsides with increased exudate formation, with an onset of dyspnea due to compression of the lung, which then becomes the principal symptom. The principal symptom of malignant infiltration of the pleura and exudate is dull, permanent pain.

**Diagnostics** – Reduced percussion over the base of the lungs, weakened up to disappeared respiration, weakened pectoral fremitus and bronchophony are commonly found during clinical examination. Chest radiography in two projections is an important examination. In standing position, an exudate amount of about 300 mL and higher is apparent, while an amount of about 100 mL can be recognized in the side-lying position. Monographs can be used for orientation diagnosis. When an encapsulated exudate is suspected, a CT should be performed, generally recognized as the predominant method in the diagnosis of pleural exudate, its amount and distribution. Thoracic puncture provides information on the exudate characteristics. It is performed using a closed system, with the patient in the sitting position and under local anesthesia, along the scapular line (on the level of the 8$^{th}$ or 9$^{th}$ intercostal space). Thus obtained punctuate is examined in microbiological, cytological, and biochemical tests. Performing pH assessment is also suitable as it has prognostic meaning, particularly for parapneumonic exudates, and may reveal in due time any developing empyema (pH lower than 7.0).

**Therapy** – Exudate up to 500 mL usually requires no therapy. Non-malignant exudate responds to the underlying disease treatment and resorbs spontaneously. If not, a puncture is indicated to provide relief, which can be repeated. The total amount of removed liquid should not exceed 1.000 mL/d. If the exudate is replenished constantly, chest drainage is indicated. The drain should be connected to a controlled suction system. If not even the drainage is successful and the exudate keeps being replenished, pleurodesis is indicated, which is carried out chemically (tetracycline, bleomycine) or bacteriologically (*Corynebacterium parvum*). Malignant exudates with primary or metastatic tumors of the pleura are indicated for thoracoscopic treatment, primarily without repeated punctures and drainages. Besides others, thoracoscopy provides the advantage of the possibility to collect a sample of the pleura or lung for histological assessment. Talc pleurodesis is indicated only for malignant exudates (talc is poured evenly in the thoracic cavity, causing pleural cavity obliteration). The procedure is quick, gentle and its success rate is more than 95%.

**Complications** – An extensive exudate may even lead to the development of respiratory failure. The risk of circulatory instability is associated with quick exudate releasing. Introduction of an infection and empyema development are rare complications after treatment.

**Prognosis** depends on the underlying disease.

## PYOTHORAX (THORACIC EMPYEMA)

Pyothorax (thoracic empyema) means accumulation of suppuration in the pleural cavity.

**Etiology** – Primary thoracic empyema is caused by direct penetration of bacteria in the cavity upon injury, surgery, puncture or drainage of the chest. Secondary empyema develops based on inflammatory pulmonary processes. Most commonly, it is parapneumonic or postpneumonic empyema (more than 70% of all empyemae). Furthermore, empyema may be a complication of pulmonary abscess, brochiectases, or lung tumor. In rare cases, it may be present with abdominal pathologies such as subphrenic and liver abscess, pancreatitis, when it is caused by hematogenic spreading, and rather rarely, it may be caused by direct rupture of the lesion into the chest. The numbers of specific empyemae rise with the increasing number of TBC diseases. The spectrum of infectious agents that cause an empyema is variegated and includes staphylococci, streptococci, bacteroides, *E. coli, Proteus,* and *Klebsiella.*

The disease develops in three phases:
- Exudative
- Fibroproductive – initial days
- Organizational: this phase onsets on day 7 to 10, passing to the chronic stage usually in week 6, with manifestations of a chronic septic condition.

**Symptomatology** – Ranges from creeping signs of an inflammation up to a rapid development of sepsis. The most commonly present symptoms include high fever, chills, shivers, pleural pain, productive cough, tachypnea to dyspnea, tachycardia, and circulatory and respiratory failure in peracute forms.

**Diagnostics** – Medical history data on an inflammatory pulmonary disease are important. The physical finding is identical to that of fluidothorax, while febricities are also present. Laboratory assessment shows a rise in FW, leukocytes, CRP, bilirubin, liver tests, and later a decrease in values of the red blood count, and coagulation disorders. As for imaging methods, radiography in two projections is carried out, as well as CT, which is important for accurate localization, differentiation from a pulmonary abscess, providing the possibility of targeted puncture or drainage. Exudate puncture and bacteriological as well as cytological examinations are used to confirm the diagnosis, and to determine the phase of the disease and the etiological agent.

**Therapy** – The provoking cause must be eradicated; for an empyema following after a pulmonary infection, antibiotics should be administered according to their sensitivity. Thoracic drainage with active suction is performed locally. When suppuration has been evacuated, the empyema cavity can be flushed with an antiseptic solution. The drain should be left in place until obliteration of the cavity is completed. If the empyema persists even with proper drainage, surgical revision is indicated. The surgery consists in decortication of the lung and in lavage of the thoracic cavity with subsequent drainage. This solution is sufficient in the vast majority of cases and leads to permanent healing. If not, pleurostomy (opening of the pleural cavity at the place of the inflammatory lesion on the outside) is indicated first, and if the condition is not healed, thoracoplasty is performed subsequently, i.e. resection of the ribs and pleura.

**Complications** – In rare cases, a suppuration rupture into the thoracic wall occurs – necessitated empyema. Other complications include: septic shock development, formation of septic metastases, formation of bronchopleural fistulas.

**Prognosis** – Postpneumonic empyema offers the best prognosis, usually healed with no further consequences. Other types show a more severe course and their prognosis is serious. Surgical lethality is about 2%.

### HEMOTHORAX

Hemothorax is described in Section 2.5.4.

### CHYLOTHORAX

This is a rare type of exudate, accumulation of lymph in the pleural cavity. Based on etiology, it is classified as congenital, traumatic and obstructive. More than one half of chylothoraces are of traumatic origin with the predominant representation of iatrogenic peroperative lesions from surgeries of the esophagus, lungs and descending aorta. Symptomatology is identical to that of another fluidothorax. As for diagnostics, puncture is of decisive importance. The punctate shows a high concentration of triacylglycerols, the finding of chylomicrons, and a large number of T lymphocytes. The therapy is conservative at the beginning: limitation of oral intake, parenteral nutrition, thoracic drainage. If lymph production does not decrease within 14 days, surgery is indicated where the thoracic duct is located and ligated, with subsequent pleural abrasion. The procedure can also be performed using thoracoscopy. The prognosis is always serious.

## 2.2.4  Pleural Tumors

- **Benign tumors** are rare; they include lipomas, fibromas and hemangiomas. Among benign tumors, benign fibrous pleural tumors (formerly benign mesothelioma) occur most commonly in the pleura. The tumors are asymptomatic, and a CT of the chest is used as the diagnostic method. Therapy consists in radical excision. They should always be operated due to concerns about turning malignant. The prognosis is excellent, with no need of additional measures.
- **Malignant tumors** may be primary pleural mesotheliomas or secondary tumors; the latter include metastatic involvement of the pleura, most commonly with pulmonary carcinoma, breast carcinoma and ovarian tumors.

### DIFFUSE PLEURAL MALIGNANT MESOTHELIOMA

As for etiology, the exposure to asbestos has an undoubted effect, although it is not the only cause of the tumor development. Diffuse mesotheliomas are highly malignant, locally invasive tumors. TNM classification and Butchart's classification based on TNM, and the disease stage taking into account potential resectability are important for determining the surgical strategy.

**TNM Classification:**
- T1 – The tumor is limited to ipsilateral pleura
- T2 – Besides pleural infiltration, the ipsilateral lung or diaphragm or pericardium is also affected
- T3 – Infiltration of the thoracic wall or mediastinum including organs and tissues

# THORACIC SURGERY

- T4 – Tumor in the contralateral pleura, lung or peritoneum and in abdominal organs
- N1 – Ipsilateral peribronchial or hilar lymph nodes are affected
- N2 – Ipsilateral mediastinal lymph nodes are affected
- N3 – Contralateral lymph nodes are affected
- M0 – Distant metastases are not present
- M1 – Distant metastases are present

**Symptomatology** – Malignant mesothelioma is manifested by chest pain, subfebriles, formation of exudate and dyspnea.

**Diagnostics** – Radiography, CT of the thoracic and abdominal cavity, NMR of the diaphragm, cytological examination of the exudate obtained through puncture usually is not beneficial for the diagnostics. Thoracoscopy or pleuroscopy with targeted pleural collection for histological assessment determines accurate diagnosis in 98% of cases. Histological diagnosis is difficult due to possible confusion with adenocarcinoma. Therefore, immunohistochemical assessment of the collected sample is necessary.

**Therapy** is complex and very aggressive during initial stages and in patients in an outstanding clinical condition, which are the only cases where permanent recovery can be considered. Based on the most recent knowledge, stages I and II (T1, T2, max. N1, T3 being the borderline) are indicated for surgical treatment. The radical procedure consists in pleuropneumonectomy with resection and replacement of the diaphragm and pericardium and with removal of ipsilateral mediastinal lymph nodes. Subsequently, system therapy and biological treatment are applied. Palliative oncological treatment is indicated for higher stages. Malignant exudates are resolved through thoracoscopic talc pleurodesis.

**Prognosis** – For the diffuse form, the average survival period is 18 months from making the **diagnosis**. In patients who have undergone the surgery, even a 30% 5-year survival can be found in the literature depending on the stage of the disease, histological type of the tumor, and radicality of the procedure.

## 2.3 Lungs

### 2.3.1 Anatomical Notes

The lungs are divided into lobes and segments, both anatomically and functionally. Ten segments are found on the right and usually 9 on the left (segment 7 is missing or is merged in segment 8). The right lung is larger and takes about a 54% share in ventilation. The lungs have a double circulation. 97% of blood passing through the lung flows through the pulmonary artery. The rest falls on bronchial arteries, which represent the nutritional circulation of the lungs. Venous blood flows out of the lungs exclusively via the pulmonary veins. Lymphatic drainage is very abundant; the lymph flows from the intrapulmonary lymph nodes to the hilar ones and further to mediastinal and cervical nodes.

### 2.3.2 Examination Methods

1. Medical history and physical examination
2. Radiography in two projections is the first-choice method
3. CT with contrast agent administration is the most precise method. The resolution capacity is 3 mm and less. This method provides precise localization of any pathology and its relationship to the surrounding structures. It describes the size of the lymph nodes, which is of high importance for determining operability of the pulmonary carcinoma. In pleural exudates, this method can be used to determine their content based on density measurement. Puncture of peripheral lesions in the lungs or targeted drainage are performed under CT guidance
4. NMR assessment in diagnostics of the pulmonary processes does not offer any higher benefit compared to CT. It is not used as the standard, with the exception of the need to distinguish whether soft tissues in the area – the diaphragm, pleural cupula and adjacent neurovascular bundles, the axilla, pericardium, thoracic wall – have been affected by the primary pulmonary process
5. Angio CT or digital subtraction angiography (DSA) are used for the diagnostics of arteriovenous malformations, congenital anomalies, pulmonary embolism. Spiral CT is carried out in order to assess the details – the relationship of the pulmonary carcinoma to blood vessels
6. Bronchoscopy is performed using a flexible or rigid apparatus. The bronchial tree can be viewed directly up to the level of subsegmental orifices. This method allows for collecting material directly from the pathological lesion, for performing bronchial lavage with the possibility of further examination of the obtained liquid and cells. Bronchoscopy is used to perform a puncture of the pulmonary tissue or peribronchial nodes. It is also an important therapeutic method (extraction of aspirated objects, suction after lung surgeries). Rigid bronchoscopy can be used to insert a stent in the respiratory pathways. Isotope examination is important for the diagnosis of pulmonary embolism. The ventilation/perfusion scan is performed before pulmonary resection with borderline values of ventilation functions
7. Spirometry or the body-test determines the values of pulmonary volumes and capacities and their ratios, which can be used to determine the maximum possible extent of resection
8. Mediastinoscopy with sample collection from paratracheal nodes is important for determining the scope of cancer in pulmonary tumors. It is performed when large (over 10 mm) nodes are present in the mediastinum, visualized by CT

THORACIC SURGERY

9. Thoracoscopy provides a morphological view of the thoracic cavity with targeted collection of pathological tissue. Thoracoscopy can be used to perform all types of pulmonary resections using the VATS method (video-assisted thoracoscopy)
10. PET – positron emission tomography is used for the diagnostics of pulmonary carcinoma, and also to determine the stage of the disease, particularly to determine N/M involvement, and furthermore to observe the course of the disease after completed complex therapy of bronchogenic carcinoma
11. Tumor markers CEA, NSE, CYFRA 21-1 are used especially as part of observing the process dynamics in the course of and after the treatment of pulmonary malignancies.

### 2.3.3 Lung Tumors

■ BENIGN LUNG TUMORS

These tumors are rare and represent 1–2% of all pulmonary tumors. They stem from respiratory pathways in the vast majority of cases. They include: **polyps, papillomas, adenomas, hamartoma.** These tumors are asymptomatic and are normally found accidentally based on radiography performed for another indication. In rare cases, hemoptyses or obstructions of the bronchi may be the cause. However, no focal finding can be concluded as a benign lesion without histological diagnosis, and therefore all these tumors are indicated for surgical removal. The operation means definitive healing.

A special unit is represented by the so-called **"coin lesions"**. These are solitary, peripheral and well circumscribed, coin-shaped lesions. They originate either from granulomatous inflammation or are the manifestation of a primary or metastatic tumor. "Coin lesions" are indicated for surgical removal given the possibility of their cancer etiology (up to 30%).

The resection can often be done using thoracoscopy; if malignity is found, the procedure is converted and a lobectomy is performed.

■ MALIGNANT LUNG TUMORS

Currently, lung carcinoma is the second most frequent malignity after colorectal cancer (CRC) in the Czech Republic.

**Etiology** – Nicotine abuse is a demonstrable cause (up to 80%), while the risk of cancer depends on the number of smoked cigarettes, on the age at starting to smoke and on the period that the habit has lasted. Other factors include exposure to aromatic hydrocarbons, and heavy metals. Another risk factor is alpha-radiation of radon, which is present in the soil in some localities. Higher occurrence has been found in patients with chronic lung inflammation where the carcinoma develops in scars present in the pulmonary parenchyma. Hereditary factors cannot also be neglected.

**Pathological anatomy** – In the vast majority of cases, bronchogenic carcinoma stems from bronchial epithelium; in 2% of cases the carcinoma is of alveolar origin and sarcomas represent less than 1%. Exact histological classification is of crucial importance for the treatment strategy and is also an important prognostic factor.

According to WHO, bronchogenic carcinoma is classified as follows:
1. Epithelial malignant tumors:
    - a) Epidermoid
    - b) Adenocarcinoma
    - c) Adenosquamous
    - d) Large cell carcinoma
    
    Taken together, they represent about 75% of all lung carcinomas.
    - e) Small cell – oat cell – about 20% of all carcinomas
    - f) Malignant carcinoid about 1%
    - g) Bronchial gland carcinoma
2. Non-epithelial tumors (fibrosarcoma, leiomyosarcoma, neurofibrosarcoma)
3. Malignant mesotheliomas
4. Rare primary tumors (pneumoblastoma, carcinosarcoma, malignant lymphoma, etc.)

Besides the histological type, the malignity grade is also assessed, the so-called **grading** (G1–G3).

The scope of the tumor is determined based on TNM classification (**staging**).
- T1 – Tumor smaller than 3 cm; does not exceed the lobar bronchus or visceral pleura
- T2 – Tumor larger than 3 cm or showing invasion in the visceral pleura or infiltration of the main bronchus in a distance of 2 cm and more from the carina
- T3 – Any size of the tumor; invasion in the thoracic wall, diaphragm, pericardium, in the main bronchus in a distance of less than 2 cm from the carina
- T4 – Any size with infiltration of the heart or esophagus or large blood vessels, vertebrae, carina, or malignant exudate
- N0 – No involvement of lymph nodes
- N1 – Involvement of intrapulmonary or homolateral hilar nodes
- N2 – Involvement of homolateral mediastinal nodes
- N3 – Involvement of contralateral mediastinal nodes or homolateral supraclavicular or scalene nodes
- M1 – Distant metastases

The TNM combination is used to determine the stage of the disease (I, II, IIIA, IIIB, IV) based on which the method of therapy is determined, taking into account the histological type.

# THORACIC SURGERY

Bronchogenic carcinoma develops hematogenic metastases in the liver, skeleton, adrenal glands and the brain. Lymphatic spreading is also common, particularly for adenocarcinoma.

**Symptomatology** – In the vast majority of cases, bronchogenic carcinoma remains asymptomatic for a long time. In this phase, it is discovered as an accidental finding in a radiographic scan. Relapsing pneumonias on the basis of obstruction of respiratory pathways are an alarming and often omitted symptom. Therefore, in adulthood, every case of pneumonia should be an indication for making a scan before and after treatment. Typical symptoms of lung carcinoma, however not early, include dry irritating cough, hemoptysis, pain in the chest and dyspnea. Every occurrence of dry cough lasting longer than 3 weeks should be examined in detail. Other symptoms: the superior vena cava syndrome, the Horner syndrome, paresis of the recurrent nerve, diaphragm, and spine pain. These symptoms are the manifestation of local growth of the tumor and usually mean that the tumor is inoperable. Special symptoms are caused by hormonal production as part of the paraneoplastic syndromes: Cushing syndrome, pseudohyperparathyroidism, gynecomasty and relapsing phlebothrombosis.

**Diagnostics** – The aim is to obtain accurate TNM classification and to find out about the histological type of the tumor. As for medical history, information on risk factors is important. The clinical finding is poor and if present, it is usually a manifestation of an advanced finding – atelectasis, alar pneumonia, exudate. Special examinations are described in Section 2.3.2. CT is important for determining the stage when any areas possibly affected by the tumor are deduced from lymph node sizes. Nodes up to 10 mm are considered as benign, nodes over 10 mm are considered as potentially malignant. When enlarged nodes are present in the mediastinum, mediastinoscopy is carried out with collection of the nodes for histological assessment which allows for exact evaluation of the N stage, also in the peroperative period. Sonography of the liver, scintigraphy of the skeleton, abdominal CT are performed as part of the search for any metastases, and also CT or NMR of the skull and bone marrow puncture in the case of small cell carcinoma. The histological type of the tumor is determined from the material obtained from a bronchoscopy or transthoracic puncture under CT guidance or using thoracoscopy. Pulmonary functions must be examined before approaching the surgical solution; this examination makes it possible to determine the maximum possible extent of resection. Cardiology examination is applied in patients with cardiac history given that lung surgeries pose increased demands on the cardiovascular apparatus and respiratory functions.

**Therapy** shows decisive dependence on the following factors:
- TNM or the stage of the disease
- Histological type of the tumor
- Cardiac and respiratory reserve

- General condition of the patient
- Local operability of the tumor and experience of the surgeon

Surgical treatment is of decisive importance in the therapy. However, radical operability of the tumor is very low – about 15%. This is due to the locally advanced stage of the tumor, presence of metastases, limitation of cardiorespiratory functions, associated serious diseases.

Stages I and II (T1, T2, N0, N1) are indicated for resection treatment for a non-small cell carcinoma. In stage IIIA (T3 or N2 M0), the operation is preceded by neoadjuvant or concomitant chemoradiotherapy. Additional oncological treatment follows after the operation. Exceptionally, also a T4 tumor with no nodal or metastatic involvement may be indicated for resection. Stages IIIB (T4 or N3) and IV (M1) are generally a contraindication for surgical treatment. Only T1 or T2 N0 M0 are indicated for resection for a small cell carcinoma. Combined oncological treatment always follows. Another precondition for the fulfillment of indication criteria is represented by sufficient cardiopulmonary reserve and general condition of the patient that allows for performing the demanding surgical procedure.

If the operation is contraindicated, oncological treatment is applied: chemotherapy, external radiotherapy, brachytherapy, local laser recanalization of the bronchus obturated by the tumor.

**Complications of surgical treatment** are the following: operative or post-operative bleeding, pneumothorax, insufficient expectoration after the surgery with development of atelectasis and pneumonia, furthermore post-operative arrhythmia, cardiac or respiratory insufficiency. A serious complication is the development of a bronchopleural fistula, which usually occurs on day 7 to 12, and which is very difficult to resolve, particularly after a pneumonectomy. Operative lethality is below 1% for lobectomy, and up to 6% for pneumonectomy.

**Prognosis** shows decisive dependence on the stage of the disease, on the histological type and operability of the tumor. For non-small cell carcinomas, the 5-year survival in stage I is 75–85%, in stage II it is 30–40%, and less than 5% in higher stages. The recovery rate is 5 to 10% for a small cell carcinoma. Further dispensing of the patient is necessary, initially at an interval of 3 months, later 6 months, and this includes physical examination, radiography of the heart and lungs, CT of the chest, sonography of the liver and bronchoscopy.

### 2.3.4 Inflammatory Diseases of the Lungs

Diagnostics and conservative therapy of these diseases falls in the field of pneumology; this section mentions only indications for surgical treatment.

## LUNG TUBERCULOSIS

- A primary complex or solitary lesion that cannot be reliably distinguished from a carcinoma
- A residual lesion after successful **conservative therapy** – tuberculomas, cavernas, atelectases
- Bleeding not manageable by conservative therapy
- Persisting bronchopleural fistula

## BRONCHIECTASIS

**Bronchiectasis** – Conservative therapy failure with the precondition of localized changes.

## PULMONARY ABSCESS

**Pulmonary abscess** – drainage under CT guidance and further conservative therapy is the method of choice. Surgical procedure can be considered provided that this therapy has failed and in the case of lung gangrene.

### 2.3.5 Types of Surgical Operations

Two types of resections are recognized in pneumosurgery: **atypical and typical**.

Atypical Resections
- Wedge
- Marginal
- Enucleation of the lesion

Typical Resections
- Segmental resection
- Lobectomy
- Bilobectomy
- Pneumonectomy
- Extended pneumonectomy – removal of structures near the lung, such as the diaphragm, pericardium, the thoracic wall
- Cuff resection – usually a lobectomy with resection of the adjacent part of the central bronchus, with subsequent anastomosis of the central and peripheral bronchial stub

A lobectomy is the least radical procedure in the surgery of lung carcinoma. Segmental resections are used on a less common basis, and they are indicated for: bronchiectases, benign tumors, metastases. Atypical resections are reserved for benign pulmonary lesions, metastases and pulmonary tissue collections for diagnostic histology.

## 2.4 Mediastinum

### 2.4.1 Anatomical Notes

From the point of view of anatomy, mediastinum is an exactly defined space whose borderlines are formed by the sternum in the front, by the chest spine in the back, by mediastinal pleura on both sides, and by the upper thoracic aperture on the upper side. In terms of surgery, further division of this space is important. The anteroposterior plane, passing through the sternal angle in the front and through the body of the 4$^{th}$ vertebra in the back, separates the superior and inferior mediastinum. Inferior mediastinum is further subdivided to the anterior part – from the sternum to the anterior area of the pericardium, the middle part – the pericardium with the heart, and the posterior part – between the posterior area of the pericardium and the spine (Fig. 2.2).

### 2.4.2 Acute Mediastinitis

This is a serious and rapidly progressing disease, burdened with high mortality even today.

**Etiology** – The most common causes include esophageal perforation, infection transfer from neighboring organs – the lungs, pleura, spine, perforation of the tracheobronchial tree, and also odontogenic inflammations and throat infections. Penetrating traumas and early infections of sternotomy represent relatively rare causes.

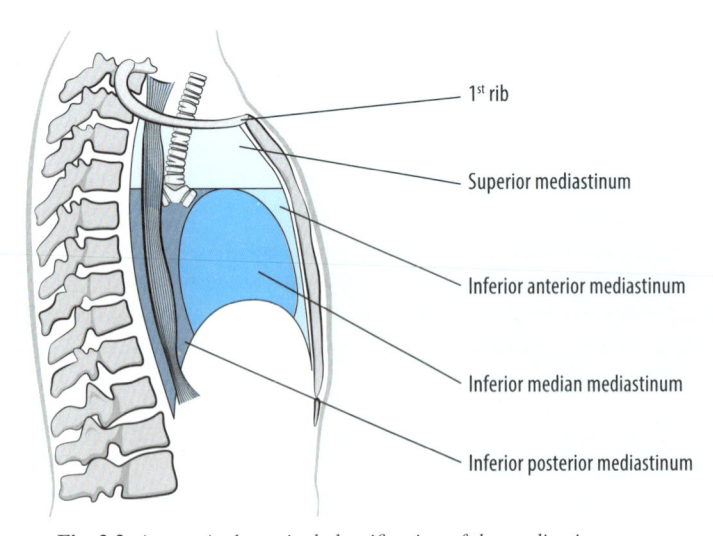

**Fig. 2.2** *Anatomical-surgical classification of the mediastinum*

**Symptomatology** – The clinical image is dominated by a generally serious condition with fever, tachycardia and septic shock development. Patients complain of chest pain and neck pain; signs of inflammation may be apparent locally in the area of the jugulum, and possibly subcutaneous emphysema.

**Diagnostics** stem from medical history (instrumental examination, injury, tumor, infection) and the clinical finding. Radiography shows unclearly circumscribed and expanded mediastinum. Spiral CT assessment is necessary, furthermore endoscopic examination of the esophagus and respiratory pathways. Complete laboratory assessment supplements the diagnosis (inflammatory signs). If esophageal endoscopy is negative and perforation in this area is suspected, esophagogram can be performed using water solution of a contrast agent in order to determine the localization and size of the perforation.

**Therapy** – For perforation mediastinitis, surgical revision and suture of the defect should be performed in the first 6 hours after the injury. A longer time interval gives no hope for the suture healing. From general measures, the important ones include circulatory resuscitation in the case of signs of shock, administration of broad spectrum antibiotics, enteral nutrition, and a nasogastric probe. The mediastinum should be drained using a thick drain, from jugular or paravertebral access or transdiaphragmatically based on the process localization.

**Prognosis** – Based on severity of the inflammation and of the underlying disease, mortality reaches up to 40%.

### 2.4.3 Mediastinal Tumors

These tumors are a very inhomogeneous group of diseases in terms of their etiology, symptomatology, course, therapy, and prognosis. There are many classifications of mediastinal tumors (**the department, where the author of this text is active, uses modified Diviš classification**). The term "tumors" includes benign and malignant tumors.
1. Thyroid tumors
2. Parathyroid tumors
3. Thymic tumors
4. Heteroplastic dysembryomas – teratomas and dermoid cysts
5. Homoplastic dysembryomas – bronchogenic, pericardial, pleural, esophageal and lymphatic cysts
6. Neurogenic tumors
7. Mesenchymal tumors
8. Primary sarcomas
9. Primary carcinomas
10. Pseudotumors
11. Vascular tumors

**Symptomatology** – Most tumors, particularly the benign ones, are asymptomatic. Symptoms such as pain in the chest, respiratory problems and inspiratory stridor, hoarseness, dysphagia, singultus (hiccups), diaphragmatic paresis, superior vena cava syndrome or the Horner syndrome tend to be present in huge benign tumors. The symptoms above follow from compression or penetration of the tumor in appropriate structures. The symptoms of myasthenia gravis are present in some thymic tumors.

**Diagnostics** – Radiography of the chest in two projections, CT or NMR. Endoscopic examination methods: laryngoscopy, bronchoscopy, esophagoscopy. Other examinations: ORL, neurological and cardiological. From imaging methods: radiography, esophageal passage, DSA (suspicion for aortic aneurysm, highly vascularized tumor). From laboratory assessments: tumor markers (AFP, HCG, CEA, NSE, TPA), blood count and differential count of white blood cells, and possibly hematological examination with bone marrow puncture. In addition, surgical methods with the possibility of tissue sample collection are used in the diagnostics: thoracoscopy, mediastinoscopy, parasternal mediastinotomy and puncture under CT guidance. Individual examination methods depend on the localization of the tumor and expected etiology.

**Therapy** – All mediastinal tumors which meet the following criteria are an indication for surgical revision and tumor removal: local operability of the tumor, patient tolerability of thoracotomy or sternotomy, and in malignancies, absence of distant metastases.

**Complications of surgical treatment** – Peroperative bleeding, heart rhythm disorders, iatrogenic injury to large respiratory pathways, esophagus, large blood vessels, and the thoracic duct. In the post-operative period, the complications include pneumothorax, infection, continued bleeding which requires urgent revision. Worsening of myasthenic manifestations occur in patients with the symptoms of myasthenia gravis if their preoperative immunosuppressive preparation was not sufficient.

**Prognosis** – Very good after radical removal of benign tumors, with no need for further therapy, only dispensing. The initial tissue and advancement of the tumor are factors that matter in malignancies. Relatively good prognosis has been seen in thyroid, parathyroid and thymic tumors.

### 2.4.4 Mediastinal Emphysema

This is the pathological accumulation of air in the mediastinum. This condition is caused by perforation of large respiratory pathways in the mediastinum or esophageal perforation.

Subcutaneous emphysema dominates in the clinical image, manifested by local swelling and fulmination with the most found in the neck, in the head and upper limbs, with fast progression to the whole body. Dyspnea occurs and if the condition continues, it leads to cardiac failure due to reduced venous return. Radiography is important for the diagnosis – pneumomediastinal image, and endoscopic examination.

**Therapy** is surgical and consists in the suture of the perforated organ, mediastinal drainage and other measures similar to those in mediastinitis.

## 2.5  Thoracic Trauma

These traumas may occur separately or as part of polytraumas. Up to 30% of fatally injured persons die of thoracic trauma. In polytraumatized patients, the most risky combination is represented by an injury to the chest and head, associated with up to 80% mortality. On the contrary, even a relatively small injury may cause serious complications in patients of higher age due to a primary cardiac or respiratory disease. Based on their mechanism, traumas are classified as follows:
- Blunt trauma
- Open trauma

In open traumas, it is important to distinguish whether they are:
- Penetrating
- Non-penetrating

The borderline between these types is formed by parietal pleura whose injury is caused by penetration. Therefore, careful revision is important in the treatment of a wound in the chest, during which the type and seriousness of the trauma are classified.

**Symptomatology** depends on the type and extent of the injury to the chest organs. Pain in the affected side is present, which worsens with movement, cough and respiration. Dyspnea, tachypnea, cyanosis and circulatory complications are usually symptoms of serious injury to the thoracic wall or intrathoracic organs. Pneumothorax, hemothorax or both, subcutaneous emphysema, and paradoxical movement of the thoracic wall are usually present in these types of traumas. Arrhythmia and circulatory instability are present in mediastinal traumas. Local signs of trauma are expressed in skeletal fractures in the chest: hematoma of the thoracic wall, swelling, crepitations, pathological configuration of the affected area; subcutaneous emphysema may be present. In most serious injuries, the clinical image is dominated by hypovolemic shock and global respiratory insufficiency.

**Diagnostics** – Medical history and careful clinical assessment. Thorough revision of the wound is necessary in open traumas, and deciding on whether it is a penetrating or non-penetrating trauma. Radiography is the basic assessment in

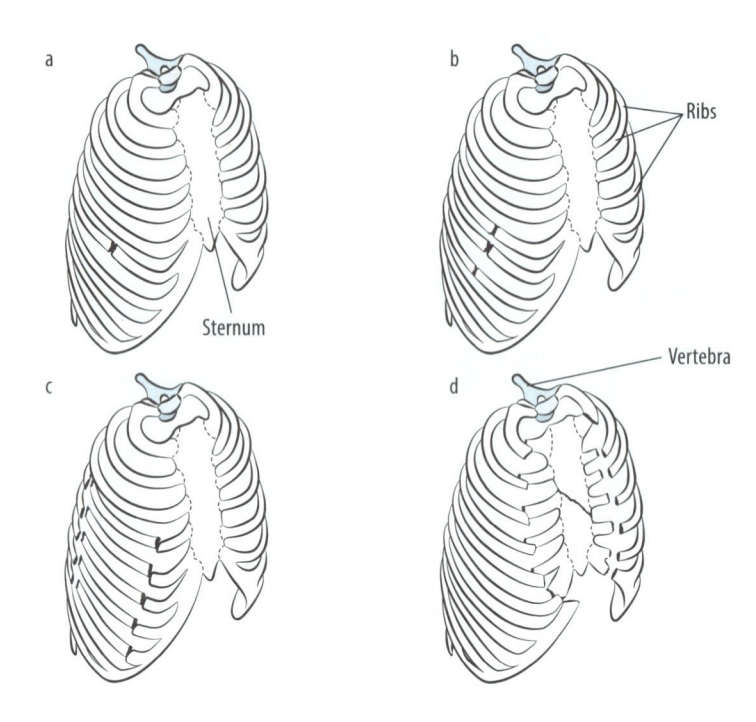

**Fig. 2.3** *Types of rib fractures: a) Simple rib fracture; b) Serial rib fracture; c) En bloc rib fracture; d) En bloc fracture with sternal break and fracture*

all types of injuries. Spiral CT is today's standard in serious thoracic traumas and polytraumas, and possibly other special examinations based on the findings (bronchoscopy, esophagoscopy, ECHO, contrast radiography, NMR and others). From laboratory assessments, the tests performed include a blood count, blood gases, basic biochemical screening, ECG. Invasive monitoring of circulatory parameters, diuresis and pulse oxymetry are necessary in severe traumas. Urgent bronchoscopy is indicated in mediastinal emphysema with suspected rupture of the tracheobronchial tree.

## TYPES OF THORACIC TRAUMA
- Injury to soft tissues of the thoracic wall
- Rib fractures
- Sternal fractures
- Hemothorax
- Pulmonary contusion

## 2.5.1 Injury to Soft Tissues of the Thoracic Wall

Injuries to soft tissues of the thoracic wall include a whole scale of types from simple circumscribed contusion of the thoracic wall up to open trauma wounds. Localized pain and local findings predominate. The treatment is symptomatic – analgesics, resting regimen, or causal – treatment of the local finding.

## 2.5.2 Rib Fractures

1. Simple fractures – fracture of 1 to 2 ribs at a single place
2. Serial fractures – fractures of 3 and more ribs at a single place
3. En bloc fractures – double fracture of two and more ribs with an instable central fragment ("flail chest" – cf. Fig. 2.3)

**Therapy** of simple fractures is usually outpatient and symptomatic. Serial fractures require hospitalization, monitoring of cardiorespiratory functions, and regular radiography check-ups to exclude any other complications. The therapy is based on good oxygenation ($O_2$ therapy), perfect analgesia, such as using an epidural catheter, respiratory rehabilitation and care of good expectoration to prevent pulmonary complications. En bloc fractures are the most serious type of injuries to the chest skeleton, and for the patient they mean a risk of immediate respiratory and cardiac failure. Besides measures listed for the therapy of serial fractures, invasive monitoring must be included in the therapeutic scheme. Artificial pulmonary ventilation is indicated in the event of any signs of developing respiratory insufficiency. Fractures associated with a serious intrathoracic trauma, compound injuries to the chest and abdomen, and substantially dislocated fractures are an indication for surgical treatment and stabilization of the chest by using splints.

## 2.5.3 Sternal Fractures

Sternal fractures are rare and are treated symptomatically. They are indicated for surgery only in the case of substantial dislocation, intolerable pain, and fractures associated with another intrathoracic trauma.

## 2.5.4 Hemothorax

Hemothorax is caused by a more extensive trauma of the thoracic wall, injury to pulmonary parenchyma or blood vessels of the pulmonary and systemic circulation. It may also occur as iatrogenic, after chest surgeries, chest drainage or central venous cannulation. The physical finding is identical to that in fluidothorax,

and hypovolemic shock develops upon higher blood loss. Hemothorax is classified as follows, based on the amount of blood in the thoracic cavity:
- Small – up to 500 mL
- Medium – 500 to 1500 mL
- Large – more than 1500 mL

**Therapy** depends on the blood loss volume. In case of weaker bleeding, a sufficient measure includes chest drainage in the 4$^{th}$ or 5$^{th}$ intercostal space along the middle axillary line, using a sufficiently thick drain (32 Ch), regular checking the blood count, ABR, vital functions; radiography check-ups and monitoring of waste materials from the drain are a matter of course. The patients must be placed in the intensive care unit. Massive bleeding usually necessitates artificial pulmonary ventilation, invasive monitoring, blood loss replacement, thoracic cavity drainage and urgent surgery. Loss through the drain of more than 300 mL/h for 3 hours, progression of the radiography finding with the above-mentioned loss in one hour, single loss higher than 1,500 mL, persisting hypotension and hypovolemia with adequate volume replacement represent indications for surgical revision. The aim of the surgery is to find the bleeding source and provide treatment (suture, lung resection, etc.).

### 2.5.5 Pulmonary Contusion

Pulmonary contusion occurs with blunt injuries to the chest through a direct mechanism or the mechanism called "contrecoup". In the pulmonary contusion, small focal bleeding in the interstitium occurs, reflected in the radiographic scan as a blurred focus, or up to the formation of infiltrates, depending on the extent of the injury.

Therapy of simple contusions is symptomatic – observation, oxygenation, respiratory rehabilitation and prevention of complications. In large contusions associated with respiratory insufficiencies, artificial pulmonary ventilation with the PEEP and CPAP regimen is necessary. The prognosis of these patients is very serious. A surgery is indicated exceptionally, upon development of septic complications that cannot be handled in a conservative manner as well as upon fibrotization of the lung. The decision to perform pulmonary resection in the contused lung is very complicated and its indication is determined exclusively by the thoracic surgeon in cooperation with the anesthesiologist.

Other types of thoracic traumas are rare. This topic is highly specialized and exceeds the scope of this publication. Thus only an overview is presented below:
- Tracheal and bronchial trauma
- Heart contusion
- Penetrating cardiac trauma
- Blunt and penetrating injury to large blood vessels

- Injury to the thoracic duct
- Inhalation trauma of the tracheobronchial tree
- Esophageal trauma

### 2.5.6 Complications of Thoracic Trauma

Complications of thoracic traumas are relatively common. Primary or secondary infection may lead to development of thoracic empyema, mediastinitis or early complications. Insufficient treatment and evacuation of hemothorax lead to development of fibrothorax with subsequent limitation of respiratory functions. Another associated intrathoracic injury (most commonly the esophagus, thoracic duct) or injury to abdominal cavity organs may be overlooked during surgery due to massive bleeding. Development and non-recognized cardiac tamponade, continued post-operative bleeding or formation of a bronchopleural fistula represent very serious complications.

## 2.6 GI Surgery Using a Thoracic Approach

The opening of the thoracic cavity and the procedure form part of the surgical procedures applied in the treatment of some diseases of organs found in the upper part of the abdominal cavity. In most cases, the so-called two-cavity approach is applied; in the first period, laparotomy (usually upper median laparotomy) is used to open the abdominal cavity, the abdominal phase of the surgery is performed, and when closed and upon changing the patient's position, the second phase of the operation is carried out. This second phase entails opening the appropriate hemithorax, usually using a posterolateral thoracotomy. The thoracic phase of the surgery follows; the thoracic cavity is drained and closed. Disadvantages of this combined approach include the laboriousness, the need to change the patient's position, and the fact that it is impossible to explore both cavities at the same time. The so-called thoracophrenolaparotomy can be opted for in some cases, i.e. upper median laparotomy extended to the necessary side of the hemithorax up to the $7^{th}$ or $8^{th}$ intercostal spaces, up to the level of the middle to posterior axillary line, together with intersecting the diaphragm. This approach entails the disadvantage of disrupting diaphragm continuity and its innervation.

The vast majority of procedures concerned include surgical diseases of the esophagus and of the area of the gastric cardia. Tumors of the distal part of the esophagus and of the gastric cardia are treated using the two-cavity approach. During the abdominal phase of the surgery, the affected part of the esophagus or stomach is loosened together with the tumor, and replacement of the resected part of the upper gastrointestinal tube is prepared. A tubulized stomach, a part of the small or large intestine on the vascular graft can be used as replacement.

Subsequently, the affected part of the gastrointestinal tube in the chest is loosened, it is resected, and a sentinel lymphadenectomy is performed. The procedure is completed by reestablishing the continuity of the gastrointestinal tube. If the resected part of the esophagus is replaced with the stomach, the only anastomosis is present in the chest or in the mediastinum. When replaced with the intestine, proximal anastomosis is present in the chest. A total esophagectomy with cervical anastomosis is necessary in the case of tumors in the middle and upper third of the esophagus. In this case, the chest is opened only for dissection of the upper part of the esophagus, subsequently completed with lymphadenectomy. This part can be left out in some cases, performing blunt extirpation of the esophagus using the cervical and abdominal approach. Another solution consists in performing the thoracic phase of the surgery using thoracoscopy.

From other diseases of the esophagus, epiphrenic diverticula and achalasia can be tackled using a thoracic approach. Mini-invasive surgery is being used even more frequently for the management of these diseases.

A thoracic approach from a thoracotomy is one of the possibilities how diaphragmatic hernias can be handled.

Other indications for opening both cavities, in this case usually from thoracophrenolaparotomy, include liver surgeries, particularly right-sided or extended right-sided hemihepatectomy: then the thoracic cavity is opened in order to gain access to the inferior vena cava.

All these procedures are technically demanding and burdensome for the patient, and are associated with a number of risks in the peroperative and especially post-operative periods.

# 3 MAMMARY GLAND SURGERY

*3.1 Introduction*
*3.2 Classification of Breast Diseases*
*3.3 Diagnosis of Breast Diseases*
*3.4 TNM Classification of Breast Cancer*
*3.5 Breast Cancer Therapy*
*3.6 Prognosis of Patients with Breast Cancer*
*3.7 Complications of Surgical Treatment*
*3.8 Medical Surveillance after Breast Cancer Therapy*
*3.9 Breast Reconstruction after Mastectomy*

## 3.1 Introduction

According to various statistics, benign breast diseases affect 50–90% of female population in advanced countries. Breast cancer is the most common malignant disease in women, and as a cause of death due to malignant disease it ranks second after lung cancer. According to data from the year 2005, breast cancer accounts for 21% of all malignities. This also points to the severity of this issue and the need of its thorough knowledge. High incidence of benign diseases requires from the examining physician high proficiency in differences between benign and malignant lesions, both during clinical examination and in the assessment of other diagnostic methods. This is why breast disease centers are designed as multidisciplinary sites where the surgeon, gynecologist, radiodiagnostician, oncologist, and pathologist cooperate in making the diagnosis and choosing the most effective therapy.

## 3.2 Classification of Breast Diseases

### 3.2.1 Inflammatory Diseases

1. Mastitis
    - During puerperium and lactation (puerperal mastitis)
    - In non-lactating women (be careful about erysipeloid carcinoma)

- Silicone mastitis (granulomatous inflammation as a response to an implant or paraffin injection for cosmetic reasons)
- Specific types of mastitis (particularly tuberculous)
2. Breast abscess
3. Fat necrosis of the breast (after a trauma or irradiation)

### 3.2.2 Fibrocystic Breast Disease (Synonyms: Mastopathy, Mammary Dysplasia, Fibrocystic Mastopathy, Chronic Mastitis)

A heterogenous group of conditions characterized particularly by cysts and periductal fibrosis. The following terms are used based on the extent to which individual morphological structures are represented: simple cyst, epitheliosis, adenosis or radial scar. In terms of cellular proliferative activity and its relation to the risk of breast carcinoma development we distinguish three types:
- Simple mastopathy without proliferation (breast cancer risk 0.5 to 1.3%)
- Proliferating mastopathy (breast cancer risk 1.9 to 3.4%)
- Proliferating mastopathy with atypias (breast cancer risk 5 to 11%)

### 3.2.3 Benign Tumors

1. Benign epithelial tumors
   - Intraductal papilloma
   - Nipple adenoma
   - Mammary gland adenoma
2. Fibroepithelial tumors
   - Fibroadenoma
   - Cystosarcoma phyllodes

### 3.2.4 Malignant Tumors

1. Non-invasive – called *in situ* carcinomas; premalignant changes originating from epithelial cells of the ducts or lobules after tumorous transformation, which may precede formation of an invasive tumor by even more than 10 years
   - Ductal carcinoma in situ
   - Lobular carcinoma in situ
2. Invasive carcinomas
   - Ductal (occurrence approx. in 84%)
   - Lobular (occurrence approx. in 15%)
   - Less common variants (1%) – medullary, mucinous, papillary, cribriform, tubular, comedonal, Paget's carcinoma of the nipple and others

- Erysipeloid (inflammatory) carcinoma – very aggressive form of dedifferentiated carcinoma
3. Sarcomas – rare
   - (Stromal sarcoma, leiomyosarcoma, liposarcoma, lymphangiosarcoma and others)
4. Malignant lymphomas – rare
   - (Leukemic infiltrates, Hodgkin's and non-Hodgkin's lymphoma)

### 3.2.5 Accessory Breast

Accessory breast is not a tumor in the proper sense but rather a developmental deviation. It may be localized anywhere along the milk line. Most commonly, it is found in the axilla. Accessory breast is subject to the same hormonal influences and pathological processes as the normal mammary gland, including malignization. From the clinical point of view, it is important that the accessory breast can mimic breast cancer (lump in the axilla) or can appear as painful inflammation of the lymph node associated with marked pain and bound to the premenstrual period or pregnancy. Its diagnosis can be specified more exactly by sonography or histology of an excisional biopsy specimen. In the case of malignization, the therapeutic strategy is identical to that in a normally located mammary gland. If the mammary gland is located away from milk line, it is an aberrant mammary gland.

### 3.2.6 Gynecomasty

Gynecomasty means unilateral or bilateral enlargement of the mammary gland in men, conditioned hormonally by androgen deficit or estrogen surplus, due to paraneoplasty (bronchogenic carcinoma), related to liver cirrhosis (hormone degradation disorder) or drugs. Endocrinological and urological examinations (germinal testicular tumor) should also be done as part of differential diagnosis. Male breast carcinoma occurs rarely (0.1% of all tumors in men), and therefore it is usually diagnosed in a late stage. Its diagnosis and therapy are identical to those of breast cancer in women.

## 3.3 Diagnosis of Breast Diseases

### 3.3.1 Medical History

Important factors that increase the breast cancer risk:
- Family history of breast cancer (women whose mothers or sisters have had breast cancer, particularly before menopause, are at a higher risk for the disease)

- Hereditary disposition to breast cancer (related to mutations in suppressor genes BRCA1 and BRCA2) is diagnosed in 5 % to 7 % of breast cancer patients
- No childbirth or the first child at 35 years of age or older
- Women who have not given birth or who gave birth for the first time after 35 years of age
- Early menarche (before 12 years of age) and late menopause (after 50 years of age)
- Mammary dysplasia
- Personal history of unilateral breast cancer
- Uterine body carcinoma
- More than 10 years of using hormonal contraceptives with high or moderate estrogen dosage
- Long-term use of estrogens in the postmenopausal period (hormone replacement therapy)

Menstrual cycle problems, previous breast disease, its duration or recurrence and nipple discharge also play an important role.

### 3.3.2 Clinical Examination

The patient (both female and male) is first examined in standing possition by visual inspection in order to detect any breast asymmetry and to evaluate skin condition. Subsequently, the patient is examined in the supine position with the hands behind the head (the breast stretches over the chest wall and becomes all accessible for palpation).

All quadrants (Fig. 3.1) one by one and the central part of the breast with the areola and nipple (discharge, Paget's disease) are examined. Finally, the breast is examined in the sitting position with contraction of the pectoral muscles.

A breast lump larger than 1 cm can be detected by palpation, but it is important to take into consideration the relation of the lump to the breast size, lump location and the quality of the mammary gland itself. Examination is completed with palpation of the lymph nodes in the axilla, supraclavicular and infraclavicular regions. If findings of the physical examination are uncertain, the examination should be repeated, preferably immediately after menstruation. The patient should be instructed as to the importance of breast self-examination.

■ SYMPTOMATOLOGY

#### Breast Lump
Besides pain, the lump is the most common reason why women come for an examination. Breast lumps may be found accidentally while washing the body

# MAMMARY GLAND SURGERY

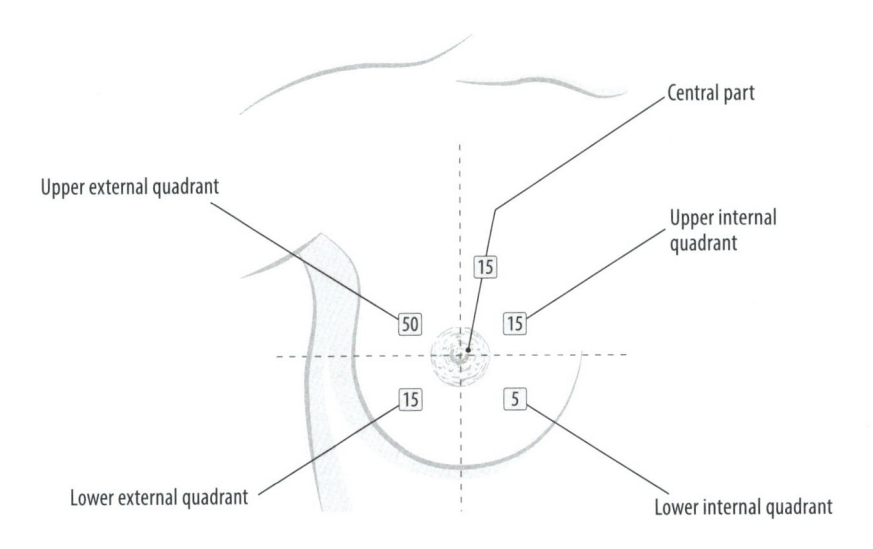

**Fig. 3.1** *Schematic division of the breast in quadrants with carcinoma incidence frequencies (percent)*

or during self-examination. Sometimes, it may be found after mild contusion of the breast as a hematoma residue and/or it may be a coincidence. The lump may be smooth, rigid, well circumscribed, loosely movable (fibroadenoma, cyst), or hard, uneven, fixed, pulling in the skin (cancer). In fibrocystic mastopathy, lumps are characterized by uneven edges and are more or less tender to palpation.

## Deformation
In the case of malignity, deformation is a late manifestation. The skin over the lump is pulled in, fixed, usually not painful. A nipple pulling inward due to cancer should be distinguished from a true inverted nipple which is usually present from birth, often bilaterally, and may interfere with breastfeeding.

## Reddening and Edema
In the case of malignity, these may be either late manifestations or signs of rapidly progressing erysipeloid cancer. The skin may look like an orange peel. An edema of the arm (lymphedema) may also be present due to tumorous obstruction of the lymphatics. In the case of inflammatory breast diseases, the skin is usually smooth, red, warm, painful on palpation, with possible fluctuation.

## Pain
Pain is not a typical manifestation of malignity. Benign mastodynia is usually caused by hormonal changes in the premenstrual period and it usually subsides

TEXTBOOK OF SURGERY

with the beginning of menstruation. In terms of differential diagnostics, it is necessary to exclude vertebrogenic difficulties, intercostal neuritis, etc.

### Discharge (not during Lactation)

Discharge may be serous, whitish, grey-green, brownish, bloody, unilateral or bilateral. This condition is most commonly caused by intraductal papilloma (rarely by intraductal carcinoma), mammary dysplasia, hormonal disorders (prolactin), use of hormonal contraceptives and some drugs. Bloody discharge may be the first sign of malignity.

## 3.3.3 Imaging Methods

Imaging methods are of crucial importance in the diagnosis of breast pathologies. However, it should be emphasized that an optimal diagnostic results (in relation to long-term survival of cancer patients) can only be achieved by combining clinical examination, including risk assessment based on medical history, with the choice of a suitable imaging method. When the finding is uncertain, the diagnostic process should be continued with needle biopsy or surgical excision of the lesion.

### ■ MAMMOGRAPHY

Mammography (MG) is the basic imaging method used to find early (also non-palpable) stages of breast cancer. It is also used as a screening method. The mammogram is assessed for the breast architecture and the presence of shadowing and microcalcification. If the mammographic finding is positive yet no lesions are clinically palpable, needle biopsy is done under radiographic control (stereotaxis) or the lesion is marked, with subsequent excision and histological assessment. The diagnostic yield for mammography in combination with clinical examination is up to 90 % in the case of malignancy. When used as a single assessment method (screening), its yield achieves about 40%, while the number of false positive findings is about 60%.

### ■ ULTRASONOGRAPHY

Ultrasound (US) is used particularly to differentiate cystic and solid lesions. The success rate of differentiating benign from malignant lesions has been permanently rising as well. When a cyst is suspected, ultrasound-guided cyst aspiration can be performed and fluid cytology done.

### ■ DUCTOGRAPHY

In nipple discharge, the specific discharging duct orifice is identified and, after contrast material has been injected, it is X-rayed. The radiograph is examined for filling defect indicating the presence of intraductal papilloma or carcinoma.

## MAMMARY GLAND SURGERY

### ■ MAGNETIC RESONANCE MAMMOGRAPHY (MRM)

The main indications for MRM with use of a paramagnetic reagent include suspected breast cancer in women with breast implants, patient's age under 25 years, and exclusion of a multifocal breast cancer.

### ■ COMPUTED TOMOGRAPHY (CT)

CT is used to determine the relationship of a malignant lesion to the thoracic wall or the pectoral fascia and for radiotherapy planning.

### ■ POSITRON EMISSION TOMOGRAPHY (PET)

PET, possibly in combination with CT (PET CT), is not a standard preoperative examination. It is used to differentiate between the malignant and the benign etiology of MG and US findings in very dense breasts, in postoperative scar tissue and after radiotherapy, for staging or restaging (detection of local or distant recurrence) and monitoring of the therapeutic response.

### 3.3.4 Biopsy and Cytology

Needle biopsy or cytology is used to collect tissue for histological assessment. Both examinations require an experienced specialist due to the risk of false negative results (5%). Surgical excision of the lesion is performed for a reliable histological verification in the event of clinical or mammographic suspicion of malignity and negative aspiration biopsy.

### 3.3.5 Histopathological and Immunohistochemical Assessment

When the material of a suspected lesion has been collected, it is assessed microscopically to determine the following: size of the tumor, histological type and its grade, dissemination into the circulation and lymphatic systems, perineural invasion, and presence of necroses. In the case of surgical extirpation, the safety border is assessed, which separates the malignant lesion from the healthy tissue. During axillary lymphadenectomy, the number of nodes affected by metastases is assessed. Immunohistochemical examination is used to determine presence/absence of hormonal estrogen and progesterone receptors, cell proliferation markers (Ki-67, PCNA) and c-erb-B2 oncogene expression (Her-2/neu).

### 3.3.6 Laboratory Assessments

Changes in tumor marker values (Ca 15-3, TPS, CEA) are used particularly for early determining of a relapse or tumor generalization. Of decisive importance is the dynamics of changes in their levels. The result of a single examination is of little value. The normal finding does not exclude the presence of a tumor.

## 3.4 TNM Classification of Breast Cancer

Tis – carcinoma *in situ* (non-infiltrating intraductal or lobular carcinoma *in situ* or Paget's disease of the nipple, with no concomitant palpable or radiological breast tumor
- T1 – Tumor smaller than 2 cm
- T2 – Tumor 2–5 cm
- T3 – Tumor larger than 5 cm
- T4 – Tumor of any size, infiltrating through the thoracic wall or skin; erysipeloid carcinoma
- N0 – No axillary nodes involved
- N1 – Metastasis to movable ipsilateral axillary lymph node(s)
- N2 – Metastasis in fixed ipsilateral axillary lymph node(s)
- N3 – Metastases in nodes along the ipsilateral internal mammary artery
- M0 – No demonstrable distant metastases
- M1 – Demonstrated distant metastases including bilateral involvement of the breast or nodes

Table 3.1 Clinical stages of breast carcinoma

| Stage | | | |
|---|---|---|---|
| 0 | Tis | N0 | M0 |
| I | T1 | N0 | M0 |
| IIA | T0 | N1 | M0 |
| | T1 | N1 | M0 |
| | T2 | N0 | M0 |
| IIB | T2 | N1 | M0 |
| | T3 | N0 | M0 |
| IIIA | T0 | N2 | M0 |
| | T1 | N2 | M0 |
| | T2 | N2 | M0 |
| | T3 | N1, N2 | M0 |
| IIIB | T4 | Every N | M0 |
| | Every T | N3 | M0 |
| IV | Every T | Every N | M1 |

## 3.5 Breast Cancer Therapy

Therapy of breast cancer is multidisciplinary and involves participation of the surgeon, oncologist, radiodiagnostician, sonographist, and pathologist. Especially the survival period of the patient depends on a properly chosen procedure. Only then comes the "cosmetic" result; which is, nevertheless, also very important for the patient. Principal therapeutic modalities consist of the surgical procedure, radiotherapy, chemotherapy, hormonal therapy and biological treatment (targeted therapy using monoclonal antibodies). The order of individual therapeutic modalities is given by the stage of the disease. In general, at the early stages of disease (Tis, stages I and II), surgery is the first therapeutic step while therapy for more advanced stages (III and IV) usually begins with one of the oncological treatment modalities and surgery follows after its course has been completed. If surgery is indicated as the primary procedure, the other therapeutic modalities become adjuvant therapies and their choice depends on the result of histological and immunohistochemical assessments of the tumor and lymph nodes.

In the past 100 years, the surgical treatment of breast carcinoma experienced substantial development. The original super-radical surgery (Halsted) was replaced with modified radical mastectomy, and the breast-preserving surgery can now be performed (in indicated cases) thanks to the development of oncological therapeutic methods in the recent decades. This trend arises especially from the understanding that breast cancer, even at its early stages, can be a systemic disease, and thus loco-regional treatment may have only a limited effect on the length of survival. This fact has been confirmed by multicentric randomized studies.

Axillary lymphadenectomy (axilla exenteration) is a necessary part of the surgical procedure. In view of the fact that axillary nodes are not affected in almost

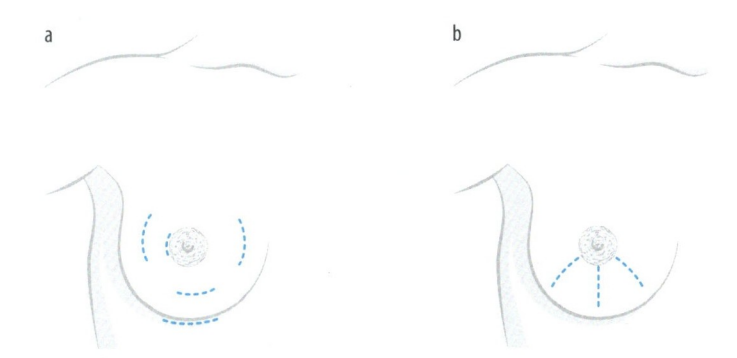

**Fig. 3.2** *Direction of incisions in the breast: a) Semicircular incision (for example, periareolar, submammary); b) Radial incisions may also be considered in the lower half of the breast*

2/3 of operated patients, the radicality of this axillary procedure is now getting reduced as well (in indicated cases) from axillary lymphadenectomy of levels I and II to sentinel lymph node dissection.

Incisions for intraoperative harvest of biopsy tissue, tumorectomy or removal of a benign lesion should, for cosmetic reasons, be made in Langer's lines (Fig. 3.2) as semicircular periareolar or submammary skin incisions or radial incisions in the lower half of the breast.

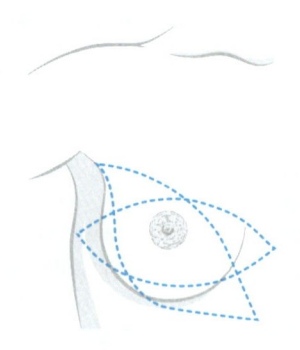

**Fig. 3.3** *Modified radical mastectomy – dermal incisions*

**Halsted radical mastectomy**, Halsted radical mastectomy, no longer used today, involves removal of the entire breast, chest muscles, and all of the lymph nodes under the arm. It was a very disfiguring operation. Today, the same results are achieved with less radical surgery followed by postoperative radiotherapy.

**Modified radical mastectomy** (Fig. 3.3) includes removal of the breast with exenteration of level I and level II axillary nodes or with sentinel lymph node dissection. It spares the chest muscles.

**Breast Conserving Surgery** (breast preservation treatment) removes only the cancerous area in healthy tissue as in tumorectomy, lumpectomy or quadrantectomy. It is always associated with relevant axillary node dissection (Figs. 3.4, 3.5, 3.6) and followed by postoperative radiation therapy of the remaining breast tissue. The results of studies on breast conserving surgery have shown the same length of survival in these patients as found in breast cancer patients after

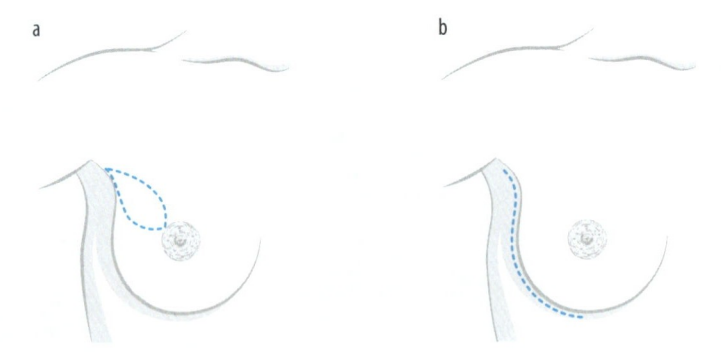

**Fig. 3.4** *Partial mastectomy with axilla exenteration in continuity: a) Surgery according to Criley; b) Surgery according to Bardenhauer*

# MAMMARY GLAND SURGERY

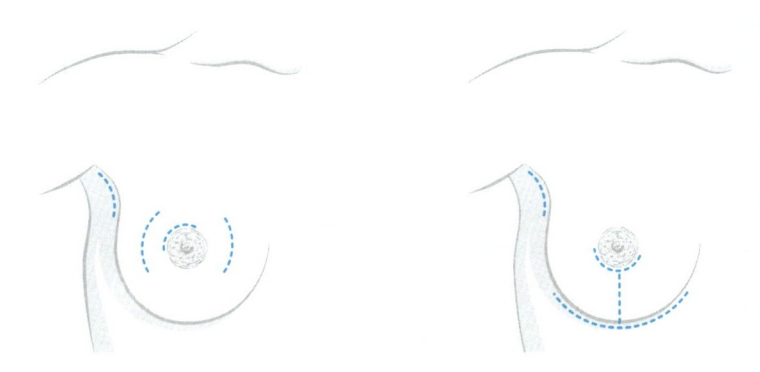

**Fig. 3.5** *Partial mastectomy with axilla exenteration in discontinuity*

**Fig. 3.6** *Centroinferior hemimastectomy with axilla exenteration in discontinuity*

radical modified mastectomy. In patients under 40 years of age, the incidence of local tumor recurrence may be more frequent. Multicentric breast cancer is a contraindication to breast conserving surgery.

**Exenteration of the axilla** is particularly of prognostic importance in terms of advancement of the disease. As a therapeutic procedure it is in the events of metastatic affection of lymph nodes. Axillary adipose tissue with lymph nodes are dissected along the lateral edge of the minor pectoral muscle up to the level of the axillary vein (level I and II). Exenteration of the axilla can be performed through the same incision as used for primary tumor removal (exenteration in continuity) or a new incision must be made (exenteration in discontinuity). A hope for five-year survival decreases with an increasing number of metastatic lymph nodes.

**Sentinel lymph node dissection** (SND) is an alternative to axilla exenteration in which, using Patent blue or lymphoscintigraphy, the sentinel node, the first one "standing guard", is identified, dissected and examined for the presence of metastasizing cancer. If it is affected, level I and II axilla exenteration is performed. This technique

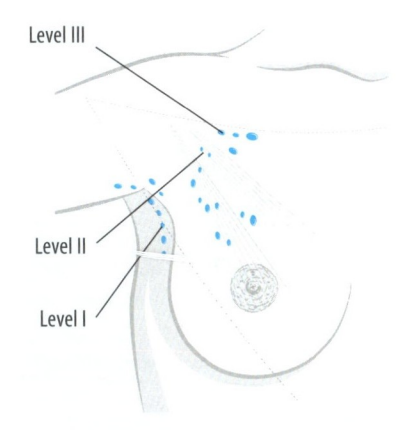

**Fig. 3.7** *Individual levels of lymph nodes in the axilla; Level I – nodes located externally from the small pectoral muscle up to the height of the axillary vein; Level II – nodes beyond the small pectoral muscle insertion up to the level of the axillary vein; Level III – nodes located medially from the small pectoral muscle insertion*

is taken into consideration in patients with negative clinical findings in the axilla (N0) and tumor size classified as T1 or T2.

## 3.6  Prognosis of Patients with Breast Cancer

Breast cancer causes death in 50% of the affected women. Prognosis of the disease depends on the size of the tumor, involvement of lymph nodes at the time of diagnosis, biological characteristics of the tumor, patient's age and her age of menopause, expression of hormonal receptors on the tumor cell, and also on the presence of distant metastases. In general, it can be said that the larger the tumor and the higher the number of affected axillary lymph nodes, the lower is the hope for five-year survival.

Determinative criteria for the 5-year period of survival are as follows:
- Tumor size
  - T1 = 85%
  - T2 = 75%
  - T3 = 35%
  - T4 = 10%
- Lymph node affection (the higher the number of affected axillary nodes, the worse is the prognosis)
  - N0 = 75%
  - N1–3 = 40–50%
  - N > 3 = 20–30%
- Tumor grading (histological type and malignity grade)
  - G1 – well differentiated
  - G2 – moderately differentiated
  - G3 – little differentiated
- Worse prognosis is associated with the infiltrating ductal carcinoma, absence of hormonal receptors, aneuploidy, higher number of tumor cells in the S-phase, and some oncogenic translocations.

## 3.7  Complications of Surgical Treatment

Complications of surgical treatment can be divided into early and late ones. While early complications (wound suppuration, hematoma, seroma, healing by second intention) require immediate surgical treatment, those late complications (postmastectomy pain syndrome and lymphedema) may appear several months or even years after the comprehensive therapy of breast cancer has been completed. The therapy of postmastectomy pain syndrome and lymphedema should be the responsibility of specialists (neurologist, physiotherapist, lymphologist). Symptomatic therapy involves administration of analgesics or non-steroid antiphlogistics and has an entirely supportive role.

### 3.7.1 Postmastectomy Pain Syndrome (PMPS)

According to various authors, the syndrome develops after comprehensive oncosurgical treatment for breast cancer in 22 to 72 % of the patients. Its major causes in relation to breast surgery include:
- neuropathic disorders manifested as phantom pain, intercostobrachial neuralgia or neuroma pain
- tight chest due to scar tissue presence
- pectoral muscle retraction due to the surgical procedure and breast and/or axilla radiotherapy
- antalgic position of the upper limb or shoulder girdle resulting in muscular dysbalance

Untreated PMPS may even disable the patient due to severaly restricted shoulder motion subsequently leading to cervicocranial or cervicobrachial syndrome. This may eventually produce a change in the respiratory stereotype, affect the statics and dynamics of the spinal column, particularly at the C/Th junction, and interfere with rib mobility at the sternocostal joints.

### 3.7.2 Neurological Disorders

Neurological disorders originate particularly from axilla exenteration and/or radiotherapy. Most commonly, sensitivity disorder is diagnosed on the dorsomedial side of the arm and below the axilla due to impairment of intercostobrachial nerves. This complication, however, does not markedly affect the shoulder girdle range of motion or the patient's quality of life. Informing the patient of the insignificant nature of this symptom is usually sufficient to make her accept the condition and get adapted to it in the long term.

Pectoral muscles atrophy appears in consequence of the surgical damage of the lateral pectoral nerve. Injury to the long thoracic nerve leads to a winged scapula (scapula alata). Injury to the thoracodorsal nerve causes denervation of the latissimus dorsi muscle. Postradiation brachial plexitis can also be found. Injuries to the aforementioned nerves affect the mobility of respective muscle groups to various extent, with consequences especially for shoulder girdle mobility. Quite exceptionally, the brachial plexus may also be injured during the surgery, with all its consequences.

Adverse effects of chemotherapy and radiotherapy may include peripheral neuropathy, plexopathy and plexitis. The consequences may be transient or permanent according to the extent of injury.

### 3.7.3 Lymphatic Insufficiency – Lymphedema

Lymphatic system insufficiency is the sign of a serious disorder of lymph flow in the axilla after lymphadenectomy and/or radiation therapy for breast cancer. Unless adequate therapy is initiated in time, lymphatic insufficiency leads to irreversible damage of the lymphatic system and tissues devoid of lymphatic drainage, with subsequent complications such as recurrent dermal and subdermal inflammatory diseases, fibrotization and induration of tissues. A clinically apparent lymphedema may occur very shortly after surgery or during radiotherapy. However, it may also appear after several years due to a gradual decrease in the lymphatic system transport capacity in the given area.

The Comprehensive Decongestive Therapy is today the gold standard of lymphedema management; it includes manual and mechanical lymph drainage, compression bandages and sleeves, and special exercises), completed with a long-term enzyme therapy with Wobenzym. If this does not produce satisfactory results, in strictly indicated cases, surgical management can be considered, such as liposuction, lymph-venous, or respectively lymphonodal-venous anastomosis may be considered in precisely indicated cases. If left untreated, lymphedema may gradually lead to the development of edema, which may cause considerable restriction of upper limb mobility, and may grow up to form of elephantiasis.

Lymphedema of the upper limb as a sequela of the comprehensive breast cancer treatment is recorded in up to 40 % of the patients. The diagnosis of its early (latent) stage, characterized by indefinite pain, tension, pressure or heavy feeling of the arm, and its immediate treatment is the best option for the patient. Compared to the ipsilateral extremity, the limb may get easily tired. On clinical examination, however, no edema is apparent. Lymphatic insufficiency can be diagnosed by lymphoscintigraphic examination.

**Non-extremity lymphedema** can be diagnosed in up to 10% of treated patients. The most common localities include residual breast tissues after conservative surgical procedure, the scar and anterior thoracic wall, the area of axilla and scapula on the same side, and the epigastrium. Suspected non-extremity lymphedema can be verified using lymphscintigraphic examination of the affected area.

## 3.8 Medical Surveillance after Breast Cancer Therapy

During the first year after completion of the therapy, the patients should be followed up every 3 months (tumor on the other side, local relapse). In the subsequent period, the follow-up interval should be extended to 6 months. The primary aim is to seek for any local relapse and lymph node metastasis as a mark of cancer progression. The control includes mammographic examination (tumor in the other breast), sonography of the scar after the surgery and of sentinel lymph nodes. The clinical examination is no less important; it is focused on the post-mastectomy pain syndrome, motor apparatus disorders (particularly the shoulder girdle on the same side) and signs of lymphatic system insufficiency in the sentinel area (latent or clinically apparent lymphedema, respectively).

## 3.9 Breast Reconstruction after Mastectomy

Indications for reconstruction should be consulted with the oncologist, and this option should be offered to the patient before surgery, particularly for psychological reasons. The reconstruction procedure does not increase the risk of relapse. The most common method of breast reconstruction is a pedicled transverse rectus abdominus myocutaneous (TRAM) flap. If this cannot be used, prosthetic materials are considered (saline-filled and silicone-filled implants).

# 4 SOFT TISSUE TUMORS IN ADULTS

4.1 *General Characteristics*
4.2 *Incidence and Localization of Soft Tissue Sarcomas*
4.3 *Symptoms of Soft Tissue Sarcomas*
4.4 *Diagnostics and Surgical Treatment*
4.5 *Conclusions for Clinical Practice*

## 4.1 General Characteristics

Soft tissue tumors represent a non-homogeneous group of benign and malignant tumors that originate in the **mesenchymal tissue with the exception of bone and reticuloendothelial tissue**. Generally speaking, benign processes, especially in the limbs and trunk, are more common than malignant ones (5:1); however, in view of the serious prognosis of patients suffering from malignant tumors (sarcomas), these processes should always be thoroughly considered and properly diagnosed and treated. **Benign tumors**, most often represented by lipomas, fibromas, neurofibromas and hemangiomas, are not of a locally invasive growth character and after being radically extirpated they neither recur nor metastasize. The real biological nature of the tissue can only be reliably assessed by means of a histological examination of the whole structure and thus should always be indicated. In case of clinical doubts about the tissue nature, the tumor should be treated as potentially malignant.

The exact **histological classification, grading and staging** are the basic preconditions for the selection of the further therapeutic strategy of sarcomas. The exact classification and evaluation of tumor margins is the task of a pathologist. Over 100 subtypes of sarcoma can be distinguished based on their morphology, growth aggressivity, system of metastatic processes or chemotherapy and radiotherapy response. Not even the histological assessment of a tumor's biological nature is always simple and unambiguous, and apart from the classic histological sample staining, immunohistochemical (expression of specific proteins), cytogenetic and hybridization (to prove changes in the gene level) methods are also used. While in children the most frequent sarcoma is **rhabdomyosarcoma**, in adults it is usually **liposarcoma, malignant fibrous histiocytoma** or **leiomyosarcoma.**

## 4.2 Incidence and Localization of Soft Tissue Sarcomas

The incidence of soft tissue sarcomas in children under 15 years of age is 4–7 cases per 1 million; more than half of them manifest before the age of 6. In adults, sarcomas are more frequent, with an incidence of 2–3 cases per 100,000 persons per year. It is thus quite a rare malignant disease that statistically represents approximately **1 % of the malignant processes in adults and 7 % of malignancies in children**.

The disease emerges most often after the third decade of life and is more frequent in males. **Predilection localizations,** where more than 60 % of these tumors can be found, **are in limbs**. The most frequently afflicted is the region of the thigh comprising more than half of all limb sarcomas. The remaining 40 % of soft tissue sarcomas develop in the **trunk and retroperitoneum**. Sarcomas at this localization represent a different diagnostic and therapeutic problem.

## 4.3 Symptoms of Soft Tissue Sarcomas

The symptoms of the disease are principally affected by tumor localization and size. If they appear in limbs, the patient usually seeks medical help due to a **palpable mass** that is often thought to be related to a previous injury. Pain and impaired function are less frequent symptoms. Due to the higher frequency of other processes in limbs (fibroma, lipoma, etc.), poor symptomatology can result in underestimation of the finding.

The symptoms of tumors situated in the trunk and especially in the retroperitoneum are also often atypical. Since the growth is slow, the surrounding tissues and organs adapt for a long time to the expansion, and therefore even extensive tumors can be found accidentally in a patient examined for another disease. The most commonly reported symptoms are **pressure, abdominal pain, abdominal pressure, impaired voiding, back pain and weight loss or a palpable mass**. In about one quarter of cases the primary retroperitoneal tumor is found accidentally in an asymptomatic patient. Another quarter of patients have neurological symptomatology due to compression of spinal nerves and nerve plexuses. On the contrary, signs of ureter obstruction or hematuria are rather rare.

## 4.4 Diagnostics and Surgical Treatment

Soft tissue tumors **in extremities** often represent a complicated differential diagnostic problem for an attending physician. Although benign tumors are approximately 5 times more frequent in this localization, the finding should not be underestimated. A possibility of malignancy should be considered if the clinical examination reveals signs frequently found in soft tissue sarcomas. Suspicion should be raised by findings such as **mass localized in the groin, popliteal and cubital fossa, fast growing and painful tumors, tumors growing in deep tissue and exceeding 5 cm in diameter**. The clinical examination is followed by an ultrasound (US) examination that in superficial processes reliably informs about the localization, size and topography of the process. If suspicion of a malignant process persists, a **magnetic resonance imaging** (MRI) is indicated. This examination provides the most reliable information about the infiltration of surrounding structures, exceeded compartment borders, and, with certain caution, information about the nature of the process.

As has already been stressed, only a **histological examination** provides reliable information about the structure and biological nature of the tumor which is essential for selection of the correct therapeutic procedure. It naturally requires obtaining a representative sample of the neoplastic tissue. A sample of about 2 cm$^3$ is sufficient for the final processing. The value of findings obtained peroperatively by freezing technology is interpreted with some controversy. Alternatively, a tissue sample can be obtained by a puncture technique administered with an ultrasound; however, an insufficient amount of the representative tissue may cause problems upon detailed examination. A suspected lesion on an extremity must be approached with the utmost caution by a surgeon well aware of the task. **Tissue excision for further examination** is indicated, and not just attempts for a non-radical extirpation. This applies above all to tumors larger than 3 cm and situated in deeper tissues. During the sample collection it is necessary to be aware of the possible further steps and to not worsen the conditions for subsequent radical procedures. It is appropriate to perform the incision in the direction of the long axis of the limb, penetrate the tumor in the shortest possible manner and not open another compartment. Thorough hemostasis and drainage (if opted for) through the wound ends are important. Hematoma in tumor surroundings and drains via contra-incisions can contribute to tumor cell dissemination from the focus. **The procedure of definitive resection** is aimed at complete elimination of the tumor in the healthy tissue with the attempt to maximally preserve functionally important structures. A rim of 2–4 cm of healthy tissue from the tumor margin is required to achieve radicality. Resection of the whole musculofascial compartments or even exceeding them thereafter requires complicated reconstructions from free tissue transfer and plastic surgery up to tendon and nerve transfers and transfers of tissues by the technique of microsurgery. This is why these procedures belong in the hands of experienced and specialized plastic surgeons that are capable of reaching the required radicality and performing a subsequent functionally acceptable reconstruction.

# SOFT TISSUE TUMORS IN ADULTS

Sarcomas of the retroperitoneum originate in the connective tissue of this region. In view of the fact that they do not originate in the organs of retroperitoneum, they are called primary retroperitoneal tumors. **80–90 % of these tumors are of a malignant nature**, and leiomyosarcoma is found in more than half of these cases. Fibrosarcomas and liposarcomas are the next most common types.

Primary retroperitoneal tumors comprise about 55 % of tumors in this localization and in a number of cases it is not easy and sometimes not even possible to distinguish them from tumors of retroperitoneal organs even if modern imaging methods are used. Depending on the localization, the pathological processes of the kidneys, suprarenal glands and pancreas, tumors originating in the lymph tissue but also inflammatory changes (abscesses), degenerative changes (e.g. pseudocysts) and, rarely, spontaneous retroperitoneal hematoma (e.g. on dicoumarin medication) should be considered. In terms of frequency, primary retroperitoneal tumors are followed by lymphomas and metastases of other tumors into retroperitoneal lymph nodes. In these cases tumors are usually multiple and diagnosis can be made by a biopsy of accessible lymph nodes situated even outside the retroperitoneum.

Neuroendocrine tumors constitute a particular group. They are localized most often in the parenchyma or in close proximity to the suprarenal gland or pancreas. In more than half of the cases hormonally active substances (noradrenaline, insulin, glucagon, gastrin, etc.) are produced. This results in the typical symptomatology, characteristic for each of the above mentioned hormones. The diagnosis is confirmed by biochemical evidence of high levels of the corresponding substance in the serum. Imaging methods serve to localize the process. Hormonally active tumors can also be present in places other than the retroperitoneum, e.g. in the mediastinum or the chest.

If a retroperitoneal process is suspected, the most important methods of examination are the modern imaging techniques. An ultrasound examination is mandatory; however, completion of the examination with a CT scan and/or MRI is usually necessary. These examinations provide principle information necessary for planning the surgical procedure: the size and localization of the tumor, its demarcation and relation to the surrounding organs, vascular structures or intestines.

The aim of the surgical treatment is **radical tumor removal** in the sense of R0-resection. In contrast to carcinomas, a regional lymphadenectomy is not usually indicated as it has no impact on the occurrence of local relapse or survival time. Only in rarely found rhabdomyosarcomas and synovialosarcoma is a regional lymphadenectomy beneficial. If the preoperative findings indicate the performance of a R0-resection improbable due to the tumor extent, infiltration of adjacent structures, metastatic process or multiple occurrences, a neoadjuvant therapy is indicated. The purpose of this treatment is to achieve tumor reduction that would thereafter enable a radical surgical treatment.

A surgical procedure can also be **indicated for palliative purposes**. This applies especially to extensive primary or recurrent retroperitoneal tumors or to metastatic stages of advanced tumors. In these situations surgery aims to relieve symptoms, first of all pain and GI voiding impairment. A palliative resection may also contribute to higher effectiveness of subsequent radiation therapy/chemotherapy.

A technical precondition for the accomplishment of an R0-resection is the attempt for **en bloc** resection which, depending on the finding, can possibly be extended to adjacent organs. This can be achieved only in cases of solitary processes, especially well demarcated ones. In this sense, whether the tumors are of cystic or solid structures does not play any significant role. Nevertheless, the situation is different in multiple occurrences of retroperitoneal tumors. Then, a radical procedure is not technically possible and if the diagnosis cannot be otherwise obtained, a probatory excision of a suitable lesion via laparotomy or laparoscopy is indicated. Further systemic treatment is selected on the basis of the histological findings; in the case of multiple occurrences of primary retroperitoneal tumors, the prognosis is usually poor. Due to the large heterogeneity of the histological types of these tumors it has not been conclusively proven which individual patients will possibly benefit from systemic chemotherapy.

## 4.5 Conclusions for Clinical Practice

Soft tissue sarcomas are relatively rare malignant diseases. Poor symptomatology can result in the **underestimation of the severity of the process**, mainly in extremities. On the other hand, a large finding on a CT scan or MRI can lead to surgical nihilism, rejecting the option of resection. Exact and detailed **histological classification and specification** (staging, grading) are preconditions for rational use of **neoadjuvant or adjuvant systemic chemotherapy and/ or radiation therapy**. Although soft tissue sarcomas are generally considered chemoresistant, a close interdisciplinary collaboration is needed to improve the therapeutic outcomes. The prognosis is usually serious.

# 5 MALIGNANT MELANOMA

*5.1 Introduction*
*5.2 Classification, TNM Classification and Staging*
*5.3 Risk Factors, Causes*
*5.4 Diagnostics*
*5.5 Therapy*
*5.6 Prognosis*

## 5.1 Introduction

Malignant melanoma is a malignant tumor originating in melanocytes. The melanocytes are localized mainly in the skin but also in the mouth mucosa and in the eye. It is a less common type of skin cancer but most deaths (75%) from skin tumors are associated with malignant melanoma. The incidence of malignant melanoma in the Czech Republic as well as worldwide has been increasing. While in 2000 it was 10.2/100,000 persons, in the year 2007 it was 13.7/100,000 persons (data from the National Oncological Register for the Czech Republic). The risk of developing malignant melanoma is associated mainly with exposure to sun rays and with skin phototype. Differences in the rate of incidence between males and females are not significant. In spite of intensive research for new options of non-surgical treatment, radical surgical excision still remains the main therapeutic method.

## 5.2 Classification, TNM Classification and Staging

Melanomas can be divided into several basic types.

**Lentigo maligna** – planar superficial lesions limited only to the upper skin layer. The risk of occurrence increases with age. These can be found especially in areas with continued exposure to sun rays (i.e. the face).

**Superficial spreading melanoma** – SSM – is the most common form of melanoma (70 %). It is characterized by horizontal growth; its originally smooth

**Table 5.1** Clark Classification of Malignant Melanoma

| Clark I | Invasion confined only to the epidermis |
|---|---|
| Clark II | Invasion into stratum papillare, without penetration to the junction otf stratum reticulare |
| Clark III | Invasion into the junction of stratum reticulare |
| Clark IV | Invasion into to the stratum reticulare |
| Clark V | Invasion into the subcutaneous tissue |

**Table 5.2** TNM Classification of Malignant Melanoma

| T0 | Melanoma not detected | | |
|---|---|---|---|
| Tis | Melanoma *in situ* | | |
| T1 | Breslow up to 1 mm | T1a | 0.75 mm, without ulceration |
| | | T1b | over 0.75 mm or ulceration |
| T2 | 1–2 mm | T2a | without ulceration |
| | | T2b | with ulceration |
| T3 | 2–4 mm | T3a | without ulceration |
| | | T3b | with ulceration |
| T4 | More than 4 mm | T4a | without ulceration |
| | | T4b | with ulceration |
| N0 | regional lymph nodes negative | | |
| N1 | 1 regional lymph node involved | | |
| N2 | 2–3 lymph nodes involved | | |
| N3 | 4 or more lymph nodes involved | | |
| M0 | without metastases | | |
| M1 | skin metastases and metastases to distant lymph nodes | | |
| M2 | lung metastases | | |
| M3 | all other metastases | | |

borders become irregular. Due to the small depth of invasion the prognosis of this type of melanoma is very good.

**Nodular melanoma** – NMM – is the second most frequent form of melanoma (20%), characterized by early vertical growth. It is a serious form of melanoma as

■ Table 5.3 TNM stages of Malignant Melanoma

| Ia  | T1a, N0, M0    |
| --- | -------------- |
| Ib  | T1b–2a, N0, M0 |
| II  | T2–4, N0, M0   |
| III | T1–4, N1–3, M0 |
| IV  | M1             |

the disease prognosis strongly depends on the depth of invasion. Nodular melanoma can arise on intact skin as well as by transformation of a pigment nevus.

**Acral lentiginous melanoma** – this type of melanoma is localized on skin areas lacking hair follicles, i.e. on the sole of the foot, the palm and in the area of the nails. Prognosis of this type of melanoma is the worst of all.

**Mucosal melanoma (of rectum, vulva), eye melanoma, soft-tissue melanoma** – rare but highly dangerous forms and localizations of malignant melanoma.

TNM classification of malignant melanoma is based on the **depth of invasion** in millimeters (Breslow), regional lymph node involvement and the presence of distant metastases. Clark classification evaluates the depth of melanoma invasion on the basis of infiltration of individual skin layers. Considering the depth of invasion in melanoma (T), the essential information is whether the tumor exceeds 1 mm and also the presence of ulceration. In lymph node involvement (N) the number of involved regional lymph nodes is assessed. In metastases (M) their localization is evaluated. Stages I and II are referred to as early stages where no lymph node involvement is present. Late stages are characterized by lymph node and metastatic involvement.

## 5.3   Risk Factors, Causes

**Exposure to UV radiation** is the most significant risk factor for developing malignant melanoma. The important factors are, primarily, sun ray intensity and the time of exposure. The latest studies have also clearly proven an association between higher risk of developing melanoma and tanning in sun beds. Especially patients with a low skin phototype (so called melanoma phenotype) carry a higher risk of developing melanoma. Genetic factors which predispose to development of skin melanoma have also been identified. In consanguineous relatives of patients suffering from malignant melanoma the risk is higher by up to 10%. Patients with a family history of melanoma and/or with multiple dysplastic nevi should be screened by a dermatologist on a regular basis, at least once a year. Melanoma development also endangers patients with long-term immunosuppression. In addition to UV radiation causes, malignant melanoma can also arise in areas with chronic irritation. Intensive research is being conducted with the goal to identify genetic disorders responsible for the development of malignant melanomas. The aim is to identify "high risk" patients who are expected to develop malignant melanoma even before detection of visible lesions.

## 5.4 Diagnostics

A visual examination of risk nevi is the fundamental diagnostic tool as well as the primary form of prevention. The **ABCDE rule** is a worldwide accepted principle:
- *A: Asymmetry* – skin nevi of irregular shapes constitute a risk for development of malignant melanoma
- *B: Border* – malignant melanoma has irregular borders in relation to its surroundings, "blurred" margins, unclear transition to healthy skin
- *C: Color* – brown, black, white, blue, red color of the lesion
- *D: Diameter* – a relative criterion as the nodular melanoma does not need to be large; lesions larger than 6 mm are usually considered risky. Planar large lesions are typical for lentigo maligna and SSM
- *E: Enlarging* – lesions that change in size are risky. If they are growing, nodularities appear but nodularities can also appear if lesions are reducing in size

Other melanoma signs include bleeding or lesion ulcerations. Acral lentiginous melanoma usually begins as a blue or dark spot in the predilection area. In addition to visual assessment of lesions, dermatoscopic examination is one of the basic examination methods. The dermatoscope magnifies the lesion up to 10 times and enables thorough inspection. Digital dermatoscopes can detect a risk lesion by means of computer evaluation of the criteria.

Lesions evaluated as hazardous can be excised for histological analysis. The excision must extend into at least 1–2 mm of healthy tissue. At the same time the excision for biopsy should not be too extensive, the length of the scar should not exceed 3 cm. In the case of a long scar, it is difficult or even impossible to complete the examination of sentinel lymph node (SLN) if indicated on the basis of the histological examination. In highly probable or macroscopically evident melanomas the excision should be radical including the examination of SLN during one surgical session.

**Examination of regional lymph nodes** plays an important role in diagnosing malignant melanoma. Evaluation of possible lymph node involvement by palpation or by an ultrasound examination as a part of preoperative staging is necessary for selection of the correct therapeutic procedure.

A set of "minor symptoms" like weight loss, loss of appetite or even cachexia are signs of generalized, advanced disease; another sign can be the presence of subcutaneous metastases.

The first sign of malignant melanoma can simply be lymphadenopathy or, unfortunately, even generalization without detecting the primary lesion. The original primary melanoma can undergo a complete regression before the advanced disease is diagnosed.

Diagnostics of ocular or vulvar melanoma lies beyond the scope of general surgery. On the other hand, the rare but highly malignant rectal melanoma can be revealed during anoscopic or rectoscopic examination.

Within preoperative and postoperative staging, PET/CT has a high sensitivity for malignant melanoma and its metastases.

## 5.5  Therapy

**Radical surgical excision** is the fundamental malignant melanoma therapy. In stages Tis and T1a of skin melanoma, a rim of 1 cm of healthy tissue is considered sufficient. In stages T1b–T3 a rim of 2 cm and in stage T4 2–3 cm. Mapping and **SLN examination** has an indispensable role in standard therapy protocol of malignant melanoma. Collection and examination of SLN including immunohistochemical examination of micrometastases is indicated in histologically proven malignant melanoma larger than 1 mm according to Breslow classification. In large planar lesions of more than 1.5 cm in diameter and lesions with ulceration, regression or nodularity (stages Ib–IIc), a simultaneous examination of SLN during primary excision is indicated. An essential requirement for examination of SLN is a preoperatively negative examination of regional lymph nodes and absence of distant metastases N0, M0. Mapping of the drained lymphatic region with the use of radionuclides and patent blue is irreplaceable mainly in melanoma localizations with uncertain lymph drainage such as the trunk (axilla, groin) or head.

If the presence of (micro) metastases in the SLN is confirmed, completion of a **radical regional lymphadenectomy** is indicated. This includes dissection of axilla, ilioinguinal dissection and neck lymphadenectomy.

If the rectum is involved, a radical resection or abdominoperineal amputation of the rectum is indicated.

Radical excision or resection of malignant melanoma metastases depends on decisions regarding the optimal procedure within multimodal antineoplastic therapy. It is always necessary to evaluate the therapeutic options for a particular patient individually.

In indicated cases, subcutaneous metastases can be extirpated; liver, lung or even CNS metastases can be resected.

Use of chemotherapy, immunotherapy and radiotherapy within the scope of adjuvant or palliative treatment of melanoma is, despite certain success, still rather limited. The basis of adjuvant therapy lies in the long-term application of interferon. Other drugs used include dacarbazine, and interleukin IL-2; current studies focus on possible usage of melanoma vaccines. Radiotherapy in locally advanced or metastatic melanomas can improve the quality of life, and slow progression; nevertheless, they do not increase the overall survival rate.

Follow-up examinations consist of physical examinations, i.e. searching for possible satellite or subcutaneous and lymph node metastases, and require available paraclinical imaging methods (ultrasound, CT, MRI, PET). An increased level of lactate dehydrogenase can indicate possible liver metastases.

## 5.6 Prognosis

The prognosis of malignant melanoma depends on the stage of the disease. While in stage Ia the 5-year survival is almost 100%, in patients with lymph node involvement it declines to 35% and in metastatic melanoma the median survival time is 6–12 months with a 5-year survival below 10%. Negative prognostic criteria constitute the depth of invasion, presence of ulceration, signs of regression, perineural spread, regional lymph node involvement and, obviously, the presence of satellite or distant metastases.

# 6 ABDOMINAL WALL AND HERNIAS

*6.1 Hernias*
*6.2 Inflammations and Tumors*
*6.3 Developmental Defects*

## 6.1 Hernias

### 6.1.1 Definition, Incidence, Pathogenesis

Hernia means a pouch of the parietal peritoneum due to a preformed or secondarily developed defect in the abdominal wall. Hernias may include any organ of the abdominal cavity, most often the omentum or intestine. The crevice, through which the pouch passes, is called the hernial orifice.

Hernias are among the most common surgical diseases in general: 5–10% of the population is affected.

Inguinal hernias occur most commonly. They develop predominantly in men (up to 90%). Hernias in scars, umbilical and femoral hernias are more common in women.

Hernia development is conditioned by the presence of areas of physiological or pathological weakening of the abdominal wall, umbilicus and the groin, semilunar line, lumbar trigone area or a scar after laparotomy. Chronic elevation of intra-abdominal pressure is added to this predisposition through the following: obesity, chronic cough, ascites, pregnancy, increased physical strain, working in a bent-forward position.

### 6.1.2 Classification

If the hernial sac projects outwards through the abdominal wall, it is an **external hernia** (Fig. 6.1); if found inside the abdominal cavity, it is an **internal hernia**.

The most common types of external hernias include inguinal hernias, femoral hernias, umbilical hernias, epigastric hernias and hernias in scars. Hiatal hernias and Treitz's hernias are examples of internal hernias.

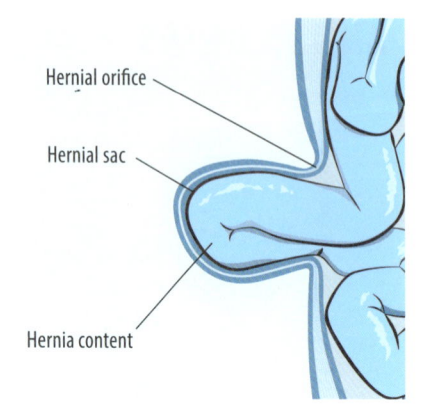

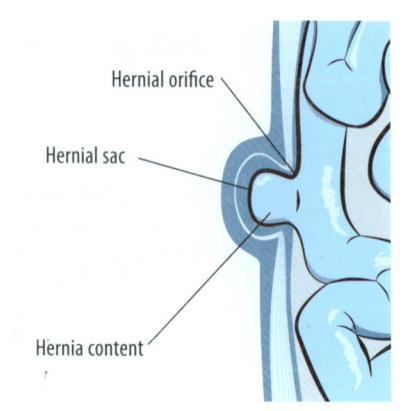

**Fig. 6.1** *External hernia*

**Fig. 6.2** *Hernial incarceration of the wall*

Congenital and acquired hernias are categorized according to the time of the first manifestation. **Congenital hernias** are present at birth. **Acquired hernias** develop later on in life. Hernias can be loose, **reponible**, if its content can be easily reintroduced to the abdominal cavity, or **irreponible** if the opposite is true. In case that an organ is included in the hernial sac, for example the urinary bladder wall or sigma wall, it is called a **sliding hernia**.

### 6.1.3 Clinical Aspects, Complications

Typically, a hernia does not cause any problems for the patient except those esthetical ones. It may cause pain, less commonly also passage disorders. **Hernia incarceration** is a serious complication. This occurs upon sudden shifting of the hernial sac contents without the possibility of repositioning back into the abdominal cavity. This condition involves the risk of ischemia of the hernial sac contents. Subjectively, the patient complains of intensive pain in the area of the hernia, and vomiting may be present. If a passage disorder develops, gas and stool blockage occurs. Painful irreponible hernia is found during a clinical assessment, slowed peristalsis or peristalsis with obstruction phenomena based on auscultation. In intestinal perforation, signs of peritoneal irritation are also found in rare cases. Native radiography of the abdomen may be helpful for the diagnosis, as signs of an ileus condition may be present in the abdomen, and possibly sonography of the area with the hernia.

Only a part of the intestinal circumference may be incarcerated (**Richter's incarceration** of the wall, Fig. 6.2). In this case, a risk is posed by necrosis of the intestinal wall, but no passage disorder is present. Two or more intestinal ansae may be incarcerated, with necrosis of the part turned away from the hernial sac towards the abdominal cavity (**W-shaped Maydl's incarceration**, Fig. 6.4). In

# ABDOMINAL WALL AND HERNIAS

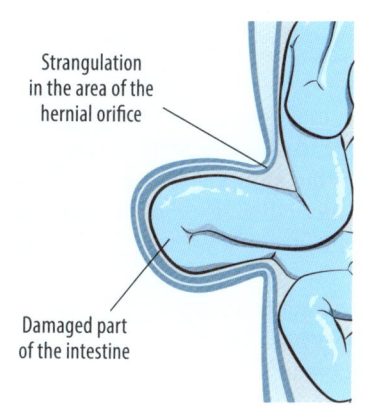

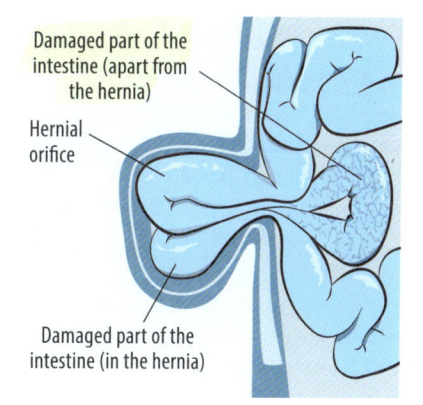

**Fig. 6.3** *Incarcerated hernia*

**Fig. 6.4** *"W-shaped" incarceration*

this case, the intestine is perforated into the free abdominal cavity. If the contents cannot be repositioned in the abdominal cavity due to its fixation to the hernial sac and no vascular supply disorder is present, this condition is called **accreted** hernia. Sometimes it may be difficult to distinguish between an acutely incarcerated and an accreted hernia.

## 6.1.4 Therapy

The therapy is surgical. The procedure is performed electively, with only incarcerated hernia requiring acute surgery. The surgery consists in releasing the hernial sac, repositioning its content in the abdominal cavity, and closing the hernial orifice. Visceral vitality, for example, vitality of the intestine, must be evaluated in incarcerated hernias. Resection becomes necessary if visceral vitality is impaired. The hernial orifice may be closed by mere suture or, more commonly, using a plasty where individual tissue layers are overlapped. This enhances the strength of the suture. Another possibility is offered by using a grid. The mesh is used to cover the hernial orifice and is fixated at the edges. Prolene, nonabsorbable grids are used in most cases. However, absorbable grids are also available, and possibly also non-wetting grids which prevent adherence, for example, of the small intestine. The important fact is that all plasties should be sutured without tension, i.e. **tension free plasty**. The surgery can be performed using both the open and laparoscopic approach. The surgery is done under general anesthesia, conduction-spinal anesthesia or possibly conduction-epidural anesthesia or under local infiltrative anesthesia.

After the procedure, the patient should avoid any heavy physical strain for at least 5 weeks. Conservative therapy, which means that the patient wears a hernial band, can be considered only in patients who are not able to undergo surgery due to serious comorbidities.

### 6.1.5 Inguinal and Femoral Hernia

In order to understand the therapy of hernias found in the inguinal region, the anatomy of the inguinal region should be mentioned. The inguinal ligament, passing from the anterior superior iliac spine to the pubic tubercle, separates the more cranially located inguinal canal from the more caudally located vascular and muscular lacuna. The inguinal canal through which the spermatic funicle passes in men and the round ligament of the uterus in women is circumscribed by the following 4 walls:
- Ventrally – by the aponeurosis of the external oblique muscle
- Dorsally – by the transversal fascia, transversal muscle and peritoneum
- Cranially – by the edge of the internal oblique muscle
- Caudally – by the inguinal ligament

The dorsal wall of the inguinal canal is divided by inferior epigastric blood vessels into the lateral part (lateral inguinal fossa; spermatic funicle or round ligament of the uterus project here) and the medial part (medial inguinal fossa). A hernia protruding through the lateral orifice is called an **indirect inguinal hernia** (Fig. 6.5a) (the hernial orifice over the inguinal ligament is located laterally from epigastric blood vessels; in men, the hernial sac in the seminal cord is covered by the cremaster muscle). A hernia protruding through the medial orifice is called a **direct inguinal hernia** (Fig. 6.5b) (the hernial orifice over the inguinal ligament is located medially from epigastric blood vessels). A lateral inguinal hernia runs through the entire inguinal canal, therefore it is called indirect, while a medial hernia is oriented directly outwards (into the external orifice of the inguinal canal), and thus it is called direct. In men, an indirect hernia may reach all the way into the scrotum (**scrotal hernia**), or into the large labia in women. The hernial orifice of a **femoral hernia** (Fig. 6.5c) is located below the inguinal ligament and over the cranial edge of the two pubic bones, in the area of vascular lacuna. The hernial sac protrudes medially from femoral blood vessels to the subcutis.

Indirect inguinal hernias and particularly femoral hernias have narrow orifices, and thus they show a higher tendency to incarceration than direct inguinal hernias. The inguinal sac of a male indirect hernia may be congenital. The connection between the peritoneum and the scrotum is open in the

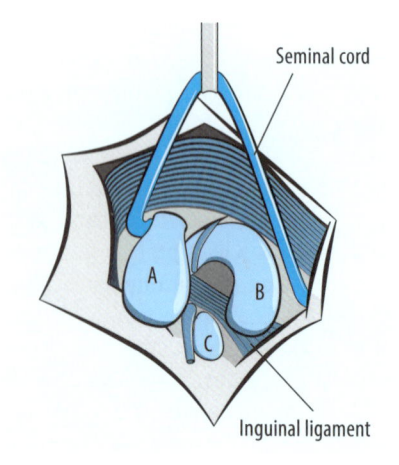

*Fig. 6.5 Hernias in the abdominal area: Direct (A) and indirect (B) inguinal hernia, femoral hernia (C)*

fetal period, i.e. the vaginal process of the testis. It obliterates before birth, but it may also close spontaneously as late as 2 years of age. An indirect inguinal hernia develops later through protrusion of the visceral content in one half of cases where the vaginal process of the testis remains open in its entirety or partially.

In **differential diagnostics** of palpable resistances in the groin, the following diseases should be considered: lymphadenopathy, great saphenous vein varices, undescended testicle; upon differentiation of scrotal hernias, the diseases may include hydrocele, orchitis, epididymitis, testicular tumor, and testicular torsion. Hernia surgery is indicated only upon exclusion of other serious diseases whose treatment would have higher priority.

A medical history and physical examination are usually sufficient to confirm or exclude a hernia in the inguinal area. Sonography may be completed if anything remains unclear.

Inguinal and femoral hernias are treated using surgery. A number of plasties have been created. Their classification is based on their relationship to the spermatic cord; therefore the plasties are classified as ventral, pre-funicular, and dorsal, retro-funicular.

**Anterior plasties** include the plasty according to Maydl-Kukula, which is of historical importance and represents a Czech contribution to surgery worldwide. Today, it is no longer used due to the weakness of the suture of the internal abdominal oblique muscle to the inguinal ligament in front of the funicle.

**Posterior plasties** are used to **strengthen the posterior wall of the inguinal canal using transverse fascias**. Technically, the following solutions are used: simple closure (suture) of the defect, multiplication (strengthening) of the ligament layer or closure of the defect by inserting an artificial implant (mesh).

Two approaches can be considered when laparoscopy is chosen: **TAPP** – transabdominal preperitoneal plasty and **TEP** – total extraperitoneal plasty. Their joint disadvantage consists in the need of general anesthesia and the risk of organ injury particularly in the intraperitoneal approach. They bring the advantage of lower post-operative pain and faster convalescence. In terms of the number of relapses of the disease, there is virtually no difference between the open and laparoscopic approaches according to the most recent data.

## 6.1.6 Umbilical Hernia

Umbilical hernia occurs as acquired in newborns, and it may also be congenital. The hernial orifice is found in the area of umbilical annulus. Umbilical hernias in adults have a tendency to incarcerate. They should be treated surgically. Upon removal of the hernial sac, the hernial orifice is sutured using direct suture of the white line, or possibly a circumflex plasty is created using Mayo surgery. If possible, the umbilicus should be reconstructed, which is important from the cosmetic point of view. However, the patient should be informed before the surgery that under certain circumstances it may not be possible to preserve the umbilicus.

### 6.1.7 Hernias in Scars and Ventral Hernias

After laparotomy, **wound healing impairments**, for example due to an infection or early physical exertion, may lead to development of hernias in the scar (incisional hernia). A hernia in a scar should be treated surgically.

Hernias of the semilunar line and hernias in the white line can be ranked among ventral hernias; however, these hernias are rare.

In terms of differential diagnosis, ventral hernias should be distinguished from a **diastasis of direct muscles**. This is not a hernia; the white line is only loosened and both recti muscles are more distant from each other. The reason to operate a diastasis of direct abdominal muscles is only cosmetic.

### 6.1.8 Rare Hernias

- Spiegel's hernia (the hernial orifice is found immediately lateral to the external edge of the direct muscle sheath, at the point of its division to the anterior and posterior parts, more commonly in the lower abdomen)
- Obturator hernia (obturator foramen orifice)
- Ischiadic hernia (ischiadic foramen orifice)
- Lumbar hernia (lumbar trigone orifice)
- Perineal hernia (ischiorectal fossa orifice)

These hernias are not often manifested before incarceration. A surgical solution is used.

### 6.1.9 Internal Hernias

The same also applies to a relatively rare group of internal hernias whose diagnoses, in almost all cases, are determined only upon surgery indicated due to incarceration:
- Foramen of Winslow hernia
- Treitz's hernia
- Perivesical hernia

A special group of internal hernias is formed by diaphragmatic hernias, which are discussed in Section 7.2.

## 6.2 Inflammations and Tumors

Inflammations of the abdominal wall are rare in adults. **Omphalitis** is an acute inflammation in the area of the umbilicus. Poor hygiene and obesity are major predisposing factors. The inflammation is manifested by reddening of the umbilicus and the nearest surrounding area, pain, swelling and fever. Conservative therapy is applied (antibiotics as general, compresses as local) and if the problems continue, surgical incision and drainage are performed.

# ABDOMINAL WALL AND HERNIAS

Chronic inflammation – **Schloffer tumor** – composed of fibrous tissue and granulation tissue around foreign bodies (suture residue); the tumor is most likely to develop in scars after surgery. It may be difficult to distinguish it from a hernia in the scar. Surgical extirpation is the form of therapy.

**Benign tumors** are common; however, they are of little clinical importance given that the dimensions of lipomas, hemangiomas and fibromas are usually small and do not cause problems. Surgical extirpation is indicated if they keep growing or for cosmetic reasons.

A **desmoid** (sometimes also called fibromatosis) is a rare benign tumor. It affects young women in most cases. A desmoid forms a solid, slowly growing tumor, which relapses. Due to its infiltrative growth, it may sometimes be considered as semimalignant. Broad excision of the tumor is the form of therapy.

Malignant tumors are uncommon; primary tumors may stem from any layer of the wall. They include sarcomas (fibrosarcomas, rhabdomyosarcomas). Broad excision with subsequent adjuvant therapy is the form of therapy (cf. Section 4.4).

Secondary tumors of the abdominal wall, most often carcinomas of intra-abdominal origin, typically occur in the umbilicus or in scars after abdominal surgeries. Extirpation is the form of therapy (no surgery is indicated if generalization of the basic tumor is present).

A special situation is represented by **intra-abdominal tumors** that grow through into the abdominal wall and are palpable as tumors of the abdominal wall. This may be the first manifestation of the tumor. This situation should always be taken into consideration, and when a palpable tumor is present, its origin should be excluded or confirmed using a targeted examination, most often using imaging methods.

## 6.3 Developmental Defects

Developmental defects of the abdominal wall, if causing problems, fall into the field of interest of pediatric surgery. If they persist until adult age, they may become a reason for surgical treatment.

A **persistent omphaloenteric duct** may remain preserved until postnatal life, either in its entirety or some of its parts (umbilical fistula, cyst along the course of the original duct, Meckel's intestinal diverticulum). It usually causes no problems, and eventual symptoms are invoked by complications – fistula secretion in a scar, gradually growing resistance exerting pressure on the surrounding areas, signs of acute abdomen in presence of bleeding, perforation or acute inflammation of the Meckel's diverticulum. Surgical removal of the pathological tissue is the form of therapy.

**Persistent urachus** is a fistula between the urinary bladder and the skin. If only a part remains preserved, cysts are formed and they may get infected. Surgical extirpation of the fistula is the form of therapy.

# 7 ESOPHAGUS AND DIAPHRAGM SURGERY

7.1 *Esophagus*
7.2 *Diaphragmatic Hernias*

## 7.1 Esophagus

The esophagus is a hollow tubular organ approximately 25 cm long, which connects the pharynx and the stomach and is used for food transporting. The esophagus runs through the posterior mediastinum, includes three physiological stenoses and is lined with squamous epithelium, which is not acid-resistant. Only about 2 cm of the distal abdominal esophagus are covered with cylindrical epithelium. The circular smooth musculature of the esophagus is thickened at the entry in the superior thoracic aperture, forming the superior esophageal (Killian's) sphincter; the musculature is also multiplied distally, at the entry in the stomach, forming the inferior esophageal sphincter. External longitudinal muscles are cross-striated in the upper third, while smooth muscles are found in the two lower thirds. The esophagus is not covered with serosa but only with thin adventitia, therefore some diseases (inflammations, malignancies) spread to surrounding areas at hazardous speeds.

This anatomical situation is of crucial importance for esophagus surgeries given that a layer very important for healing – the serosa – is missing. Only a short intra-abdominal part of the esophagus beyond passage through the diaphragmatic hiatus is covered with serosa.

### 7.1.1 Esophageal Motility Disorders

**Cricopharyngeal dysfunction** is seen very rarely, caused by poor coordination of the superior esophageal sphincter dilatation with concurrent pharyngeal contraction. It may lead to the development of Zenker's diverticulum. **Diffuse esophageal spasm** is characterized by painful contractions of the esophagus outside the act of swallowing, often in emotionally labile patients. The therapy of these diseases should be as conservative as possible.

# ESOPHAGUS AND DIAPHRAGM SURGERY

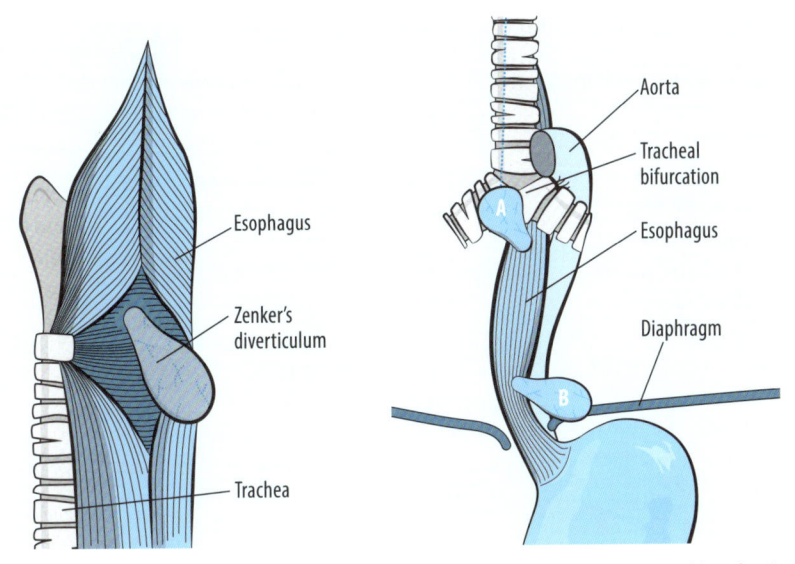

**Fig. 7.1** *Zenker's parapharyngeal diverticulum of the esophagus*

**Fig. 7.2** *Parabronchial traction (A) and epiphrenic (B) diverticulum of the esophagus*

## 7.1.2 Diverticula

Esophageal diverticula can be categorized either as true, if the herniation is formed by all layers of the wall, or false, thus a herniation of the mucosa and submucosa through weakened musculature. Furthermore, the diverticula can be categorized as pulsion or traction, based on their development mechanism.

The juxtasphincteric **pulsion** diverticulum develops on the basis of functional disorders of sphincter relaxation. Chronic undulating elevation of intraluminal pressure leads to herniation of the epithelium through the weakened part of the muscle layer. Most commonly, such a diverticulum is found in the cervical area (70%), the so called **Zenker's** diverticulum (Fig. 7.1). It is usually manifested by dysphagia, vomiting of undigested food, irritable cough, oral malodor and sometimes also a palpable resistance in the neck on the left, which subsides after vomiting. **Epiphrenic** diverticulum is relatively rare and usually symptom-free. Dysphagia, food regurgitation and pain beyond the sternum may occur if the diverticulum is of larger dimensions.

**Traction** diverticulum is formed by all layers of the wall, and thus it is a true diverticulum. It develops through a retractive process in the surroundings of the esophagus, usually due to a lymph node modified by inflammation. Most commonly, it is localized in the central part of the esophagus and is connected with the name of Rokitansky (Fig. 7.2).

The therapy of symptomatic diverticula usually consists in surgical resection of the diverticulum.

### 7.1.3 Achalasia – Idiopathic Esophageal Dilatation

This disease is characterized by a **neuromuscular disorder** of the distal part of the esophagus and is conditioned by relaxation disorders of the distal esophageal sphincter. The condition is caused by ganglion cell destruction of the myenteric plexus; however, its etiology remains unknown. An exception is formed by the so called **Chagas disease**, with the etiological agent being the parasite **Trypanosoma cruzi**.

Initially, peristalsis remains normal, but it is weak and the lower esophageal sphincter fails to relax. The musculature may show transient compensatory hypertrophy; over time, however, the dilatation progresses with flabbiness of the whole esophagus with the sphincter constricted, making the impression of a spasm (the so called decompensated stage – Fig. 7.3).

Problems may develop on the basis of an emotional insult, with dysphagia usually being the first symptom; the dysphagia may be paradoxical (worse swallowing of liquids than solid food). Other symptoms may include retrosternal pain after a meal, oral malodor, regurgitation, respiratory problems caused by aspiration, and finally severe dysphagia that renders swallowing both liquids and solid food impossible and is associated with weight loss.

Contrast radiography shows dilated esophagus (megaesophagus) with smooth walls and with a smooth distal stenosis having the shape of a bird beak. Unlike achalasia, the dilatation over the obstruction is not as large in tumors, and the stenosis is often longer and shows an irregular shape. Samples should be taken for biopsy during an upper endoscopy in order to exclude malignancy. The diagnostics includes esophageal manometry.

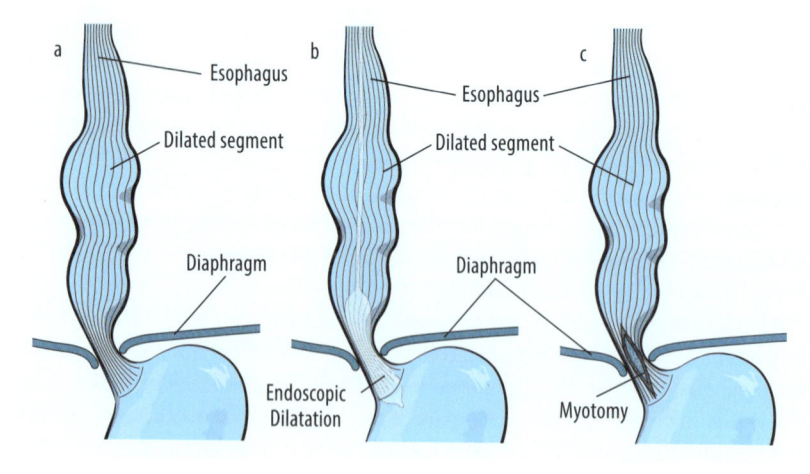

*Fig. 7.3 Esophageal achalasias: a) Decompensated stage; b) Endoscopic dilatation; c) Myotomy according to Heller*

# ESOPHAGUS AND DIAPHRAGM SURGERY

**Conservative therapy** (endoscopic dilatation, local botulinum toxin administration, general medication using nitrates or nifedipine) usually fails to provide a longer lasting effect, therefore **surgical treatment** is applied. Longitudinal extramucous myotomy of the distal esophagus and gastric cardia approximately 5–6 cm long according to Heller is the classic surgery. Today, the procedure is performed using laparoscopy with good results (Figs. 7.3b, 7.3c). Achalasia can also be operated on using a thoracoscopy from thoracic access.

Note: According to some opinions, achalasia is associated with an increased risk of tumor development!

## 7.1.4 Esophageal Injury

Esophageal injury occurs through instrumental examination such as upper endoscopy, endoscopic sonography, etc., as a consequence of pathologically changed tissue, for example, due to a carcinoma or diverticulum. Less commonly, esophageal perforation may be caused by swallowing a foreign body, unintentionally (for example, a bone or part of a dental prosthesis) or intentionally, the so called "anchors" seen in self-harm by prisoners. In rare cases, esophageal injury may be caused due to an open injury to the neck or chest, i.e. stab or gunshot wounds. These conditions may lead to **esophageal perforation**. Another rare affection is Boerhaave's syndrome, i.e. spontaneous rupture of the esophagus after strenuous vomiting, mainly after excessive alcohol consumption.

**Acute mediastinitis** is the main risk of esophageal perforation, which progresses very rapidly and quickly leads to fatal **sepsis** if left untreated.

Medical history data (vomiting, a swallowed foreign body, previous instrumentation procedures or even dysphagia) are helpful in determining the **diagnosis**. Symptoms observed in objective examination include dyspnea, cyanosis, sometimes fever, hematemesis, and tachycardia. Subcutaneous emphysema is palpable and mediastinal emphysema is visible in the native chest scan. The diagnosis can be confirmed by contrast radiography of the esophagus using water solution of iodine-based, not barium-based contrast medium. An endoscopy is not always conclusive.

The **therapy** for perforation is surgical and urgent, with some exceptions. The sooner the patient is operated the better the subsequent prognosis will be. Surgical solution consists in mediastinal drainage from a thoracotomy. An attempt to suture the perforation may be undertaken during the initial 6 hours. Later, this approach is rendered impossible due to inflammation with an edema and considerable fragility of esophageal tissue. Additional measures are applied with surgical treatment: insertion of a nasogastric probe, administration of broad-spectrum antibiotics, correction of the internal environment using infusion therapy, prevention of organ failures, and general sepsis therapy at the department of resuscitation. If primary surgical treatment of the finding in the esophagus cannot be applied or if the surgical treatment fails considering that a long time has elapsed from the onset of the first symptoms, cervical esophagostomy should be established, with passive chest drainage and nutrition gastrostomy or jejunostomy. Alternatively, a self-expandable metallic stent can be introduced via endoscopy, with chest drainage of the affected hemithorax, in cases of rather small defects of the esophageal wall and suitable anatomical localization. However, the prognosis is unfavorable in cases of developed sepsis, and the lethality rate with mediastinitis is about 50%.

### 7.1.5  Burns in the Esophagus

Burns in the esophagus are caused by swallowed acid or alkali. Hydroxide burns cause deep coliquation necrosis, while acid burns lead to coagulation necrosis. Predominant symptoms include pain in the throat, dysphagia, retrosternal pain, and sometimes also septic fever or signs of shock development. (Attention must be paid to acute dyspnea when glottic edema is present!)

**Assessments** performed include thoracic radiography or possibly radiography with contrast water solution; early endoscopy is important to determine the damage rate of the tissue.

Neutralizing substances (milk, lemon juice) are administered as first aid; it is not recommended to evoke vomiting due to the risk of aspiration. **Therapy**: broad-spectrum antibiotics, corticosteroids, analgesics, anti-shock measures.

Esophageal stricture develops in about 10% of injured persons within 2 weeks, which is more common after hydroxide digestion. Dilatation is performed in this case, about 4 weeks after the injury. If it fails, a surgical solution should be considered – resection of the stenotic segment of the esophagus.

Note: An increased risk of carcinoma development is present in patients with esophageal stricture after a burn!

### 7.1.6  Bleeding

Bleeding in the esophagus is mainly caused by esophageal varices and Mallory-Weiss syndrome (cf. Chapter 19).

### 7.1.7  Reflux Disease (GERD) – Gastroesophageal Reflux, Reflux Esophagitis

Gastroesophageal reflux (GER) is described as an entry of the gastric contents into the distal esophagus. Reflux may also be physiological (during the night), and its effects are counteracted by the self-cleaning action of esophageal peristalsis. Pathological GER is prolonged, shows higher frequency and does not occur only during the night. It usually depends on reduced tone of the lower esophageal sphincter (LES). Reduced LES tone may be caused directly by the following fac-

# ESOPHAGUS AND DIAPHRAGM SURGERY

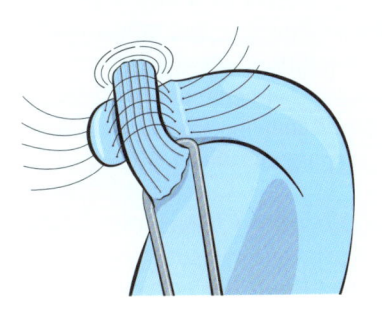

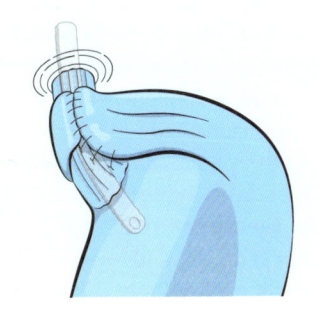

**Fig. 7.4** *Fundoplication preparation procedure*

**Fig. 7.5** *Fundoplication – resulting condition*

tors: fatty diet, chocolate, caffeine, theophylline, cocoa, alcohol, smoking, and also progesterone, nitrates, some anticholinergics, and antirheumatics (NSAID). Some other factors which take part in reflux development are: low self-cleaning ability of the esophagus, aggressive acid content of the stomach, elevated intra-abdominal pressure, reduced evacuation of the stomach, His angle disturbance (particularly after some surgeries), and NG probe insertion. The effect of presence of a sliding hiatal hernia on GER has been discussed. Hiatal hernias certainly impair antireflux mechanisms of the distal esophagus and are present in some patients with GER. On the other hand, there are persons with hiatal hernias who have no symptoms of GER (cf. Section 7.2).

The refluxate is mostly acidic; it may be alkaline in exceptional cases. **Reflux esophagitis** may develop on the basis of mucosa irritation associated with GER. The scope and severity of this inflammation may vary; the inflammation is classified according to Savary and Miller using 4 grades:
1. Presence of sporadic erosions
2. Longitudinally merging erosions
3. Erosions occupying the whole circumference of the esophagus (circular erosions)
4. Scarring, strictures, chronic ulcer

Both erosions and ulcers may heal with metaplastic cylindrical epithelium; this condition is called **Barrett's esophagus**. An ulcer localized in the junction area in the metaplastic epithelium is called Barrett's ulcer. These cases of metaplasia and subsequent dysplasia are precancerous conditions and may provide the basis for the development of adenocarcinoma of the esophagus.

GERD symptoms include mainly heartburn, burning retrosternal pain, and possibly regurgitation or certain respiratory problems caused by aspiration. Dysphagia or odynophagia (painful swallowing) are symptoms of an advanced finding, usually a stenosis or Barrett's esophagus.

The prominent **assessment method** is endoscopy, which is used to determine the gravity of esophagitis, to confirm the diagnosis by biopsy, and to exclude malignancy. Furthermore, contrast radiography is performed, which is the best method to demonstrate the presence and extent of a hiatal hernia. Reflux can be best demonstrated by a 24-hour pH-metry with insertion of the thin pH-meter probe in the esophagus. Normally, pH values of 4 to 7 are present in the esophagus. Esophageal manometry is completed before a contemplated surgical solution, with evaluation of the tone of the lower esophageal sphincter. Performing a reflux scan is another possibility.

The **therapy** of reflux disease is conservative initially. Conservative therapy consists in dietary and regimen measures that form an integral part of the therapy – frequent meals of low volumes, the elimination of fats, sweet and acidic meals, yeast pastries, coffee, chocolate, cocoa, alcohol and smoking. It is recommended to sleep in a half-sitting position, avoid heavy labor and forward bends. Antacids are administered in mild cases, or **anti-secretion therapy** in more severe cases with reflux esophagitis, i.e. $H_2$-receptor blockers (ranitidine, famotidine), while, recently, proton pump inhibitors (omeprazole) are preferred. Prokinetics (cisapride, methoclopramide, etc.) may be added to the medication. The therapy takes at least 6 weeks, sometimes even longer, until the esophagitis is healed. As a safety measure, anti-secretion medication should be administered in reduced doses long term.

**Surgical treatment** is indicated for esophagitis grades 3 to 4 and where conservative therapy has failed and the patient suffers from repeated relapses of the disease. The patient's refusal to take medication – proton pump inhibitors, prokinetics – permanently is another indication. Various **antireflux surgeries** are based on the same principle: increase the LES tone by creating a cuff from the gastric fundus around the distal esophagus (Figs. 7.4, 7.5). If a sliding hernia is present, the distal esophagus is repositioned below the diaphragm again. The cuff may circumscribe the esophagus to various degrees; abdominal access is usually used for the surgery, exceptionally thoracic access. 360-degree fundoplication according to **Nissen-Rossetti** is most commonly used in the Czech Republic; when a broad hiatus is present, the fundoplication is completed with suture of the crura. In almost all cases, surgery is performed by laparoscopy, with very good results. No additional medication is needed after a successful surgery. The rate of complications is low; more serious conditions may occur in exceptional cases: bleeding or perforation in the esophagus, which should be kept in mind, and if these conditions do occur, they should be diagnosed and resolved in a timely manner in the postoperative period. Dysphagias may occur after the surgery; despite the fact that they are transient, the patient should be warned about them.

### 7.1.8 Tumors

**BENIGN TUMORS**

Benign tumors of the esophagus are rare; **leiomyoma** is the most common, located **intramurally** and present in about 2/3 of cases. A lipoma, fibroma or

ESOPHAGUS AND DIAPHRAGM SURGERY

**hemangioma** may also be localized intramurally. Epithelial tumors grow in the **intraluminal** localization: pedunculated polypus, mural papilloma or adenoma.

Benign tumors are usually symptom-free, and dysphagia may occur when they have grown to larger dimensions. Endoscopy and contrast radiography are used as assessment methods, completed with endosonography, and also CT if any doubt remains. Surgical treatment is applied, and enucleation or resection of the esophagus in the case of intramural tumors.

### MALIGNANT TUMORS

Although considered as rather rare diseases in the area of the esophagus, the occurrence of malignant tumors has been rising in the last decade. The lowest occurrence has been associated with the white population, higher in the black population, and substantially higher in Asians, particularly in the Chinese and Japanese.

The etiology is unknown. Several risk factors have been reported – male sex, over 60 years-of-age, poor nutrition with hypovitaminosis, alcohol and tobacco abuse and poor dental hygiene. Consumption of hot beverages and spicy meals is another risk factor. The tumors develop from achalasia precanceroses, structures after a burn, scleroderma, reflux esophagitis and epithelial dysplasia (Barrett's esophagus). Malignant tumors are localized mainly in the lower and middle thirds of the esophagus, less frequently in the upper third.

The **squamous cell carcinoma** is most common, representing about 60% of all findings. **Adenocarcinoma** occurs in about 40% of cases and is localized in the distal esophagus. It often develops on the basis of Barrett's esophagus. A melanoma, mucoepidermoid carcinoma, adenoid cystic carcinoma, undifferentiated carcinoma, leiomyosarcoma, malignant lymphoma and small cell carcinoma may occur in rare cases.

TNM classification is used for staging, based on which:
- T1 – the tumor infiltrates the mucosal tunic or submucosa
- T2 – infiltration of the muscular tunic
- T3 – adventitial infiltration
- T4 – adjacent organs are also affected

Metastases in regional lymph vessels around the esophagus are common, marked as N1. Infiltrations of cervical, supraclavicular, mediastinal nodes distant from the esophagus and celiac or perigastric nodes are considered as distant metastases. Presence of distant organ metastases is marked as M1; metastases in the liver and in the lungs are most common, but also in the bones and eventually in the brain.

The **diagnostics** are associated with the problem of the absence of early symptoms. The most common symptoms include **dysphagia** and **odynophagia**, which only occurs with 50% stenosis of the esophageal lumen. This is why all people over 50 years of age who have swallowing problems must be examined to exclude esophageal malignancy. Additional but late symptoms include weight loss, retrosternal pain, regurgitation, hoarseness, cough, back pain.

In order to establish proper **therapy**, not only the type and localization of the tumor should be diagnosed, but also its extent and staging. Standard assessments include upper endoscopy with biopsy and contrast radiography of the esophagus, which can demonstrate an irregularly shaped stenosis (the so called saw shape); furthermore, CT assessment of the chest and upper part of the abdomen to exclude metastases and to evaluate how the tumor is related to the surrounding structures. PET CT is the most recent assessment method. Esophageal endosonography contributes to determining the extent of the tumor and any potential involvement of the surrounding lymph nodes. Bronchoscopy is another method, and mediastinoscopy in exceptional cases; however, these procedures are not routinely performed. Marker assessment is used for checking the course.

Only **radical surgery** leads to recovery. All patients with a circumscribed tumor (T1, T2, T3) without distant metastases are indicated for this therapy. Patients with T4 finding are indicated for preoperative radio- and chemotherapy aimed at reducing the size of the tumor or its full eliminating. Further therapy depends on the response to oncotherapy. Radical surgery consists in resection of the esophagus in a sufficient distance from the tumor (subtotal or total esophagectomy) given that submucosal growth of the tumor is often also present. The procedure always includes abdominal D2 lymphadenectomy, mediastinal lymphadenectomy, and also cervical lymphadenectomy in tumors of the central and thoracic third of the esophagus. The surgery is carried out from transthoracic and abdominal access. It is a burdensome, two-cavity procedure, associated with a higher number of complications and also higher mortality. Another option is offered by blunt dissection of the esophagus from the abdomen and neck without opening the thoracic cavity. Intrathoracic dissection of the esophagus and thoracoscopic lymphadenectomy can be performed in unadvanced findings. Reconstruction of GIT continuity after the resection is most commonly achieved by pulling a tubulized stomach up to the chest (Fig. 7.6). The large intestine is also a suitable replacement (Fig. 7.7). The possibility of using a jejunal loop is limited by the length of its suspension with blood vessels. The reconstruction takes place in the esophageal bed, retrosternally or subcutaneously in exceptional cases. Postoperative complications include cardiovascular complications, pneumonia, and bleeding. In terms of surgical complications, anastomotic failure is most feared, with subsequent development of a fistula in the pleural cavity or in the mediastinum, with the development of mediastinitis.

According to the definitive histological finding, particularly taking into account the radical nature of the procedure and involvement of the lymph nodes, further oncological therapy is indicated. Palliative resection is not indicated in patients who cannot undergo radical surgery due to the high risk of this proce-

# ESOPHAGUS AND DIAPHRAGM SURGERY

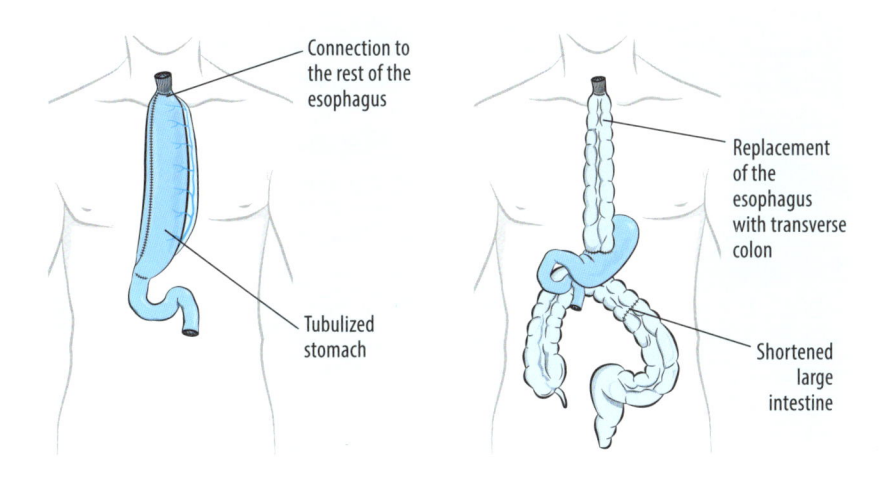

**Fig. 7.6** *Replacement of the esophagus with tubulized stomach*

**Fig. 7.7** *Replacement of the esophagus with large intestine*

dure. Formerly, only palliative actinotherapy was applied, completed with surgical gastrostomy for food intake, or Häring's plastic esophageal prosthesis was inserted. Currently, palliative actino- and chemotherapy is completed with mini-invasive surgery in inoperable tumors in order to restore patency of the esophagus. Endoscopic reduction of the tumor mass using a laser and/or endoscopic insertion of an esophageal stent is also possible. Usually, a self-expandable metallic stent is used, covered with a thin plastic foil, which makes the tumor growth through openings in the stent more difficult. Where gastrostomy is needed, some mini-invasive methods can be used (laparoscopy or percutaneous gastrostomy).

The prognosis of patients with esophageal carcinoma is very serious and depends on the stage of the disease. Operable findings represent about 50%, with 5-year survival of about 20%. The mean survival rate of patients with an inoperable finding is about 9 months. Five-year survival of all esophageal tumors is about 5%.

## 7.2 Diaphragmatic Hernias

So called **hiatal hernias**, i.e. the shift of a part of the stomach in the thoracic cavity, are the most common diaphragmatic hernias. **Sliding hiatal hernias** (Fig. 7.8) are usually associated with GER. The symptoms and therapy are described in Section 7.1.

**Paraesophageal hernias** (Fig. 7.9) are gastric fundus herniation into the chest through the hiatus along the esophagus. His angle is preserved, the lower esophageal sphincter is competent, and thus no GER is present. The symptoms follow

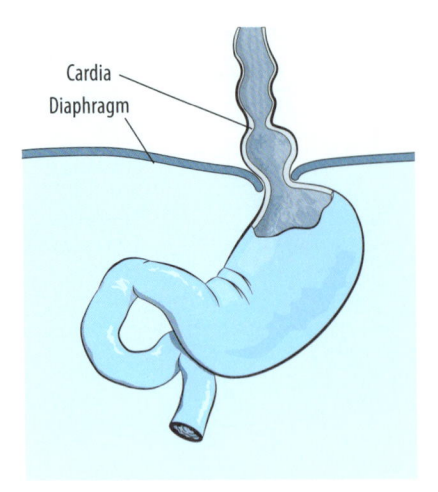

**Fig. 7.8** *Sliding hiatal hernia*

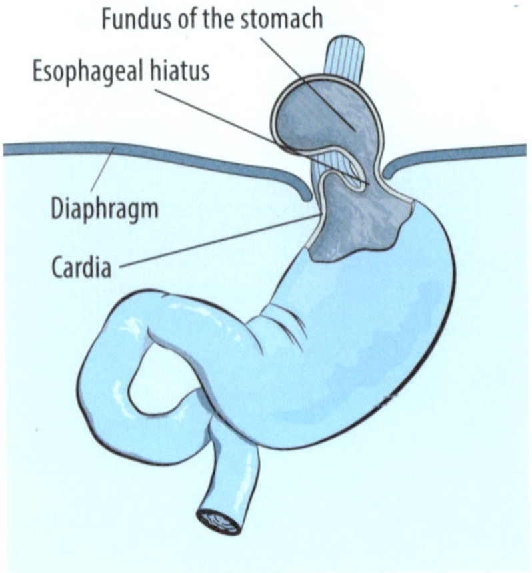

**Fig. 7.9** *Paraesophageal hernia*

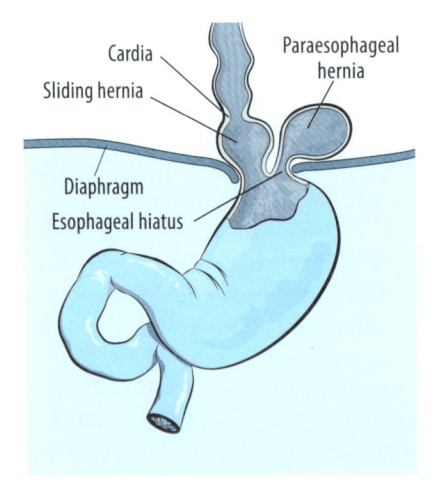

**Fig. 7.10** *Mixed hiatal hernia*

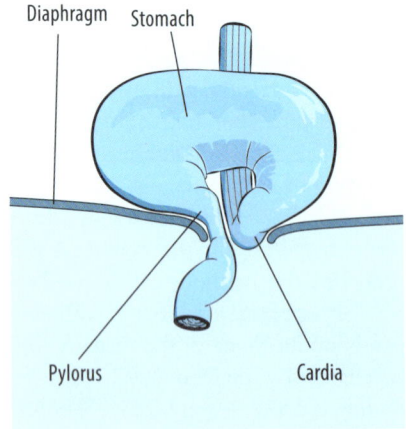

**Fig. 7.11** *Upside down stomach*

from incarceration of the tissue in the hiatus and from pressure exerted on the surrounding organs. Retrosternal pain is usually present as well as respiratory or cardiac problems such as palpitations and arrhythmia. The diagnosis is determined using endoscopy and contrast radiography. Surgical treatment is applied – reposition and fixation of the fundus with hiatus suture. Both types may also be combined in a **mixed hernia** (Fig. 7.10). The so called "upside down stomach" (Fig. 7.11) is also connected with hiatal hernia, which is explained in more detail in Section 8.4.4 – Volvulus of the stomach.

# 8 GASTRIC AND DUODENAL SURGERY

- 8.1 Introduction – Anatomical and Physiological Comments
- 8.2 Symptomatology of Gastroduodenal Diseases
- 8.3 Examinations of the Gastroduodenum
- 8.4 Gastric and Duodenal Diseases
- 8.5 Gastroduodenal Surgical Procedures

The stomach and the duodenum form a functional unit. Their relationship is apparent in some diseases such as the peptic ulcer, while other diseases, for example, malignant tumors, actually differ.

## 8.1 Introduction – Anatomical and Physiological Comments

The stomach is a sac-shaped organ where the following parts are recognized: cardia (transition between the esophagus and the stomach), fundus, body, antrum (the exit part) and pylorus that separates the stomach from the duodenum and functions as a sphincter. The stomach has an abundant vascular supply. It is innervated not only by sympathetic fibers, but especially by the gastric branches of both vagus nerves. Vagus innervation has direct influence on HCl secretion, gastric motility and pyloric relaxation. The stomach serves as a food reservoir; it finishes the mechanical processing of the food, and Fe and Ca are absorbed through its mucosa. The digestive effect is ensured by pepsin that splits proteins, and by hydrochloric acid that splits cellulose and provides an antiseptic effect. The formation of the intrinsic factor is important, which facilitates $B_{12}$ vitamin absorption in the small intestine.

These functions are derived from the structure of the epithelium and its glands where the following cells are found:
- **Chief cells** – secernate pepsinogen and cathepsin, **pepsin** precursors. These cells are present particularly in the fundus and in the body.
- **Parietal cells** – produce **HCl** and the intrinsic factor. These cells are also found in the fundus and in the body of the stomach.

- **Mucous cells** – produce mucus that forms the gastric barrier and prevents reverse diffusion of H⁺ ions. Most of these cells are found in the cardia and in the pylorus.
- **G cells** – are located in the antrum and produce gastrin. These cells respond to vagal stimulus upon chemical and mechanical irritation of the antrum. Gastrin together with direct vagal stimuli (cholinergic impulses) stimulates the secretion of chief and parietal cells.

The duodenum is the initial part of the small intestine; it circumscribes the pancreatic head and is partially located in the retroperitoneal region. The duodenum is divided in four sections:
- D1 – Extended bulb beyond the pylorus and a short horizontal section up to the superior duodenal flexure
- D2 – Descending part up to the lower flexure
- D3 – Horizontal part
- D4 – Short ascending part that passes into the jejunum at the Treitz's ligament

Brunner's glands are found in the proximal part of the duodenum and produce alkaline mucin. Pancreatic and biliary ducts empty into D2 at the papilla of Vater; this secretion neutralizes acidic chyme. Pancreatic juice includes other digestive enzymes such as amylase and lipase; carbohydrates, water-soluble vitamins and also Fe, Cu and Mg are absorbed in the duodenum.

## 8.2   Symptomatology of Gastroduodenal Diseases

The course of some diseases may be **asymptomatic**, such as the early stage of malignant tumors, rather small benign tumors including adenoma, and chronic gastritis.

More commonly, gastroduodenal diseases are **symptomatic**. The **upper dyspeptic syndrome**, i.e. a set of minor symptoms (vague mild pain in the epigastrium, the pain is indistinctive, more like pressure, with a loss of appetite, flatulence, etc.) is most commonly a sign of so-called functional problems, but it may also be a manifestation of a more severe chronic gastritis, ulcerous disease or gastric carcinoma.

Typical symptoms of gastroduodenal diseases include **nausea, vomiting and pain**. Vomiting of acidic gastric juices is typical for a gastroduodenal ulcer and acute gastritis, while profuse vomiting with the presence of undigested food is typical for an obstruction in the pyloric region. As for gastric carcinoma, vomiting as well as pain and weight loss are usually late symptoms of advanced disease.

GASTRIC AND DUODENAL SURGERY

Epigastric pain dependent on meals can be observed in ulcerous diseases, usually after a meal when gastric ulcer is present and in a fasting condition when a duodenal ulcer is present.

Various gastroduodenal diseases may also be associated with bleeding in the GIT, while microscopic bleeding is manifested by **anemia**, macroscopic by **hematemesis** or **melena,** in exceptional cases by **hematochesis** in massive bleeding.

## 8.3  Examinations of the Gastroduodenum

The diagnosis of gastric and duodenal diseases is usually determined using endoscopy, with concurrent examination of the esophagus. **Esophagogastroduodenoscopy** is performed using flexible gastroscopes with pro-grade optics. Biopsy is performed as a rule. In indicated cases, diagnostic endoscopy may become therapeutic endoscopy. Polyps can be removed using the electrocoagulation loop, a so-called **polypectomy**. **Endoscopic hemostasis** is an option when bleeding is present. Methods of endoscopic hemostasis are described in Chapter 19. Today, a premalignant lesion or a small early carcinoma can be removed using a modern endoscopic method – **mucosectomy** or **submucous resection**.

Besides biopsy, the staging of malignant tumors is performed using **endoscopic sonography** and **CT** assessment. These methods are used to determine the extent and infiltration of the tumor, its relationship to the surrounding organs and possibly any involvement of lymph nodes. Contrast radiography is also carried out in indicated cases.

## 8.4  Gastric and Duodenal Diseases

### 8.4.1  Inflammations of the Stomach (Gastritis)

**Acute gastritis** is caused by irritable poison, alimentary in most cases, or alcohol abuse. Other causes may include drugs such as corticoids, cytostatics and nonsteroidal antirheumatics (NSAID – Acylpyrin, Brufen, etc.). The symptoms include vomiting and pain in the epigastrium. The diagnosis is determined based on the clinical findings or upper endoscopy in more severe cases. The therapy is conservative, incorporating dietary measures and eliminating the provoking poison.

**Chronic gastritis** is a common disease after 50 years-of-age, characterized by chronic inflammatory infiltration in the region of the proper lamina and often also by mucosal atrophy, and sometimes by mucosal metaplasia. Etiology is not exactly defined; a part of the disease is caused by autoantibodies, while the effect of *Helicobacter pylori* (Hp) has been assumed in other parts.

**Chronic diffuse gastritis** (formerly called type A gastritis or chronic hypertrophic-atrophic gastritis) occurs in the whole stomach except the antrum. It is associated with hypoacidity up to achlorhydria. Hp is not present but antibodies against parietal cells are found in the serum. Vitamin $B_{12}$ absorption is also considerably reduced, and pernicious anemia may develop.

**Chronic gastritis** localized in the **antrum** (formerly type B) is more common; this type of gastritis is caused by metabolism of the present Hp. Serum antibodies are not present; however, this type of gastritis is one of the causes of the development of peptic ulcers. **Focal atrophic gastritis** develops with normal acidity or mild hypoacidity, in the presence of Hp in the antrum. This type of gastritis causes mucosal metaplasia of the intestinal type, which may become the basis for the development of gastric ulcers. Marked acidity and the presence of Hp cause **diffuse antral gastritis,** with potential metaplasia of the duodenal epithelium, causing the development of an ulcer in the duodenum.

**Pangastritis** is a combination of both types. Chronic inflammation associated with achlorhydria or mucosal metaplasia is considered as precancerosis.

Chronic gastritis is often asymptomatic. The symptomatic form is manifested by the upper dyspeptic syndrome. The therapy is conservative (symptomatic), including Hp eradication if present.

### 8.4.2  Gastroduodenal Ulcer Disease

Ulcer disease is a specific human disease that causes a mucosal defect through peptic corrosion of the epithelium. The defect is understood as superficial **erosion** not reaching beyond the muscular mucosa, or a deeper **ulcer** with inflammation of the surroundings, localized in the stomach or in the duodenum. Formerly, a **polyetiological** nature of this disease was assumed, particularly based on association with some factors. Intrinsic factors include genetic disposition, blood group 0 (in the duodenal ulcer), and diseases such as the Zollinger-Ellison syndrome (tumor from hormonally active G cells, localized particularly in the pancreas, which causes gastrin hyperproduction resulting in permanent severe hyperacidity), hyperparathyroidism (increased supply of $Ca^{2+}$ ions stimulates G cells). Extrinsic factors includes stress, alcohol abuse, smoking, drugs such as NSAIDs, corticoids, cytostatics, and also *Helicobacter pylori*, i.e. chronic gastritis with metaplasia caused by this agent. Currently, precisely the *Helicobacter pylori* infection with its consequences is considered to be the main etiological factor. Pathological influence of NSAIDs on the gastric mucosa is considered to be the second serious factor for ulcer development.

**Acute stress ulcers** develop after major surgeries, burns or polytraumas, and are caused particularly by reduced mucosal microcirculation. Often they are multiple.

In terms of peptic ulcer **pathophysiology**, the imbalance between aggressive and protective actions exerts opposing effects. **Aggressors** include hyperacidity (no ulcer can develop without the presence of acid), *Helicobacter pylori* which is present in 90% of duodenal ulcers, duodenogastric reflux, microcirculation disorders and ulcerogenic drugs. Particularly Aspirin and all NSAIDs are hazardous, which reduce the levels of endogenic prostglandins. An ulcer is formed if aggressive actions predominate or if protective actions become weaker.

**Gastric ulcer** is usually localized in the mediogastric region, in the small curvature, or in the antrum; subcardial localization is another possibility.

Gastric ulcer occurs more often in higher age groups, more commonly in men of lower social classes, and it tends to show a seasonal course. Pain in the epigastrium is the **major symptom**, following immediately or within several hours after a meal. The pain depends on the ulcer localization and on the type of meal. Other symptoms include vomiting, nausea, and heartburn. The patient is therefore afraid of eating and becomes cachectic.

**Duodenal ulcers** occur more commonly than gastric ulcers. They are usually localized in the bulb in the anterior or posterior wall, 5% of findings are postbulbar. Duodenal ulcers affect younger individuals, and are often related to hyperacidity and Hp infection. They show a characteristic seasonal course with exacerbation in spring and autumn. Epigastric pain in a fasting condition is a **typical symptom**, which subsides after a meal but then returns again. The patient is often woken up by pain in the early morning (so-called night hunger pain). Vomiting and heartburn may be present, and relief is provided by alkalies.

Complications may be the first symptom of an ulcer disease. The objective finding is usually poor; palpation pain in the epigastrium is usually present. Upper endoscopy is the predominant examination, while contrast radiography has been subsiding. Besides determining the diagnosis, a test for Hp is also carried out during the endoscopy, and a **biopsy** is always performed in **gastric** ulcers, in order to exclude malignancy, given that about 10% of gastric lesions are of malignant origin.

Currently, the **therapy** of ulcer disease is mainly **conservative**. It consists in regimen adjustment – resting regimen with sick leave, non-irritating diet, elimination of alcohol, smoking and ulcerogenic drugs. Medication functions on the principle of aggressor inhibition, stimulation of protectors, or it provides a combined effect. Recent drugs of choice include **proton-pump inhibitors** (Omeprazole, Pantoprazol, and Lanzoprazole) and they are always used for resistant and recurrent ulcers. Other alternatives include **H$_2$-receptor blockers** (Ranitidine, Famotidine), pirenzepine, sucralfate, antacids, and synthetic prostaglandins. When the finding of Hp is positive, eradication using the so-called triple combination is performed: a proton pump inhibitor combined with two ATBs of choice – amoxicillin, clarithromycin, and metronidazole. Bismuth salts provide lower efficacy and thus are no longer used.

**Surgical treatment** on non-complicated ulcer disease is indicated only if the conservative therapy fails, thus for resistant and relapsing ulcers. Surgery is also needed for gastric ulcers suspected of malignancy despite a negative biopsy.

These are ulcers that fail to heal within 3 months, are larger than 2 cm and localized in the great curvature.

**Gastric resection** is the basic procedure applied for both gastric and duodenal ulcers: two-thirds resection with type I anastomosis is the procedure of choice. Another variant that can be considered for duodenal ulcers is **vagotomy**, most commonly proximal, superselective, with the advantage of performance as a laparoscopic procedure. The numbers of surgeries performed for this indication have decreased thanks to very good results of conservative therapy.

Prognosis of an ulcer disease is usually good; however, the numbers of complicated forms have been rising recently.

**Ulcer disease complications** include bleeding, penetration, perforation, and stenosis. The potential of malignant reversal of a peptic ulcer has not been confirmed by research; when a malignancy is found, a tumor has been present from the beginning.

**Bleeding** from ulcers is described in detail in Chapter 19.

**Penetration** means covered perforation of the deep peptic ulcer into surrounding organs. Most commonly, ulcers of the posterior wall of the duodenal bulb penetrate into the pancreas. Gastric ulcers of the small curvature may penetrate into the liver. Penetration is manifested by marked, permanent pain. Surgical treatment is applied in cases where conservative therapy has failed.

**Perforation** of the peptic ulcer is classified as an acute abdomen. As a rule, ulcers localized in the anterior wall of the stomach or duodenum are found to penetrate, while perforation is most commonly seen in ulcers localized in the area of the pylorus. Initially, chemical peritonitis develops. In the course of time, the content of the abdominal cavity becomes infected and the finding changes to suppurative, usually diffuse peritonitis. Severe diffuse bacterial peritonitis is a serious result of this process.

Typically, the patient reports a sudden onset of strong up to shocking **pain in the epigastrium**, which may shoot into one or both shoulders (phrenic symptom). Subsequently, the pain moves to the whole abdomen; vomiting need not be present as a rule.

An **objective assessment** is dominated by exhaustion of the patient who adopts the antalgic position on their back with bent lower limbs. Tachycardia is usually present. Local findings in the abdomen include restricted advancement of the respiratory wave, board-like contraction of the abdominal wall (muscular defense), marked pain upon palpation and percussion mostly found in the epigastrium, painful response to the shaking of the peritoneum, disappearing peristalsis. *Per rectum* examination may cause pain and possibly reveal the arching of the Douglas space.

Native imaging of the abdomen in the standing position with evidence of pneumoperitoneum is the basic **examination** method. If there are doubts, gastroscopy can be performed with subsequent repeated native sonography of the abdomen or diagnostic laparoscopy.

The **therapy** of a perforation is always **surgical** and consists in treatment of both the perforation and the peritonitis. As a rule, suture of the perforation is performed with omentoplasty. Gastric localization of the ulcer necessitates excision of the edge for histological examination in order to exclude any malignancy. Peritonitis is treated by repeated flushes of the abdominal cavity with the cleaning of all peritoneal recesses. The procedure can be carried out **laparoscopically**.

Mortality still remains at 6 to 10%, caused by developed peritonitis with multiple organ failure, usually due to late diagnosis.

Scarring of the ulcer localized in the pylorus or duodenum may lead to **stenosis**. The patient exhibits symptoms of gastric evacuation disorder, suffers from pain in the epigastrium, from nausea, with repeated vomiting of undigested contents. The stomach is dilated and can be tapped and sometimes also palpated. A splashing sound is heard upon percussion. The diagnosis can be performed using upper endoscopy and/or contrast radiography. The **therapy** is **surgical** and consists in resection of the stomach; before the surgery, the stomach must be emptied and toned by inserting an NG tube with repeated flushes. The inner environment is corrected using infusion therapy; hypochloremia usually dominates.

### 8.4.3 Gastric Tumors

**Benign tumors** of the stomach are rare. Fibromas and neurofibromas are usually asymptomatic. Gastrointestinal stromal tumors – **GIST** occur most commonly. Although located in the wall, they may bleed into the lumen, often causing anemia. A voluminous GIST may induce symptoms of a stomach evacuation disorder, i.e. pressure, dyspepsia, pain, vomiting. The diagnosis is determined using endoscopy. The therapy is surgical; the tumor is removed by limited resection, sometimes also mere extirpation in healthy tissue. Mucosal **polyps** are either superficial hyperplasias or **adenomas** that are precanceroses. This is why adenomas must be removed – by endoscopic polypectomy.

**Malignant gastric tumors** are very serious surgical diseases, despite the fact that their number has been declining in the Czech Republic. Up to 95% of these tumors are **adenocarcinomas** (papillary, tubular, mucinous, signet ring cell cancer), or in exceptional cases adenosquamous carcinomas, small cell carcinomas, undifferentiated carcinomas, malignant GIST or malignant lymphomas.

The etiology is unknown; however, **dispositional** and **eliciting factors** do exist. Tumors develop more in men, higher age groups, blood group A, and a higher occurrence can also be seen in certain geographic regions. **Precanceroses** such as polyps (adenoma), achlorhydria, and chronic gastritis with metaplasia add to these dispositional factors. Risk factors include **carcinogens** such as benzopyrenes, nitrosamines in food (baked, smoked meats) and some food dyes.

Gastric carcinoma may be polypous, bowl-shaped, ulceriform or infiltrating (plastic linitis). **Gastric carcinoma classification** according to Laurint is important for the extent of the resection, which recognizes the intestinal type carcinomas and their diffuse forms. Diffuse types with infiltrative growth are associated with very poor prognosis.

TNM classification is used for staging, which is determined as follows:
- T1 – tumor infiltrating the proper lamina or reaching even into the submucosa
- T2 – tumor infiltrating the musculature
- T3 – tumor penetrating the serosa
- T4 – infiltration of neighboring structures and organs
- N1 – lymph node metastases with infiltration of not more than 6 nodes. N2 is classified as the infiltration of 7–15 nodes; N3 is used for the infiltration of more than 15 nodes.
- M1 – presence of distant metastases, particularly in non-regional nodes (for example, supraclavicular, the so-called Virchow's node) and the liver, but also in the lungs, bones, brain or mural peritoneum with the formation of malignant ascites

Metastases of the signet ring cell carcinoma in the ovaries are known as a Krukenberg tumor.

A considerable number of these tumors initially grow as asymptomatic or cause only minor problems: dyspepsia, pressure in the stomach, nausea, the so-called **set of small symptoms**, and therefore it is often diagnosed late. The disease should be revealed at the earliest stage for a better prognosis. **Early cancer** may take the arched form – type I, superficial flat form – type II, or excavated form – type III. It is always a small lesion in the mucosa, reaching not further than into the submucosa, with no involvement of the lymph nodes – T1, N0.

Aversion to meat, pain, wearisomeness, anemization may occur in more advanced forms. Loss of weight, vomiting (in the case of blockage in the pylorus) and dysphagia (associated with cardiac localization) are usually late symptoms.

The **clinical finding** is usually poor; in more advanced conditions, the tumor may be palpable, dilatation of the stomach may be found, as well as Virchow's lymph node or ascites.

**Upper endoscopy** with biopsy is the main **diagnostic** method. Every lesion in the stomach should be examined histologically, and patients at risk should be distinguished and examined on a regular basis. Double contrast radiography is used, particularly in infiltrating carcinomas, which may spread underneath the mucosa and are not readily visible. Radiography of the lungs and sonography of the liver are performed in order to exclude any metastases; endosonography and CT imaging of the abdomen are performed to determine the depth of mural infiltration and any possible involvement of the nodes. Markers are used to control the course of the therapy.

The **therapy** is fundamentally **surgical**, the curative procedure being **radical surgery: total gastrectomy** with resection of the small and large omenta with regional lymphadenectomy of the 1$^{st}$ and 2$^{nd}$ compartments, as well as splenectomy if nodes in the splenic hilum are infiltrated. In proximal tumors of the cardia, a part of the distal esophagus is also resected. **Subtotal gastrectomy** is indicated for intestinal type tumors of the distal third of the stomach. GIT reconstruction is performed by creating Roux-en-Y anastomosis in the jejunal loop or a jejunal interponate between the esophagus and the duodenum. Actinotherapy and chemotherapy are not very significant for gastric carcinoma if the resection is curative (R0). Neoadjuvant chemotherapy can be used in the preoperative period in UICC stage III.

For inoperable findings, the treatment should restore GIT passage – by endoscopic introduction of a stent or by GEA establishment. In locally operable tumors with distant metastases, simple palliative resection can be carried out. The purpose is to reduce the tumor mass and maintain food passage or to remove the source of repeated bleeding.

Exceptionally, in early forms of carcinoma, excision or resection is sufficient and today, endoscopic methods (mucosectomy, submucous resection) can also be applied.

Early diagnosis is important for the prognosis, given that early forms are associated with a rate of 95% of 5-year survival. However, radical resection is possible only in about one half of all tumors found on average. Survival depends on the extent and grading, while a 15–40% 5-year survival of operated patients has been reported.

Primary lymphomas are associated with a relatively good prognosis; in terms of therapy, chemotherapy is primarily indicated in the lymphomas. MALT lymphomas respond favorably to Hp eradication with one-time irradiation.

**Duodenal tumors** are very rare, particularly malignant tumors do not occur virtually at all. **Benign** tumors include lipoma, adenoma, and villous adenoma; in terms of **malignant** tumors, primary **adenocarcinoma** may develop in exceptional cases. A carcinoma may grow into the duodenum from the pancreatic head. If operable, the appropriate radical procedure is Whipple duodeno-pancreatectomy (cf. Chapter 13).

## 8.4.4 Volvulus of the Stomach

Volvulus of the stomach may develop along the transverse or longitudinal axis with loose suspensions. Also, the stomach may rotate along both axes (the so-called "upside down stomach"); this condition is often associated with diaphragmatic hernia. Acute volvulus is manifested particularly by severe epigastric pain, while chronic volvulus is associated with vomiting, sometimes also pressure pain in the epigastrium. The diagnosis is determined using contrast radiography. Endoscopy usually does not provide much benefit in this case. The therapy is surgical and consists in derotating and fixating the stomach.

### 8.4.5 Bezoars

Bezoars are masses formed in the stomach from swallowed hair – **trichobezoars**, or from food residues, particularly fruits and vegetables – **phytobezoars**. Gastric concrements are developed from swallowing paraffin or chewing gum. They may be indicated by nausea, vomiting, pain in the epigastrium and weight loss. The diagnosis is determined using endoscopy. The therapy of symptomatic bezoars consists in endoscopic or surgical removal.

### 8.4.6 Ménétrier's Disease

This is a rare disease of the gastric mucosa of unknown etiology. It is characterized by large hypertrophic cilia present in the whole stomach except the antrum. The disease is associated with high secretion of mucus and with marked hypoacidity up to achlorhydria and hypoproteinemia. It affects mostly older men, sometimes with family disposition. A broad spectrum of clinical symptoms is usually present, most commonly pain in the epigastrium, weight loss, diarrhea. Laboratory findings show anemia, hypoproteinemia and hypoalbuminemia. The diagnosis can be confirmed by contrast radiography and upper endoscopy with a biopsy. The disease is a precancerosis, and thus the patient should be distinguished and a total gastrectomy should be performed if malignant conversion is suspected.

## 8.5 Gastroduodenal Surgical Procedures

The stomach usually heals well after a surgery as it is well perfused and contains no bacterial flora thanks to HCl secretions. Single-layer seromuscular continued stitches can be used for sutures. Double-layer suturing combining Albert and Lembert stitches is sometimes used for hemostatic reasons, or the sutures are placed using staplers. Major risks of gastroduodenal surgery include bleeding and suture or anastomosis disintegration.

The basic types of surgeries are provided below for clarity.

### 8.5.1 Local Procedures

- **Gastrotomy, duodenotomy** means longitudinal or transverse opening of the stomach or duodenum (Fig. 8.1).
- **Pyloroplasty** is a longitudinal tomy in the pyloric region closed crosswise with a suture (Fig. 8.2).
- **Suture** of the perforated peptic ulcer is usually associated with excision of the edges and/or omentoplasty (Fig. 8.3).

# GASTRIC AND DUODENAL SURGERY

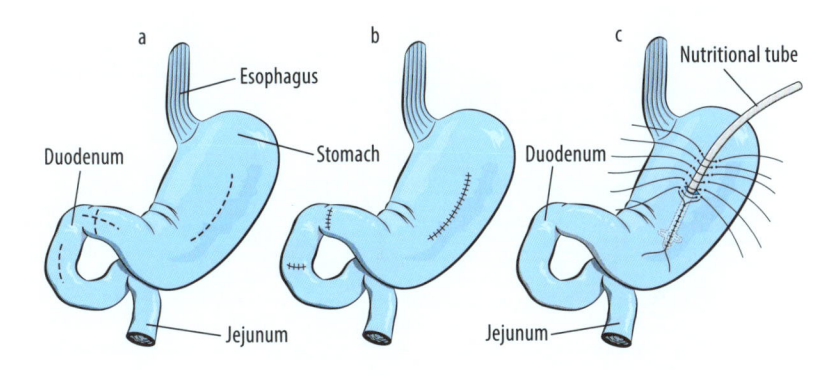

**Fig. 8.1** *Gastrotomy and duodenotomy: a) Incision; b) Sutures; c) Witzel gastrotomy*

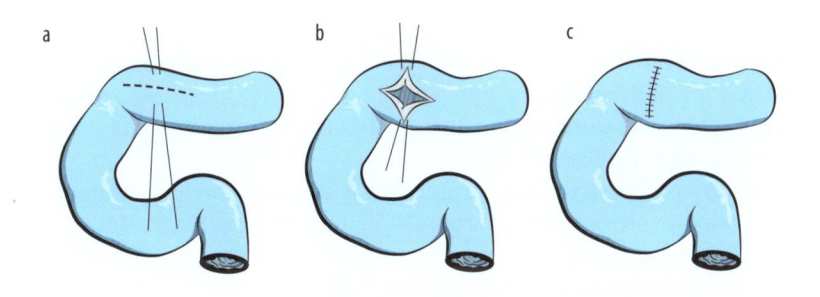

**Fig. 8.2** *Heinecke-Mikulicz pyloroplasty*

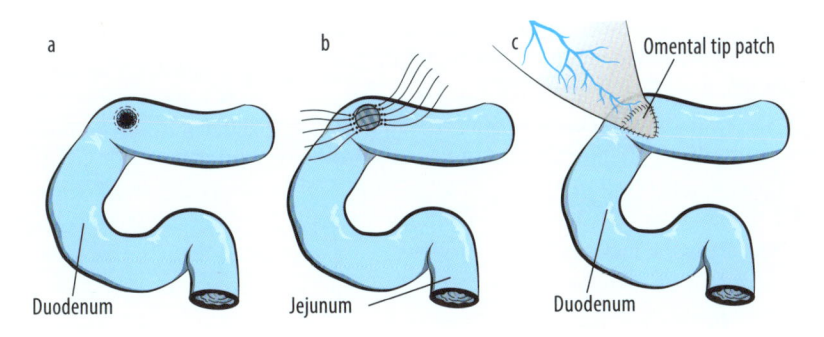

**Fig. 8.3** *a) Perforation of the duodenal bulb ulcer; b) Suture; c) Omentoplasty*

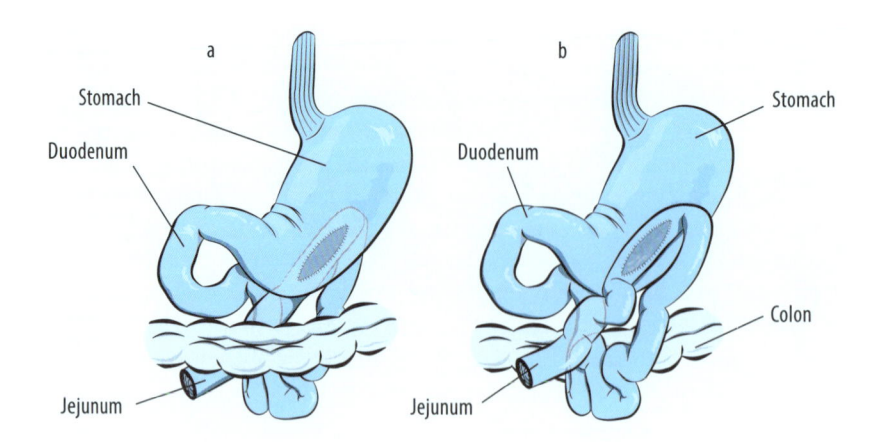

Fig. 8.4 *Gastroenteroanastomosis: a) Posterior (retrocolic) according to Hacker; b) Anterior (antecolic) according to Wölfer*

- **Surgical suture** (sewing through) of the bleeding ulcer with a blood vessel at the bottom, performed from within the tomy.
- Local **devascularization procedures**, the ligation of supply vessels, are used when bleeding is present.
- The purpose of **gastrostomy** according to Witzel is to provide nutrition when an unmanageable obstruction is present in the esophageal and cardiac region (Fig. 8.1c). Endoscopic insertion of an intraluminal stent is the method of choice; if failed, a gastrostomy is performed, which is inserted using the laparoscopic or percutaneous (PEG) methods.

### 8.5.2 Gastroenteroanastomoses

Gastroenteroanastomosis means connection of the stomach with the first jejunal loop. It is performed when an obstruction is present in the pyloric or duodenal region which cannot be resolved otherwise. More commonly, gastroenteroanastomosis is established on the posterior wall of the stomach according to Hacker (posterior GEA), or anterior anastomosis according to Wölfer (anterior GEA) in exceptional cases (Fig. 8.4).

GEA may also be established using laparoscopy, but the procedure is more complex from the technical point of view.

### 8.5.3 Resection Procedures

Gastric resection procedures have been carried out since the second half of the 19th century. The surgery was developed for the therapy of ulcer diseases, but soon it began to be used for the treatment of tumors as well.

# GASTRIC AND DUODENAL SURGERY

In principle, the various types of resection differ according to their extent and the way GIT continuity is restored (Fig. 8.5). Resection usually means that the lower two thirds of the stomach are removed including the pylorus, thereby eliminating a large part of secretory epithelial cells of the stomach and the antrum with gastrin production. GIT continuity is restored after tubulization of the stub. Resection procedures are related to many famous names, particularly the name of Billroth. The term **type I gastric resection** is used in current surgery, with the anastomosis sutured end-to-end between the stub of the stomach and the duodenum (Fig. 8.6). This type of anastomosis is more physiological, functionally better, and therefore it is preferred whenever it is feasible. **Type II gastric resection** consists in making a blind closure of the duodenum and in attaching the

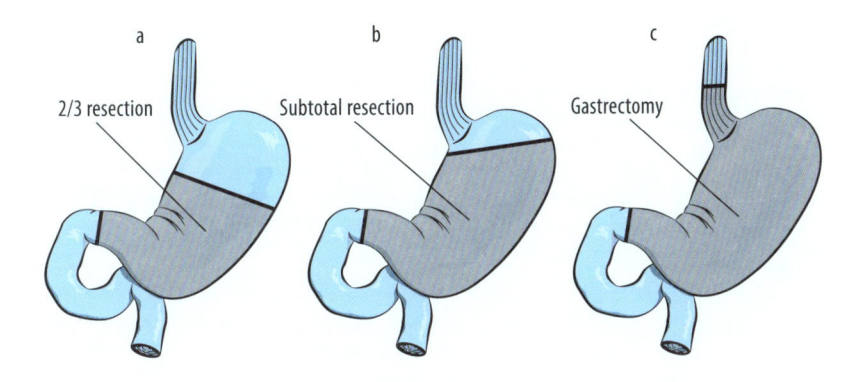

**Fig. 8.5** *Gastric resection – resection line*

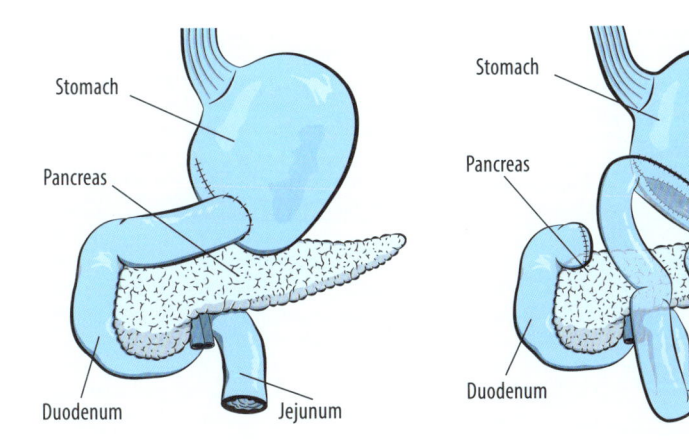

**Fig. 8.6** *Type I gastric resection with anastomosis*

**Fig. 8.7** *Type II gastric resection with anastomosis*

stub of the stomach to the first jejunal loop (Fig. 8.7). This type of anastomosis is less physiological and is associated with the risk of post-operative insufficiency of the duodenal stub and with the potential of the stub of the stomach being irritated by alkaline secretion. Occurrence of the so-called dumping syndrome is more common after Type II resection. Roux-en-Y anastomosis is an alternative to

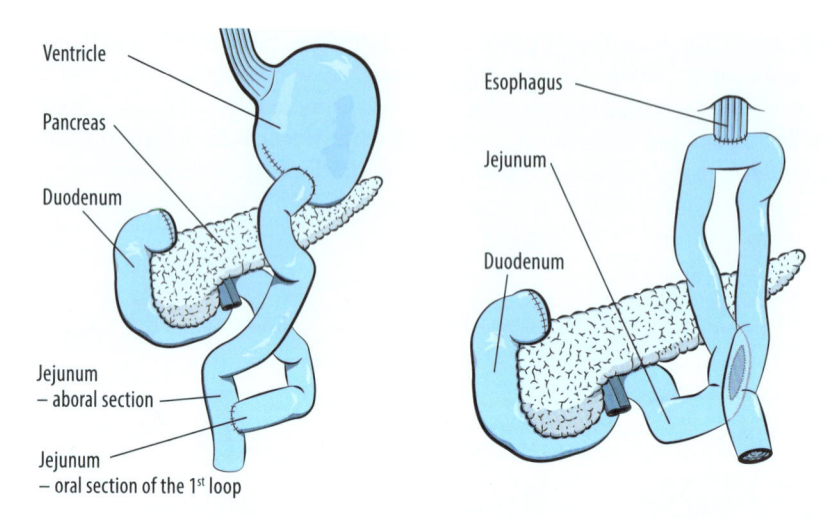

**Fig. 8.8** *Gastric resection – Roux-en-Y anastomosis*

**Fig. 8.9** *Condition after total gastrectomy – anastomosis using the omega loop with EEA according to Braun*

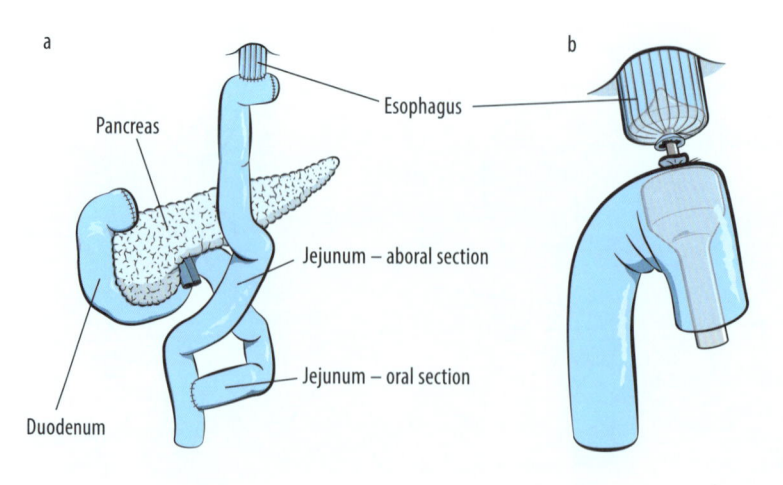

**Fig. 8.10** *Status after total gastrectomy: a) Anastomosis according to Roux; b) Esophageal anastomosis using the circular stapler*

## GASTRIC AND DUODENAL SURGERY

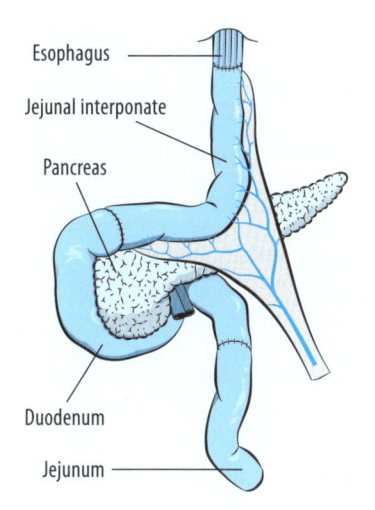

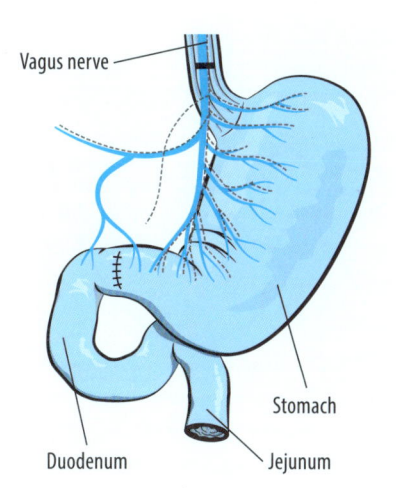

**Fig. 8.11** *Condition after total gastrectomy – use of interponated jejunum to connect the esophagus and the duodenum*

**Fig. 8.12** *Truncal vagotomy with pyloroplasty*

Type II resection (Fig. 8.8). Type II gastric resection can also be achieved using laparoscopy; in this case, the anastomosis is established using a linear stapler.

**Total gastrectomy** – removal of the entire stomach – is usually indicated for a carcinoma. Anastomosis with the esophagus is more risky considering that the esophagus has no serosa. **Subtotal gastrectomy** is performed in indicated cases and this means that a small edge of gastric tissue is left around the cardia. This procedure is indicated in intestinal type tumors localized in the distal third of the stomach. Attachment using the so-called omega loop used to follow after a gastrectomy, corresponding in essence to Type II resection. However, Braun's entero-enteroanastomosis (EEA) had to be performed due to the long afferent loop (Fig. 8.9). Currently, the Roux-en-Y anastomosis is used (Fig. 8.10) or a modification of Type I resection using an interponate of the proximal jejunum between the esophagus and the duodenum (Fig. 8.11).

### 8.5.4 Vagotomy

The purpose of vagotomy is to reduce gastric HCl secretion by gastric denervation.

**Truncal vagotomy** means separation of the trunk of both vagus nerves at the lower esophagus. The denervation is usually perfect, but it also affects other organs (the gallbladder, the intestines), and the surgery must be completed with pyloroplasty in order to remove pylorospasm (Fig. 8.12).

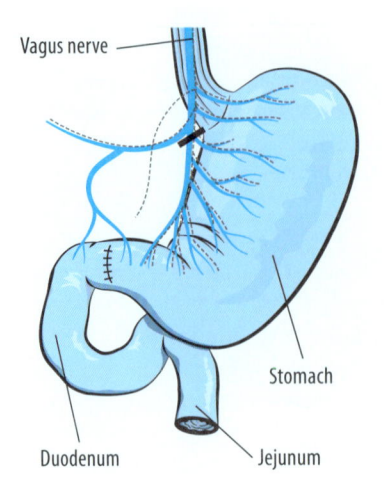

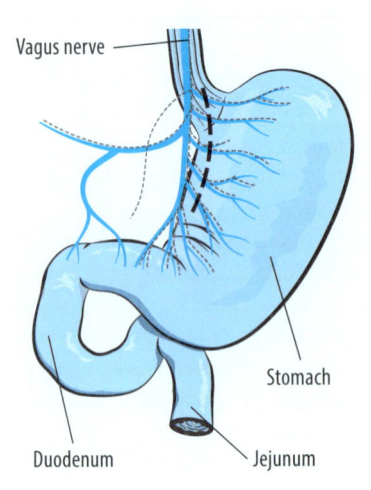

**Fig. 8.13** *Selective vagotomy with pyloroplasty*

**Fig. 8.14** *Superselective vagotomy*

**Selective vagotomy** means separation of both vagus nerves below the point of division of organ branches, and thus it is associated with fewer negative effects. Pyloroplasty is also necessary in this case (Fig. 8.13).

**Superselective vagotomy** (proximal vagotomy) means that the motor supply of the pylorus is left out (so-called crow's foot), and thus no pyloroplasty is needed. Individual secretion branches for the stomach are interrupted; the procedure can also be performed as a seromyotomy. The procedure is associated with few side effects; however, the reduction of acidity is not as high. The use of peroperative pH metry is recommended to ensure that the denervation is perfect (Fig. 8.14).

Vagotomy can also be carried out using laparoscopy; anterior superselective (seromyotomy) and posterior truncal vagotomies are combined in this case.

### 8.5.5 Specific Complications after Gastroduodenal Surgeries

**Postprandial diarrhea** occurs frequently after vagotomies during the first year. As a rule, it subsides after dietary and regimen measures.

**Anastomosis blockage** (efferent loop syndrome) is caused predominantly by the swelling of the anastomosis and reduced peristalsis after surgery, usually after a Type I resection. It is manifested by the removal of high amounts of liquids through the tube and vomiting after meals. The therapy is conservative: NG tube insertion with flushes and suction, parenteral nutrition, endoscopic dilatation of the anastomosis.

## GASTRIC AND DUODENAL SURGERY

**Afferent loop syndrome** may occur after a Type II resection. It is caused by congestion in the afferent loop, which is long or partially compressed. The symptoms include pressure up to pain in the epigastrium after meals, nausea and the vomiting of the contents with bile, with subsequent considerable relief. The solution is surgical: the compressed loop is cleared, entero-enteroanastomosis is carried out for a long loop, and conversion to Type I resection or Roux-en-Y anastomosis follows.

The **dumping syndrome** develops after a Type II resection and its **early** and **late** forms are distinguished. The early syndrome is caused by fast progression of hypertonic chyme to the jejunum which becomes distended and absorbs liquid, leading to relative hypovolemia. The late dumping syndrome is caused by reactive hypoglycemia, which may follow after quick absorption of sugars and subsequent hyperinsulinemia. The **symptoms** of the early dumping syndrome include pressure in the epigastrium after meals, pain, nausea, lightheadedness, palpitations, diarrhea, sometimes fainting with decreased pressure. Late dumping syndrome is manifested by hypoglycemia developing about 1–3 hours after a meal. The **therapy** is conservative, dietary and regimen-based. It is recommended to observe a diet with restricted sugars, predominance of protein, small portions, no drinking during the meal, and resting on the right hip after the meal. In exceptional cases, the condition necessitates a surgical solution, conversion to a Type I resection or antiperistaltic interposition of a short section of the jejunum.

**Alkaline reflux gastritis** develops in about 25% of patients after resection procedures, particularly after a Type II resection. Patients with alkaline reflux gastritis should be distinguished and regularly monitored.

These complications are rare given that the number of patients after gastric resection and particularly after a Type II resection have decreased.

# 9 SURGERY OF THE SMALL AND LARGE INTESTINES, RECTUM AND ANUS

9.1 Anatomical and Functional Notes
9.2 Symptoms of Intestinal Diseases
9.3 Diagnostic Notes
9.4 Small Intestine
9.5 Large Intestine
9.6 Rectum and Anus

Surgical diseases of the small intestine, colon, rectum and anus are understood as a broad scale of conditions whose management and healing require surgical (operative) treatment or where operation is one of the components of a more complex therapy. The most common surgical diseases in adults include: a) acute and chronic inflammations for the small intestine; b) tumors, diverticular disease and non-specific intestinal inflammations, ordered according to frequency, for the colon; and c) hemorrhoids, inflammations and tumors, found in all injury localizations of the anorectum.

## 9.1 Anatomical and Functional Notes

The **small intestine**, about 3.5–5 m long, is the longest part of the digestive tract. The first part of the small intestine, the duodenum, is classified in the same category as the stomach in terms of its anatomy, function and diseases. A large part of the duodenum is found in the retroperitoneal localization; the other two compartments of the small intestine, the jejunum and ileum, are localized only intraperitoneally, suspended by **mesentery**. The mesentery fixates the small intestine to the posterior abdominal wall, and **blood and lymph supply** is brought to the intestine through the mesentery. Arterial blood supply is provided almost exclusively by the superior mesenteric artery. The non-obliterated omphaloenteric duct – Meckel's diverticulum – is found approximately 80–100 cm from the ileocecal (Bauhin's) valve in about 2–5% of persons.

# SURGERY OF THE SMALL AND LARGE INTESTINES, RECTUM AND ANUS

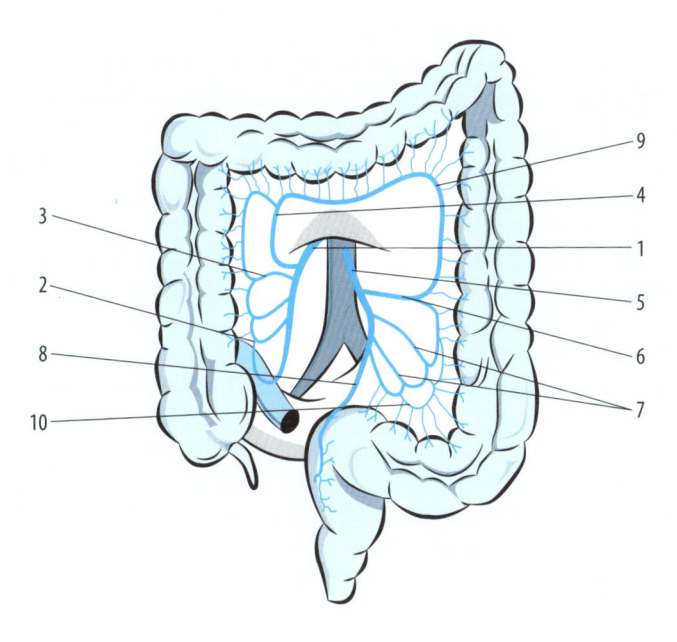

**Fig. 9.1** *Arterial supply of the large intestine: 1) superior mesenteric artery; 2) ileocolic artery; 3) right colic artery; 4) middle colic artery; 5) inferior mesenteric artery; 6) left colic artery; 7) sigmoid arteries; 8) superior rectal arteries; 9) large anastomosis of Riolan; 10) Drummond anastomosis*

The **large intestine** is 1.2–1.4 m long. The cecum, transverse colon and the sigmoid loop are located intraperitoneally, the ascending and partially also descending colons are located retroperitoneally.

The serosa – one of the four layers of the intestinal wall – is missing in the retroperitoneal segments. In a similar manner to the small intestine, the large intestine is suspended by the **mesocolon**, through which blood and lymphatic vessels are brought to the intestine. The ascending colon is characterized by the widest diameter, while the sigmoid loop is the narrowest part; the lumen of the intestines and the nature of their contents participate in the symptoms of their diseases.

**Vascular supply** is ensured by several arteries (Fig. 9.1), the right half of the colon up to the splenic flexure is supplied by the right colic artery and middle colic artery (branches of the superior mesenteric artery), while aborally from the splenic flexure, the colon is supplied with blood from the left colic artery, from the inferior mesenteric artery. The colon segment between the middle colic and left colic arteries is supplied by an arterial duct, the large anastomosis (Halleri, Riolani). The rectum is supplied with arterial blood by the superior rectal artery from the cranial side, and by hemorrhoid arteries from the caudal side.

The intestinal **lymphatic system** is formed by lymph nodes and lymphatic vessels. Lymphatic vessels run along arteries and veins forming plexuses where lymph nodes are integrated. Based on localization, the nodes are divided into groups where the nearest ones are found near the intestine and the most distant ones are found at the orifices of large blood vessels (three levels of the nodes in the small intestine and four in the large intestine). In the small intestine, the lymphatic system starts as the Peyer's patches (lymph nodules) and ends in the chyle cistern. Epicolic nodes are found within the shortest distance from the colon, while that of the paraaortic nodes is the longest.

In terms of surgical treatment, knowledge of the vascular supply of the intestines is necessary for surgeries (to preserve nutritive blood vessels, to use the vessels as points of reference while removing lymph nodes, particularly in surgeries due to a tumor), and also in terms of diagnostics and therapy of diseases caused by damage to the vascular supply of the intestines (for example, ischemic colitis, embolism and thromboses).

Digestion is the **main function of the small intestine**. Digestion is composed of three different activities: digestion of the content (chyle) in the intestinal lumen using digestive enzymes, absorption and transport.

This function is irreplaceable; the removal of the whole small intestine or leaving less than 50 cm of the intestine is (with exceptions) incompatible with survival. Only segments of the small intestine can be removed (resected) with no damage; if the resection is more extensive, typical disorders develop depending on localization.

Resection of the jejunum is better tolerated thanks to the higher adaptive capacity of the ileum than ileal resection. It causes resorption disorders of iron, calcium and water-soluble vitamins. An extensive resection of the ileum causes a disorder of the resorption of water, electrolytes, vitamin $B_{12}$ and conjugated bile acids. Removal of extensive segments of the small intestine with subsequent malabsorption and maldigestion leads to numerous other metabolic disorders that take part in the development of short bowel syndrome. The small intestine also fulfills an immunological function, particularly IgA synthesis.

The **main function of the large intestine** is to thicken the intestinal content and transport it toward the rectum. This purpose is fulfilled by resorption to thicken the liquid content and transform it to formed stool, motility to ensure mixing of the content and movement in the aboral direction, and secretion, including mucus secretion that facilitates the passage of the formed stool through distal intestinal segments. While in the right half of the colon, the intestinal content is still liquid, it is formed in the left part. Unlike the small intestine, rich bacterial flora is present in the large intestine, which participates in the synthesis of biotin, folic acid and vitamin K, in the metabolism of bile salts to bile acids, and also in urea hydrolysis to ammonia.

The **main function of the rectum and anus** is continent emptying. The rectum, particularly the rectal ampulla, functions as a stool reservoir, while stool continence depends especially on the competence of the sphincter apparatus.

SURGERY OF THE SMALL AND LARGE INTESTINES, RECTUM AND ANUS

Stool emptying at a suitable moment is the result of a complex interplay between the CNS and numerous reflexes that lead to the relaxation of the sphincters, contraction of smooth muscles of the rectum, and an increase in the intra-abdominal pressure through contraction of abdominal muscles. Continence is not only about the ability to hold stool, but also about the ability to distinguish whether the defecation can be postponed, what the nature of the emptied content will be, and possibly to release gas but hold in the stool.

The large intestine, the rectum and the anus are not life-critical and can be removed to various extents. The consequences depend on the localization and extent of the removal and cause reduction of the resorption area of the intestine, shortening of the transition time, lowering of the capacity of the colon as a reservoir, and also fecal incontinence if the anorectum and the sphincter apparatus are removed. Long-term survival after the removal of the whole large intestine including the rectum and anus is possible; usually disturbed only by the present ileostomy (small intestine outlet, see below) after initial adaptation.

## 9.2 Symptoms of Intestinal Diseases

Intestinal diseases can be asymptomatic as well as symptomatic. **Asymptomatic diseases** are those that remain free of any symptoms, for example, intestinal polyps, early tumors, and diverticula.

**Symptomatic diseases** are accompanied by one or several symptoms that may be different or complementary in their forms, manifestations and time, or also in the urgency and seriousness of the symptoms.

The most common **manifestations** include digestive and emptying problems, weight loss, presence of pathological admixtures in stool, and change in the defecation process, tenesmus, blood loss anemia, palpable resistances in the abdomen or in the rectum, pain, continence disorders, fever, and/or a "set of small symptoms". These manifestations may persist weeks and months, while acute manifestations – most commonly absence or impairment of intestinal passage, peritonitis or blooding in the lower digestive tract – last tens of minutes up to hours. About 20% of intestinal diseases are manifested as an acute abdomen. Usually, digestive problems are an expression of maldigestion or malabsorption. Defecation problems tend to be caused by an obstruction in the intestinal lumen, most commonly a tumor. Pathological admixtures in stool include blood, mucus, tissue fragments and/or undigested gastric content.

The majority of intestinal diseases are accompanied by bleeding in the intestines. Chronic bleeding from higher intestinal segments is not visible to the eye and can be demonstrated only in the laboratory. Chronic bleeding from lesions localized in the colon distally from the splenic flexure is usually evident as thin filaments of blood on/in stool, and/or may be registered in the bowl as blood. In the event of lesions in the rectum and anus, the patients notice red blood flow during defecation or even without defecation. Bleeding not visible to the eye is denoted as occult, while visible bleeding is denoted as manifest.

Mucus on/in stool or mucus defecation in amounts that almost replace the volume of stool is another common admixture.

Changes in the defecation process are important signs, such as onset of diarrhea instead of constipation, urge followed by inadequate volume and characteristics of stool, or transient stabilization of a new process.

It should be emphasized that other intestinal diseases, particularly those of infectious and alimentary origin, as well as unsuitable eating and emptying habits, may be accompanied by the aforementioned symptoms as well.

## 9.3 Diagnostic Notes

The diagnostic procedure should evolve from basic to special examinations, from simple to complex ones, and from non-invasive to invasive examinations. **Medical history** is the fundamental part of examinations, focused on information on digestion and defecation, and **physical examination** – general examination, examination of the abdomen and **per rectum**. Any signs of weight loss, nutrition disorders and hydration, palpable resistances in the abdomen, palpable tumors **per rectum**, and the condition of the anal sphincter are explored during the general examination, and stool residues and any admixtures on the glove are examined at the end of the examination. When an **acute examination** is performed, any signs of localized or diffuse peritoneal irritation are looked for, as well as signs of obstruction, e.g. narrowing of the small intestine loops visible to the eye, obstruction phenomena (or silence) during auscultation, tympanic percussion, atonia of the sphincter, hypotonia of the rectal ampulla, absence of intestinal content in the rectum, and presence of blood should be confirmed in the event of bleeding. The collection of a medical history and physical examination must always precede any further examinations, which include imaging, endoscopic and laboratory methods.

Native **radiography** is the **basic imaging method**, performed in the standing position using a horizontal x-ray beam; in intestinal diseases, this method can be used to assess gas distribution in the intestine, sometimes to reveal the nature of the filling material (for example, stagnating scybala), and especially to confirm the presence of levels in the intestine as a sign of absence of intestinal passage, and possibly the presence of air in the free abdominal cavity in the event of perforation. **Passage through the small intestine under radiographic control** is used for planned radiography, with oral contrast administration, and **enteroclysis**, i.e. contrast application in the duodenum using an introduced tube. Double contrast **irigography** is used for radiographic examination of the large colon, which consists in monitoring the contrast filler instilled in a retrograde manner through the rectum in the colon after emptying, later completed with air insufflation. A contrast that sticks to the mucosa can be used to display not only the contours of the intestine, but also small details of the mucosa when the examination is successful, for example, polyps. The so-called **defecography** is a special variant of the contrast examination of the colon, thus a radiographic record of defecation. This examination is used for defecation disorders.

**Angiography** is a less common contrast examination, used in the search for vascular intestinal events, for example, for embolism or thrombosis of the superior mesenteric artery, ischemic colitis, etc.

**Ultrasound examination** plays a role in the diagnostics of intestinal diseases in the detection of abdominal resistances (tumors, inflammatory infiltrates, abscesses, for example, in the event of the Crohn's disease), in liver examination (to look for metastases of colorectal tumors), or in the diagnostics of periproctal abscesses and fistulae. **Endorectal sonography** is carried out on a frequent basis using a special tube, while endoluminal sonography of higher parts of the colon is performed in exceptional cases. The examinations are used to assess the depth of the invasion of any present neoplasias and to evaluate the structure found near the intestine, particularly lymph nodes.

Ultrasound can also be used to assess intestinal motility, and thus to diagnose, for example, absence or impairment of intestinal passage.

**Endoscopy** is the fundamental examination of the colon and rectum – **anoscopy** for anal examination including the anal channel and its internal orifice, **rectoscopy** for examination of the segment of 25 to 30 cm from the edge of the anus depending on the anatomical situation and length of the tube of the device, sigmoideoscopy and **colonoscopy** to examine the whole colon. These last two examinations are performed using a flexible device that can pass through the intestinal flexures. Colonoscopy reaching as far as in the cecum is successful in more than 90% of patients. The endoscopic examination includes collecting samples for histological assessment, **biopsies**. Endoscopic examination of the small intestine, enteroscopy, requires special examination techniques that allow for an examination using a special endoscope. Endoscopic examinations provide the advantage of direct diagnostics of mucosal findings, eventually joined with biopsy collections, as well as that of converting the diagnostic procedure to a therapeutic one, e.g. **polypectomy**, **sclerotization** or **coagulation** of bleeding lesions, endoluminal dilatation. Disadvantages include the necessary preparation of the intestine and the risks associated with the examination.

The importance of **CT assessment** comes to the fore in the diagnostics of advanced findings, for example, of tumors, together with the assessment of their dimensions including any involvement of lymph nodes, relationship to other structures, the assessment of resectability, or in complications of intestinal diseases (for example, complications of the diverticular diseases of the colon).

Advanced examinations include three-dimensional (3D) **CT assessment**, which makes it possible to obtain computer-based reconstruction of the intestine and virtual imaging including small mucosal lesions.

**Magnetic resonance imaging** or **immunoscintigraphy** are usually used only as targeted methods in the diagnostics of intestinal diseases. MRI may be substantially beneficial, for example, in the diagnostics of anorectal malformations, complicated fistulae or for tumor staging, while immunoscintigraphy is used, for example, to examine non-specific intestinal inflammations or bleeding.

**Demonstration of occult bleeding**, usually using Hemoccult, is used for early detection of colorectal tumors. In the Czech Republic, screening is available for the whole population over 50 years of age. It allows identification of asymptomatic individuals with a positive test result, and ensures colonoscopic examination for them. Currently, $3^{rd}$ generation, semi-quantitative tests are available, which can be used to differentiate a normal finding in the intestine, adenomas and tumors.

As for **laboratory methods**, **bacteriology** confirming any microbial and/or parasitary cause is important for the diagnostics of intestinal diseases, **histology** to determine the nature of biopted lesions, and **biochemistry** to determine **tumor markers** and other phenomena. In the diagnostics and follow-up of patients with colorectal cancer, carcinoembryonic antigens proved useful as its markers – **CEA** and/or **CA 19-9**. Determination of tumor markers is important particularly for long-term follow-up. Any rise in the values informs of a recurrence of the diseases and/or of the presence of metastases.

Other examinations are also used in the diagnostics of functional intestine disorders, for example, intestinal "transit time", EMG of the sphincters and lower pelvic region, anorectal manometry and other highly-specialized examinations.

## 9.4 Small Intestine

### 9.4.1 Congenital Anomalies of the Small Intestine

The main congenital anomalies of the small intestine include:
- Conditions following from disorders of various phases of the intestine rotation during intrauterine development, the so-called intestinal malrotations – omphalocele, nonrotation, congenital volvulus of the small intestine, Ladd's syndrome, external closure of the duodenum, counterclockwise rotation, subhepatic cecum and mobile cecum and retrocecal appendix
- Atresias and congenital intestinal stenoses, Meckel's diverticulum, intestinal duplicatures and cysts
- Meconium ileus

These conditions require early solutions that fall in the field of pediatric surgery; only some of them can be seen in adults.

The so-called counterclockwise intestinal rotation, mobile cecum or cecum in the subhepatic region, respectively, or appendix in the retrocecal position are likely to cause no problems to their carriers and may be revealed accidentally during an examination or surgery. However, these anomalies should also be kept in mind in the diagnostics of manifested as an acute abdomen, particularly if associated with any non-typical finding. Intestinal duplicatures and cysts are also asymptomatic with rare exceptions and are usually revealed on an ad-hoc basis. Meckel's diverticulum is the most common anomaly of the small intestine.

## 9.4.2 Meckel's Diverticulum

Non-obliterated departure of the omphaloenteric duct can be found in 2–5% of persons in a distance of approximately 100 cm orally from the Bauhin's valve. The diverticulum is 2 to 10 cm long, and is localized on the antimesenteric side of the intestine. As a rule, Meckel's diverticulum is found accidentally during surgery, especially during appendectomy surgeries. Clinically, the diverticulum is manifested only by its complications: inflammation, bleeding or perforation of the peptic ulcer of ectopic gastric mucosa, absence or impairment of intestinal passage and tumors. The diverticulum can be demonstrated only in exceptional cases without surgery; it can be found based on contrast radiography of the small intestine, US or CT assessment.

**Meckel's diverticulum** cannot be clinically differentiated from acute appendicitis. Therefore, any present (and inflamed) diverticulum should be looked for during an appendectomy where the finding in the appendix does not explain the patient's problems. Diagnostic help may be provided by sonography identifying the inflamed diverticulum.

**A peptic ulcer** may develop in Meckel's diverticulum if ectopic gastric mucosa is found in the diverticulum. It is manifested by severe bleeding in the gastrointestinal tract, apparent as melena on the outside, or by perforation and perforation peritonitis.

**Absence of intestinal passage** may develop upon torsion and strangulation of the diverticulum, by invagination caused by the insertion of the diverticulum in the ileal lumen, or possibly by adhesion, stemming from the diverticulum, to other visceral structures or to the abdominal wall.

**Tumors** of Meckel's diverticulum are rare; a carcinoid is concerned in the majority of cases.

**Therapy** is exclusively surgical and consists in the resection of the diverticulum.

Besides Meckel's diverticulum, the so-called **Graser's diverticula** occur in exceptional cases in the small intestine, on the mesenteric side of the intestine. These are false diverticula given that they are formed only by the mucosa. They are most commonly localized in the jejunum.

### 9.4.3 Crohn's Disease

Chronic granulomatous inflammation of the small intestine (regional granulomatous enteritis) was described as early as in 1932 and called Crohn's disease after one of the authors. Although the inflammation may affect all segments of the digestive tract, the intestine is its common localization, while the terminal ileum is most commonly the first to be affected.

**Etiology** of the inflammation is not exactly known; four ranges of co-acting etiopathogenetic factors have been recognized during the recent decade: immunological, genetic, infectious factors and factors of the external environment. Autoimmune diseases, autoimmune reactivity disorders and dysregulations of mucosal immunity are considered as immune factors. The disorder named last is thought to be associated with the development of an inadequately intensive and permanent immune response to common antigen stimulations, which remain without a response in healthy persons. Currently, immune system disorders are assumed to play a significant, however not dominant, role in pathogenesis of the inflammation, despite the recent understanding. The genetic effect has been confirmed by high familial incidence, association with racial and ethnic factors, and by occurrence together with other genetically evoked syndromes. No mode of inheritance is known. Manifestation of the inflammation on the genetic foundation seems to develop due to factors of the external environment. In familial manifestation of Crohn's disease, the probable place of the disorder is the pericentromeric region of chromosome 16 and its genes 12, 3 and 7. The hypothesis of its primarily infectious origin assumes the effect of *Mycobacterium paratuberculosis*, paramyxoviruses and *Listeria monocytogenes*, and/or *Yersinia enterocolica* infection as the cause. Also, an inadequate immune response to normal intestinal flora is a potential cause, including a disorder of the barrier function of the intestine. As for external influences, composition and preparation of food has been discussed (high portion of refined sugars, low consumption of non-absorbable fibers and unsaturated fatty acids), smoking and hormonal contraception.

The disease affects young people between the $2^{nd}$ and $4^{th}$ decades, often also children; the disease causes growth disorders if developed before the growth is finished. The incidence of the disease has also been rising in the Czech Republic in a similar way compared to countries of the western hemisphere; currently, 2–3 new diseases develop per 100,000 inhabitants in the Czech Republic, and the prevalence is approximately 25.

In terms of **pathology and anatomy**, Crohn's disease leads to acute and chronic changes that may occur concurrently and be accompanied by additional complications, e.g. stenoses, fistulae and abscesses. The basic finding is an inflammatory infiltrate formed by cellular granulomas, which affect the submucosa at first, later the whole intestinal wall, adjacent mesenteric lymph nodes and the mesentery. The affected segments may be up to 20 cm long, well circumscribed against healthy tissue, and they may represent a single disorder or be distributed in multiple steps. The terminal ileum or the ileocecal area are the typical **localizations**; other common localizations include the large intestine and the anorectum.

**Clinical manifestation** depends on the localization, extent and form of the disease. Major forms of the disease are the acute and chronic form; according to more recent opinions, the form is related to the type of the disease: the perforating type of Crohn's disease leads to frequent complications, need for surgery with frequent relapses, while the non-perforating type usually does not involve perforations but shows a tendency to the development of stenoses.

The **acute form** is accompanied by symptoms almost identical to those of acute appendicitis: pain in the right lower abdomen, fever, sometimes diarrhea. Therefore the patients are usually operated on and the actual nature of the disease is revealed only during the surgery (no finding in the appendix, thickened wall of the terminal ileum or cecum, and possibly any infiltrate, enlarged lymph nodes, or exudate). In an acute state, the disease manifests in about one tenth of patients. Appendectomy is usually the surgical procedure undertaken (histological confirmation), which is not accepted without reserve due to the risk of the development of a fistula when the cecum is affected or due to unnecessary removal of the appendix if not affected. Conservative therapy is applied when Crohn's disease has been confirmed. In the preoperative period, information on prolonged typical problems, palpable resistance and/or sonographic finding may call attention to the disease.

The **chronic form** typically manifests by an alternation of calm periods (remissions) and acute exacerbations.

Usual manifestations include abdominal pain, diarrhea, fever, weight loss, fatigue. Enterorrhagias, abscesses and fistulae may appear in the lumbar area, in the lower abdomen, near the anus, pain in the joints, vision disorders, or dermatitis (extraintestinal symptoms). An abdominal resistance, usually in the right lower abdomen, signs of weight loss and avitaminoses (vitamin $B_{12}$, vitamin D and folic acid) can be found based on physical examination; laboratory assessment may show anemia with decreased serum levels of $Fe^{2+}$, and hypoproteinemia. The **diagnosis** can be determined using contrast radiography of the intestine, using endoscopy (if the segment accessible by endoscopy is affected – cf. Section 9.3) with subsequent biopsy, using sonography and possibly CT assessment. Immunoscintigraphy and/or determination of antibodies can be used if any doubt persists. **Differential diagnostics** should differentiate a tumor, inflammatory infiltrate and abscesses (for example, TBC, actinomycosis).

In its chronic form, the disease continues for many years. Its manifestations depend on the activity of the disease, on the success of medicamentous therapy, and on **complications**, which include:

- Infiltrates and abscesses (septic conditions)
- Internal (entero-enteral, entero-colic, entero-vesical) and external fistulae (in the right lower abdomen, in the lumbar region, in the perianal region)
- Stenoses leading to absence or impairment of intestinal passage
- Bleeding
- Perforations with the development of peritonitis
- Toxic condition (toxic megaileum)
- Secondary involvement of other organs – for example, urethral stenosis

Typically, the **therapy** of Crohn's disease is conservative, while surgical treatment is necessary in the event of complications. **Conservative therapy** includes dietary measures (non-residual food rich in energy, with restricted fats, restricted milk consumption, substituting electrolytes, vitamins, $Fe^{2+}$), regimen measures (particularly reducing energy demands, hygienic measures) and medication. The purpose of medication is to calm the acute exacerbation and maintain remission of the disease. Glucocorticoids and aminosalicylates (sulfasalazine, mesalazine) are administered, and also immunosuppressives in refractory conditions (azathioprine, mercaptopurine) and biological therapy active against TNFα. **Surgical therapy** should be reserved for the treatment of complications of Crohn's disease, and also for the event that conservative therapy is not sufficient to manage the disease.

Resection of the affected intestinal segment with restoration of intestinal continuity by an anastomosis is the basic surgical procedure in Crohn's disease. When multiple stenoses are present the resection of which would cause the removal of too large a part of the intestine, the so-called stricturoplasty is the method of choice (Fig. 9.2), which dilates the affected segment and leaves its tissue in place. Where the affected segment cannot be removed, intestinal bypass or intestinal ostomy is indicated. The number of relapses at the site of surgery or in another

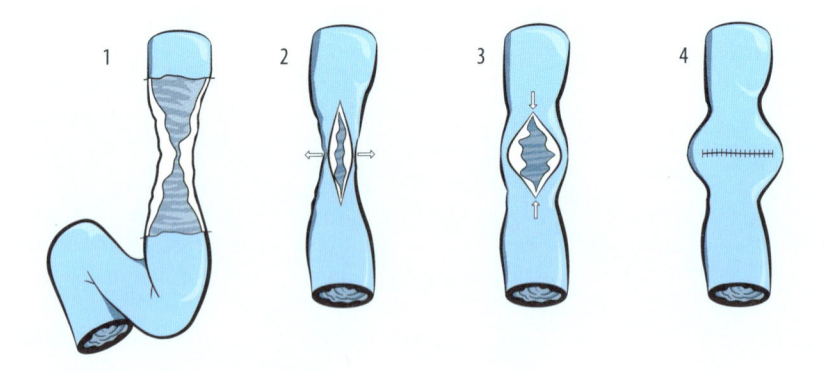

**Fig. 9.2** *Stricturoplasty with Crohn's disease*

# SURGERY OF THE SMALL AND LARGE INTESTINES, RECTUM AND ANUS

GIT segment is high and cannot be reduced by extending the resection. Long-term conservative therapy is also needed after the surgery. The manner of treatment of other surgical complications depends on their nature (for example, incision and drainage of the abscesses, including the administration of antibiotics).

Apart from exceptional cases, the **prognosis** of Crohn's disease is determined by its lifelong course, a high number of relapses and reoperations, the need for long-term medication with its consequences, and a higher risk of intestinal neoplasias.

## 9.4.4 Small Intestine Tumors

Small intestine tumors are rare affections (about 1.5% of tumors of the gastrointestinal tract). Major manifestations include bleeding and absence or impairment of intestinal passage. The tumors may initiate from all layers of the intestinal wall and can be classified as benign and malignant based on their characteristics.

**Benign tumors** occur more frequently than malignant (a 4:1 ratio). Assessed based on the initial tissue, the tumors may be **epithelial** – adenomas; **mesenchymal** – leiomyomas, fibromas, angiomas (hemangiomas and lymphangiomas), neurinomas; and/or **heterotopic tumors** – endometriosis, aberrant pancreas. As a rule, these tumors are manifested only by their complications or are revealed by chance during surgeries for another cause. Absence or impairment of intestinal passage, ileus condition, is usually a complication, which may be complete (acute condition) or incomplete (chronic condition), or possibly intermittent, or invagination (in pedunculated tumors in both cases).

The **symptoms** are typical for a mechanical ileus: stoppage of gas and stool passage, nausea and vomiting, colicky abdominal pain. Bleeding is another symptom, which occurs due to erosion of blood vessels of the tumor, particularly in hemangiomas, and tends to be intense.

Benign tumors of the small intestine include polyposis, typically accompanied by abdominal pain, vomiting, intestinal obstruction (including invagination) or bleeding. Besides polyps in the small intestine, patients often have polyps in the colon and dotted pigmentation around the mouth, on the lips and on the buccal mucosa. The signs described belong to the inherited Peutz-Jeghers syndrome.

**Diagnosis** of a benign tumor is usually accidental or follows from the management of an acute condition. Before surgery, it can be revealed by contrast radiography of the small intestine, and/or by US or CT, enteroscopy (not performed as a process), and by angiography in the event of heavy bleeding.

**Therapy** consists in the removal of the pedunculated tumors or in intestinal resection if the tumor is sessile.

**Malignant tumors** of the small intestine, which are clinically significant, include adenocarcinomas, sarcomas and carcinoids. They occur more commonly in men than in women.

A carcinoma occurs most commonly in oral segments of the small intestine, and it causes no problems (no impairment of passage of the liquid content). It is therefore usually revealed only at an advanced stage when it becomes the cause of acute obstruction, bleeding or a generalized malignant disease (metastases, ascites).

Sarcomas affect younger patients and children. The patients become anemic and cachectic more rapidly than in cancer, and bleeding and perforations are more frequent than obstructions. Considering the volume of the tumor, sometimes the sarcoma can be found also by palpation during the examination of the abdomen. Diagnostics is not different from the above. Surgical **treatment** consists in radical surgical removal of the affected intestinal segment including the appropriate mesenteric segment. Further management of the patient and **prognosis** of the disease depend particularly on whether all affected tissue has been completely removed, and on sensitivity of the tumor to subsequent oncotherapy (chemo-, and/or radiotherapy, based on the type of the tumor).

**Carcinoid of the small intestine** represents almost 20% of small intestine tumors. It is benign based on histology but develops metastases. The carcinoid stems from endocrine argentaffin cells forming part of the APUD system; these cells produce serotonin, calicrein, histamine and prostaglandins. Except the esophagus, these cells are present in the entire digestive tract. They are most abundant at the base of crypts of Lieberkühn in the terminal ileus and in the appendix, therefore the carcinoid is found most commonly in these localizations.

Carcinoid **symptoms** follow from its endocrine activity, thus from excessive production of the above hormones. Their manifestations are described as the **carcinoid syndrome** and include:
- Paroxysmal reddening of the skin of the cheeks and upper half of the body
- Diarrhea and abdominal pain caused by serotonin-provoked increased peristalsis
- Bronchial asthma with dyspnea
- Oligurias and edemas, heart weakness
- Pain in the joints, malabsorption

The **diagnosis** follows from histological assessment of the removed appendix where a carcinoid, which had been asymptomatic, is found, or from examinations performed due to the above symptoms.

Demonstration of serotonin in the blood and examination of 5-hydroxyindoleacetic acid (serotonin metabolite) in the urine (over 10 mg in 24 h) confirms the diagnosis. US and CT assessments and/or contrast radiography of the small intestine may also contribute in terms of diagnostics. Given that carcinoids establish metastases, they should be looked for – liver and abdomen assessment using US, and CT, respectively.

**Therapy** is surgical. Carcinoid of the appendix is treated using an appendectomy; carcinoid of the cecum is resolved by ileocecal resection or right-sided hemicolectomy based on the extent of the carcinoid. Additional examination is needed to ensure whether the tumor was removed completely, such as histology of the edges of the resecate, laboratory assessments to exclude persistent hormonal activity, and US and CT to exclude any metastases. Metastases should be removed by surgery; cytostatics are administered for locally inoperable findings or multiple metastases.

## 9.4.5   Small Intestine Adhesions

Adhesions are typical affections of the small intestine. Adhesions develop for numerous reasons, while most of them do not originate in the intestine; for example, due to a trauma, peritonitis or previous surgery. Adhesions may be solitary, taking the form of a single strip, multiple or even areal, and they may bind the viscera and especially the intestines to each other, to other organs, or to the abdominal wall. While in the event of circumscribed intra-abdominal affections, for example, inflammations or perforations, adhesions prevent the spreading of the pathological process in the abdomen and play a protective role, they themselves become the cause of complications, adhesive ileus, in most cases. For the sake of completeness, it should be mentioned that even an extensive presence of adhesions may be quite asymptomatic while the presence of even a single adhesion may become the cause of ileus, volvulus or strangulation.

**Diagnostics**: Prior to an operation, the presence of adhesions can only be estimated from scars after previous operations, whether they provide evidence of complicated or uncomplicated healing, based on the nature of the problems, sometimes based on a radiographic finding, and in exceptional cases based on evidence of fixation or motility disorder of the intestine in contrast radiography of the small intestine. Adhesions are commonly found only during an operation (laparotomy or laparoscopy).

**Therapy** of adhesions consists in their disruption and in the releasing of **all** viscera, careful treatment of all, even small injuries in the serosa of the peritoneal cavity, and careful arrangement of the viscera after returning it to the abdomen at the end of surgery.

**Prevention** of adhesions formed spontaneously is not yet possible. Post-operative adhesions can be prevented using sparing surgical techniques, atraumatic instruments and sutures, suitable drainage, and by preventing any types of post-operative complications. Use of flushing solutions including the solutions of hyaluronidase or corticoids has not led to reduced formation of adhesions.

Use of a foil (Seprafilm, Genzyme) is rare; this foil is inserted in the abdomen before its closure, and gradually releases hyaluronidase. The same is true for Adept solution which temporarily modifies the adhesiveness of the mesothelium.

### 9.4.6 Appendicitis

Acute appendicitis (inflammation of the appendix) is the most common inflammatory cause of acute abdomen, affecting persons of all age groups. In terms of **etiology**, it is an infection caused by microbes of the intestinal flora. The reasons for development of the inflammation have not been sufficiently explained (coprostasis in the narrow appendix, parasites, reduced defensive capacity).

In terms of **pathology and anatomy**, appendicitis is classified as:
1. Catarrhal
2. Phlegmonous
3. Gangrenous

**Clinical picture**: Appendicitis usually develops from full health and manifests by pain around the stomach, which moves to the right lower abdomen in the course of several hours. It is accompanied by nausea, vomiting, stoppage of passing gas and stool. The pain increases upon movement or shaking of the abdomen. Progression of an untreated inflammation causes gangrene of the wall of the appendix (including nerve terminations) and the pain subsides temporarily, which can lead to false conclusions. The pain returns after several hours, but this time as a sign of peritonitis. The duration of this development of changes in time varies from tens of minutes (Foudroyant course) up to tens of hours.

**Symptoms** of appendicitis: anamnestic data described, tachycardia (HR 100 and higher), rather low fever. Palpation and percussion pain in the right lower abdomen, with the maximum at the so-called McBourney's point (the boundary between the external and middle third of the line connecting the umbilicus and ventral iliac spine). When the inflammation spreads to the peritoneum, signs of peritoneal irritation appear:
1. Muscle contraction
2. Painful percussion in the appendical region (Plenies sign)
3. Painful shaking of the peritoneum (Blumberg and Rovsing sign)
4. Pain in the Douglas space during examination *per rectum* or *per vaginam*
5. Laboratory non-specific signs of inflammation – leukocytosis, elevated CRP, FW

Ultrasound examination shows inflammatory thickening of the appendical wall, appendical rigidity, and pain upon its compression.

Diagnostic problems occur in **special forms** of appendicitis caused by:
1. **Atypical position of the appendix**
   – Pelvic position – appendicitis irritates the urinary bladder, adnexa and rectum with signs of irritation of these organs; muscle contraction may be missing
   – Laterocecal position – considerably lateral localization of pain, possibly in the lumbar region

- Retrocecal position – the appendix is covered by the cecum; pain in the abdomen is often not expressed; signs of ileum predominate over peritoneal signs; irritation of the ureter may cause colicky pain, and irritation in the retroperitoneum to psoatic symptoms
- Mesoceliac position (the appendix is covered by the loops of the small intestine) – pain around the umbilicus, muscle contraction is missing, signs of the ileus predominate
- Subhepatic position – similar to cholecystitis
- Left-sided appendicitis with inverted position of the internal organs
- Appendicitis in the 4$^{th}$ and subsequent months of pregnancy – the appendix is covered and pushed out cranially by the uterus
2. **Modified response to the inflammation**
3. **Modified defensive capacity**
    - Newborn and pediatric appendicitis
    - Senile appendicitis where the typical subjective problems and the objective finding are missing, including tachycardia and leukocytosis
    - Appendicitis with immunosuppressive therapy (corticoids, immunosuppressives)
    - On antibiotic therapy

**Complications of appendicitis** depend on how quickly the inflammation develops and on the ability to circumscribe the inflammation. Major complications include **perforation of the appendix** (with circumscribed or diffuse peritonitis), periappendicular infiltrate and periappendicular abscess. The symptoms of peritonitis mentioned above become more pronounced upon perforation. An **infiltrate** is manifested as painful resistance in the right lower abdomen; signs of peritoneal irritation need not be apparent, and tachycardia may be unconvincing. The infiltrate is absorbed or coliquated, leading to **periappendicular abscess** with septic manifestations. Also the abscess may absorb, or diffuse peritonitis develops if its delimitation is insufficient.

**Therapy** of appendicitis is conservative and surgical. Conservative therapy consists in a resting regimen in bed, limited oral intake of liquids, abdominal compresses, and possibly application of antibiotics. **Conservative therapy** may be sufficient in cases without any threatening or present perforation. Since it is difficult to rule out those cases where perforation would never occur, and given the minimum surgical risks of an appendectomy, surgery is indicated in all cases.

**Surgical treatment** of appendicitis consists in the revision of the abdomen and removal of the appendix. Currently, the procedure can be performed as conventional or laparoscopic. The major advantage of laparoscopic APE is the possibility of diagnostic laparoscopy at the beginning of the surgery.

Therapy of the infiltrate is conservative (in line with the above), while the development of peritonitis is a reason for surgery. Abscesses must be emptied, by puncture under US or CT guidance, or using a surgical procedure.

Peritonitis is a clear indication for surgery. The procedure will typically include APE, cleaning of the abdominal cavity, and drainage.

**Prognosis** – local complications after appendectomies due to uncomplicated appendicitis do not exceed 5%, and general complications occur in 1 per mille of cases. Perforated appendicitis, particularly with diffuse and inveterate peritonitis, is burdened with both types of complications, with lethality of up to 10%.

**Differential diagnostics** should exclude affections that cause similar symptoms:
- Mesenteric lymphadenitis – often occurs after a virus, after a common cold. Affection of lymph nodes is indicated by the presence of palpable lymph nodes also in other localizations. US is useful to differentiate the condition
- Acute gastroenteritis – diarrhea, vomiting and fever without peritoneal irritation, acute cholecystitis – confusion is possible with a subhepatic position of the appendix; differentiation – positive biliary history, propagation of pain, US
- Perforation of the gastroduodenal ulcer – peritonitis; pneumoperitoneum is shown in the radiography scan but missing in appendicitis
- Crohn's disease – acute manifestation – palpable resistance, US finding
- Meckel's diverticulum or sigmoid diverticulitis – these affections cannot be differentiated virtually at all; US assessment provides differentiation in exceptional cases
- Affection of the right kidney and the ureter
- Affection of the right adnexa in women including extrauterine pregnancy

## 9.5 Large Intestine

### 9.5.1 Congenital Anomalies

**Atresia** and stenosis of the colon are rare conditions; narrowing of the colon lumen with atresias of the small intestine, microcolon, is more common. **Rotation disorders** were described above (cf. Section 9.4.1). **Hirschsprung's disease** (colonic aganglionosis, congenital megacolon) is a disorder resulting from the absence of ganglia in the myenteric plexus and in the submucous plexus, leading to a permanent spasm of the aganglionic segment of the colon and rectum. It is discussed in detail in pediatric surgery as a disease that affects children starting from newborns. It should be noted that a rare incomplete affection may escape attention until adulthood. It causes stubborn constipation not responding to therapy. The diagnosis can be determined using all assessments of the large intestine described including functional examinations, and confirmed by deep biopsy of the intestinal wall reaching up to the submucosa.

Therapy is surgical. If feasible, resection of the affected aganglionic segment is the solution, and resection of the segment devastated due to long-lasting dilatation.

**Idiopathic megacolon** is considered as a false megacolon, most probably on a congenital basis, caused by immaturity of ganglion cells of intestinal plexuses. This is apparently the cause of reduced propulsive activity and subsequent obstipation and dilatation of the intestine.

## 9.5.2 Diverticular Disease of the Large Intestine

Many conditions are understood as a diverticular disease; this is the presence of diverticula on the intestine that they have in common. Congenital, or true, diverticula have a wall with all intestinal layers, while acquired, or false, diverticula are much more common; their wall is formed only by the mucosa that pushes intestinal musculature aside and causes bulging of the serosa. The diverticula may affect the whole intestine, while the sigmoid loop and the descending colon are their typical **localizations**, the transverse colon and its right half are affected less commonly. Multiple diverticula occur as a rule in the left half of the colon, and solitary diverticula in the right half. Diverticular affection of the intestine with no manifestations of inflammation is called **diverticulosis**, and diverticular inflammation is called **diverticulitis**. Diverticulitis may lead to perforation and peritonitis rapidly, or to the formation of a circumscribed inflammation around the intestine, **pericolic infiltrate**, pericolitis, or perisigmoiditis based on the most common localization.

**Development** of the disease seems to be **caused** by long-term increased intraluminal pressure due to hypertonia of intestinal musculature. Consumption of food with low content of residues (particularly of fibers) means that the volume of the intestinal content is insufficient, and propulsion of such content causes strenuous muscular contractions ("idle contractions"), a rise in the pressure and subsequently prolapse of diverticula through the intestinal wall.

**Incidence** of the disease rises with age; this disease is exceptional in the 3$^{rd}$ decade and the highest between the 6$^{th}$ and 9$^{th}$ decades.

**Symptoms** depend on the nature of the affection. Diverticula are present in approximately 60% of 60-year-olds, while only a fraction suffers from any problems resulting from them, most commonly constipation or abdominal pain. Clinical symptoms of the disease are manifested only after complications occur. The deceptive nature of the disease consists in the fact that peritonitis upon perforation of a single diverticulum may be the first sign, while in other cases, extensive affection by diverticula may not necessarily cause any significant complications.

**Complications** of a diverticular disease include diverticulitis and its complications: bleeding and disorders arising from post-inflammatory fibrous scarring, especially absence or impairment of intestinal passage.

**Diverticulitis** develops most probably from an infection from stool stasis in the diverticulum where it cannot be emptied through the narrow neck, and whose pressure leads to decubital necrosis in the diverticulum. In this phase, the inflammation is manifested by abdominal pain (usually in the left hypogastrium), nausea, vomiting, stoppage of passing gas and stool, fever and tachycardia. Besides painful palpation, painful cylindrical resistance can also sometimes be palpated, and/or signs of circumscribed peritonitis. Laboratory assessment reveals leukocytosis, elevated C-reactive protein, and high FW.

**Pericolic infiltrate** develops upon passage of the inflammation into the surroundings, well demonstrable by palpation. Coliquation of the infiltrate or covered perforation of the diverticulum causes **pericolic abscesses** and fistulae or intra-abdominal and/or retroperitoneal abscesses. They are manifested by the above-mentioned symptoms and manifestations of sepsis. Inflammatory infiltrate may induce purulent inflammation of the peritoneum, or **purulent peritonitis**. If perforation of the diverticulum occurs, circumscribed or diffuse **perforation peritonitis** develops; stercoral (fecal) peritonitis occurs when the intestinal content empties into the abdomen. The symptoms follow from the extent of the affection, i.e. peritoneal signs dominate with muscle contraction, tachycardia, hypotension, with a rapid onset of septic shock. The level of inflammatory involvement of the intestine and abdominal cavity can be classified according to Hinchey (I–IV based on the surgical finding) and according to Hansen and Stock (I–III based on CT).

Other acute complications of a diverticular disease include **intestinal obstructions and bleeding**. Obstruction is caused by fibrous stenosis of the segment affected by the diverticulitis. Bleeding is usually not intense, leading to chronic anemization, or acute and intense, which requires immediate treatment. **Fistulae** are a common complication of a diverticular disease, usually leading into the urinary bladder or vagina. They are often caused by a single diverticulum, which perforates into the wall of the urinary bladder or vagina with inflammation. In the first case, the fistula is manifested by pneumaturia and fecaluria (and symptoms of urinary infection), while the second condition is manifested by uncontrolled escape of gas and stool through the vagina.

All examination methods of the large intestine find their place in the **diagnostics**. Irigography is the sovereign method of determining the disease. Besides physical examinations, the methods used to diagnose complications include radiography including contrast radiography, ultrasound, and CT with high precision. As for **differential diagnostics**, other affections of the large intestine must be differentiated, particularly tumors, non-specific inflammations, and especially adnexitis and renal colic among other than intestinal diseases.

**Therapy** of a diverticular disease depends on its origin. Asymptomatic diverticulosis requires no therapy. High residue diet is advisable, especially fibrous meals. The therapy of inflammatory complications is **conservative** at first, consisting in limited oral intake, administration of infusions, application of antibiotics and/or clysmata with a non-absorbable antibiotic, and physical rest. Surgical treatment may be acute and elective. **Acute** surgery is necessary in peritonitis or intestinal obstruction and in bleeding. The solution consists in resecting the affected intestinal segment or its elimination by ostomy and usually drainage (cf. Section 9.6.8). Depending on the conditions at the hospital, abscesses can be currently treated in the first period using CT navigated puncture; bleeding can be treated by embolization under angiographic guidance, or also operated on if this option is not available. **Elective** surgery is applied in fistulae, stenoses or cases after two and more attacks of complications of diverticular disease including diverticulitis.

The **prognosis** of the disease cannot be fully foreseen. The diverticula do no disappear, but the disease can be maintained without progression by suitable diet and defecation habits. A surgical solution should not be postponed in symptomatic persons; the risk of complications rises in time and with age. A diverticular disease does not increase the probability of tumor development.

## 9.5.3  Non-Specific Inflammations of the Large Intestine

### CROHN'S DISEASE OF THE LARGE INTESTINE

The condition that Crohn's disease would be limited to the large intestine is rare. Most common localizations include the cecum where the granulomatous inflammation extends from the ileum, and the rectum in exceptional cases. Symptoms of the disease show no principal difference from its symptoms in the small intestine, i.e. tenesmus, diarrhea, fever, weight loss, and sporadically blood in stool. Conclusive examinations include particularly colonoscopy and biopsy. Other examinations including laboratory ones do not differ from those used for the affection of the small intestine. Conservative therapy is also identical, with the addition of clysmata or suppositories with corticoids when the rectum is affected. Surgical treatment of Crohn's disease is reserved for the treatment of complications. Resection is the solution for solitary segmental affection of the colon, or proctocolectomy for diffuse affection or severe proctitis.

### IDIOPATHIC PROCTOCOLITIS (IPC, ULCERATIVE COLITIS)

IPC is a non-specific inflammation of unknown etiology, which affects the large intestine exclusively. Apart from exceptional cases, the inflammation starts in the rectum and spreads orally, and it may affect the whole large intestine. In terms of **pathology and anatomy**, it is a chronic inflammation of the mucosa – initially edematous, hyperemic, granular, with rapidly developing ulcerations. The ulcerations merge, and destruct the mucosa; hypertrophic infiltrated mucosas, or pseudopolyps, tend to be present between the ulcers. The inflammatory affection can typically be demonstrated only in the mucosa, while other intestinal layers are affected only in severe forms of IPC. IPC **incidence** shows two peaks: the first at about the age of 20 and the second in about the 6$^{th}$ decade; approximately 7 cases per 100,000 inhabitants exist in the Czech Republic, identically for men and women.

Based on its **clinical course**, the disease is classified as follows:
a) Chronic relapsing form
b) Acute fulminant form
c) Chronic stationary form of IPC

Blood in stool, watery stool with admixture of blood and abdominal pain linked with defecation are characteristic for the first form. The course of the disease shows spontaneous variations and may transform to the other two forms. The acute fulminant form affects approximately 5% of patients with IPC. This form is manifested by fever, bloody watery diarrhea, dehydration, and later by paralytic ileus. Progression of the disease to all layers of the intestinal wall paralyzes motility of the colon, causing stasis of its content, deepening the septic condition (the inflammation results in **toxic dilatation of the colon**) toxic megacolon, or leading to stercoral peritonitis due to perforation of the colon. This last form is associated with frequent stools with an admixture of blood, abdominal pain, and weight loss; the problems last for years and cause gradual destruction of the colon. Shortening and straightening of the intestine is typical, as well as rigidity, and ulcerations and pseudopolyps persisting in the mucosa.

Long-lasting duration of the disease increases the risk of cancer up to 30 times.

IPC **complications** are local and general. Local complications include toxic dilatation of the colon, perforations, stenoses, bleeding, and tumors. General complications include dermal (purpura, erythema nodosum), hepatic (steatosis and cirrhosis), articular (arthralgia and arthritis), ophthalmological (iridocyclitis) manifestations, disorders of nutrition and of the internal environment.

**Diagnosis** is determined based on symptoms, clinical examination and examination of the large intestine, including biopsy. Rectoscopy is an important examination given that the rectum is always affected by colitis due to the distribution of inflammatory changes.

**Therapy** of proctocolitis is mainly **conservative** and consists in adherence to a dietary regimen (well digestible food rich in energy, with limited residues), limited physical activity and application of medicaments. Chronic forms are treated using aminosalicylates (sulfasalazine, mesalazine), prepared in a manner to act as late as possible in the large intestine; corticosteroids, and possibly immunosuppressives. **Surgical treatment** is indicated based on complications, e.g. upon development of a tumor, in severe forms of IPC that cannot be managed by conservative therapy, including acute operations due to toxic megacolon, upon perforation, massive bleeding and upon obstruction. The basic procedure entails the removal of the whole large intestine (colectomy), possibly including the rectum (proctocolectomy) with the establishment of an ileostomy. Currently, restorative proctocolectomy is viewed as the procedure of choice, with an ileal reservoir and ileoanal anastomosis (cf. Section 9.6.8).

**Prognosis** depends on the form, extent and duration of the inflammation, while especially the risk of tumor development is present with a long-lasting course of the disease. The prognosis in patients after proctocolectomy is excellent, burdened only by the ostomy; in persons after restorative surgeries, the prognosis is burdened by complications of this technically demanding solution, including inflammation of the ileal reservoir, so-called "pouchitis".

### ISCHEMIC COLITIS

Ischemic colitis is caused by a **perfusion disorder** of the colon. The splenic flexure and the sigmoid loop of the colon are reported as the most common **localizations**. When caused by vascular closure, the ischemia is assessed as an occlusive type, or non-occlusive type in cases where no evidence of closure is found (for example, perfusion disorder due to shock). Ischemia may take three **basic forms**:
- Acute and complete ischemia leading to gangrene of the intestine
- Transient and incomplete ischemia with manifestations of hemorrhagic colitis
- Postischemic stenosis

The manifestations depend on the characteristics of the affection. The first two types are manifested by abdominal pain, tenesmus with diarrhea and bleeding (from the mucosa affected by ischemia), and gangrene by development of peritonitis. Postischemic stenosis is manifested with a delay after a ischemic attack, and its manifestations include partial or complete intestinal obstruction.

The **diagnosis** is often difficult and the condition may be explained by an endoscopic finding of mucosal affection in the ischemic segment of the intestine, and irigography when stenoses are present. Gangrene of the intestine is usually an unexpected finding during operations indicated for peritonitis.

**Therapy** depends on the scope of the ischemia. Conservative therapy entails the elimination of oral intake, administration of infusions, and/or also antibiotics and vasodilatants. Surgical therapy is indicated acutely when gangrene is present in the intestine (early after ischemia), upon intestinal obstruction (delayed if any stenosis develops); as a rule, it consists in the resection of the affected intestine segment.

### 9.5.4 Tumors of the Large Intestine

**Benign tumors** occur in up to 50% of persons. Mesenchymal tumors, e.g. lipomas, lymphomas, leiomyomas, hemangiomas, and fibromas, are less common; more frequent are epithelial tumors, i.e. polyps. Polyps are further classified as adenomas, hyperplastic and inflammatory polyps and hamartomas, or as solitary polyps and multiple polyps (polyposes) according to their number (and structure).

**Adenomas** (neoplastic polyps) represent up to 90% of all polyps. They occur in aboral segments of the intestine, most commonly in the rectum and sigmoid. They may be **pedunculated** (usually the tubular adenoma) or attached to the mucosa – **sessile** (villous adenoma). The risk of **malignant degeneration** is associated with polyps; the risk rises with the size of the polyp. Malignant reconstruction, cancerization of the polyp, has several phases starting from cellular atypias of epithelial cells, carcinoma *in situ* i.e. with no invasion through the mucosal propria lamina, up to invasive carcinoma that grows through the lamina propria. Clinically, they are manifested by bleeding, sometimes tenesmus, and they may be silent.

Villous adenomas spread areally on the mucosa, often reaching a considerable size. They are usually manifested by mucus on the stool surface or by diarrhea with mucus; they may cause dehydration and hypokalemia.

The **diagnosis** is **determined** based on a medical history, indagation and endoscopic examination. The **therapy** consists in endoscopic removal of the polyps, surgical removal from colotomy or the resection of the affected part of the intestine.

**Polyposis** affects the entire colon and usually also the rectum. **Familial adenomatosis** (FAP – familial adenomatous polyposis) is an autosomally inherited disease. There are tens to hundreds of polyps in the intestine and their number increases in an aboral direction. From the point of view of histology, they are tubular adenomas, which deteriorate into cancer. The disease has three phases: latent, in the first decade of life, when the polyps are not visible in the intestine; asymptomatic, in the second decade when the polyps can be found but do not yet cause any symptoms; symptomatic, manifested by diarrhea, bleeding and hypoproteinemia. The **therapy** is surgical. A total colectomy should be carried out in time, i.e. before the development of cancer. When no polyps are present in the rectum, it can be preserved for the sake of natural defecation and continence, establishing an ileorectal anastomosis; if the rectum is affected as well, restorative proctocolectomy must be performed with an ileal reservoir and ileoanal anastomosis. The **prognosis** depends on the advancement of the disease at the time of therapy initiation and on careful endoscopic monitoring used also for immediate removal of any polyps in the rectum.

Other polyposes include **Gardner's syndrome** (diffuse adenomatosis associated with presence of mesenchymal tumors – desmoids, osteomas and cysts), and **Turcot's syndrome**, which is a combination of polyposis and CNS tumors.

**Hyperplastic polyps** develop based on an irritation of the mucosa. **Inflammatory polyps** are associated with intestinal inflammations; they are formed by clusters of inflammatory hyperplastic mucosa. **Hamartomatous polyps** occur most commonly in the small intestine (**Peutz-Jeghers** syndrome). They tend to relapse more often but do not malignize.

**Mesenchymal tumors** of the colon are usually asymptomatic and their occurrence is sporadic. As a rule, they are manifested only with the onset of complications such as bleeding or obstruction. Based on the initial tissue, they may be lipomas, lymphomas, hemangiomas, neurofibromas, and possibly endometriosis. The therapy is surgical and consists in resecting the affected intestine segment.

**Malignant tumors of the large intestine** are all carcinomas with rare exceptions. Their **incidence** has been rising steadily (45 cases per 100,000 persons), and they are the most common GIT tumor in both men and women. Their incidence reaches its maximum at the end of the 6th decade. Their **etiopathogenesis** has not yet been fully explained, and their formation is obviously associated with multiple factors. About 10% of the tumors develop as **hereditary**, others as **sporadic** (i.e. develop accidentally). According to current knowledge, a genetic disorder can be found in the background of not only a hereditary but also a sporadic colorectal carcinoma. In affected persons, it causes:
a) Sequential accumulation of molecular changes
b) Gradual accumulation of genes associated with tumorous transformation ("cancer-related genes": the APC oncogene, the KRAS tumor suppressor gene, the DCC gene – deleted in colorectal carcinoma, the tumor suppressor gene p53)
c) Changes in the function and regulation of the expression of genes which are important for tumorous transformation by affecting key proteins of **signaling pathways**, for example, growth factors, EGFR and VEGF growth factor receptors.

**Exogenous** influences (lack of fiber in food, excessive amounts of animal fat and meat) and **endogenous** influences (hereditary, tumors in other localizations, familial form of breast cancer) have been considered among the causes of development. In terms of hereditary causes, familial adenomatous polyposis (**FAP**) and hereditary nonpolyposis colorectal cancer (**HNPCC**) are the most important. FAP has been described in detail. HNPCC is an autosomal dominant disease characterized by early development and manifestation of the carcinoma, often related to carcinomas of other localizations. The disease affects blood--related family members and relatives, is known as Lynch syndrome, and the familial affection is reported as a family cancer syndrome. The genetic defect responsible for this affection can be demonstrated in 80% of patients; it is advisable to make use of genetic counseling in the examination of affected families due to the high risk of cancer development.

The **risk level** of colorectal carcinoma development is evaluated as **low** (in healthy asymptomatic persons without risk factors where no tumors occur among their immediate blood relatives; about 70% of persons); **medium** (colorectal carcinoma in an immediate blood relative, or cured colorectal carcinoma in the personal history, respectively; about 25% of persons); and **high** (FAP, HNPCC, long-lasting history of non-specific intestinal inflammations, particularly IPC).

Based on **localization**, tumors in the rectum occur most frequently (50%), in the sigmoid (25%), in the cecum and the ascending colon (15%), as well as in the transverse and descending colons (about 10%). Endophytic growth of the tumors into the intestinal lumen predominates in the right half of the colon, while infiltrative growth is seen mainly in the left half.

The **manifestation** depends on localization. Tumors in the right half of the colon are associated with no problems for a long time, causing occult or manifest bleeding (in exceptional cases), and they lead to anemia. Anemia and palpable resistance in the right half of the abdomen are common findings. In the left half of the colon, the tumor is manifested by intestinal passage disorders, i.e. obstipation and change in the defecation process, presence of mucus and blood in stool, with the first manifestation being acute intestinal obstruction in about 20% of patients. Besides the symptoms referred to above, rectal tumors also cause tenesmus, urge, and feelings of insufficient emptying, while tumors of low localizations are manifested by ribbon-like stool and continence disorders.

In terms of **pathology and anatomy**, adenocárcinoma is most common – 90%. Carcinomas are classified as differentiated, transient and non-differentiated (anaplastic) based on tumor differentiation. The differentiation level is expressed by "**grading**".

Tumors spread in the following ways:
1. Infiltratively through the intestinal wall
2. Through the lymphatic system with involvement of lymph nodes on various levels
3. Within the blood stream (in the liver and lungs)
4. Through implantation (in the intestinal lumen or along the peritoneum)

Tumors in the colon and rectum metastasize in the aforementioned ways of spreading; their metastases are most commonly found in sentinel nodes, and distant metastases are found in the liver and lungs.

The progression grade of the tumor, "**staging**", is expressed by its classification, which evaluates the level of its growth through the intestinal wall (T), involvement of lymph nodes (N), and presence of distant metastases (M). The **international classification TNM** is commonly used in the Czech Republic, replacing the formerly used classification according to Dukes (Fig. 9.3); in summary, the extent of the disease is expressed by stages I–IV.

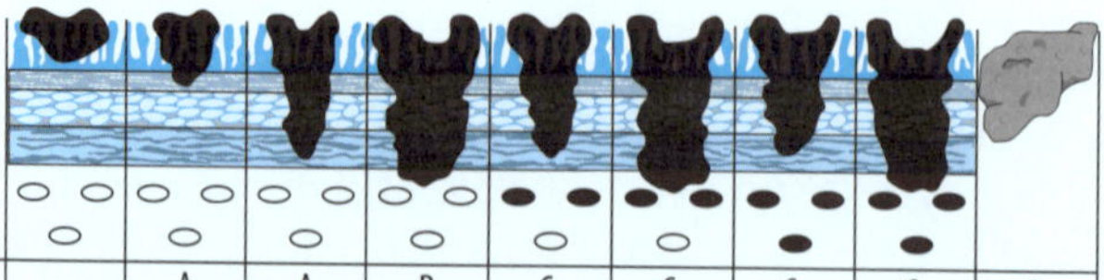

| Dukes | - | A | A | B | $C_1$ | $C_1$ | $C_2$ | $C_2$ | D |
|---|---|---|---|---|---|---|---|---|---|
| TNM | $T_{is}N_0$ | $T_1N_0$ | $T_2N_0$ | $T_3N_0$ | $T_2N_1$ | $T_3N_1$ | $T_2N_2$ | $T_3N_2$ | $M_1$ |

**Fig. 9.3** *Brief classification of tumors of the large intestine according to Dukes and TNM*

## SURGERY OF THE SMALL AND LARGE INTESTINES, RECTUM AND ANUS

The **diagnostics** has been discussed generally, but two methods should be mentioned in particular. Examination of **occult bleeding** (FOBT – Hemoccult) is important as a screening assessment to detect asymptomatic persons in an early phase of the disease. The examination has been gradually improved, and currently, it is available as a semi-quantitative examination capable of distinguishing various types of affection in the intestine. Persons with positive test results undergo another examination, a colonoscopy.

Determination of tumor markers, CEA and/or CA 19-9, is suitable for long-term monitoring of patients after colorectal tumor therapy. If the tumor has been removed completely, marker levels normalize, and they rise in the case of a relapse or metastases.

The **therapy** of tumors in the colon is surgical. This consists in the removal of the intestinal segment with the tumor, together with the adjacent mesocolon containing sentinel lymphatic vessels, and in the restoration of intestinal continuity by an anastomosis (cf. Section 9.6.8 for the types and scopes of the procedures). The current terminology distinguishes **curative performances,** when all tumorous tissue is removed with no demonstrable residues of the tumor, the so called "R0-resection"; performances after which some surgically irremovable residues remain – palliative resection (R1 – microscopic, R2 – macroscopic residues); and **palliative procedures** where the surgically irremovable tumor is left on site, but intestinal passage is opened through an intestinal outlet, ostomy or intestinal bypass, and/or the manifestations of the tumor are alleviated. Surgical removal of the colonic tumor is the basis of therapy and is irreplaceable. Its use and the strategy of further oncological therapy, usually chemotherapy, depend on the stage of the disease.

Presence of metastases in the liver or lungs does not eliminate the possibility of resection (palliative resection). **Metastases of colorectal cancer** are usually multiple. Their surgical removal, particularly when the liver has been affected, improves both the quality and period of survival. The current possibilities of multimodal therapy of metastasizing colon cancer use a combination of several lines of chemotherapy, biological therapy, chemoembolization of the liver, anatomical and extra-anatomical resection of the liver, and RFA (radiofrequency ablation), which have helped to improve the prognosis and survival. Five-year survival can be achieved in up to one third of patients.

An **acute complication** occurs in about 20% of patients with colorectal cancer, i.e. acute intestinal obstruction, perforation of the intestine or bleeding. **Intestinal obstruction, ileus state**, has typical symptoms whose intensity depends particularly on whether the intestinal closure is complete and on its localization (cf. Chapter 16 for the symptoms and diagnostics). The therapy is surgical, while releasing the obstruction in the intestine (resection of the affected segment, ostomy, and bypass) is a lifesaving task, and the removal of the tumor is only the subsequent goal. The operation is complicated by the presence of high amounts of stagnating content. Under favorable conditions, a procedure identical to the extent of the planned operation can also be performed in an acute setting.

**Intestinal perforation** is manifested by peritonitis (cf. Chapter 17). The point of perforation is either the tumor (disintegration) or the intestine above the obturating tumor (diastatic perforation). The therapy is surgical. In an acute operation, the site of perforation should be closed or – better – removed by resection; subsequently, the abdomen is cleaned and drainage is established. Perforation cannot be treated in this way in all situations. Derivative ostomy located orally above the site of perforation and drainage of the abdominal cavity are usually the solution. The postoperative and therapeutic results depend particularly on the duration of peritonitis and on the level of contamination.

**Bleeding** is caused by erosion of the tumor vessels. In addition to operation and resection of the intestinal segment with the tumor, acute angiography can be performed based on the capacity of the department and bleeding can be stopped by the embolization of the supply arteries, removing the intestine with the tumor soon, after due preparation.

**Prognosis** of colorectal tumors expressed as 5-year survival depends on the stage of the disease and on the possibility of removing the tumor by surgery. 90% of patients in stage A, about 70% in stage B, and about 50% of stage C survive for 5 years. The 5-year survival of stage D was an exception as recently as at the turn of the millennium. The prognosis of patients operated on due to a tumor with an acute complication is worse. Given that a relapse or metastases develop in up to one half of radically operated persons, the patients are usually followed-up for 5 years. This is carried out with the help of a protocol that includes examinations identical to those at the primary determination of the diagnosis. Death is usually caused by local relapses, distant metastases and generalization of the tumor.

## 9.6 Rectum and Anus

The rectum and anus, or anorectum, functions as the stool reservoir and the organ of continence.

The rectal ampulla and anal channel are distinguished. The ampulla is about 15 cm long; its upper third is intraperitoneal, while the distal two thirds are in the extraperitoneal position where the serosa is missing. The ampulla is of entodermal origin and its mucosa is covered with cylindrical epithelium; three cilia are prominent in the lumen transversally – Kohlrausch's plica and Houston's plicae. The anal channel is of ectodermal origin, about 3–5 cm long. It has a double lining, covered with cylindrical intestinal epithelium over the dentate line, and by squamous epithelium below this line, gradually changing into skin at the external orifice of the anus. Their differentiation is important particularly for tumors. The musculature of the channel is composed of the external and internal sphincter

SURGERY OF THE SMALL AND LARGE INTESTINES, RECTUM AND ANUS

and the puborectal muscle, both of which ensure closure of the anus. The internal hemorrhoid plexus is found in the submucosa round the internal orifice of the anal channel, and external plexus round the external orifice. Their function is to ensure a precise sealing of the anal sphincter. Anal glands, important in the development of abscesses and fistulae, are found below the mucosa of the anal channel and in the space between the internal and external sphincters.

## 9.6.1  Congenital Anorectal Malformations

Anorectal malformations, e.g. stenosis and atresia of the anus, atresia of the anus and rectum, and atresia of the rectum, belong to the most common congenital disorders. Treatment of these conditions falls in the domain of pediatric surgery or that of adult surgery if reconstruction surgeries have not been successful in restoring the function or if they were not possible at all.

## 9.6.2  Hemorrhoids

Hemorrhoids are varicosely dilated veins of the hemorrhoid plexuses, i.e. external and internal hemorrhoids, and intermediate hemorrhoids between them. Constitutional influences take part in their development (especially insufficiency of the connective tissue), as well as provoking influences (constipation and defecation habits, disproportionate increase of intra-abdominal pressure, pregnancy, portal hypertension). Hemorrhoids are present in at least one half of the adult population. They may be problem-free, and apparent intermittent bleeding may be their only symptom. Given that every plexus has its own vascular supply, the blood is usually of clear red color, and internal hemorrhoids are usually the source. Based on their extent, **internal hemorrhoids** are categorized in three grades (Fig. 9.4):
1. Enlarged internal hemorrhoids
2. Externally prolapsed hemorrhoids with spontaneous reposition
3. Hemorrhoids with permanent prolapse

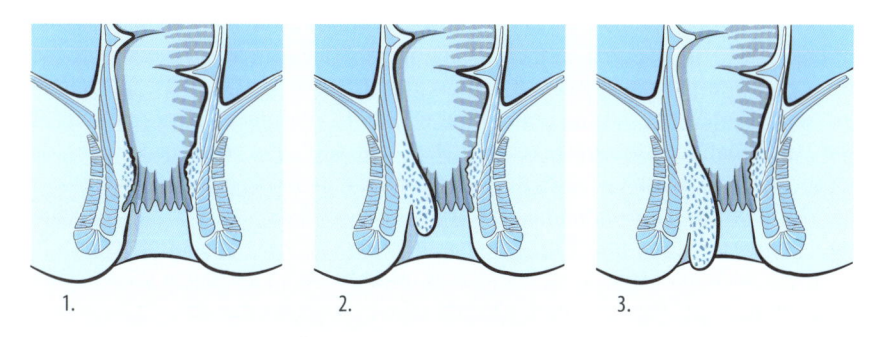

**Fig. 9.4** *Hemorrhoids of grades 1, 2 and 3*

Acute inflammation (thrombophlebitis of the hemorrhoid plexus) is the most common **complication**, associated with the distention of the hemorrhoid and considerable pain, and a prolapse up to the incarceration of the plexus, which may even result in gangrene. When the inflammation has subsided, patients usually have a feeling of "wet anus", burning sensation, and pain when passing stool. **External hemorrhoids** form nodules around the anus, which complicate hygiene; they become a cause of considerable problems upon inflammation and thrombosis.

**Diagnosis** is determined by aspection, indagation and ano-(recto-)scopy; in terms of differential diagnostics, it is most important **to exclude a different cause of bleeding, especially a tumor**.

**Therapy** is conservative, semi-invasive and surgical. **Conservative** therapy includes resting in bed in the acute stage, and both general and local application (ointments, suppositories) of antiflogistics and venotonics. Subsequently, in the calm stage, therapy includes an adaptation of defecation, regimen, and venotonics. **Semi-invasive therapy,** for example, ligation of the plexuses (Barron's technique), sclerotization, infrared coagulation, "DG-HAL" – ligation of the supply vessels navigated by Doppler endosonography. **Surgical therapy** includes extirpation of the hemorrhoid plexuses using various surgical techniques, destruction of the plexuses using cryotherapy, hyperthermia, and stapler surgery of the hemorrhoids (mucosectomy of the distal third of the rectum, while interrupting the supply vessels).

### 9.6.3 Perianal and Periproctal Abscesses

Perianal abscesses are most commonly caused by an inflammation of the perianal glands. Infection enters the glands from the Morgagni crypts in the dentate line of the anus into which the perianal glands empty. Other causes of abscesses (injury of the rectal or anal wall, infection transferred from other organs) are exceptional. Depending on where the infection reaches, a submucous abscess develops or an abscess in deeper spaces between the sphincters or in the area of the pelvic base. Abscesses perforate spontaneously on the outside or into the intestine, or they must be incised and drained. If the resulting defect fails to heal, a fistula remains.

Subcutaneous, submucous, intermuscular, ischiorectal and pelvirectal abscesses are distinguished based on their **localization**. Subcutaneous abscesses are the most common – about 50–60%. Intermuscular abscesses (between the sphincters) are important as the starting point of an infection, causing abscesses of both of the aforementioned localizations (Fig. 9.5). The so-called horseshoe abscess is a special form, which encircles the intestine along its whole circumference.

**Manifestations** of an abscess are typical: high fever, shivers, tachycardia, pain in the anus accentuated by stool passage, impossibility to sit. Bulges visible on the outside, infiltrate with fluctuation, sometimes an erythema on the skin. The diagnosis is supported by US examination (external or endorectal) and trial puncture under general anesthesia.

**Therapy** is surgical – timely incision and evacuation of the abscess, and drainage. No problems are usually encountered in superficial abscesses; revealing and treating abscesses of high localizations is more complicated (ischiorectal and pelvirectal). More extensive affections also require antibiotic therapy.

### 9.6.4 Fistulae

Most commonly, fistulae are residues of abscesses; they occur less commonly with Crohn's disease and idiopathic proctocolitis, and rarely after injuries or with tumors. Complete fistulae have two orifices, incomplete fistulae have only one. Internal fistulae open into the anus or rectum and are asymptomatic. External fistulae cause difficulties by mucus or even stool secretion, and eczemas develop upon irritation of the surrounding skin. Retention in the fistula is manifested by pain and fever, similar to an abscess.

Based on **localization** and relationship to the sphincter, fistulae are distinguished as submucous and subcutaneous, and also as extra-, inter- and transsphincteric (Fig. 9.6).

One or more orifices of the fistula are visible during physical examination, and infiltration along the fistula can sometimes be found by palpation. The finding can be specified closer using a tube, applying a dye in the fistula, contrast radiography – fistulography, and also US, CT or MRI assessment in exceptional cases.

**Therapy** of the fistulae is surgical and includes three basic modes: discision of the fistula on the tube (**fistulotomy**), excision of the fistula and healing **per secundam** (**fistulectomy**) and gradual cutting through the fistula using ligatures

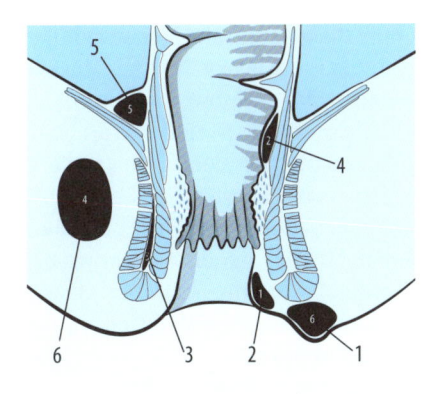

**Fig. 9.5** *Perianal and periproctal abscesses: 1) marginal subcutaneous abscess; 2) submucous abscess; 3) intermuscular abscess; 4) ischiorectal abscess; 5) pelvirectal abscess; 6) perianal subcutaneous abscess*

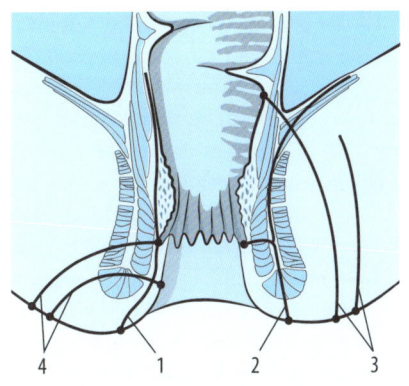

**Fig. 9.6** *Perianal and perirectal fistulae: 1) intrasphincteric fistula; 2) intersphincteric fistula; 3) extrasphincteric fistula; 4) transsphincteric fistula*

(**tracking ligature**, **Hippocratic elastic ligature**). It is always important to find the internal orifice of the fistula; without treatment the fistula is almost certain to relapse.

**Perianal hidradenitis** is a special form of affection with multiple fistulae around the anus, stemming from a chronic inflammation of apocrine glands found in this localization.

### 9.6.5 Other Benign Affections of the Anus

**Proctalgia fugax (anal cold)** is a painful disease manifested by spasmodic pain of the anus that occurs at rest, with no known provoking cause. Examinations show no organic finding; sedatives are particularly helpful in the therapy. **Pruritus ani (anusitis)** is manifested similarly; organic causes of irritation should be excluded. The symptoms collide with symptoms of organic disease, and thus they should be kept in mind as part of differential diagnostics.

**Anal fissure** is a painful disease which develops most commonly after an injury during passage of rigid stool. As a rule, it develops as an acute problem and if left untreated, a chronic fissure develops. It is manifested by pain in the anus accentuated by defecation, and by bleeding and the blood has a clear red color. Indagation demonstrates increased sphincter tone (protective spasm) and a palpable fissure, which is visible by anoscopy.

Therapy of an acute fissure requires rest, adaptation of defecation, and spasmo-analgesics. The purpose of therapeutic measures is to reduce the sphincter tone, in the medicamentous mode, by divulsion of the anus using surgery or by partial sphincterotomy.

**Anal prolapse** is partial when it affects only the mucosa, and complete if the whole wall of the anus is prolapsed. This condition is caused by weak suspension of the rectum, contributed to by defecation difficulties, sitting on the toilet in children, and also hemorrhoids, pregnancy and parturition. Besides the prolapsing part of the intestine, usually noticed by the patients, this condition is usually associated also with pain, bleeding and problems with continence.

Reposition is the therapy of an acute prolapse. Chronic prolapse in children can be managed by adaptation of defecation and by fixating the anus using adhesive plaster; anal cerclage, Thiersch's procedure, is usually helpful in adults.

Resection of the prolapsing intestine, reinforcement (reconstruction) of the pelvic base and rectopexis represent more radical solutions.

**Anal sphincter incontinence** is a consequence of mechanical damage to the sphincters (particularly the internal anal sphincter muscle) – motor incontinence, or a consequence of a perception disorder (paraplegia, diseases and denervations after surgeries in the small pelvis) – sensory incontinence. Three grades are distinguished:

1. The patient cannot retain gas
2. The patient cannot retain gas and loose stool
3. The patient cannot retain even formed stool

The current diagnostics includes, in addition to common intestinal examinations using pelvic CT and MRI assessment, US assessment of the sphincter, EMG of the sphincter, and anorectal manometry.

The therapy depends on the cause: the methods used include physiotherapy and rehabilitation techniques, surgical treatment (anal cerclage, sphincter-plasties, autologous replacement of the sphincters including electrical stimulation implants, an artificial anal sphincter or possibly an ostomy).

### 9.6.6 Tumors of the Rectum and Anus

**Benign** tumors are rare; they may stem from all tissues: adenomas, hemangiomas, lymphangiomas, and fibrolipomas.

**Malignant** tumors are represented by adenocarcinoma in more than 90% of patients. Rare tumors include **sarcoma**, **malignant melanoma** and **malignant lymphoma**.

With an incidence of 35/100,000, **rectal carcinoma** is more common than anal carcinoma. On the macroscopic level, it is manifested as a polypous or exulcerating carcinoma. It spreads in the same way as colon cancers, by infiltration, through the lymphatic path in the nodes and through the venous path. In principle, the diagnostics and therapy are identical to those of colon tumors. Given that this is a common disease, the following should be kept in mind:
- The symptoms (particularly bleeding) do not differ from other benign affections
- Indagation – examination **per rectum** – reveals the finding in more than one half of the patients
- Rectal cancer does not exclude the possibility of a synchronous tumor in the intestine
- Hemorrhoids do not exclude the possibility of rectal cancer

**Surgical removal** is the **basis of the therapy** of rectal tumors, while the choice of the procedure depends on the distance from the anus. Resectable (removable) tumors of the upper third of the rectum can be resolved by resection with an anastomosis; a tumor in the middle third is usually resolved by resection or amputation of the rectum depending on technical feasibility, and rectal amputation and terminal colostomy are usually performed when the tumor is localized in the lower third. Surgery due to a rectal tumor includes the removal of the mesorectal tissue (TEM) that contains the nearest lymph nodes. Besides localization, the extent of the procedure depends on the stage of tumor progression.

T1 tumors can be removed by a local procedure (transanal access, posterior rectotomy, surgical rectoscope); T2 and T3 tumors can be removed by resection or amputation of the rectum. T4 tumors – infiltrating the surrounding tissues and not removable due to local causes – can be reduced in size or recanalized (cleared) by cryodestruction, electrical coagulation, laser, and introduction of a stent. When a rectal tumor is not removable, a solution is offered by establishing an ostomy (cf. Section 9.6.8), which may help to maintain intestinal passage and reduce any disturbing symptoms (tenesmus, bleeding, mucus discharge).

Depending on the stage, additional methods are used in the therapy of rectal carcinoma, such as radiotherapy potentiated by chemotherapy. The best results of the therapy of advanced rectal tumors – T3, T4 – can be expected upon sequential use of **multimodal therapy in this order**: neoadjuvant (preoperative) radio- and chemotherapy → operation → adjuvant (postoperative) chemotherapy (depending on the definitive classification of the tumorous affection and circumstances of the operation). Multimodal procedures require exact pre-therapeutic classification before initiation of therapy. In some patients this approach allows for reducing the tumor in size or its staging; more favorable conditions for an operation are the result, as well as a higher hope for retaining the sphincter and the possibility of natural defecation and continence and a lower rate of local relapses. In a small number of patients, radiochemotherapy may even result in the tumor disappearing completely. The presence of tumor residues, demonstrable only with difficulty, is usually the cause of an early relapse of the tumor. Operation to the standard extent has always been indicated due to this risk.

**Malignant anal tumors** – carcinoma and melanoblastoma. These carcinoma originate from the layered anal epithelium. They are classified as follows:
- Basaliomas – slow growing, no metastases, therapy by local excision
- Bowen's and Paget's carcinoma, treated by local excision or cryodestruction
- Epidermoid carcinoma – localized at the edge of the anus, highly malignant, metastazing in inguinal lymph nodes
- Cloacogenic carcinoma – from the residues of the embryonic cloaca, highly malignant and fistulating in the surroundings. Epidermoid and cloacogenic carcinomas are treated by rectal amputation.

Note: Long-term irritation, for example, due to an inflammation or chronic perianal fistula, may lead to development of epidermoid carcinoma.

**Melanoblastoma** is manifested as a small tumor at the boundary of the mucosal and dermal part of the anus, and it may be pigmented or with no pigment – amelanotic. The tumor is highly malignant and its development of metastases does not respect the usual lymphatic flow. Therapy: wide excision, anorectal amputation.

### 9.6.7 Acute Diseases and Conditions of the Small and Large Intestines, and of the Rectum and Anus

Absence or impairment of intestinal passage caused by an obstruction, intestinal perforation, intense bleeding and injury are major acute surgical diseases of the intestines. The principles of treatment, and the conditions they lead to are discussed in appropriate chapters (Chapters 15–17).

For the sake of completeness, other acute conditions should be mentioned: **volvulus**, **incarceration** of the intestines in both external and internal hernias, **strangulation** and **invagination**; besides mechanical obstruction, vascular supply of the intestine is always affected, as well.

**Intestinal vascular events** are serious, fortunately rare, conditions – mesenteric embolism and mesenteric thrombosis. The superior mesenteric artery is affected by **embolism** more often than the inferior.

This is manifested by sudden, sharp pain in the abdomen, accompanied by tachycardia, hypotension and even collapse, nausea, sometimes vomiting, followed by an urge and abundant defecation. Most of the symptoms become reduced before the patient is examined. The findings of the physical examination, radiography and laboratory assessment are usually poor and not adequate for the patient's problems. Anamnestic information on previous embolisms and the finding of cardiac fibrillation may be a guide. The condition of the patient worsens again in the course of several hours; peritoneal irritation leads to an indication for surgery.

Ischemic (and gangrenous) small and large intestines are found during the surgery, in the extent corresponding to the loss of arterial supply. Procedure: embolectomy, resection of the gangrenous intestine, most often only laparotomy (the finding is insolvable). Survival is exceptional.

**Thrombosis** develops gradually and has less striking symptoms. Indication for surgery is identical; thrombectomy or establishment of an aortomesenteric bypass using a vascular prosthesis can be achieved only rarely due to the advanced finding of intestinal ischemia. The lethality rate is high.

Urgent selective angiography and/or Doppler ultrasonography are dominant examinations in the **diagnostics** of intestinal vascular events.

### 9.6.8 Basic Surgeries in the Intestines, Rectum and Anus

Surgeries in the intestines can be classified schematically as follows: resections, bypasses and ostomies.

In the small intestine, the extent of resection corresponds to the extent of affection; in the case of tumors, the mesentery is resected together with the affected

**TEXTBOOK OF SURGERY**

intestine, in the range of the sentinel region of the affected segment. Dilatation of stenotic segments in Crohn's disease – stricturoplasty is a special procedure carried out in the small intestine. Erosion of adhesions – adhesiolysis is the most frequent procedure in the small intestine.

Resections of the affected segment of the intestine and of the adjacent mesocolon in standard extents that suit oncosurgical requirements and anatomical accesses have stabilized in procedures in the large intestine. The choice of rectal surgery depends on whether intestinal continuity can be restored by an anastomosis and continence preserved after removing the affected segment.

Individual types of surgical procedures are shown schematically in Figs. 9.7 to 9.16.

Basic resection procedures include:
- Right-sided hemicolectomy (Figs. 9.7a, 9.7b)
- Transverse colon resection (Fig. 9.7c)
- Left-sided hemicolectomy (Fig. 9.8a) and extended left-sided hemicolectomy (Fig. 9.8b)
- Sigmoid resection (9.8c)
- Rectal resection (9.9a) terminated by restoration of intestinal continuity by an anastomosis (9.9b) or blind closure of the rectal stub and sigmoideostomy

Complete removal of both the rectum and anus (abdominoperineal resection) always requires establishment of an ostomy (9.10).

Currently, all surgeries of the intestines can be performed from laparotomy or in the laparoscopic mode. Gaining the possibility to perform a proper procedure in the affected segment of the intestine should be the main reason for choosing surgical access.

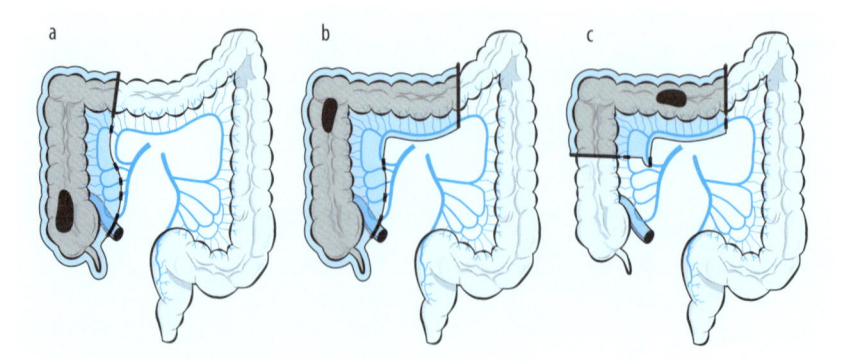

**Fig. 9.7** *Extent of resection for a tumor of the cecum, ascending colon and transverse colon: a), b) Right-sided hemicolectomy; c) Transverse colon resection*

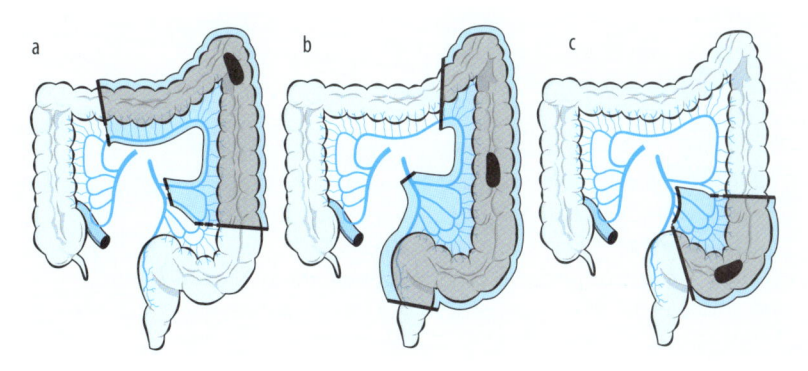

# SURGERY OF THE SMALL AND LARGE INTESTINES, RECTUM AND ANUS

**Fig. 9.8** *Extent of resection for a tumor of splenic flexure, descending colon and sigmoid: a) Left-sided hemicolectomy; b) Extended left-sided hemicolectomy; c) Sigmoid resection*

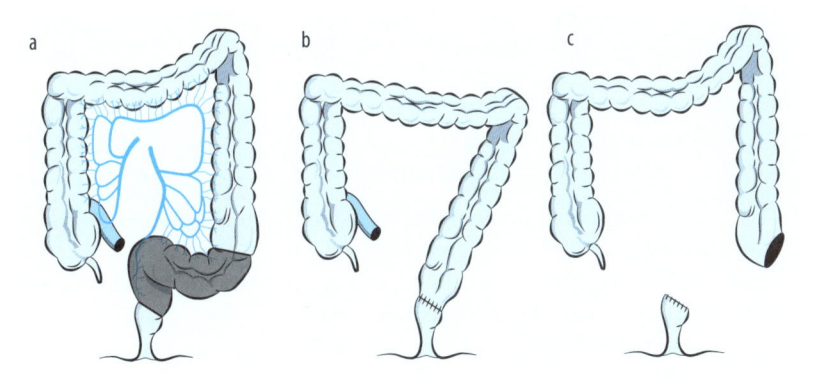

**Fig. 9.9** *Resection: a) due to rectal tumor; b) with intestinal continuity restoration by an anastomosis; c) or with blind closure of the rectal stub and sigmoideostomy*

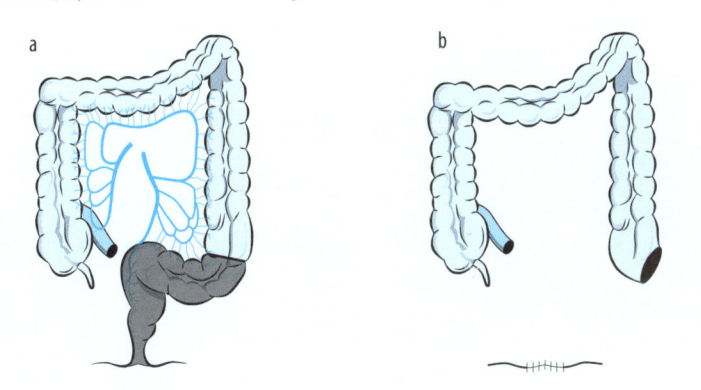

**Fig. 9.10** *Abdominoperineal resection of the rectum*

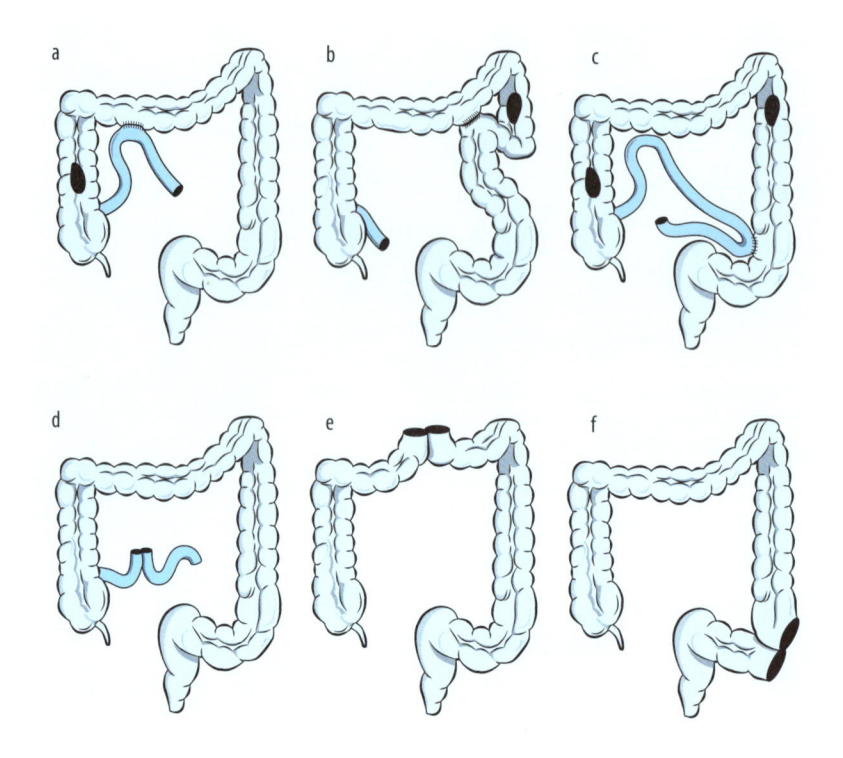

**Fig. 9.11** *Schematic illustration of possible intestinal bypasses and ostomies: a) Ileocolic (ileotransverse) anastomosis; b) Colocolic anastomosis; c) Ileosigmoid anastomosis; d) Double-barrel ("loop") ileostomy; e) Transversostomy; f) Sigmoidostomy*

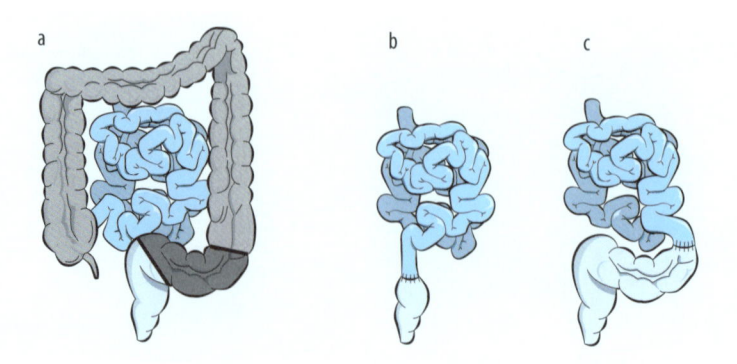

**Fig. 9.12** *a) Subtotal colectomy; b) Subtotal colectomy with ileorectal anastomosis; c) Subtotal colectomy with ileosigmoid anastomosis*

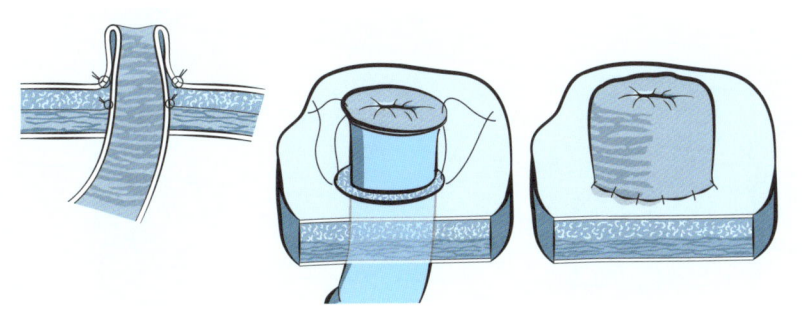

**Fig. 9.13** *Scheme of ileostomy establishment according to Brook*

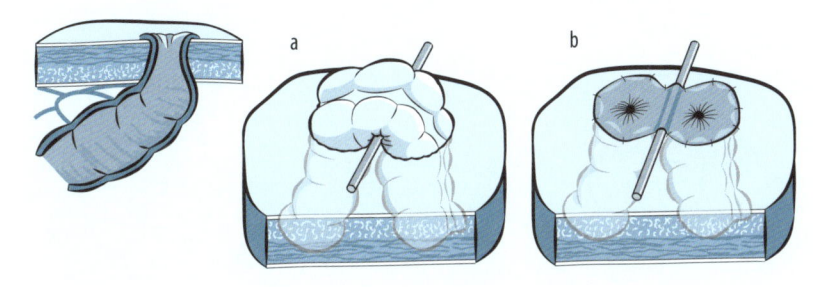

**Fig. 9.14** *Scheme of establishment of a single-barrel and double-barrel ostomy*

Endoluminal stapler

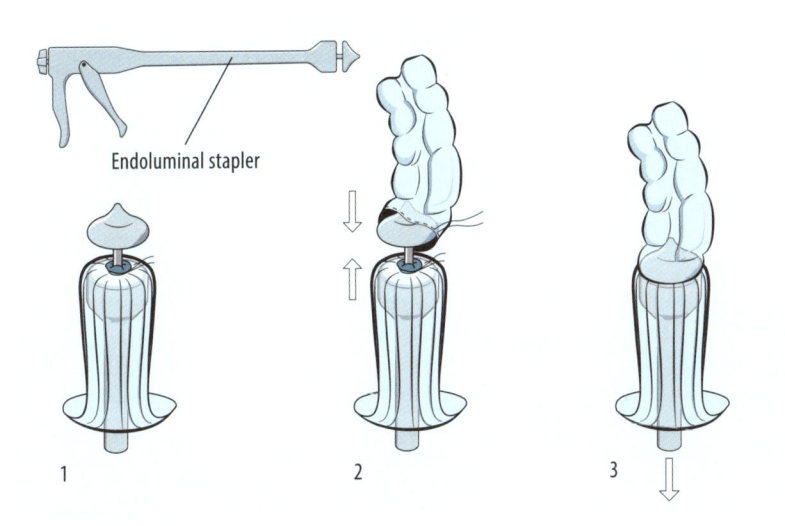

1   2   3

**Fig. 9.15** *Endoluminal stapler – suturing device – for the intestine and for establishment of an anastomosis (schematic)*

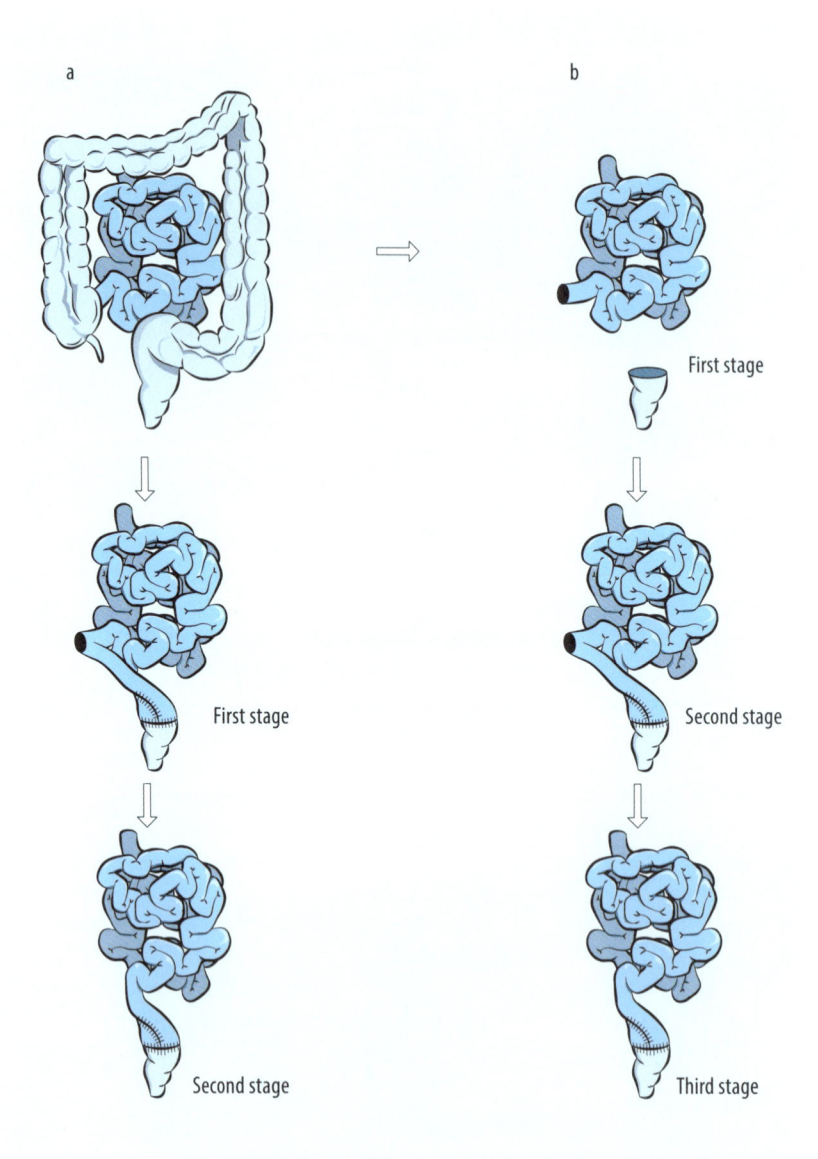

**Fig. 9.16** *Possibilities of surgical procedures in colectomy due to complications of idiopathic proctocolitis: a) Colon removal, formation of an ileal reservoir and establishment of ileoanal anastomosis with protective ileostomy in the first surgical period, and closure of the ileostomy in the second surgical period; b) Colon removal, blind closure of the rectum and establishment of ileostomy in the first period; finishing the of resection of the rectum and establishment of an ileal reservoir in the second period, and closure of the ileostomy in the third surgical period*

# 10 LIVER SURGERY

10.1 Symptomatology of Liver Diseases
10.2 Clinical Findings
10.3 Paraclinical Assessments
10.4 Benign Focal Liver Diseases
10.5 Malignant Liver Diseases

The liver is the largest parenchymatous organ of the abdominal cavity. It is the place of numerous crucial biochemical processes of the organism. The most substantial part of plasma protein synthesis takes place in the liver, the supplies of readily usable energy sources are stored or, on the contrary, processed in the liver, and detoxication or elimination of many metabolic products or exogenous toxins also occurs there. The functional reserve of a healthy liver is large, ten times exceeding the common need.

The majority of diseases and disorders of the liver tissue are treated conservatively, while focal hepatic processes are suitable for surgery. In addition to progress in intensive medicine, expansion in the knowledge of the functional anatomy of the liver in the 1950's and 1960's was a particular prerequisite for the development of modern surgical treatment of hepatic diseases. Segmental division of the liver that respects the supply of individual regions (segments) of the "portal triad", i.e. terminal branches of the hepatic artery, portal vein and the bile duct (Fig. 10.1), allows for performing even extensive anatomical resections of the liver tissue. Expansion of experience from transplantation medicine has considerably influenced the development of this field of surgery.

## 10.1 Symptomatology of Liver Diseases

**Icterus (jaundice)** is of crucial importance in the symptomatology of liver diseases, and in the event that it is of infectious origin, it may be associated with **signs of sepsis. Pressure, pain in the upper abdomen, weight loss and general loss of will** are more common symptoms than icterus in malignant hepatic processes. Any long-term use of medicaments (toxic damage, hyperplasia), alcohol

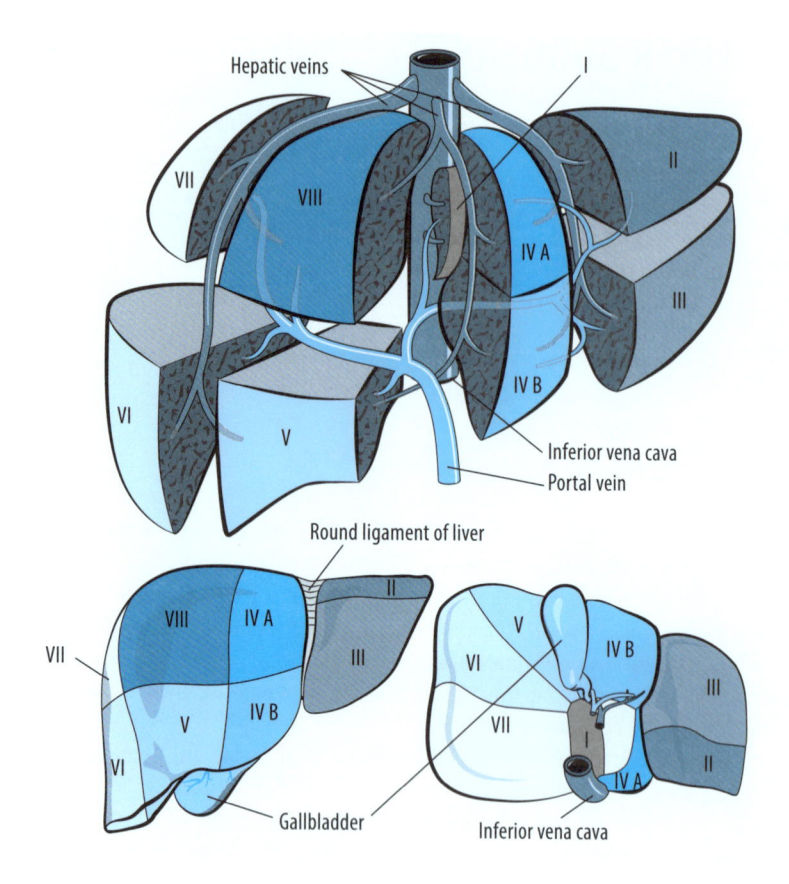

Fig. 10.1 *Surgical anatomy of the liver*

(cirrhosis), previous liver diseases (infectious hepatitis) and treatment due to malignancy (metastasis) should be explored in the history of patients with suspected liver disease. Information on any stay in foreign countries (parasitary disease) is also important, particularly with inflammatory constellation of the findings.

## 10.2 Clinical Findings

The clinical finding should focus not only on the examination of the liver (size and consistency, palpable resistance, pain), but also on any presence of ascites and signs of portal hypertension (splenomegaly, dilated subcutaneous veins around the umbilicus, "caput medusae", or the palm tree sign).

Table 10.1 Child-Pugh classification of severity of liver disease

| Parameter | Score 1 | Score 2 | Score 3 |
|---|---|---|---|
| Nutritional status | Very good | Good | Poor |
| Ascites | None | Low | High |
| Encephalopathy | None | Mild | Severe |
| Albumin (g/l) | Over 35 | 34–30 | Below 30 |
| Bilirubin (µmol/l) | Up to 34 | 35–51 | Over 51 |
| Quick (%) | Over 70 | 50–69 | Below 50 |

Child A score 6, Child B score 7–9, Child C score 10 and higher

## 10.3 Paraclinical Assessments

Paraclinical assessments are of extraordinary importance in the diagnostics of liver diseases. Laboratory diagnostics are crucial for the functional diagnosis, and imaging methods for the localization and assessment of focal changes.

### 10.3.1 Basic Laboratory Assessments

Basic laboratory assessments include particularly serum bilirubin level including direct, i.e. conjugated bilirubin. Elevated indirect bilirubin provides evidence of hemolysis or Gilbert's disease, but it may also be found in infectious hepatitis. Elevated transaminases (ALT, AST) are the consequence of parenchyma damage of inflammatory or ischemic origin. Elevated ALP signalizes cholestasis. Serum albumin assessment and the Quick test (synthetic hepatic function) form part of the basic evaluation of the functional state of the liver; more complex classification according to Child (Table 10.1) provides a better picture.

Laboratory diagnostics are not reliable for distinguishing the biological characteristics of a lesion found in the liver. Only the dynamics of a rise in alpha-fetoprotein in patients with cirrhosis indicates hepatocellular carcinoma; tumor markers (CEA) are increased when liver metastases are present, especially those of colorectal cancer.

### 10.3.2 Imaging Methods

**Ultrasonography (US)** is the first method of choice in the examination of liver diseases. US examination can be used to identify the majority of lesions over 1 cm in diameter. US provides basic information on the width of both intra- and extrahepatic bile ducts and on lithiasis, width of the portal vein trunk, and also on flow in the portal stream when the Doppler modification is used.

**CT assessment** provides spatial depiction of focal and diffuse changes in the parenchyma, and it can be used for differential diagnostics of some lesions after contrast application. While metastases can be demonstrated using contrast CT assessment in up to 90% of cases, the sensitivity for hepatocellular carcinoma covers lesions smaller than 3 cm in less than 50% of cases. **MRI assessment** seems to provide somewhat higher sensitivity for the detection of primary tumors of the liver (about 80%). Liver **scintigraphy** has generally lost its diagnostic privileges; however, it does occupy a special position for the demonstration of metastases of endocrine GIT tumors in the liver (octreotide scintigraphy for the gastrinoma, MIBG for the feochromocytoma). The need for **angiography** (an invasive procedure) has also declined with the development of spiral CT; today, angiography has remained important particularly for demonstrating variants in arterial supply of the liver when establishing an interaarterial port for chemotherapy is planned. **Targeted punctures with biopsy** under US or CT control are associated with a non-negligible risk of complications (bleeding, biliary peritonitis or a fistula, arteriovenous fistula), and thus they are indicated only for principal therapeutic consequences. Higher safety is offered by collecting materials using a puncture under **laparoscopic control**, possibly in combination with **peroperative laparoscopic US**. And finally, **ERCP or PTC assessment** is indicated for depicting any changes in intrahepatic bile ducts. However, it should be noted that even with the use of the entire scale of the assessments above, **explorative laparotomy** to evaluate resectability cannot be avoided in some cases of focal lesions in the liver. In particular, this applies to the scope of affection of the liver hilum and the dorsal side of the liver.

The functional reserve of the parenchyma should be examined before making a decision on liver resection because in patients with significantly limited function (CI, chronic hepatitis, metabolic disorders) no more extensive resections can be planned. Also, surgical treatment is usually not indicated for multiple affections in both lobes, and alternative therapeutic methods should be considered.

## 10.4 Benign Focal Liver Diseases

### ■ LIVER CYSTS

Liver cysts are a congenital disease with an incidence rate below 1%. The disease often has an asymptomatic course and requires no treatment. Therapy is indicated when symptoms of pressure in the surrounding area are present. Puncture evacuation of the serous content is of diagnostic importance; communication with the biliary tree or vascular stream cannot be demonstrated. The puncture has no long-term effect and the cyst must be fenestrated using the omental flap as filler. The procedure can also be done laparoscopically.

### LIVER CYSTADENOMA

Liver cystadenoma are relatively large (usually over 10 cm) encapsulated tumors, mostly in middle-aged women. The cause of their development is unclear; their symptomatology is given predominantly by oppression of the surroundings, e.g. icterus if the bile ducts are oppressed, or stomach evacuation disorder. In rare cases, they may manifest by bleeding into a cyst; cancerization leading to the development of a cystadenocarcinoma is also rare. The method of choice is resection of the lesion in the healthy tissue.

### LIVER ABSCESS

Liver abscess develops most commonly on the basis of ascending cholangitis or iatrogenically after surgical or instrumental procedures in the area of the liver or in bile ducts. In terms of microbiology, they are most often associated with *E. coli*, *Staphylococcus aureus* and streptococci. Clinically dominant symptoms include, other than sepsis expressed in various modes, especially pain in the right upper abdomen and symptoms of compression of the surroundings. Besides antibiotics, the therapy includes targeted drainage by puncture under US or CT control, less commonly operative evacuation and drainage.

### INTRAHEPATIC CHOLANGIOLITHIASIS

Intrahepatic cholangiolithiasis (Caroli's syndrome) develops as a consequence of biliary stasis in cystically dilated intrahepatic bile ducts, while relapsing inflammations (Caroli's disease) are typical alongside of lithiasis. Stenosis of the bile duct after a surgical injury in the bifurcation region or stenosis after biliodigestive anastomosis may be another cause. In both cases, clinically dominant symptoms include pain in the epigastrium and upper abdomen, relapsing obstruction icterus and signs of sepsis. Multiple abscesses may also form in the affected area, and secondary biliary cirrhosis develops when the condition lasts for a longer period. Besides the general antimicrobial therapy, effective drainage should be provided in this case, too. In some patients with bile duct stricture, this can be achieved by endoscopic drainage (stent) or through percutaneous transhepatic access (PTC and drainage); in some patients surgical drainage is necessary with intrahepatic lithiasis removal, and the only solution in other patients is to resect the affected segment of the liver tissue.

### PARASITARY CYSTS

Parasitary cysts are most commonly solitary cysts due to *Entamoeba histolytica* or *Echinococcus granularis* infection. While amebiasis is often treated conservatively with success (metronidazole) and only complications occurring during the therapy (perforation with formation of purulent peritonitis) or resistance to therapy require interventional or surgical treatment and drainage of the lesion, echinococcal cyst is often indicated for surgical treatment. Two layers of the wall are characteristic for the echinococcal cyst, and the diagnosis can be confirmed by serological determination of specific antibodies. Intermittent pain in the right epigastrium and subfebriles often dominate among the symptoms. Surgical treatment is required for echinococcal cysts over 4 cm in diameter and cysts localized near the sheath (the risk of rupture into the free abdominal or pleural cavity). The risk of an anaphylactic reaction due to parasitary dissemination is present also peroperatively, and therefore the surgical field should be carefully covered with cloths saturated with 20% NaCl before opening the cavity; when the content of the cyst has been removed by suction, 20% NaCl solution should be instilled. Subsequently, the cyst including its internal sheath is excised or, preferably, resected with the edge of the surrounding tissue.

## LIVER HEMANGIOMA

Liver hemangioma – the incidence rate of larger hemangiomas has been reported at about 5%, while solitary lesions are present in 90% of cases. The hemangioma is often asymptomatic and commonly affects younger women. Symptoms due to obstruction are clinically dominant, as well as pain due to pressure exerted on the sheath and rarely rupture into the abdominal cavity. Only growing hemangiomas, those over 6 cm in diameter, and symptomatic hemangiomas are indicated for surgery. Other cases are only followed (US, CT) given that the risk of resection exceeds the risk of spontaneous course in these cases.

## LIVER CELL ADENOMA AND FOCAL NODULAR HYPERPLASIA

Liver cell adenoma and focal nodular hyperplasia (FNH) – focal proliferation of liver cells particularly affects women of reproductive age. The cause is unknown; the disease may be associated with hormonal influences and with contraception. The symptoms may vary – compression of the surroundings, bile duct obstruction, pain due to tension in the sheath or bleeding. About 30% of lesions develop as multiple; biopsy is always indicated when FNH is suspected. Considering that cancer lesions have also been demonstrated in the resecates of these lesions in rare cases, a trend toward more generous indication of resection therapy can be seen today.

Surgical treatment of benign liver diseases is associated with the principal **risks** of bleeding, both perioperative and postoperative, infections (subphrenic abscess, early infection), and complications in the bile ducts (biliary fistula, biliary stenoses and strictures). Liver failure rarely occurs with proper indication. The prognosis after successful surgical treatment is usually very favorable and the life of the patient does not usually have any special limitations.

## 10.5 Malignant Liver Diseases

### 10.5.1 Primary Liver Malignoma

Primary liver malignoma are quite rare in Central Europe, representing about 3% of all malignant tumors. Their occurrence is up to 30 times higher in developing countries and Eastern Asia.

**Hepatocellular carcinoma (HCC)** develops from hepatocytes and its potential relationship to some cases of FNH has been mentioned. Hepatitis type B and C, cirrhosis based on hepatitis, metabolic disorders (hemochromatosis) and irradiation are described as predisposing factors. Alcohol in itself is not an apparent predisposing factor; however, incidence of HCC in alcoholic cirrhosis is 4 times higher compared to the normal population. HCC diagnostics is difficult and usually delayed; its resectability is low also given that 3/4 of HCC diseases occur in our conditions in cirrhotics, and thus the possibility of more extensive resection is excluded due to insufficient functional reserve. The effect of adjuvant therapy has not been generally demonstrated; alternatives of surgical treatment, providing results sometimes even comparable to resections, include separate chemoembolization or local intraarterial cytostatic perfusion, instillation of 90% alcohol and cryotherapy or radiofrequency ablation of the lesions. Liver transplantation can be considered in small, centrally localized lesions; however, long-term results are better than in the resection.

**Cholangiogenic carcinoma** stems from epithelium of intrahepatic bile ducts. The etiological relationship of its development with primary sclerosing cholangitis (relatively common in patients with idiopathic proctocolitis) has been reported, as well as fibrous cystic changes in the bile ducts (Caroli's syndrome), but also with the use of anabolic steroids. The possibilities of surgical treatment are limited similarly as in HCC, and the prognosis is even worse. The principle of resection therapy consists in the removal of the lesion, in a minimum distance of 1 cm in the healthy tissue (bisegmentectomy, lobectomy, and extended lobectomy in rare cases). Major contraindications include bilateral lesions, infiltration of large vascular trunks and distant metastases (the lungs, skeleton).

### 10.5.2 Liver Metastases

The liver is the most common place for distant metastases of other malignant tumors; liver affection is present in more than 1/3 of patients who die of any malignancy. More than one half of liver metastases originate in tumors from the portal venous basin. In terms of practice, surgical treatment is meaningful only for metastases of colorectal cancer and endocrine GIT tumors. The number of resections of a solitary liver metastasis, both synchronous (together with radical surgery of the primary tumor) and metachronous (metastasis diagnosed during follow-up of patients after radical surgery of the primary tumor) has been rising particularly in connection with **colorectal cancer**, currently the most common malignoma in the Czech Republic. Removal of the liver lesion is associated with significant extension of the mean time of survival, although only 5% of the resections are actually curative, i.e. leading to definitive healing of the tumor.

**Metastases of endocrine tumors** are associated with considerably better prognosis than metastases of other GIT tumors. Resection of the solitary metastasis as an addition to radical removal of the carcinoid or endocrine active pancreatic tumor leads to good results in the long term. Multiple year survival has been reported even for non-resected metastases of these tumors.

On the contrary, liver metastases of other tumors are indicated for surgical treatment only exceptionally. In particular, metastases of gastric and pancreatic carcinoma are quite infaust in terms of their prognosis. Individual cases of small and solitary metastases of breast cancer, malignant melanoma, hypernephroma or sarcoma are indicated for resection in exceptional cases, particularly if their metachronous development occurs after a longer time interval. However, the benefit of liver resections for long-term survival has not been statistically demonstrated for these tumors.

Current possibilities and indications for liver transplantation are discussed in the chapter on transplantation (Chapter 21).

# 11 GALLBLADDER AND EXTRAHEPATIC BILE DUCTS

> 11.1 Symptomatology of Gallbladder and Bile Duct Diseases
> 11.2 Clinical Findings
> 11.3 Paraclinical Assessments
> 11.4 Therapy of Gallbladder and Bile Duct Diseases
> 11.5 Basic Surgical Procedures in Gallbladder and Bile Ducts
> 11.6 Prognosis of Patients with Gallbladder and Bile Duct Diseases

Diseases of the gallbladder and extrahepatic bile ducts, particularly cholelithiasis and associated complications, are among the most frequent gastrointestinal tract diseases in Central Europe.

Extrahepatic bile ducts carry **bile formed in the liver to the duodenum** into which they open at the place of the papilla of Vater, together with the pancreatic outlet. The main closing mechanism – the muscular valve called sphincter of Oddi – is also found at this place, which allows for regulation of bile outflow. The gallbladder forms a reservoir where bile concentrates and is emptied based on neurohumoral stimulations of gallbladder contractions (synergy with relaxation of the closing mechanism of the papilla – Fig. 11.1).

The bile plays an important role in the digestive process by **emulsifying fats**. Vitamins A, D, E and K, which are soluble in fats, cannot be absorbed when no bile acids are present in the intestine.

A substantial part of gallbladder and bile duct diseases is causally related to the formation of stones. Concrements are formed predominantly in the gallbladder. Under the conditions of bile concentration, the stability of the solution becomes disturbed and cholesterin crystals are formed. Subsequently, concrements are formed around the crystals by apposition. The causes of the disturbed stability of the bile solution apparently consist in different representations of some of its components; in addition to genetic and hormonal influences (women are affected more commonly) dietary habits have an impact as well. Formation of stones in bile ducts is rare and occurs especially in the event of cholestasis and infection, which is often associated with it (stenoses and strictures of bile ducts, cysts in bile ducts).

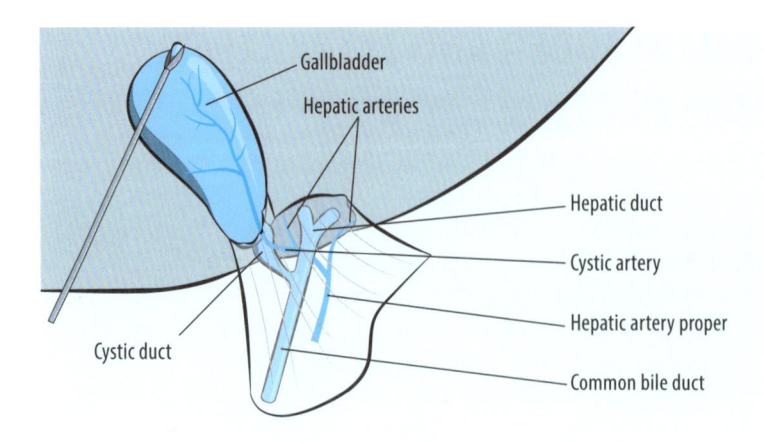

Fig. 11.1 *Anatomy of gallbladder and extrahepatic bile ducts*

Gallbladder stones (**cholecystolithiasis**) may be clinically silent, they may obstruct gallbladder emptying (**biliary colic**), or they may pass to the bile ducts (**choledocholithiasis**) and obstruct bile outflow to the duodenum, leading to the development of an **obstruction icterus**. Rarely, a stone may pass out from the gallbladder to the adjacent duodenum or colon through a fistula and cause a picture of intestinal passage impairment (**biliary ileus**). Small stones may spontaneously leave the gallbladder naturally through bile duct and the papilla of Vater, and **biliary pancreatitis** may develop in a small portion of these cases.

Cholelithiasis is often associated with the infection of stagnating bile and with the inflammation transferred to the organ wall (**cholecystitis, cholangitis**). Inflammatory affection of the wall may even cause perforation of the gallbladder and the discharge of its content into the peritoneal cavity (**biliary peritonitis**).

Besides cholelithiasis and inflammations, **tumors** are the most serious diseases of the gallbladder and bile ducts. The vast majority of them are malignant tumors – adenocarcinomas. Their prognosis is highly unfavorable.

**Stenoses** and **strictures** are another group of bile duct diseases; however, most often of iatrogenic origin.

## 11.1 Symptomatology of Gallbladder and Bile Duct Diseases

**Pain** and **jaundice** dominate in the symptomatology of gallbladder and extrahepatic bile duct diseases. Sudden colicky pain in the right upper abdomen or epigastrium, irradiating into the back and below the scapula, accompanied by nausea and vomiting is typical for biliary colic. When associated with fever and signs of inflammation, the symptoms signalize acute cholecystitis, and in these cases the pain changes from colicky to permanent. When yellow color of the skin and sclerae appear together with dark urine in connection with biliary colic or immediately after it, the symptomatology is typical for bile duct closure due to a stone. The risk of infection of the stagnating bile (cholangitis) rises in connection with the obstruction, with the following clinical manifestations: icterus, pain in the epigastrium and fever with shivers (Charcot's triad). On the contrary, painless development of icterus with the finding of palpable enlarged gallbladder often indicates malignant obstruction of bile duct (Courvoisier's sign).

## 11.2 Clinical Findings

**Pain in the right upper abdomen and middle epigastrium** is found most commonly by clinical examination. Palpable, painful, spherical **resistance** is sometimes found corresponding to a filled, hydropic gallbladder. Depending on the progression of inflammatory changes, **muscle contraction** may be found, circumscribed in the right upper abdomen (pericholecystitis) or diffuse muscle contraction of the abdominal wall with signs of peritoneal irritation (biliary peritonitis). **Varying signs of the small intestine obstruction**, together with pain in the right upper abdomen, must raise suspicion of biliary ileus (blockage of the small intestine due to a large gallstone, reaching the intestine through the cholecystoduodenal fistula in most cases).

In certain cases, even advanced inflammation of the gallbladder may be accompanied by a poor clinical finding, which makes the diagnostic procedure much more complicated. This applies particularly to acute cholecystitis in elderly and generally weakened persons and to acalculous cholecystitis in critically ill patients (where it is an organ manifestation of MODS with a genesis similar to that of a stress ulcer). In such event, this risk should be at least considered and the diagnostic help of imaging methods should be used.

## 11.3 Paraclinical Assessments

Laboratory assessments and the whole scale of imaging methods are applied in paraclinical diagnostics of gallbladder and bile duct diseases.

### 11.3.1 Laboratory Assessments

Laboratory assessments performed as standard include serum bilirubin levels including the ratio of direct (conjugated) bilirubin, transaminases ALT and AST, ALP and GMT (laboratory differentiation of obstruction and parenchymatous icterus), and facultative activity of amylases in serum and urine, and HBsAg (Australia antigen). The laboratory findings also include general parameters of inflammation. Other assessments to complete and specify the diagnosis are chosen based on the clinical finding and evaluation of the basic laboratory results.

### 11.3.2 Imaging Methods

**Ultrasonography (US)** has a privileged position among imaging methods. US examination is non-invasive and generally widely available. It provides basic information in respect of the evidence of stones in the gallbladder and bile ducts, and allows for measuring relatively accurately the width of the bile duct (normal width 6–7 mm). The thickness and condition of the gallbladder wall can be determined with relative precision (inflammatory affection, suspected malignancy), as well as any presence of loose liquid in the surroundings (inflammation). Last but not least, the examination also includes information on the structure of the liver tissue (metastatic lesions, abscess and nodular reconstruction).

**Endoscopic examination** (endoscopic retrograde cholangiopancreatography – **ERCP**) is indicated in the presence of clinical or laboratory suspicion of choledocholithiasis or bile duct obstruction of another origin. Besides high diagnostic value in terms of demonstrating the cause and localizing the obstruction, this examination is especially valuable given that the therapeutic component is linked directly to the examination – stone extraction, cutting of the stenotic papilla (endoscopic papillotomy – **EPT**), drainage through the stenosis using a plastic stent. Endoscopy can also be performed using an introduced sonographic tube (endosonography – **EUS**). This method offers special sensitivity also for small lesions obturating bile ducts and is suitable for preoperative staging of tumor processes.

**CT assessment** is most often indicated to complete the staging procedure for suspected malignant origin of the bile duct obstruction or gallbladder tumor. On the contrary, CT assessment is not suitable for demonstrating cholecysto- or choledocholithiasis – and compared to US, it provides lower yield for a higher price and radiation load for the patient.

In the cases of obstruction icterus where ERCP is not feasible for technical reasons (unsuccessful tube insertion, conditions after gastric resection with B II anastomosis, etc.), the non-invasive examination using **magnetic resonance (MRCP)** is the method of choice today. Compared to ERCP, its disadvantage is the impossibility of concurrent therapeutic intervention. On the contrary, such intervention is allowed by **percutaneous transhepatic cholangiography (PTC)** with the possibility of both external and internal drainage through a stent. The disadvantage of this method is the invasive examination with a certain risk of complications, particularly bleeding and biliary peritonitis.

**Native radiography of the abdomen** can be used to demonstrate a contrast shadow in the area of the gallbladder only seldom, and in the diagnostics of gallbladder and bile duct diseases it is valuable particularly in the event of the suspicion of biliary ileus. Besides the ileus finding of levels in the small intestine, air in bile ducts – pneumobilia – is apparent in about 30% of patients.

## 11.4 Treatment of Gallbladder and Bile Duct Diseases

Not only conservative methods and endoscopic and intervention radiology procedures, but often particularly surgical treatments are used in the therapy of gallbladder and extrahepatic bile duct diseases.

### 11.4.1 Therapy of Cholelithiasis and Complications

**Asymptomatic cholecystolithiasis** (accidental finding based on US examination) requires no therapy. Cholecystolithiasis symptoms are typically manifested as **biliary colic**. The therapy is conservative, with the use of **spasmolytics and diet**. In most cases colics occur repeatedly with various frequencies, and the risk of other complications rises with the duration of problems. Surgical removal of the gallbladder with stones – **cholecystectomy (CHE)** is the most effective and permanent therapy. Conservative therapy (**spasmolytics, antibiotics, infusion therapy and diet**) are indicated in most cases in the event of **inflammatory gallbladder disease**. If the problems and the clinical finding progress or if the response to therapy is insufficient within 24–48 hours, surgical treatment is indicated (**CHE** using laparoscopy or conventional surgery). Urgent surgery (usually using conventional laparotomy) is required in the event of biliary peritonitis with hidden or free perforation of the gallbladder. Besides CHE, **lavage of the abdominal cavity** is also performed, and usually also the postoperative **drainage** of the right half of the peritoneum. Urgent surgery is also required in the event of **biliary ileus**. In this case, removal of the obstruction in the intestine (**enterolithotomy**) is a fundamental part of the therapy; the primary disease of the gallbladder can be concurrently resolved only rarely due to the serious general condition of the patient and usually a severe inflammatory change in the subhepatic region. However, CHE often need not be indicated, or even postponed, given that most patients pass their (often solitary) stones and have no further biliary problems. The therapy of all patients with urgent surgery obviously includes intensive care according to current criteria – removal of the inflamed or perforated gallbladder or gallstone obturating the intestine is only one of the necessary preconditions for a favorable course of these serious conditions.

**Choledocholithiasis with or without cholangitis** is primarily treated using **endoscopy (stone extraction, drainage)**, and **antibiotics** are added to the therapy if inflammation is present (for example, cefalosporins, quinolones). It should be emphasized that **obstruction cholangitis** is an acute, life threatening disease (cholangiogenic sepsis), which requires, in addition to intensive system therapy,

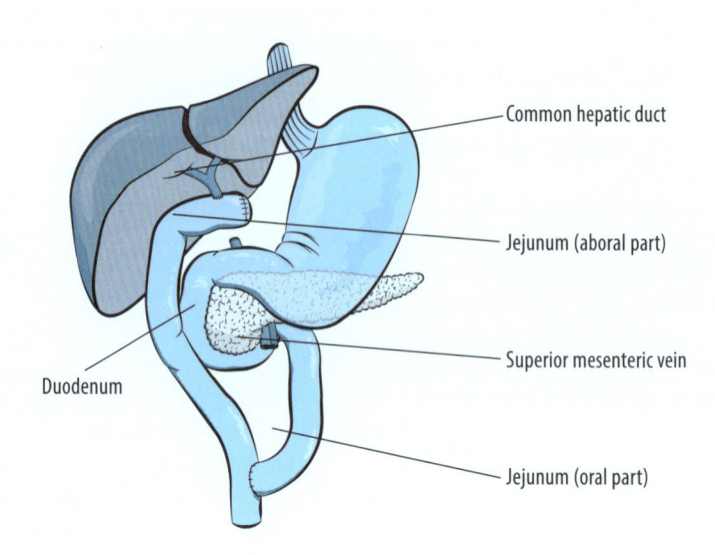

**Fig. 11.2** *Hepaticojejunoanastomosis according to Roux – the principle of excluded jejunal loop*

urgent effective bile duct drainage using endoscopy, intervention-based (PTC), or a surgical procedure (T-drain), which is seldom used today.

### 11.4.2 Therapy of Benign Strictures and Bile Duct Cysts

As for other benign causes of bile duct obstruction, **cysts of extrahepatic bile ducts** are indicated for surgical treatment – **resection of the altered bile duct and biliodigestive anastomosis** to the excluded loop of the small intestine (hepaticojejunoanastomosis according to Roux) (Fig. 11.2). Mere drainage via endoscopy or surgical anastomosis without resection entails a relatively high risk of malignant transformation. **Endoscopic dilatation and drainage** usually also provide only a temporary effect in **benign strictures** of the hepatocholedochus, which are iatrogenic in most cases (bile duct injury during CHE or bile duct revisions and drainages). Surgical revision is usually needed with the **resection of the stenotic segment and biliodigestive anastomosis (Y-Roux)**. Direct suture of the bile duct can be carried out only rarely.

### 11.4.3 Therapy of Gallbladder and Extrahepatic Pathway Tumors

Tumorous diseases of gallbladder and extrahepatic bile ducts can be radically resolved only using surgery. However, a predominant part of patients come for therapy in advanced stages when only palliative therapy can be considered.

# GALLBLADDER AND EXTRAHEPATIC BILE DUCTS

Endoscopic therapy is preferred to surgical in palliative treatment of malignant bile duct obstruction for lower morbidity and mortality. Adjuvant therapy of gallbladder and bile duct tumors generally provides a low effect and the prognosis is very poor in these patients.

**Adenocarcinoma** prevails among gallbladder tumors. The possibility of radical removal is limited by the extent of the disease, and surgical treatment is not indicated in cases where the tumor has grown into the surrounding structures and distant metastases have developed. The following applies based on the **international TNM classification** for gallbladder carcinoma:
- T1 – Tumor limited to the mucosa with no infiltration of the muscular lamina
- T2 – Tumor growing into the muscular lamina
- T3 – Tumor growing into the adjacent structures (liver, duodenum, large blood vessels)

CHE is sufficient in UICC stage I (T1 N0 M0), and CHE extended by gallbladder bed resection or resection of the 4$^{th}$ and 5$^{th}$ liver segments with lymphadenectomy of the hepatoduodenal ligament region in stage II (T2 N0 M0).

Malignant tumors (adenocarcinoma) predominate also **among tumors of extrahepatic bile ducts**, and benign adenomas are rather exceptional. Tumors of the upper third of the bile duct, i.e. in the area of the common hepatic duct and the right and left hepatic ducts, are called **Klatskin tumors** and are classified based on the level of obstruction in the liver hilum. In this case, the radical procedure involves **resection of extrahepatic bile ducts with the tumor, blind closure of the supraduodenal segment of the bile duct, and hilar biliodigestive anastomosis** to the excluded jejunal loop. However, a major part of patients are treated in an inoperable stage; the palliative procedure ensures **drainage of intrahepatic bile ducts to the intestine** (using the endoscopic or more rarely surgical technique) or at least temporarily to the outside (via PTC). Carcinomas of the middle and lower thirds of the bile duct are radically removed using **partial duodenopancreatectomy** with **standard lymphadenectomies**, similarly as the pancreatic head carcinoma. Compared to the ductal carcinoma of the pancreas, the prognosis in these cases after radical surgery is somewhat better. Radical surgery is possible in both these groups of extrahepatic bile duct carcinomas only in the UICC stages I–III, i.e. T1 N0 M0, T2–T3 N0 M0 and T1–T2 N1 M0.

## 11.5 Basic Surgical Procedures in Gallbladder and Bile Ducts

Operation in the gallbladder and bile ducts is one of the most common procedures in visceral surgery. In recent years, **laparoscopic CHE** has gained preference to the traditional **conventional cholecystectomy** using laparotomic access.

A short incision made below the umbilicus is used to puncture the abdominal cavity using the Veress needle and $CO_2$ is instilled in the cavity (capnoperitoneum). The same incision is then used to insert a trocar, which serves to introduce a laparoscope with a camera in the peritoneum. The entire abdominal cavity is inspected and additional 2–3 operative entries are made in the epigastrium using the trocar. A clear view of the Calot's triangle is obtained by pulling on the gallbladder and cutting the peritoneum partially, and the cystic duct and cystic artery are prepared. Both structures are double clipped using a clamp and interrupted. The gallbladder is then removed from its bed in the retrograde and subserous mode, bleeding is coagulated, and the gallbladder is extracted after flushing the operative field. Securing drainage of the subhepatic region may be left out in many cases; suture of the fascia is necessary in middle entries. Peroperative cholangiography is not performed as a standard; ERCP with possible extraction of the stone is performed in the preoperative period when choledocholithiasis is suspected.

**Complications of laparoscopic CHE:** injury to the bile duct or hepaticus due to unclear operative situation or anatomical variants; peroperative or postoperative bleeding requiring operative revision; biliary fistula (frequently, this can be resolved by ERCP and temporary drainage of the bile duct using a stent;

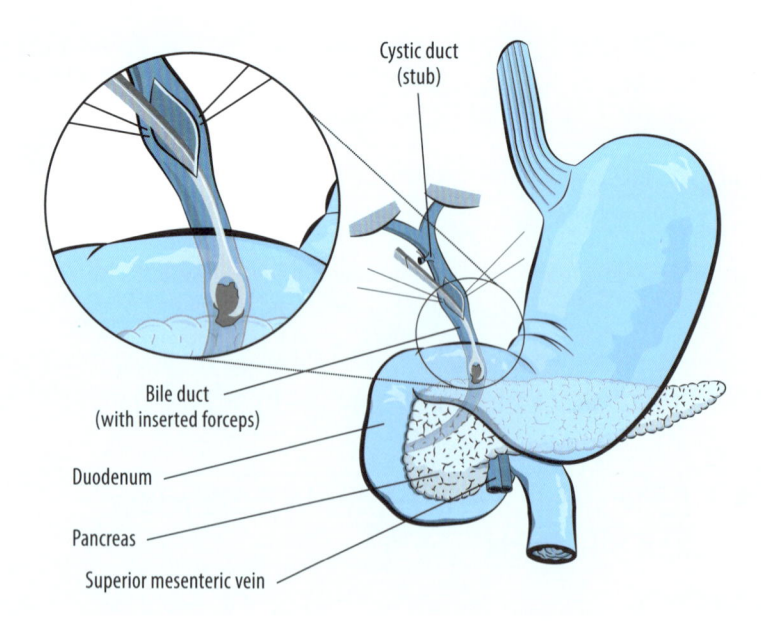

**Fig. 11.3** *Instrumental revision of the bile duct and stone extraction from bile duct using forceps*

operative revision and treatment of the injury is needed when a lesion has been demonstrated in the gallbladder wall with the stenosis). These complications apply also to conventional CHE, while their frequency is somewhat lower for conventional access. Complications specific to the laparoscopic access include an injury to intra-abdominal organs while introducing the pneumoperitoneum or trocars, loss of the stone from the gallbladder in the abdominal cavity, and an elevated risk of venous thrombosis caused by an increase in intra-abdominal pressure due to the capnoperitoneum. On the contrary, the occurrence of early infections is lower, and any hernias in the scar occur to a minimum extent.

**Bile duct surgical revision** is indicated rarely considering today's expansion of endoscopic diagnostics and therapy. These are the cases when concrements cannot be removed completely using endoscopy, or conditions inaccessible to endoscopic examination (conditions after gastric resection with B II type anastomosis, etc.). The exploration is most commonly performed from subcostal or medial laparotomy. If the gallbladder has not yet been removed, CHE is performed and the bile duct is identified. The duodenum is mobilized from the lateral side (Kocher maneuver), which makes it possible to also examine the terminal (retroduodenal) part of the bile duct. Instrumental revision of bile ducts is performed from longitudinal choledochotomy. Forceps are used to remove stones (Fig. 11.3), and both hepatic ducts and the bile duct are tubed and flushed, and the passage to the duodenum through the papilla is tubed. If a concrement is wedged or a short stenosis is found in the papilla, longitudinal duodenotomy is performed over the palpable papilla, and the papilla is incised with a sphincter (**transduodenal papillosphincterotomy**). Free tubing and extraction of the stones are thus achieved. Edges of the duodenal mucosa are sometimes fixated using fine sutures to the bile duct wall at the place of incision (**plasty of the papilla**). The duodenotomy is then closed in the transverse or longitudinal mode; choledochotomy is closed based on the anatomical situation and the finding, either using direct suture (primarily) or after insertion of the T-drain, brought outside using contraincision. The T-drain is used for transient derivation of bile, and it also allows for postoperative radiographic control. Securing drainage of the subhepatic region is used as a standard. Peroperative radiography (cholangiography) or choledochoscopy can also be used in addition to instrumental revision for bile duct examination.

## 11.6  Prognosis of Patients with Gallbladder and Bile Duct Diseases

Uncomplicated cholelithiasis can be healed using CHE; perioperative lethality is low (below 1%) and the incidence rate of serious complications is lower than 2%. The risks of surgery significantly increase in the event of complications of cholelithiasis – biliary peritonitis and biliary ileus, while a significant risk is associated with biliary pancreatitis and cholangitis. Timely indication for CHE with symptomatic cholecystolithiasis can also be considered as a preventive measure with a view to gallbladder cancer, although no direct relationship has been demonstrated. Most patients with gallbladder cancer suffer from cholecystolithiasis and chronic cholecystitis, and the majority of patients operated with early carcinoma are primarily indicated for CHE due to cholecystolithiasis. As a rule, patients after CHE need not adhere to any special dietary regimen in their further course of life. Dyspepsia and pain in the epigastrium similar to that before CHE (the so-called **postcholecystectomy syndrome**) are not common. Problems are usually caused by another GIT disease – irritable colon, gastroduodenal ulcer disease, bile duct motility disorders. However, organic changes in bile ducts should always be excluded in the first place (laboratory, US, ERCP), especially remnant choledocholithiasis, stenoses or bile duct tumors.

In general, the prognosis of patients with malignant gallbladder and bile duct diseases is one of the worst among GIT tumors. The diagnosis is often determined late, possibilities of radical removal are limited, and adjuvant therapy provides little effect.

# 12 PORTAL HYPERTENSION

*12.1 Types of Portal Hypertension*
*12.2 Pathophysiology of Portal Hypertension*
*12.3 Symptoms of Portal Hypertension*
*12.4 Clinical Findings and Complications with Portal Hypertension*
*12.5 Diagnostics of Portal Hypertension Complications*
*12.6 Bleeding from Esophageal Varices*
*12.7 Ascites – Possible Ways of Conservative and Surgical Treatment*

Venous blood of the splanchnic area is collected through three main trunks – the superior mesenteric vein, the inferior mesenteric vein and the splenic vein, which all form the portal vein after the point of their confluence. The portal vein brings blood to the liver; having flown through the liver sinuses, venous blood flows out through the hepatic veins to the inferior vena cava (**functional hepatic circulation**).

Under proper physiological conditions, the blood pressure in the trunk of the portal vein is 3–6 mmHg (0.4 to 0.8 kPa). An increase in the portal pressure may be caused by a number of various pathological conditions, causing a dilatation of side venous connections toward the low-pressure basin of the vena cava, and leading to changes in hemodynamics.

## 12.1 Types of Portal Hypertension

Three types of portal hypertension are recognized, based on the localization of the obstruction in the portal basin.

### PRESINUSOIDAL PORTAL HYPERTENSION

**Presinusoidal portal hypertension** is characterized by an obstruction in the basin of the portal vein trunk or in one of its major tributaries (segmental p. h.). Typically, the function of the liver is not impaired, and this condition is caused by myeloproliferative processes (primary polycythemia), congenital obstruction, trauma, or chronic pancreatitis (splenic vein basin).

### SINUSOIDAL PORTAL HYPERTENSION

**Sinusoidal portal hypertension (hepatic)** is the most common type in the Czech Republic; the obstruction is found in the liver parenchyma. Fibrous reconstruction of liver tissue deforms and oppresses functional sinuses and thus the pressure rises and the blood flow is slowed down. Regulatory mechanisms (volumoreceptors, perhaps also due to reduced $O_2$ content in portal blood) cause an increased inflow of arterial blood (nutritive hepatic circulation) and thus a further rise in the portal pressure. In terms of etiology, all forms of liver cirrhosis are included – alcoholic, biliary and posthepatitic. Besides complications of portal hypertension, patients are at risk of limited functional reserve of the liver (cf. classification according to Child) with the hazard of hepatic insufficiency.

### POSTSINUSOIDAL PORTAL HYPERTENSION

**Postsinusoidal portal hypertension** occurs when an obstruction is found in the area of venous drainage of the functional hepatic circulation and is relatively rare. It is used to describe the venous posthepatitic occlusion of small hepatic veins or the thrombosis of hepatic veins (Budd-Chiari syndrome).

## 12.2 Pathophysiology of Portal Hypertension

A rise in blood pressure in the portal stream leads to venous dilatation and the **dilatation of natural connections between the portal and system venous circulation** which bypasses the obstructed point. The most important connections are the following:
1. Gastric veins – esophageal veins – azygos vein, hemiazygos vein
2. Splenic vein – spleen – short gastric veins – veins in the area of distal esophagus and the cardia
3. Splenic vein – left renal vein
4. Umbilical vein – omphalomesenteric vein ("caput medusae")
5. Inferior mesenteric vein – rectal veins (hemorrhoids)

## 12.3 Symptoms of Portal Hypertension

The symptoms of portal hypertension are usually non-specific (apathy, fatigue, lack of appetite) or are masked by symptoms of an underlying disease.

## 12.4 Clinical Findings and Complications of Portal Hypertension

Typical findings include splenomegaly and sometimes also hepatomegaly (some forms or stages of cirrhosis, postsinusoidal portal hypertension), the dilatation of subcutaneous veins in the anterior abdominal wall. Varices in the lower part of the esophagus and cardia (with the portohepatic gradient over 10 mmHg, i.e. 1.33 kPa) can be demonstrated by examination; however, quite often it happens that only **complications of portal hypertension** are manifested – bleeding in the upper GIT or ascites. Other serious risks in patients with portal hypertension include portosystemic encephalopathy and spontaneous bacterial peritonitis (apparent hematogenic or lymphogenic infection of ascitic fluid).

## 12.5 Diagnostics of Portal Hypertension Complications

The leading principle of diagnostics and treatment of portal hypertension consists in influencing the underlying disease, thus predominantly conservative therapy. In terms of surgery, the issue is focused in two principal directions: **esophageal varices** and **ascites**. Ascites can be demonstrated by clinical examination, and even very low amounts of the fluid can be objectified with high precision by **US examination**. The diagnostics of esophageal varices falls in the domain of **endoscopy**; **contrast radiography** of the esophagus is used rarely for this purpose today. An endoscopic finding of a bulging site in the wall of a varicose twisted venous cord in the distal esophagus ("cherry red spots") is a clear sign of an increased risk of bleeding, which occurs in about 5% of patients with cirrhosis in the course of one year of the disease.

US examination is important to clarify the nature of portal hypertension (size and echotexture of the liver, width of the portal vein trunk), whereas **duplex US** can be used to measure the flow through the portal stream. Other complementary data can be obtained by **CT assessments, angiography and indirect splenoportography**. Then the therapeutic plan is determined, together with the assessment of **laboratory parameters of the liver function and hepatitis serology** and in the context of the clinical findings and course of portal hypertension.

## 12.6 Bleeding from Esophageal Varices

Bleeding from esophageal varices is the most serious acute complication of portal hypertension. The bleeding may be massive, and a lethality rate of up to 30% has been reported in connection with the first attack of bleeding. Early bleeding relapses within 7–10 days contribute considerably to the lethality.

The severity of the condition depends particularly on the degree of liver disorder, on hemocoagulation disorder, the gravity of renal insufficiency, the development of encephalopathy, and the activity of bleeding at initiation of the therapy.

### 12.6.1 Nonsurgical Treatment

Patients with acute bleeding in the upper GIT must be urgently admitted to a department where **intensive monitoring and treatment of circulatory disorders** can be provided. **Urgent endoscopy** is indicated in all cases for the diagnosis and localization of the bleeding source (cf. Chapter 19). Up to 30% of patients with recognized esophageal varices bleed from another source (gastroduodenal ulcer, hemorrhagic gastropathy, etc.). Endoscopic intervention also includes **endoscopic hemostasis**, which is the basis of local treatment today. Sclerotization is successful in about 80% of cases, and complications are not frequent (ulceration at the injection site with possible bleeding or perforation of the esophagus and with the development of mediastinitis). Direct endoscopic ligation of the bleeding varices using elastic rings (Barron ligature) has been promoted more in recent years, which provides at least a comparable success rate and the technique is simpler. Should endoscopic methods fail, local hemostasis is supplemented with **balloon tamponade of the distal esophagus and subcardiac area of the stomach** by inserting a Sengstaken-Blackmore tube. However, compression using inflated balloons must not take longer than 24 hours, otherwise the risk of an injury to the esophageal wall increases. Bleeding relapses tend to be quite common after the balloon compression is removed, almost in one half of the cases.

The complex treatment of bleeding from esophageal varices but also of hypertensive hemorrhagic gastropathy also includes **vasoactive treatment** aimed at restricting blood flow through the splanchnic area. An infusion with terlipressin (Remestyp) or somatostatin and its analogs is administered in the majority of cases.

Where the aforementioned ways of hemostasis are unsuccessful and bleeding from esophageal varices continues, urgent surgical treatment is an alternative that involves the insertion of a **transjugular intrahepatic portosystemic stent shunting** which connects the hepatic vein basin with a large branch of the portal vein inside the hepatic parenchyma (**TIPSS**). This procedure reduces the portohepatic gradient significantly and stops the bleeding. Compared to the surgical procedure, TIPSS in the hands of an experienced interventional radiologist means a significantly lower burden for the patient, while the result is similar to that after surgical establishment of a non-selective portosystemic shunt with all its advantages and risks (encephalopathy).

All diagnostic and therapeutic measures must take place **under permanent intensive anti-shock therapy** (volume replacement, the correction of blood coagulability disorders, oxygen therapy and controlled ventilation as the case may be). Intestinal decontamination (lactulosis, non-absorbable antibiotics, and clysmas) has proven successful in reducing the frequency of hepatic encephalopathy. Products of bacterial disintegration of partially digested blood, absorbed from the intestine, are a significant factor that increases the incidence and gravity of encephalopathy.

## 12.6.2 Possible Surgical Treatments

In the acute phase of continued bleeding from esophageal varices, surgical treatment is burdened with high lethality (bleeding relapses, liver failure) and is indicated in exceptional cases only. In this situation, **procedures preventing the inflow of portal blood to incriminated areas** (transection of the terminal esophagus using a stapler, submucosal injections of subcardiac varices according to Tores) or the **reduction of portal pressure** by establishing a portocaval shunt are options to consider.

The establishment of a portosystemic connection finds its place in **elective procedures** after survived bleeding or as prevention of other attacks. **Portosystemic connections** are surgically established anastomoses between the high pressure basin in the portal vein and the low pressure stream in the inferior vena cava basin. Besides reduced pressure in the portal stream, they usually cause reduced perfusion of liver tissue with venous blood as well and thus a worsening in hepatic functions to the extent that splanchnic blood enters system circulation without passing through the liver. This is a major disadvantage – a connection too wide will provide sufficient reduction of portal overpressure, but will also lead to severe encephalopathy. On the other hand, a connection too narrow perishes too soon, and bleeding from esophageal varices may relapse as a consequence. Therefore, this type of portosystemic connection is called **non-selective**. The most commonly used options include the mesenteric-caval H shunt via venous interponate or vascular prosthesis, direct portocaval shunt and splenorenal shunt with splenectomy (Linton). In terms of preserving liver function, only one type is suitable, the so called **selective portosystemic shunt** – distal splenorenal shunt with azygoportal disconnection according to Warren. The principle is based on termino-lateral anastomosis of the splenic vein to the left renal vein (while preserving the spleen and ligating the outlet of the splenic vein to the portal vein), which moves the risky area of the terminal esophagus to venous drainage of the low pressure system of the inferior vena cava, without restricting the inflow of splanchnic blood to the liver. Azygoportal disconnection consists in interrupting the ventricular coronary vein, the dilated branch of the portal vein that carries blood at the lesser curvature to the subcardiac area and further to the azygos vein. This procedure removes another high-pressure source of blood inflow to the area of esophageal varices. The consequences of the selective shunt on liver function are minimal; however, it is not advisable in patients with a severe hepatic lesion (Child C). Finally, **orthotopic liver transplantation** is a very successful method in the therapy of patients with portal hypertension of hepatic origin. The technical performance may be made more difficult by any prior protosystemic connection; on the other hand, TIPSS has no effect on this aspect.

### 12.6.3 Prophylaxis of Relapses after Bleeding; Prognosis

**Conservative** measures (pharmacological reduction of portal hypertension using **beta-blockers**) and **endoscopic** measures (repeated sclerotization, rubber band ligatures of the varices) are most common in the prophylaxis of relapses after bleeding from esophageal varices. Interventional (TIPSS) or surgical reduction of pressure in the portal stream is indicated only in a limited number of cases. The causal solution, **liver transplantation,** has been gaining in importance in cases where a hepatic lesion dominates.

Patients with varices without bleeding usually are not indicated for prophylactic therapy, as it cannot be determined with reliability which esophageal varices would bleed and which would not.

The prognosis of patients with bleeding from esophageal varices is always serious; after any survived bleeding and successful therapy, the prognosis is given particular to the progression of the underlying disease.

## 12.7 Ascites – Possible Ways of Conservative and Surgical Treatment

A conservative procedure is a fundamental part of the therapy of another complication of portal hypertension – ascites. Besides influencing the underlying disease, the therapy requires **restriction of liquids** to 1.5–2 liters per 24 h, **administration of diuretics** (saluretics and aldosterone antagonists), and **relieving paracentesis** is performed in advanced stages with considerable dyspnoic symptomatology. Considering albumin losses with the punctate, the losses must be compensated with IV substitution, given that ascites recur relatively quickly in these cases. **TIPSS establishment** has been used in recent years in some cases of refractory ascites (i.e. not responding to conservative therapy). The response to diuretic therapy is usually better when portal overpressure has been reduced. Surgical treatment of refractory ascites **by introducing a peritoneovenous connection** (Denver-shunt) allows for unidirectional flow of ascitic fluid to venous blood thanks to the implanted valvular system. The results are not very encouraging; serious complications include consumption coagulopathy and cardiac decompensation. The methodology of **lymphovenous anastomosis** is also based on a similar principle; in this case, the purpose of drainage between venous blood and ascitic fluid is to establish a thoracic duct with a modified outlet to the jugular vein. This solution can be described as surgical dilatation of the thoracic duct outlet to the left jugular vein from cervical access. However, the results of this approach in ascites therapy are not favorable either.

The prognosis of patients with refractory ascites is very serious given that it is an accompanying symptom of a severe hepatic function disorder. Liver transplantation may be a solution in indicated cases.

# 13 PANCREAS

*13.1 Symptoms of Pancreatic Diseases*
*13.2 Clinical Findings in Pancreatic Diseases*
*13.3 Laboratory Assessments*
*13.4 Imaging Methods*
*13.5 Acute Pancreatitis*
*13.6 Chronic Pancreatitis*
*13.7 Cystic Processes of the Pancreas*
*13.8 Pancreatic Tumors*

The pancreas is a retroperitoneally positioned parenchymatous organ with exocrine and endocrine functions. An artificial division of the pancreas into 3 parts is used. The head, closely related anatomically to the duodenum (vascular supply) and the bile duct, passes into the pancreatic body in the area of the neck (relationship to the mesenteric vessels), while the left third of the gland found in the immediate vicinity of the splenic hilum and the left adrenal gland is called the tail. Topographic relationships to the surrounding organs have a considerable effect on the symptomatology of pancreatic diseases as well as on the possibilities of surgical treatment. Vascular supply of the pancreas is provided by the celiac artery (common hepatic artery, gastroduodenal artery, splenic artery) and by the superior mesenteric artery (inferior pancreaticoduodenal artery) and their branches form together multiple anastomoses.

Insulin secretion in the beta cells of the islets of Langerhans is the most important endocrine function of the pancreas; higher numbers of these beta cells occur in the left half of the gland. Products of exocrine pancreatic secretion enter the duodenum via the major pancreatic duct (Wirsung's duct), which runs along the longitudinal axis of the gland and together with the bile duct it opens into the papilla of Vater. The minor pancreatic duct (Santorini's duct) has a variable arrangement and is less important for pancreatic drainage. In terms of physiology, lipases are the most important parts of the exocrine function given that they are not formed at any other place besides the pancreas, and therefore, a severe disorder of the pancreas function impairs the digestion of fats. On the other hand, other parts of pancreatic secretion – proteases (trypsin, elastase) and glycolytic enzymes (amylases) – can be replaced from extrapancreatic sources. Both the amount and quality of pancreatic secretion are controlled humorally (secretin, cholecystokinin), and partially they are also influenced by vagus nerve stimulation.

## 13.1 Symptoms of Pancreatic Diseases

The major symptom of pancreatic diseases is **pain**. In typical cases, patients report permanent pain in the epigastrium, propagating in bands along both costal margins to the back. Due to the vicinity of paravertebral vegetative plexuses, back pain is usually also reported, particularly at night, from which the patients seek relief by taking up a sitting or kneeling position.

Acute pain is usually associated with **nausea or vomiting**, and with **gas elimination disorder** of varied intensity; chronic pain is often accompanied by the **lack of appetite, weight loss, flatulence and loose stools** of typically fatty appearance, containing undigested residues of food. A number of "minor symptoms" such as general malaise, weakness, fatigue, loss of appetite for meat and worsened alcohol tolerance should also be considered as potentially indicating a pancreatic disease.

Anatomical relationships of the head of the pancreas to the common bile duct and duodenum determine the most common symptoms of diseases in this area, i.e. an **obstructive icterus** due to compression or infiltration of the terminal bile duct and **stomach evacuation disorders** due to compression of the duodenum. Pathological processes in the body and tail of the pancreas are not associated with these specific manifestations, and they are thus usually diagnosed late. In some cases, they may manifest by bleeding from esophageal varices due to segmental portal hypertension caused by oppression of or thrombosis in the splenic vein trunk.

Rare, hormonally active pancreatic tumors of neuroendocrine origin are associated with quite specific symptomatology, dominated by manifestations of hypersecretion of hormonally active substances (insulin, gastrin, glucagon, somatostatin, VIP).

## 13.2 Clinical Findings in Pancreatic Diseases

In acute pancreatic diseases, **pain in the epigastrium** is one of the main symptoms included in the clinical finding, with varied expression of defensive tension in muscles of the anterior abdominal wall. The pancreas itself is not accessible for clinical examination due to its retroperitoneal position, which also applies to slim patients, and palpable immobile resistances in this area are most commonly cystic formations of the pancreas (pseudocysts, cystic tumors), or advanced solid tumors in rare cases.

# PANCREAS

Similar to clinical examinations, paraclinical examinations of the pancreas are also sometimes difficult due to its position and function, and isolated reproduction of the findings may be arduous. The diagnostics of pancreatic diseases require evaluating the clinical picture in close connection with all the available auxiliary assessments perhaps even more than in other areas.

## 13.3 Laboratory Assessments

As for laboratory methods, **determination of the activity of** external secretion **enzymes** in the serum and urine (amylase, lipase) is most widely used for acute pancreatic diseases; elevation more than three times above the normal value provides evidence of acute pancreatitis. However, the finding is not very specific. Besides the usual spectrum of serum biochemical assessments completed in the diagnostics of acute abdominal pains (blood count, bilirubin, ALT, AST, urea, glycemia, minerals), determinations of Ca, ABR and especially repeated values of the **C-reactive protein (CRP)** are of particular importance in these cases for biochemical classification of the disease severity.

The assessment of tumor markers, of which the highest specificity for pancreatic diseases is **CA 19-9,** is an auxiliary method used in the differential diagnostics of tumorous changes in the pancreas, and especially in the postoperative follow-up period of patients after resection due to a carcinoma. Recurrent elevation of values provides evidence of a local relapse or distant metastases.

## 13.4 Imaging Methods

**Ultrasonography (US)** is the basic, universally available and non-invasive assessment for pancreatic diseases. While detailed assessment of changes of the pancreas may be difficult in acute conditions (covered by gas in the intestines) and in obese patients, even indirect information obtained from the examination is valuable: increase of the pancreas, fuzzy contours, fluid in the surroundings or in the free abdominal cavity (acute pancreatitis), dilatation of extrahepatic bile ducts with no evidence of cholelithiasis or possibly with dilatation of the pancreatic outlet (the "double duct sign" – tumors at the head of the pancreas or periampullary tumors), changes in the echotexture of the liver (metastases). An experienced sonographist with a good-quality device can under favorable conditions demonstrate pancreatic lesions sized over 1 cm.

The **contrast spiral CT** assessment is currently the gold standard for the diagnostics of pancreatic diseases. In cases of an unclear clinical-laboratory finding, this method can be used to confirm or exclude the diagnosis of severe acute pancreatitis (AP), and CT findings can also be used for early classification of AP grade and for precise determination of the extent and localization of pancreatic necroses including the possibility of targeted puncture of the lesion. The spiral CT examination is the decisive method in the diagnostics of focal processes in the pancreas, and in many cases, it is also used as the basis for preoperative staging. This method also provides information on dilatation of the bile ducts and of the pancreatic outlet, as well as on any presence of hepatic metastases.

Although being an invasive assessment, **endoscopic retrograde cholangiopancreatography (ERCP)** combines a diagnostic and a therapeutic component. When any signs of a bile duct obstruction are found, this method is a necessary part of the diagnostics of the origin and localization of the obstruction, and at the same time, in biliary AP, it can be used to resolve papillary obstruction caused by a stone using endoscopic papillotomy (EPT), or by introducing a bypass stent in cases where any organic stenosis of the bile duct is present due to pressure exerted from within the surroundings (an inflammation, cyst, tumor) or due to a tumor growing through it. When obstructive icterus is present and endoscopic approaches cannot be used (states after B II gastric resection, technical obstacles), **percutaneous transhepatic cholangiography (PTC)** is an option with the possibility of external or internal drainage (a stent). Serious objections have been raised recently against PTC drainage considering its invasive nature and particularly the potential for disseminating tumor cells in the peritoneum through the puncture site. On the contrary, non-invasive diagnostic options are provided by cholangiography – **magnetic resonance (MRCP)**; however, without any possibility of a concurrent therapeutic intervention.

**Endoscopic sonography (EUS)** is the most sensitive method for the diagnostics and preoperative staging of focal processes in the area of the pancreas, particularly for lesions less than 2 cm in diameter. However, its yield significantly depends on the proficiency of the examiner.

Experience with **positron emission tomography (PET)** has appeared in recent years; based on different relationships of tumorous tissue to glucose metabolism, this method can identify and differentiate the lesions of malignant tumors and the lesions of fibrosis in chronic pancreatitis. The reliability of malignant process differentiation has been estimated at 80%.

**Angiography** of the celiac artery and of the superior mesenteric artery is usually not needed to determine the relationship of the tumor to large vessels or to demonstrate any variations of arterial supply of the liver; an indication may be the effort to localize a small neuroendocrine tumor. **Scintigraphy** with labeled somatostatin is also used in these cases.

**Functional tests** of exocrine pancreatic secretion after cholecystokinin or secretin stimulation are a combination of biochemical and endoscopic diagnostics.

## 13.5  Acute Pancreatitis

**Acute pancreatitis (AP)** is primarily an **aseptic, autodigestive process in the pancreas and in the surrounding fatty tissue, inducing generalized inflammatory response (SIRS) of different** severity. A wide scale of changes may become the pathological substrate for AP, ranging from hyperemia and interstitial edema of the pancreas to extensive necrosis of pancreatic parenchyma and of the surrounding fatty and connective tissue, often with the presence of local hemorrhages. Similar to morphological changes, the clinical picture of AP is varied, and a supplementary specification – **classification of AP severity** – must thus be added to the diagnosis itself. Simplified classification to 2 basic types has been determined for clinical needs:
1. Mild AP (80% of cases) shows an uncomplicated course and subsides without any consequences with common infusion therapy during 7–10 days.
2. Severe AP (20% of patients) is a serious disease with the occurrence of general (system) and/or local complications.

**System complications**, at least in the initial phase of AP, are the consequence of SIRS and most commonly they include circulatory failure (pancreatogenic shock), respiratory insufficiency (ARDS), renal and hepatic insufficiency, hemocoagulation disorders (DIC) and neuropsychic disorders. **Local complications of AP** occur due to necrosis of the pancreas and surrounding tissues. These complications can be categorized as **septic** (infected necrosis, pancreatic abscess), **visceral** (external and internal fistulae, erosive bleeding, obstruction of the bile ducts and GIT) and **degenerative** (postnecrotic pseudocyst).

**AP incidence** in Europe has been estimated at 10–40 cases/100,000 persons annually. Mortality has been reported at about 2%; however, it rises to 20–40% in patients with a complicated course of the disease.

AP is most likely induced by joint action of several mutually potentiating factors (**multifactorial origin**), which condition – at the same time and to a different extent – secretive stimulation of the gland (fatty food, alcohol), overpressure in the outlet system of the pancreas (for example, wedged or passage of a gallstone in the papilla) and local perfusion disorder (alcohol, neurohumoral influences). **Cholelithiasis** (40%) and **alcohol** (40%) have been reported most often among known etiological factors. Other etiological influences are rare (medicines, hormonal disorders during pregnancy or the postpartum period, hyperparathyroidism, dyslipoproteinemia, viral infections, etc.). A direct or indirect trauma may also induce AP (postoperative and posttraumatic AP), as well as iatrogenic rise in the pressure in pancreatic outlets during ERCP. The etiology remains unexplained in about 15% of cases (**idiopathic AP**).

**The pathophysiological mechanisms** leading from intraparenchymatous activation of proteolytic (trypsin, elastase) and lipolytic enzymes (phospholipase

$A_2$) in the pancreas to activation of a cascade of mediator reactions in the whole organism, resulting in SIRS have not been explained in detail. Microcirculation disorders in the splanchnic area due to circulating vasoactive substances is likely to be decisive for the switching from the edematous form to necrosis of pancreatic tissue.

**Clinically, AP is defined as a disease associated with acute pain in the epigastrium, accompanied by at least a triple rise in the activity of serum amylases.** Sudden onset after a fatty meal or alcohol is typical as well as permanent severe pain spreading in bands in the epigastrium and irradiating to the back, with nausea and repeated vomiting without relief. Gas passage is also stopped as a rule. The patient is pale, sometimes sweaty, and assumes a stiff position. Besides tachycardia and decreased system pressure, oliguria and hyperventilation are present from the beginning in severe cases. Local findings in the abdomen do not always reflect the gravity of the general condition and range from mere pain in the epigastrium and meteorism to diffuse contractions of muscles of the anterior abdominal wall (however, pain p. r. is usually missing), caused by chemical irritation of the peritoneum by pancreatogenic ascites. The finding of paralytic ileus based on auscultation is also a rule in severe cases. On the contrary, some traditional "specific" signs that depend on retroperitoneal hemorrhages (Grey Turner's sign – grey marble texture on the hips) or fatty tissue hemorrhages (Cullen's sign – periumbilical cyanosis) are rarely found (in less than 10% of severe AP cases) and usually after 3–4 days.

Increased activity of serum and urine amylases is typical in the **laboratory diagnostics of AP**; however, these are not changes completely specific for AP. Rare findings of hyperamylasemia with perforation/ penetration of a gastroduodenal ulcer, high ileus or mesenteric occlusion are most important in differential diagnostics; however, they are usually lower than three times the normal value. Unlike amylase, the determination of serum lipase activity does not provide any essential benefit; however, it may lead to a diagnosis in unclear cases, particularly after a lengthy interval from the beginning of the problems, given that increased lipase activity in the serum persists longer than hyperamylasemia.

In terms of other laboratory findings, hyperbilirubinemia over 50 to 70 μmol/l is significant, which provides evidence of biliary etiology especially with elevated ALT and AST; on the contrary, hyperglycemia in this phase of AP is more a consequence of the complex metabolic disorder under stress (catecholamines) than damage of the insular apparatus. Hypocalcemia also does not reflect with reliability the gravity of the condition. CRP level assessment is used most commonly for early classification of AP severity. In the event the level is 150 mg/l or more during the first 2–5 days, this indicates severe AP with a complicated course of the disease in more than 80% of cases.

The **significance of US and CT assessments** for AP diagnostics has already been mentioned; a CT finding may be another point of departure for early classification of AP. Last but not least, **puncture-lavage of the abdominal cavity** may be helpful in differential diagnostics to differentiate AP from an acute abdomen of another origin, and also in early classification. In typical cases, the punctate has a brick-like color, shows high activity of amylases and provides evidence of severe AP in 90% of cases.

**ERCP** is indicated within 48 hours from the beginning of the disease when biliary obstruction is suspected (bilirubin over 70 mmol/l), more with a therapeutic aim than as a diagnostic method, to remove the obstruction from the papilla and thus prevent the development of complicating obstructive cholangitis.

Where another cause of an acute abdomen cannot be excluded quickly and reliably using available methods, diagnostic laparotomy in sporadic cases is indicated even today. In an emergency situation, surgical revision is lesser evil than postponing surgery for perforation peritonitis due to a gastroduodenal ulcer, biliary peritonitis or intestinal ischemia. However, "non-surgical" diseases should also be taken into account in differential diagnostics, among which an inferior myocardial infarction can induce very similar general circulatory symptomatology as well as considerable pain in the epigastrium with vomiting.

**AP therapy** is primarily conservative; surgical treatment is required with complications of pancreatic necrosis.

Mild AP is treated with success by limiting oral intake for several days and using non-specific infusion spasmolytic-analgesic therapy. In the event that cholelithiasis is found, cholecystectomy (usually laparoscopic) is indicated after the

Table 13.1 Basic therapy of severe acute pancreatitis

| | |
|---|---|
| 1. Improvement of tissue perfusion | Volume replacement (crystalloids, colloids, plasma) |
| | Inotropic support (biogenic amines) |
| 2. Oxygenation improvement | Standard oxygen therapy ($O_2$ mask 6 l/min) |
| | Controlled ventilation (with $p_aO_2$ at 8 kPa) |
| 3. Analgesia | Strong analgesics i. m. |
| | Local anestetics in infusions |
| | Epidural continuous analgesia |
| 4. Nutritional support | Parenteral branched-chain amino acids |
| | Fat emulsions |
| | Early enteral nutrition |
| 5. ERCP and EPT | Within 48 hours in case of biliary obstruction |
| 6. Prophylactic antibiotics | Upon demonstration of necrosis to reduce the risk of septic complications |

clinical finding has calmed but while hospitalization still continues. The removal of cholelithiasis is a prevention of biliary AP relapses.

Patients with severe AP should be hospitalized at an ICU (Intensive Care Unit) or ARU (Anesthesiology and Resuscitation Unit) where continuous monitoring of circulatory and respiratory functions is ensured, as well as that of diuresis, laboratory parameters and local findings in the abdomen. Clinical parameters alone may give a false relatively favorable impression in the initial phase of AP, especially in young patients with sufficient cardiopulmonary reserve. Adequate therapy is then initiated too late, when clear signs of organ dysfunctions appear (circulatory instability, renal failure, ARDS, thrombocytopenia and DIC). However, just the initial therapy may have a significant effect on the further course of the disease.

**Basic therapy of severe AP** (Table 13.1) includes clinically proven principles of intensive anti-shock therapy aimed at improving tissue perfusion, ensuring sufficient oxygenation, removing pain, covering energy expenditure, and removing the primary cause in biliary AP.

**Supplementary therapy of AP** consists in procedures well supported by pathophysiology and often successful in experiments; however, their positive effect on lethality has not been proven by clinical studies. The procedures include a number of measures aimed at influencing secretive activity of the pancreas (nasogastric aspiration, $H_2$ blockers, glucagon, 5-fluorouracil, somatostatin), methods of targeted inactivation of pancreatic enzymes (antiprotease, phospholipase $A_2$ inhibitors) and inflammatory mediators (PAF inhibitors, peritoneal dialysis). Other procedures are still the subject of clinical studies; up to now, a positive effect on the course of severe AP has been shown by the use of modern detoxification methods (hemodiafiltration) and prophylactic administration of emipenem or quinolones with metronidazole to reduce the frequency of septic complications. However, no significant reduction of lethality among patients with severe AP has been demonstrated using these procedures.

**Surgical treatment** is indicated in patients with necrosis of the pancreas and/or peripancreatic tissues who manifest septic symptomatology (fever above 38 °C, tachycardia, tachypnea, recurrent worsening of organ function in spite of intensive therapy), and in whom bacterial contamination of the necroses has been demonstrated by targeted puncture under CT supervision. In terms of microbiology, gram-negative intestinal flora (*E. coli, Pseudomonas sp.*) is found most often. The **source of the sepsis – infected necroses** (necrectomy, "debridement") – must be **removed** under these conditions, with the maximum protection of the vital tissue, and flushing **drainage of the pancreatic area** should be ensured (omental bursa and the retroperitoneum). The method of temporary closure of the abdominal cavity with planned surgical revisions in 24-hour intervals (lavage in stages) is an alternative to continuous flushing drainage of the bursa.

Another septic complication of pancreatic necrosis, **pancreatic abscess**, also requires surgical treatment (debridement and flushing drainage). Drainage using the puncture technique under CT supervision usually provides only a temporary effect due to the presence of shreds of necrotic tissue in the cavity contents.

Visceral complications are rather rare, often occurring in connection with a prior drainage surgery and insufficient necrectomy. In particular, erosive bleeding requires an urgent solution with occlusion of the bleeding vessel.

Pancreatic pseudocysts develop 4–6 weeks after the beginning of the disease, and are usually indicated for surgery in a calm stage of the disease, with clinical symptoms of oppression (see Section 13.7).

AP even in its severe form subsides without any considerable consequences; only extensive losses of the parenchyma usually cause development of diabetes and/or exocrine insufficiency. Recently, it has been recognized that about 20% of AP cases change into chronic pancreatitis, or that they are **a priori** acute attacks of chronic pancreatitis with a picture identical to that of AP.

## 13.6 Chronic Pancreatitis

Chronic pancreatitis is a gradually progressing or occurring in repeated attacks abacterial inflammation of the exocrine pancreas that leads to reconstruction of the functional parenchyma with fibrous tissue. Thus, besides **pain** (90–95% cases), **signs of exocrine and endocrine insufficiency** of the pancreas dominate in advanced stages of chronic pancreatitis, and often also **complications due to oppression of the surrounding structures**.

In terms of **etiology**, the vast majority of cases of chronic pancreatitis in the Czech Republic are associated with excessive alcohol consumption, and rarely with metabolic disorders (hyperparathyroidism, mucoviscidosis) or genetic effects (hereditary pancreatitis). In terms of **pathogenesis** of chronic pancreatitis, it is not yet clear whether the primary lesion is a disorder of the pancreatic juice solution stability associated with the formation of precipitates or calcifications and subsequent reactive process in the outlet system of the gland (obstruction theory), or whether it is primarily represented by focal necroses in the parenchyma with subsequent scarring that deforms the outlets, and thus also leads to a pancreatic secretion drainage disorder (sequence theory). Both cases result in characteristic changes of the outlet system of the pancreas – stenoses and dilatations.

**The basic clinical symptom of chronic pancreatitis is pain**, typically localized in the epigastrium and irradiating to the back. It may be present virtually permanently or come in relapsing attacks, often clinically undifferentiable from AP. Only a small portion of patients with chronic pancreatitis have no pain. Vomiting and blocked passage may accompany acute attacks of pain; however, in interim periods, patients often report **meteorism, voluminous loose stools**

(external insufficiency) **or nausea, loss of appetite, feeling full after meals, and pressure in the epigastrium** (gastric evacuation disorder). Typical cases are men in middle age (40–50 years of age) with alcoholic history and a **bad nutritional status**. Besides acute attacks, the clinical findings in the abdomen may be poor, while **hyperperistalsis** (frequent bowel sounds) is demonstrated more commonly. Findings of free fluid in the abdominal cavity (pancreatic ascites) or a palpable pseudotumor in the epigastrium are rare even in advanced stages of chronic pancreatitis, as well as splenomegaly with segmental portal hypertension (oppression of the splenic vein). On the contrary, **icterus** of varied intensity, caused by oppression of the bile duct, is not a very rare finding in advanced chronic pancreatitis.

In addition to routine laboratory assessments, a crucial role is played by **ERCP** (imaging of the morphology of pancreatic outlets) and **CT assessment** (size, focal changes, calcifications, dilatation of the outlet) in the **diagnostics** of chronic pancreatitis. However, even simple **native radiography** of the abdomen can demonstrate calcifications in the area of the pancreas in about 50% of patients with chronic pancreatitis, which strongly support the diagnosis.

**The therapy of chronic pancreatitis** is in most cases conservative and a surgical solution is indicated only if the therapy fails or if complications occur in the further course. Causal therapy is not known. Symptomatic therapy is the basis and it is usually managed by a gastroenterologist and it is focused particularly on the **substitution of insufficient exocrine secretions** (enzyme preparations), with a **fat-restricted diet and no alcohol**. Depending on the severity of the glucose tolerance disorder (about 30% of patients), antidiabetic or insulin therapy is necessary in addition to appropriate diet. The most problematic is the **treatment of pain**, sometimes leading to dependence on strong analgesics. Pain seems to be closely related to overpressure in pancreatic outlets, and therefore, relieving the overpressure by bypassing the stenosis before the dilated outlet usually provides a good effect. This result can also be achieved using other than surgical approaches, i.e. using **endoscopy**, by transpupillarily inserted drainage of the pancreatic outlet using a plastic stent, possibly combined with the removal of any present concrements. However, the effect of this treatment is often only temporary.

**Indications for surgical treatment** of chronic pancreatitis include **progressive pain not managed by conservative therapy, stenoses of the bile duct and duodenum** caused by fibrous changes in the head of the pancreas or by pressure of pseudocysts, and the not so rare suspicion of a **malignant pancreatic tumor**. Surgery is less commonly required by complications such as bleeding in the pseudocyst, perforation into a free peritoneal cavity, internal fistulae or bleeding from esophageal varices with segmental portal hypertension due to oppression or thrombosis of the splenic vein.

The **principle of surgeries due to chronic pancreatitis** consists in relieving the overpressure in dilated pancreatic outlets often containing stones (drainage surgery), or in removal of the tissue of the head of pancreas, which not only exerts

# PANCREAS

pressure on the surroundings, but apparently also functions as an "engine" of the progressive course of chronic pancreatitis (resection procedures).

Among **drainage surgeries**, the most common procedure is the extraction of a wedge-shaped part of the parenchyma longitudinally above the dilated Wirsung's duct with pancreatojejunoanastomosis latero-laterally over the excluded jejunal loop (Partington-Rochelle).

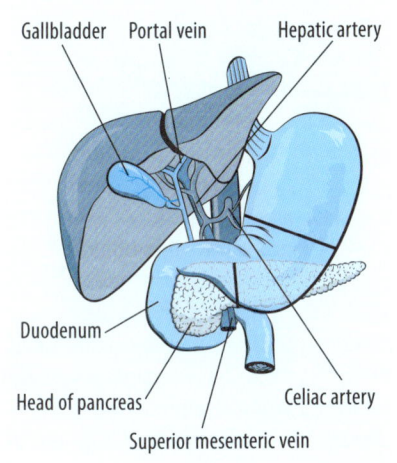

**Fig. 13.1** *Partial duodenopancreatectomy according to Whipple – scope of resection*

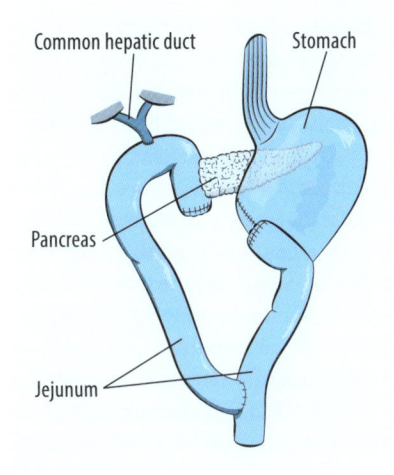

**Fig. 13.2** *Partial duodenopancreatectomy according to Whipple – reconstruction phase*

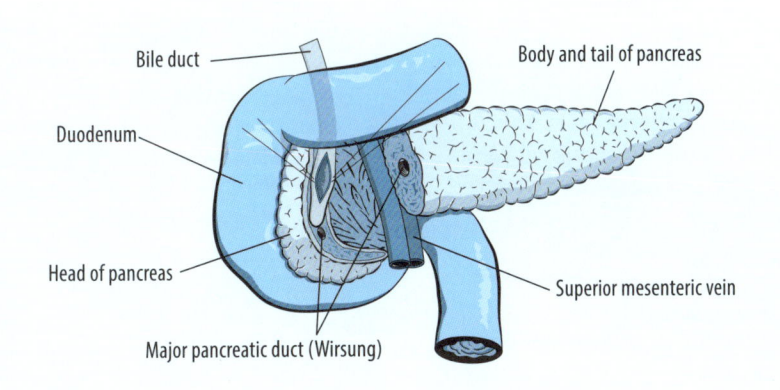

**Fig. 13.3** *Duodenum preserving resection of the head of pancreas according to Beger – scope of resection*

**Resection procedures** stem from classical partial duodenopancreatectomy (Kausch-Whipple) (Figs. 13.1 and 13.2), currently often performed in the pylorus preserving modification (Traverso-Longmire). A compromise between both types of surgeries is represented by the **resection of the head of the pancreas preserving the duodenum** (Berger) (Figs. 13.3 and 13.4) and **limited resection of the head of the pancreas** or extended drainage surgery (Fray) (Figs. 13.5 and 13.6).

With suitable indications, the results of surgical treatment are very satisfactory, especially in regards to the effect on pain. Worsening of the external or internal secretory function of the pancreas is not a rule even after resection procedures. Patients with chronic pancreatitis require permanent monitoring of the development of their disease; it is not yet clear whether the course of the disease can be stopped completely or only slowed down. Further therapy after surgery for chronic pancreatitis is also targeted only symptomatically.

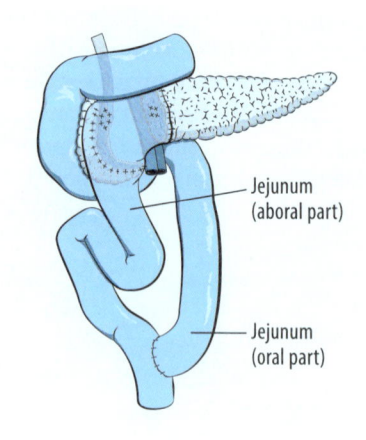

*Fig. 13.4 Duodenum preserving resection of the head of pancreas according to Berger – reconstruction using excluded jejunal loop*

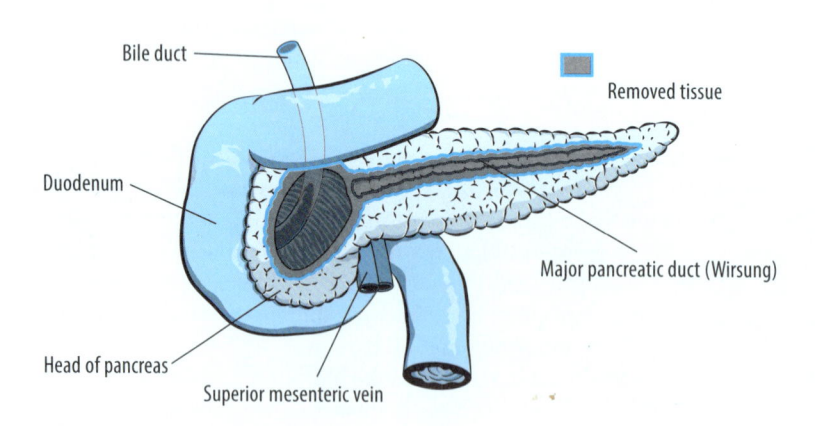

*Fig. 13.5 Limited resection of the head of pancreas according to Fray – scope of resection of pancreatic tissue*

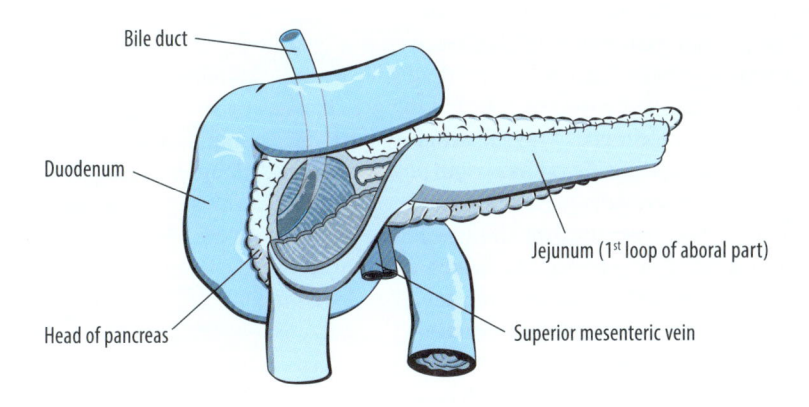

**Fig. 13.6** *Limited resection of the head of pancreas according to Fray – reconstruction using excluded jejunal loop*

## 13.7 Cystic Processes of the Pancreas

Cystic processes in the area of the pancreas are an inhomogeneous group of diseases in terms of nosology; however, their differentiation provides important consequences for the choice of the therapeutic procedure.

Besides cystic processes of the pancreas, the clinical finding of any immovable resistance in the middle epigastrium should lead to also considering the possibility of an advanced gastric tumor or abdominal aortic aneurysm as part of the **differential diagnostics**. However, only a minor portion of cystic processes reach the size accessible to common physical examination. **Imaging methods, US and CT assessments** are the basic methods for demonstrating these processes. Information essential for determining the therapeutic strategy is also provided by **ERCP examination**.

The **symptomatology** of cystic processes of the pancreas is determined especially by their localization and size – pressure exerted on the surrounding structures causes **gastric evacuation disorders** (vomiting, feeling of fullness in the epigastrium) or **bile duct obstruction**. Depending on the position, even relatively large formations may be asymptomatic, and incomparably smaller ones may give rise to obstructive symptoms. However, **pain** in the epigastrium and in the back is the most common symptom of these processes. In rare cases, symptoms based on occlusion of the transverse colon, bleeding or spontaneous rupture associated with spreading of the contents in the peritoneal cavity may occur.

As for their **morphology**, cystic formations in the pancreatic area represent quite a non-uniform group: **pseudocysts are found in 90 % cases** (cystic formations without their own epithelial lining, whose wall is formed by fibrous tissue newly created due to an inflammation) and **true cysts or cystic tumors both of a benign and malignant nature, respectively**, represent the remaining **10%**.

**Pseudocysts** are formed as a consequence of the accumulation of fluids with a necrotic portion particularly around the pancreas, away from the parenchyma itself (postnecrotic pseudocysts with AP – ERCP examination shows normal finding at the pancreatic outlets – and postnecrotic pseudocysts within the realm of chronic pancreatitis – showing changes in outlet pathways of the pancreas typical for this disease). However, retention pseudocysts are also formed in the course of chronic pancreatitis, which are characterized, besides characteristic changes in the outlet system of the pancreas, by communication with the outlets and predominantly intraparenchymatous localization in the pancreas demonstrable by ERCP examination. Pseudocysts formed in connection with AP show a clearly higher tendency to spontaneous resorption, while on the contrary longer lasting pseudocysts in the course of chronic pancreatitis are associated with a higher risk of complications.

Pseudocysts causing clinical problems are indicated for **therapy**, especially those larger than 5 cm in diameter and showing no tendency to become smaller based on US supervision. **US or CT targeted puncture** and possibly drainage are indicated as urgent measures upon an infection of the content or for diagnostic evacuation (CA 19-9 assessment for differentiation from cystic tumors); however, such a procedure is associated with a higher rate of relapses and the risk of fistulae in the puncture channel. In the event of suitable localization of the pseudocyst, its puncture-based anastomosis with the stomach or duodenum can be performed over a stent using **endoscopy**; however, the most effective are surgical procedures – **pseudocystojejunoanastomosis through an excluded Roux-loop** or **resection procedures** where multiple intraparenchymatous pseudocysts are present in chronic pancreatitis.

**Cystic tumors** of the pancreas can be categorized in a simplified manner based on their content as **serous (microcystic) cystadenomas** with very rare malignant transformation, and as **mucinous (macrocystic) cystadenomas** with frequent malignization into **cystadenocarcinoma**. The disease affects predominantly younger women, and the prognosis after **resection therapy** is incomparably better even with large sizes and malignant nature of the tumors compared to a pancreatic ductal adenocarcinoma. Five-year survival is achieved in 55 to 65% of cases.

Other cystic tumors of the pancreas are rare (papillary-cystic or solid pseudopapillary tumor, some cystic neuroendocrine tumors).

## 13.8 Pancreatic Tumors

Tumorous diseases of the pancreas, represented most commonly by adenocarcinoma of the outlet epithelium, rank among the most malignant tumors of the GIT.

# PANCREAS

Currently, pancreatic cancer occupies the 4th position among causes of death of patients with malignancy and the incidence thereof shows a rising trend. In spite of all advancements of modern medicine, the prognosis of patients with pancreatic tumors still remains very poor and the mean survival time from diagnosis is only 8 months. Very often, this is conditioned by late diagnostics given that about 90% of pancreatic tumors are revealed in an advanced stage, but also by very limited possibilities of therapy. Curative resection is possible only in approx. 2–5% of patients and various regimens of adjuvant radiochemotherapy have not brought any significant improvement of survival.

**Incidence** of pancreatic tumors in the Czech Republic is about 15 cases per 100,000 persons annually.

**Etiology** is unclear; besides genetic influences (hereditary pancreatitis), reported risk factors include cigarette smoking, fatty and meaty food, chronic pancreatitis and gastroduodenal ulcers. The disease affects more men than women (2:1) of mid to older age (55–70 years).

**Symptoms** of pancreatic tumors are linked to their relationships to the surrounding structures, while only a small portion of tumors with endocrine activity show specific symptomatology conditioned by the excessive production of hormones.

In cases where the tumor is localized in the head of the pancreas (about 80% of all pancreatic tumors), symptoms due to bile duct obstruction are predominant, while symptoms due to duodenal stenosis or pancreatic outlet stenosis are rather rare. **Icterus** associated with no pain is the most common symptom leading to diagnosis, which occurs in 90% of cases of tumors in the head of the pancreas. On the contrary, tumors in the area of the body and tail seldom cause specific problems and are diagnosed in advanced stages when they provoke **pain in the epigastrium and in the back**. Rarely, they may manifest by bleeding from esophageal varices and by splenomegaly due to occlusion of the splenic vein. A number of "minor" symptoms of tumorous diseases are often reported precisely in the history of patients with pancreatic tumors (weight loss, loss of appetite, weakness, loss of performance, etc.).

Except in cases of bile duct obstruction (ALP, bilirubin), **laboratory** assessments show no specific changes. Elevated tumor markers (CA 19-9) may provide evidence of a malignant process; glucose tolerance disorder or worsened compensation of existing diabetes may sometimes be found.

As for **examination methods**, US is of decisive screening importance; direct evidence of a tumor is provided rather rarely. CT assessment offers relatively high evidential force for focal changes in the pancreas including their relationship to the surroundings; besides the diagnostic benefit, ERCP assessment also has a therapeutic value upon temporary or permanent overcoming of an obstruction in the bile duct (drainage through a stent). Today, EUS is the most sensitive method used to demonstrate even small lesions in the pancreas and for tumor staging (size, relationship to the surroundings).

Evaluation of the **biological nature** of an expansive lesion in the pancreas by imaging and laboratory methods is not reliable. As a rule, a tumor cannot be differentiated from fibrous changes due to chronic pancreatitis using a macroscopic method in the peroperative period, either; only histological assessment can be considered as valid. Targeted puncture biopsies do provide value but only for positive demonstration of malignancy, although they are associated with a high chance of error in the collection of materials from the surroundings of the lesion. PET assessment has not fulfilled expectations either, although the differentiation of the malignant nature of a lesion is possible in about 80% of cases.

**Indication for surgery** is determined with the aim of **radical resection** of the tumor or **exploration and palliative therapy**.

Radical removal of the tumor with the surrounding structures and regional lymphadenectomy are the only therapeutic measure with a demonstrable positive effect on survival of patients with pancreatic tumors. Therefore, patients with a lesion of the tissue of unclear biological nature are also indicated for resection; as for operable processes, a tumor is present in about 70% of cases. Preoperative assessment of the extent and relationships of the tumor to the surroundings (**staging**) is a condition of correct indication. Resection is not indicated in cases where distant metastases are found (liver, peritoneum) or with infiltration of large vessels (superior mesenteric artery and vein, portal vein), given that it has no effect on the survival of the patients. Staging is then reviewed in the peroperative period and definitely upon histological assessment of the resecate. These findings are then decisive for potential indication of adjuvant therapy and for more accurate determination of the prognosis of the disease. The **TNM system with UICC classification** is used in Europe.

The following applies to pancreatic tumors:
- T1 – Tumor size up to 2 cm, limited to the pancreas
- T2 – Tumor larger than 2 cm, limited to the pancreas
- T3 – Tumor infiltrating the duodenum, bile duct, peripancreatic tissues
- T4 – Tumor infiltrating large vessels, the stomach, colon, spleen
- N0 – Regional lymph nodes without any malignant cells
- N1 – Tumor infiltration of regional lymph nodes
- M0 – Distant metastases are not present
- M1 – Evidence of distant metastases (liver, peritoneum, etc.)

Stage I – T1 and T2 N0 M0, stage II – T3 N0 M0, stage III – T1 to T3 N1 M0, stage IVa – T4 N0 and N1 M0, stage IVb T1-T4 N0-N1 M1.

The resection procedure can be considered as radical if the findings correspond to stages I and II and if R0 resection has been achieved (i.e. no residues of the tumor are left, not even microscopic). When the lymph node finding is positive, the procedure is only potentially radical, even with R0 resection with standard lymphadenectomy.

In terms of **histology, adenocarcinoma** stemming from the epithelium of pancreatic outlets occurs most frequently (**ductal carcinoma**). This most serious variant in terms of prognosis represents about 90–95% of all pancreatic tumors. The mean survival after the resection is 12–18 months in these cases. The remaining 5–10% of tumors are represented by **cystic tumors of the pancreas** (see Section 13.7) and **neuroendocrine tumors of the pancreas**. Metastasis of another tumor (Grawitz tumor of the kidney) is found relatively rarely.

Histological classification of the tumor is seldom available in the preoperative period, and thus the resection procedure strategy is standard. **Partial duodenopancreatectomy** (removal of the duodenum and right half of the pancreas together with the gallbladder and bile duct and with the distal part of the stomach – Whipple procedure, or leaving the pylorus – Traverse surgery) is performed with **regional lymphadenectomy** when the tumor is localized in the head of the pancreas. When the tumor is localized in the body or tail, **left-sided resection of the pancreas is performed with regional lymphadenectomy and splenectomy**. Limited resection or also local excision of the circumscribed tumor is possible only in a minor part of **neuroendocrine tumors** that show endocrine activity and exhibit typical symptomatology due to excessive production of the respective hormone (approx. 30% of neuroendocrine tumors). These tumors are in most cases of a benign nature. B cell **insulinomas** are most common, manifested by hypoglycemic episodes. Excessive production of gastrin with the development of relapsing and atypically localized ulcers in the stomach, duodenum and jejunum (Zollinger-Ellison syndrome) is characteristic for a **gastrinoma**. The remaining 70% of neuroendocrine tumors without endocrine activity are predominantly malignant; however, their prognosis after the resection procedure is clearly better than that of a ductal carcinoma.

Besides tumors stemming from the pancreas, **adenocarcinoma of the terminal bile duct and tumors of the papilla of Vater (ampullomas)** are also classified as tumors of the head of the pancreas. Preoperative and often also peroperative assessment of the primary originating site of the tumor is virtually impossible. The scope of the resection procedure is similar for all these possibilities. The prognosis of tumors of the bile duct and of the ampulla is after all more favorable, with approximately double the number of cases of 5-year survival after the resection compared to the ductal carcinoma (30–40%). Considering their localization in the area around the papilla, these tumors are also jointly described as **periampullary tumors** (i.e. within 2 cm from the papilla). However, they do not form a nosological unit in the real sense of the word due to their different prognoses and histological differences mentioned above.

In cases of an advanced tumorous disease (demonstration of distant metastases, local inoperability of the tumor), only **palliative** surgery is indicated to remove any bile duct obstruction and/or duodenal stenosis. Some patients with preoperative demonstration of liver metastases and in a generally serious condition are treated using **endoscopy – by inserting a stent in the bile duct through the obstruction**. This procedure is burdened with minimum complications and is associated with low hospitalization morbidity and mortality. However, clogging of the stent or dislocation occur commonly with longer survival, which requires additional repeated interventions. In addition, gastric evacuation disorders due to duodenal oppression progress in these patients sometimes, which then require surgery. Therefore, **surgical palliative therapy** is indicated in patients in a general good condition and with the perspective of survival longer than 5 months – **cholecystectomy with hepaticojejunoanastomosis through an excluded Roux-loop supplemented with gastroenteroanastomosis** (also prophylactic).

As mentioned above, the prognosis of patients with pancreatic tumors depends on the histological structure of the process and on the possibilities of radical surgical resection. In the vast majority of malignant tumors, which unfortunately to a considerable extent predominate, the prognosis is very poor. Convincing results of sufficiently large clinical studies are not yet available to establish standard adjuvant radio- and/or chemotherapy. The same applies to preoperative (neoadjuvant) chemotherapy and peroperative radiotherapy. All these procedures have been intensively explored as it is apparent that surgical resection by itself is not a sufficient measure for the majority of patients with pancreatic carcinoma.

# 14 SPLEEN SURGERY

> 14.1 Anatomy
> 14.2 Function and Physiology of the Spleen
> 14.3 Splenic Malformations
> 14.4 Spleen Surgery
> 14.5 Splenomegaly

## 14.1 Anatomy

The spleen is an intraperitoneally localized organ found under the left diaphragm, covered by the diaphragm from above, by the $9^{th}$-$11^{th}$ ribs from the front, from the side and partially from the back, and also by the spine from the back. The spleen is surrounded by serous tunic, grown together with the capsule of the spleen – the fibrous tunic. The splenic tissue is formed by dense fibrous trabeculae with splenic pulp found between them. The pulp consists of fine reticular fibrous tissue, forming a spatial grid. The pulp has two components – red, which represents about 75% of the splenic tissue, and whose sinuses are filled with blood and plasma elements; and white, representing about 25%, which is formed by lymphatic tissue. The spleen usually weighs 100 to 250 g and there is only one.

The spleen localized elsewhere is called ectopic, separated parts of the spleen are termed splenosis.

Vascular supply is ensured particularly by the splenic artery and vein, both of which branch in the splenic hilum to form vessels of lower order – segmental and trabecular. Additional vascular supply is provided by accessory vessels approaching the spleen in a non-constant mode.

## 14.2 Function and Physiology of the Spleen

The spleen is the largest organ of the reticuloendothelial system and provides hematological, immune and hemodynamic functions. Old and damaged blood elements are captured in the spleen; it is a reservoir of erythrocytes and thrombocytes, and also the site of extramedullary blood formation under pathological circumstances. Its immune function arises from the number of phagocytic cells (macrophages and reticulocytes), which capture pathogenic particles from the blood. The spleen participates in the formation of antibodies of IgM and T lymphocyte types, in the formation of autoantibodies, and in the formation of opsonins. Hemodynamic functions consist in maintaining equilibrium between circulating and deposited blood elements, and in participation in the blood coagulation process.

The spleen is not necessary for life. The highest risk following splenectomy is reduced resistance against infections, or potential reduction in anticancer immunity, and blood formation in exceptional events. Elevated spleen function – hypersplenism – leads to changes in hematopoiesis; it is characterized by splenomegaly, cytopenia in peripheral blood and escalated blood formation in the bone marrow.

## 14.3  Splenic Malformations

Congenital disorders include **aplasia** and **hypoplasia** of the spleen, **accessory spleen** (in approx. 25%), congenital splenic **cysts** and possibly **splenoptosis** ("wandering spleen").

## 14.4  Spleen Surgery

Spleen surgeries are indicated due to injuries, for hematological causes, and exceptionally for other reasons, such as the need for vascular surgery. An **injury to the spleen** is often the consequence of abdominal injuries:
- Blunt abdominal traumas, injury of the left hemithorax
- Penetrating abdominal traumas
- Ruptures of pathologically increased spleen upon minimal injury
- Iatrogenic injury to the spleen during operations in the epigastrium

An injury may affect the capsule or parenchyma of the spleen or splenic vessels upon tearing of the spleen from the hilum. **Based on the extent**, injuries to the spleen are classified as grade I to V; subcapsular hematoma is the least extensive injury and complete dilaceration of the spleen is the most extensive injury (Fig. 14.1).

**According to the clinical course**, **single-period** and **double-period ruptures** are recognized. A single-period rupture is followed by bleeding immediately after the injury. Upon dilaceration of the spleen or upon hilar vessel injuries the bleeding is intense, clinically expressed by hemorrhagic shock and hemoperitoneum – an **acute form** (classification grades 4 and 5), or a **subacute form**

# SPLEEN SURGERY

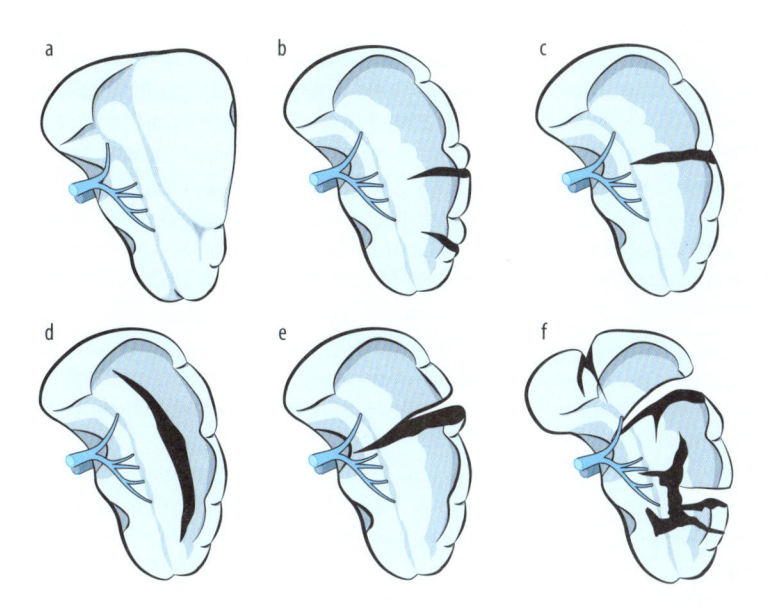

**Fig. 14.1** *Injury to the spleen: a) Subcapsular hematoma of the spleen; b) Transverse tear in the spleen; c) Deep transverse tear reaching the splenic hilum; d) Deep longitudinal tear not achieving the hilum; e) Tear that reaches the hilum; f) Multiple tears – dilaceration, fragmentation*

(grades 1–3) where the injury is less serious. Upon double-period rupture, the interval between the trauma and bleeding may last from one hour up to months.

**Symptoms** – subjective symptoms include pain in the left shoulder due to irritation of the phrenic nerve by blood in the subdiaphragm area (especially Kehr's sign), weakness up to collapse; objective symptoms include bulging of the abdomen which increases, bulging of the Douglas area upon indagation (Delbet's sign), tachycardia over HR 100/min, hypotension, decrease of the central venous pressure, decreased blood count values, leukocytosis, and decreased diuresis.

In terms of **diagnostics**, information on any prior injury is important, as well as the above-mentioned symptoms that provide evidence of intra-abdominal bleeding.

Radiography may reveal rib fractures. Fluid around the spleen and in the abdomen based on US or CT examination (the case that the fluid is blood should always be suspected upon any injury) provides evidence of an injury to the spleen; or a rupture may even be visible using these examinations. **(Diagnostic puncture and lavage of the abdomen as recommended in the past has lost meaning.)**
**Therapy** is conservative and surgical. Conservative therapy can be used to treat spleen injuries with no manifestations of circulatory instability, i.e. with

minimum bleeding (subcapsular hematomas). Intensive monitoring and the possibility to repeat the US examination to confirm that the finding does not progress are the conditions for conservative therapy. **Signs of intense bleeding** in the abdominal cavity, associated with the acute form, are an **indication for immediate surgery**. There is no time or reason to perform any other examinations in such cases given that any postponement intensifies the consequences of such bleeding.

In the subacute form, the diagnosis may be specified closer using the above-mentioned examinations.

The surgical procedure performed is a **splenectomy**; surgeries to preserve the spleen (suture, resection, hemostasis by gluing, pressure, electrocoagulation, and grid) are possible only exceptionally. Reimplantation of the splenic tissue is currently not recommended.

Iatrogenic injuries to the spleen during surgery pose no diagnostic troubles and their treatment is identical to that described above.

**Hematological reasons** for splenectomy include hypersplenism, hemolytic anemias, idiopathic thrombocytopenic purpura, primary (hemangioma, lymphangioma, sarcomas) and secondary tumors of the spleen (for example, Hodgkin's disease).

A splenectomy is indicated for **vascular reasons** only upon thrombosis of the splenic vein or when establishing a non-selective splenorenal shunt with portal hypertension.

Requirements for radical surgery are often the reason for a splenectomy **in oncosurgical procedures** in the stomach or pancreas, arising from lymphadenectomy along splenic vessels.

The main **risks of a splenectomy** include post-operative **bleeding**, post-operative **thrombosis** with a tendency to thromboses and **infections**. Thrombosis especially affects the ligated splenic vein, with a risk of spreading to the portal vein. The tendency to infections entails predominantly pneumococcal *Haemophilus influenzae* infections. The most severe manifestation of the infection is the so-called **OPSI syndrome** – overwhelming post splenectomy infection. The term OPSI syndrome is used for foudroyant sepsis with otherwise banal infections particularly of the upper respiratory pathways, accompanied by early organ dysfunction (especially DIC). The risk of OPSI syndrome in persons after splenectomy is about 1–2%; however, the lethality rate is as high as 40–70%. Prevention includes prophylactic application of PNC and vaccination.

Late complications include **splenosis**, i.e. ectopic splenic tissue clogged with the implantation of small particles of the splenic parenchyma.

## 14.5 Splenomegaly

The spleen is most commonly enlarged in the event of hematological diseases, liver diseases, autoimmune diseases and sepsis. The symptomatology arises from the underlying disease. As for surgical differential diagnostics, it is important that splenomegaly may lead to mechanical oppression in the abdomen and thus cause, for example, intestinal passage disorders, pain due to splenic infarctions or pain due to stretching of the spleen capsule.

An enlarged spleen can be demonstrated by physical examination – palpation; only extreme splenomegaly may be visible. Sonography is used for more precise examination, while absolute precision is offered by CT or MRI examinations. Doppler sonography is used to examine the flow and patency of splenic vessels. Imaging methods used to show the size of the spleen indirectly by oppression of the surrounding structures are no longer used, similar to radionuclide methods.

The aim of hematological examination of the spleen is to confirm tumorous infiltration or extramedullary hematopoiesis by splenic puncture or biopsy, respectively.

Examinations performed upon injury to the spleen have been mentioned (Section 14.4).

# 15 ACUTE ABDOMEN IN GENERAL, BASIC DIAGNOSTICS

> 15.1 Introduction and Definition
> 15.2 Classification of Acute Abdomen
> 15.3 Diagnostics
> 15.4 Differential Diagnostics

## 15.1 Introduction and Definition

Acute abdomen (AA) is defined as an abdominal process causing severe pain of sudden onset (often from full health), often requiring surgical intervention. It requires immediate diagnostics and therapy given that when left untreated they lead to serious complications including those endangering life.

For the physician, the diagnostics and therapy of AA require knowledge of and experience in differential diagnostics of diseases of abdominal cavity organs, stemming primarily from good-quality collection of the medical history, conscientious physical examination of the patient, and meaningful indication of additional paraclinical assessments. Given that AA is a contition associated with dynamic development in time, the attending physician is required to be able to continuously determine new anamnestic data and seek new symptoms of the developing disease, and the ability to analyze all new information again and again and to respond in time with suitable therapy and even to "radically" change the original therapeutic plan as the case may be. The attending physician should be well acquainted with the differences in the courses of various intra-abdominal diseases in childhood, advanced age and in pregnancy. The number of patients ventilated at ARUs, dialyzed, on antibiotics, chemotherapeutics, non-steroidal antiflogistics, cytostatics and immunosuppressives have been rising steadily. In these patients, their symptoms and the course of AA may be modified by the nature of the primary disease or its therapy. And last but not least, the doctor must not underestimate the so-called "minor symptoms", as these are often the only ones leading to proper diagnosis. Specific symptomatology, diagnostics and therapies of the diseases of individual abdominal cavity organs are described in appropriate chapters.

## 15.2 Classification of Acute Abdomen

Considering the lack of time for diagnostic circumspection and for deciding on the manner of therapy (surgical or conservative), the scheme of AA classification should be understood as a primary algorithm to be memorized by the doctor. Furthermore, it should be kept in mind that in the course of time, clinical symptomatology of an originally ileous AA may transform to inflammatory symptomatology (for example, untreated mechanical ileus caused by a sigmoideal tumor causes diffuse peritonitis after distension and perforation of the colon), and vice versa, the symptoms of an inflammatory AA may transform to ileus symptoms in the course of time (perforated appendicitis with diffuse peritonitis induces signs of paralytic ileus early on).

Classification of acute abdomen:

### NON TRAUMA BASED

1. Inflammatory
   – Inflammation limited to an organ (appendicitis, cholecystitis, diverticulitis, pancreatitis, cholangitis and gastritis)
   – Circumscribed inflammation transferred to the nearest surroundings (circumscribed peritonitis, abscesses, inflammatory infiltrates)
   – Non-circumscribed spreading of the inflammation (diffuse peritonitis)
2. Ileus
   – Mechanical ileus
     a) Obturation type
     b) Strangulation type
   – Neurogenic ileus
     a) Paralytic
     b) Spastic
   – Vascular ileus
3. Perforation events
4. Intense bleeding in the GIT

### TRAUMA BASED

1. Perforation peritonitis
2. Traumatic hemoperitoneum
3. Mixed form (perforation peritonitis + traumatic hemoperitoneum)

The knowledge of frequency with which individual organs are affected in an acute abdomen is also important because in the event of similar symptomatology, more common diseases should be excluded first and then proceed to those that are not so common. Acute abdomen occurrence based on the affected organ:

acute appendicitis 55%, acute cholecystitis 15%, mechanical ileus 10%, gastroduodenal ulcer perforation 7%, acute pancreatitis 5%, other 8%.

## 15.3 Diagnostics

### 15.3.1 Medical History

For AA, the medical history is the basis of a proper diagnosis. Especially the current development of local symptoms (pain and muscle contractions) and general symptoms (body temperature, heart rate, skin color, shivers and chills, GIT passage disorders) are emphasized, as well as previous and current diseases, surgeries, injuries, pregnancies, factors related to the occurrence of problems and their dynamics. For any observed symptoms, it is important not only whether they are or were present but also their frequency, characteristics, localization, progression, etc.

■ PAIN

- **Visceral pain** – stems from abdominal cavity organs and the retroperitoneum. It is difficult to localize and characterize for the patient (blunt, burning, pressure). In the initial phase of the disease, patients often localize the pain in the epigastrium. Diseases of individual organs are usually reflected in various areas of the abdominal wall; however, the areas do not correspond to the anatomical position of an organ (pain in the epigastrium, mesogastrium, hypogastrium, in the right or left half). Visceral pain may be colicky, may issue from hollow organs (variable, rhythmic, spasmodic, forcing the patient to move). The pain may occur suddenly in the course of several seconds (gastric perforation) or it may develop gradually. Somatic pain occurs when the inflammation also affects the parietal peritoneum (and thus surpasses the borderline of an organ).
- **Somatic pain** – stems from the parietal peritoneum and is a sign of irritation, and thus a sign of an advanced stage of the disease. It can be localized with accuracy by the patient in the area of the affected organ. Diffuse peritonitis with pain in the whole abdomen develops upon further progression of the disease.

■ GIT PASSAGE DISORDERS

**Nausea and vomiting** may be of reflexive origin, may be caused by irritation of visceral afferent nerve fibers, or may be caused by an obstruction in the GIT. The characteristics of the vomiting may provide information on the height where the GIT block is found: intense vomiting immediately after swallowing any liquid indicates high-positioned GIT block (for example, volvulus of the stomach, stenosis of the pylorus). Absence of bile in the vomit indicates a block before the papilla of Vater. On the contrary, rich admixture of bile indicates a high-positioned jejunal block. Vomiting is not an early symptom of blocks found in lower parts of the intestine (unless reflexive due to strangulation); in the event of blocks in the colon, vomiting may be of a feculent nature, or liquid showing the characteristics of stool may even be vomited (miserere). Hematemesis – the presence of a rather large amount of blood in the vomit – occurs with bleeding in upper parts of the GIT. Traces or filaments of blood are often a consequence of repeated strenuous vomiting with an injury to the mucosa in the area of the cardia (Mallory-Weiss syndrome).

- **Singultus** (or hiccups) is not a common sign of AA. It may provide evidence of developing inflammation of the peritoneum or irritation in the subdiaphramatic space (fluid, abscess).
- **Gas and stool stoppage** may be of reflex origin due to diseases of abdominal cavity organs and is an early sign in this case; or it may be caused by an obstruction in the GIT with a feeling of being bloated and with objective bulging of the abdomen, where the earliness of the symptom is given by localization of the obstruction along the digestive tract (for example, normal stool may still occur several times after incarceration of the small intestine).
- **Diarrhea** is not a typical sign of AA. Strangulation (commonly invagination in children) and bleeding in the GIT may be a cause if blood is present.

## UROLOGICAL HISTORY

Data on the frequency and urge to urinate, burning and sharp pain sensations during urination, impossibility to urinate, the color and amount of urine is important to exclude any urological problems. The urinary system may be irritated when advanced inflammatory processes are present in the hypogastrium and minor pelvis, and they could be mistaken for a urological disease.

## GYNECOLOGICAL HISTORY

Gynecological history is a necessary part of differential diagnostics in any AA, including a gynecological examination. It should be kept in mind that the woman may be pregnant even if she insists otherwise.

## OTHER ANAMNESTIC DATA

Family history may reveal some hereditary diseases important for differential diagnosis. Pharmacological history should also be detailed given that many commonly used medications (non-steroidal antiflogistics, antibiotics, immunosuppressives and corticoids) may induce an AA (gastric perforation, pseudomembranous colitis) and/or modify considerably a number of symptoms typical for a certain AA. Information on alcohol consumption and on the use of habit-forming substances is also essential (for example, bleeding from esophageal varices).

## 15.3.2 Physical Examination

The patient should be examined in the supine position, undressed from the breast nipples to the knees, with lower limbs partially bent at the knees and upper limbs held close along the trunk. The patient should be calmed before the examination. In children, the physician must gain their trust. The examination room should have adequate temperature and should be equipped with good lighting (color of the skin and sclerae).

### OBJECTIVE GENERAL SYMPTOMS

The symptoms should be evaluated as early as the patient enters the office (relief seeking position, unrest) and also while collecting the history. Skin color and hydration, paleness, sweating, characteristics of respiration and respiratory waves of the abdominal wall in connection with information on the duration of the problems may indicate the intensity of the occurring AA and lead to the first essential decision: whether the patient should be operated on immediately (for example, bleeding in the free abdominal cavity) or whether the general condition is good enough to perform additional assessments. Information on the heart rate (tachycardia with inflammatory AA), blood pressure and body temperature is very important.

### OBJECTIVE LOCAL SYMPTOMS

The examiner must know what symptoms are characteristic for any given disease in order to be able to actually find local symptoms in the abdomen. Thus the physician must know what to look for.

#### View

**Limitation of respiratory waves and/or muscle contraction** may indicate signs of peritoneal irritation. **Visible peristaltic waves, bulging in the inguinal, femoral, umbilical region** or in the **area of a scar** may indicate an incarceration, and thus an ileous AA. Venous dilatation in the umbilical region or the spider nevi indicate portal hypertension. A simple examination consists in determining the phenomena of pain caused by cough; the supine patient is asked to cough deeply and the painful reaction is observed by determining the site of pain.

#### Auscultation

**Splashing and gurgling sounds** in the abdominal cavity inform of the presence of an ileus. **Metal sounds or the falling drop phenomenon** are signs of an advanced ileus. **Dead silence** may be a sign of paralytic ileus or an advanced inflammatory AA.

#### Percussion

Percussion across all areas of the abdomen can be used to determine **pain** and also to determine one of the peritoneal irritation symptoms (Plenies sign). Vanishing of the deepened sound over the liver may be found with pneumoperitoneum. **Diffuse tympanic percussion** indicates distension of intestinal loops. Free liquid in the abdominal cavity causes **deepened sound of percussion** responding to the position of the patient.

Palpation

Upon targeted distraction of the patient's attention, the following is explored: **tension in the abdominal wall, maximum pain upon palpation, resistance and signs of peritoneal irritation**, which are characterized by muscle contractions (muscular defense) and pain upon pressure or decompression (Blumberg's or Rovsing's sign, respectively). The examination should be initiated in non-painful areas, gradually approaching the area of maximum pain. Again, the examination of the most common localizations of external abdominal hernias should not be omitted.

### 15.3.3 Per Rectum Examination

This examination is necessary in all patients suspected of AA. The Douglas space is the lowest point of the peritoneal cavity in the standing or sitting position, easily reachable **per rectum**. Pain during examination indicates the presence of peritoneal irritation (leaked inflammatory content or GIT content upon perforation). This examination also makes it possible to assess the tension of the sphincter and the extension or pliability of the ampulla. Assessment of the quality, smell and pathological admixtures in stool (mucus, blood, parasites, especially in children) is essential.

### 15.3.4 Supplementary and Auxiliary Assessments

Supplementary examinations are indicated based on anamnestic and physical examination data, which should provide closer specification of differential diagnosis. The decision on their scope depends not only on their purposeful choice, but also on the type of AA and its course. The aim is to choose those examinations that are necessary, provide high informative value for differential diagnosis, are promptly available and are not burdensome for the patient (procedure from non-invasive toward invasive examinations). Their sensitivity should be known (ability to reveal a certain deviation or disease) as well as their specificity (ability to differentiate non-pathological findings) in respect of the assumed disease, while it should be remembered that their assessment may be both false positive and false negative. The diagnosis is determined based on all information and not only based on supplementary examinations (for example, in the case of gastric perforation, pneumoperitoneum may not be confirmed by radiography). If the patient is in shock, circulatory stabilization is the primary task. Necessary examinations are performed during resuscitation. In such a case, surgery is indicated only if it resolves the immediate cause of the shock condition (for example, bleeding in the free abdominal cavity).

### ■ LABORATORY ASSESSMENTS
### Blood Count
- Leukocytosis is typical for inflammatory AA, while it may not be present in elderly or immunosuppressed and cachectic patients. It is also an early sign of blood loss, occurring before any decrease in the red blood count
- Hematocrit and erythrocyte count decrease is a manifestation of bleeding; however, it may occur with delay – after compensation of fluid volume in the blood stream
- Blood coagulability tests should be performed where a hemocoagulation disorder is suspected or before some invasive examination procedures (ERCP, PTC)
- The blood group should always be determined where bleeding is suspected and before surgery

### Biochemical Serum Assessments
- Electrolytes, urea, creatinine and glycemia provide information on the metabolic condition of the body, hypovolemia and ionic dysbalance where profuse vomiting or diarrhea is present
- CRP (protein of the acute phase) is an integral part of the system inflammatory response and in the early stage of an AA; elevated values may be significant for an inflammatory origin of the disease
- Elevated values of organ specific enzymes may indicate the cause of the AA in the event of diseases of the pancreas (amylase, lipase), hepatobiliary system (ALT, AST, GMT, ALP + bilirubin). They may be helpful for differential diagnosis in the event of acute myocardial infarction (troponin)

### Urine Assessment
- Urine assessment is important to differentiate any potential urological causes of the abdominal pain and in some metabolic disorders

### ■ IMAGING ASSESSMENTS
The same general rules apply for the indication of radiography or sonography assessments as for other supplementary assessments and the choice should not be generalized:
- **Native abdominal scan** (if not possible in the standing position, then in the lying position on the side using a horizontal beam) may indicate any presence of air in the peritoneal cavity (pneumoperitoneum); separation of gaseous intestinal content from liquid content (little levels) is a sign of an ileus condition; contrast radiography concrements in hollow organs (gallbladder and bile ducts, kidneys and urinary tract)

- **Scan of the chest easy to survey** is important as part of preoperative examinations, and it may provide information on any pathology in the chest (pseudosurgical abdominal event, volvulus of the stomach with propagation in the chest) or in subphrenic conditions (abscess, pneumoperitoneum)
- **Sonography** (US) provides information on any present solid formations, concrements, circumscribed inflammatory formations (abscesses), on thickened walls of abdominal cavity organs due to an inflammation (cholecystitis, appendicitis, sigmoiditis), as well as on any present fluid in the free abdominal cavity (inflammatory exudate, blood, ascites, etc.). Abscess cavities can be drained under US control.
- **Contrast assessment of the digestive tract** (using water solution or barium contrast medium) is indicated in the case of differentially diagnostic problems of obstruction or pseudo-obstruction
- **Elimination urography** may be indicated to confirm or exclude any suspected renal origin of the problems (ureterolithiasis)
- **Computed tomography** (CT) is ever more available and its use in differential diagnostics of AA may be essential especially where no unambiguously proper diagnosis can be determined using clinical examination combined with radiography and US assessments
- **Angiography** may provide closer specification of any suspicion of intestinal ischemia or determine the place of bleeding in the intestine. It is a highly selective assessment. It is not commonly available 24 hours a day
- **Magnetic resonance imaging** (MRI) finds application in differential diagnostics of AA only in exceptional cases and its yield in a specific situation should be consulted with a physician who assesses MRI findings

## ENDOSCOPY

- Endofibroscopy or video endoscopy has a stable position in AA differential diagnostics and therapy. It should be performed by experienced endoscopists due to the risks of complications (perforation of the esophagus and colon):
- **Esophagogastroduodenoscopy** is indicated urgently, especially when bleeding in upper parts of the GIT is present, in which case it clarifies the place of bleeding, and at the same time, it allows for treating the bleeding as well (injections, clipping, ligation, electrocoagulation, sclerotization, gluing, laser). In addition, it plays an important role in differential diagnostics of pain in the epigastrium
- **Colonoscopy** is of the same importance in colon diseases
- **ERCP** has an irreplaceable role in the diagnostics and resolution of obstructions of the biliary tree

## LAPAROSCOPY

As a mini-invasive method, laparoscopy has been finding ever broader application in differential diagnostics, and subsequently also in the therapy of AA (acute appendicitis, perforation of the gastroduodenal ulcer, gynecological acute abdomen). It is also useful in elderly and polymorbid patients where laparotomy due to hesitation may have fatal consequences.

## 15.4 Differential Diagnostics

The focus of AA diagnostics consists in high-quality differential diagnostics of pathological processes in the abdominal cavity, but also in other areas (pseudosurgical abdominal events). It follows from the knowledge of the issues of diseases of individual organs including urological and gynecological diseases, and in principle, it is a thorough analysis and subsequent synthesis of information from the medical history, physical examination and supplementary assessments. It should always be kept in mind that acute abdomen is a life-threatening condition, which must be handled by each physician at his or her level. Either successful management of the AA or a number of health-related, usually serious, complications, which may even lead to the death of the patient, may be derived from the physician's decision on further procedures (for example, referring the patient for surgical examination). The symptomatology of malignancies in the abdominal cavity usually develops gradually. They may manifest as AA especially by bleeding in the GIT, perforations in the free abdominal cavity or an ileus condition.

### 15.4.1 Differential Diagnostics of the Most Common Causes of Pain Based on Localization

Epigastrium
- Acute cholecystitis
- Acute gastritis
- Perforation of gastroduodenal ulcer
- Acute pancreatitis
- Acute appendicitis (during the first hours of the disease)
- Acute myocardial infarction
- Basal pneumonia
- Spontaneous PNO

Right Hypogastrium
- Acute appendicitis
- Acute gastroenteritis
- Acute cholecystitis
- Right-sided renal colic
- Perforation of gastroduodenal ulcer
- Mesenteric lymphadenitis

- Adnexitis
- Extrauterine pregnancy
- Crohn's disease

Left Hypogastrium
- Left-sided renal colic
- Sigmoid diverticulitis
- Acute adnexitis
- Extrauterine pregnancy

## 15.4.2 Pseudosurgical Acute Abdomen

Pseudosurgical abdominal events are diseases whose symptomatology is very similar to that of AA, but the problems do not originate from diseases of organs in the abdominal cavity. Differentiating these events from surgical AA is essential given that erroneous indication of a surgical procedure may have fatal consequences for the patient (for example, in the case of acute myocardial infarction).

In the majority of cases, pseudosurgical events originate from thoracic organs, metabolic disorders, and they may be encountered also in rheumatic diseases, in some neurological diseases, and others.

Causes in Thoracic Organs
- Acute myocardial infarction
- Pneumothorax
- Basal pneumonia

Metabolic Disorders
- Diabetic pseudoperitonitis
- Uremia
- Acute porphyria
- Hyperthyroidism

Rheumatic Diseases
- Rheumatic fever
- Henoch-Schönlein purpura

Neurological Diseases
- Cerebrospinal multiple sclerosis
- Tabes dorsalis

Other Causes
- Spinal cord injuries
- Heavy metal intoxication

# 16　ILEUS – INTESTINAL OBSTRUCTION

*16.1 Definition*
*16.2 Ileus Classification Based on Its Causes*
*16.3 Pathophysiology of the Ileus and Ileus Disease Development*
*16.4 Ileus Symptomatology*
*16.5 Ileus Diagnostics*
*16.6 Therapy*
*16.7 Prognosis*

## 16.1　Definition

**Ileus or ileus state** is a condition when stoppage of the intestinal passage is manifested clinically. An identical set of symptoms is a manifestation of complications of numerous diseases of various etiologies and prognoses.

Ileus is an acute disease – an **acute abdomen** (AA) that requires prompt diagnosis and immediate commencement of therapy, usually surgical. Untreated absence or impairment of intestinal passage leads through various pathophysiological mechanisms to the development of an **ileus disease.** It is a general affection of the organism which is characterized by the failure of vital organ systems. The extent and nature of the disease inducing absence or impairment of intestinal passage and the development of an ileus disease with organ dysfunction are the limiting factors of successful ileus treatment.

## 16.2　Ileus Classification Based on Its Causes

According to its cause ileus is classified as **mechanical, functional** and mixed.

**Obstructive ileus** is the most common form of mechanical ileus. Intestinal obstruction causes differ based on the age of the patient and on localization. Adults are affected by absence or impairment of intestinal passage more commonly than children. Various adhesions are the most common causes of the small intestinal ileus, while impairment of colon passage in adults is most commonly caused by a tumor.

# ILEUS – INTESTINAL OBSTRUCTION

**Obstruction (closure)** of intestinal lumen is caused by an obstruction:
a) Intraluminal (foreign bodies, biliary stones, parasites)
b) Intramural (tumors, inflammatory stenoses)
c) Extramural (adhesions, incarcerated hernias, extramural tumors)

**Strangulation** is a serious form of mechanical ileus, characterized by closure of the intestinal lumen, disorder of the intestinal perfusion and innervation due to the compression of mesenteric vessels and nerves. It is caused by incarcerations in an external or internal hernia, between the adhesions, by invagination or volvulus. Strangulation is an absolute indication for urgent surgical intervention.

**Functional ileus** is induced by intestinal motility disorder without any mechanical obstruction preventing the passage of intestinal content, and it is classified as paralytic and spastic.

**Paralytic ileus** is caused by intestinal motility paralysis. Intestinal motility disorder is common in inflammatory diseases in the abdominal cavity, in pancreatitis, cholecystitis, appendicitis, diverticulitis, and with peritonitis. It develops as a reflectoric condition with renal and biliary colic, high blood loss, urine retention, vertebral fractures and processes in the retroperitoneum of varied etiologies. More rarely intestinal paralysis accompanies internal environment disorders such as dehydration, diabetic acidosis, uremia, hypocalcemia.

Intestinal motility disorder may also be induced by some medications, such as tricyclic antidepressants, neuroleptics, and opiates.

The rare **spastic ileus** is a condition where spastic paresis of intestinal musculature occurs, such as, for example, after lead poisoning or porphyria.

**Pseudo obstruction of the large intestine** (Ogilvie syndrome) – dilatation of the large intestine predominantly with gas; it is a rare functional condition based on various factors. Attenuation of parasympathetic activity or metabolic abnormalities is seen as the common denominator of causes that induce pseudo obstruction. The condition is accompanied by various associated diseases in 80% of cases. Clinically, it is difficult to distinguish from mechanical ileus with an obstruction in distal parts of the colon.

**Postoperative ileus** is a separate group. The etiology of postoperative ileus is multifactorial. It is a response to surgical trauma and visceral manipulation during surgery, to the administration of anesthesiological medicines, and opiates in pain management. Postoperative paralytic ileus usually subsides within 4 days after the surgery. Long-lasting postoperative paralysis may lead to an ileus disease.

A combination of paralytic and mechanical ileus (for example, with intra-abdominal abscess or peritonitis) is called a **mixed ileus**.

**Vascular ileus** is caused by affection of the intestinal vascular supply by embolism or thrombosis.

## 16.3 Pathophysiology of the Ileus and Ileus Disease Development

Pathophysiological mechanisms participating in the development of ileus disease differ based on the height of the intestinal lumen closure. The division to small and large intestinal ileus therefore stems not only from the localization of the obstruction but also from the pathophysiology of the changes. The small intestinal ileus is further divided into a high-positioned ileus with an obstruction in the jejunum and ileus of the whole small intestine with an obstruction localized in the distal ileum.

An obstruction in the **small intestine** is the cause of the ileus in 75–80% of cases. The surface of the small intestinal mucosa is considerable, reported between 200 and 300 m². The small intestine is an organ that exerts considerable influence on the mediator-based response of the organism. Upon stoppage of passage in the small intestine which shows only weak bacterial colonization, considerable propagation of feculent bacteria occurs, particularly of *E. coli*. The rise in the number of bacteria causes hypersecretion from the mucosa and increases intestinal wall perfusion. The small intestine is dilated; however, intraluminal pressure in the small intestine does not exceed 8 cmH$_2$O (0.78 kPa) and does not exert any significant effect on perfusion of the small intestine wall.

**High level obstruction** affects approximately 20% of patients with small intestine passage impairment in which the obstruction is located in the jejunum. The patients are in danger of high losses of water and electrolytes through vomiting, causing marked hypovolemia and electrolyte dysbalance. Mediator response to high-positioned ileus is initially insignificant.

In the event of **ileus of the whole small intestine** caused by an obstruction in distal parts of the ileum, bacterial flora in the small intestine undergoes both qualitative and quantitative changes. In the early phase, bacterial toxins do not pass through the mucosal barrier, but released endotoxins are the cause of marked hypersecretion into the lumen of the small intestine, causing hypovolemia. The mucosal barrier becomes damaged early, with subsequent translocation of the bacteria. The evidence of endotoxinemia can be found from approximately day 4 after the onset of intestinal passage stoppage. The systemic inflammatory response syndrome – SIRS develops with manifestations of organ dysfunction. Untreated SIRS develops into multiple organ failure – MOF. This condition called "ileus disease" poses a threat particularly to patients with an obstruction in distal parts of the ileum, but also patients with an obstruction in the colon and with an incompetent Bauhin's valve.

Gradual development is characteristic of the **large intestine ileus**, initially characterized by an indistinctive clinical picture, which occurs in 20–25% of patients with intestinal passage impairment. Only the distension of the colon is present with a competent Bauhin's valve, which is up to 95% of cases. Unlike the small intestine the total surface area of the large intestinal mucosa is approximately only 1 m². No hypersecretion from the mucosa thus occurs in the colon, which means that hypovolemia is not an early sign of a large intestinal ileus. No release of inflammatory mediators from the large intestine wall was demonstrated. The antibacterial barrier of the colon mucosa is very efficient, and therefore, the share of bacterial translocation during the large intestinal ileus development is not so significant. On the contrary, the rising volume of gas and stool in the colon is important, which leads to a rise in intraluminal pressure values up to about 100 mmHg (13.3 kPa). Upon high intraluminal pressure and distension, particularly of the right half of the colon, ischemia of the intestinal wall develops up to its perforation. Distension of the colon and ischemia of its wall are considered as major factors causing the development of SIRS. In terms of prognosis, the development of **distension perforation** and of perforation stercoral peritonitis is highly unfavorable.

In **strangulation**, the aforementioned pathophysiological mechanisms caused by intestinal obstruction intertwine with the pathophysiology of acute intestinal ischemia. In a complete intestinal ischemia in the experiment, focal ischemia of the mucosa develops as early as within 30 minutes; when the ischemic condition lasts longer than 60 minutes, the musculature of the intestinal wall becomes affected and later also the serosa of the intestine. Gangrene of the intestinal wall can be expected within two hours of complete strangulation. Severe pains at the beginning of the ischemic condition are caused by irritation of afferent sympathetic fibers out of the spinal cord. Gradually SIRS and sepsis with MOF develop.

## 16.4 Symptoms of Ileus

The basic symptoms of ileus include **stoppage of gas and stool passage, vomiting** caused by accumulation of the contents above the obstruction or reflectoric vomiting upon strangulation, **bulging of the abdomen** and colicky **pain** at the beginning of the obstructive ileus or severe, unsoothable pain at the beginning of strangulation ileus.

Some of the major symptoms of ileus may be missing in the course of the disease. Colicky pain is missing in paralytic ileus, and vomiting when the obstruction is found in distal parts of the colon. Minimum clinical manifestations are present in connection with high-positioned ileus where, other than vomiting, basic symptoms of intestinal obstruction are also missing: bulging of the abdomen, stoppage of gas and stool passage, as well as pain.

The general symptoms of the shock begin rapidly upon strangulation. In other events of ileus, both the general symptoms and findings in the abdomen develop with varied intensity depending on the height of the obstruction in the intestine,

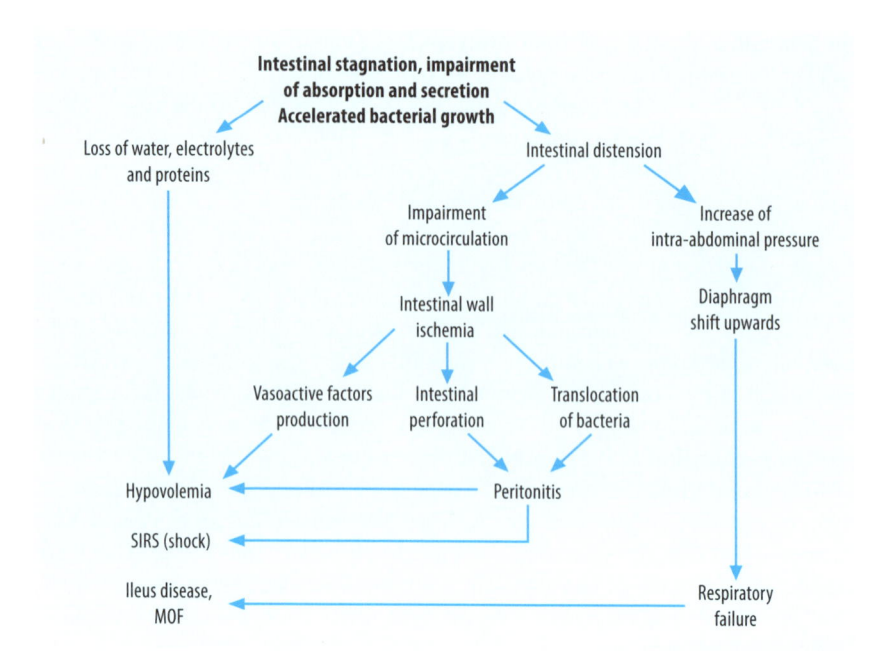

```
                Intestinal stagnation, impairment
                    of absorption and secretion
                    Accelerated bacterial growth
         ↙                                          ↘
Loss of water, electrolytes                    Intestinal distension
    and proteins                              ↙                ↘
                              Impairment                    Increase of
                           of microcirculation         intra-abdominal pressure
                                    ↓                           ↓
                             Intestinal wall                Diaphragm
                                ischemia                  shift upwards
                         ↙          ↓          ↘
              Vasoactive factors  Intestinal   Translocation
                 production      perforation    of bacteria
                         ↘          ↓          ↙
    ↓                             Peritonitis
Hypovolemia  ←                                          
SIRS (shock) ←
Ileus disease,                                          Respiratory
    MOF      ←                                            failure
```

Fig. 16.1 *Ileus – the sequence of pathophysiological disorders*

but they also depend on functionality of the Bauhin's valve, the general condition of the patient, and possibly also on advancement of a malignant tumorous disease.

The clinical manifestations of both obstruction and functional ileus of the small intestine may be similar. The clinical picture of obstructive ileus of the large intestine is almost identical when the obstruction is found in the left half of the colon, and the pseudo obstruction of the colon – the Ogilvie syndrome.

## 16.5   Ileus Diagnostics

The examination procedure should lead to prompt determination of diagnosis. This is important particularly in the event of strangulation where the vascular supply disorder poses an immediate threat to vitality of the intestine.

In the diagnostics of ileus, recognizing the **symptoms of strangulation, localizing the obstruction** (in the small or large intestine) and assessing the **cause** of ileus (obstruction or functional) are of primary importance. Examination of the patient in the ileus condition should respect the usual procedure of examination in patients with an condition of an acute abdomen. This includes anamnestic data, objective examination, assessment using imaging methods, and laboratory assessments.

## ILEUS – INTESTINAL OBSTRUCTION

### 16.5.1 Medical History and Objective Examination

As for **personal history**, important data includes the extent and number of previous surgeries in the abdominal cavity, diseases of the intestine and other organs in the abdominal cavity or symptoms thereof, use of medications and coincidence of other diseases. As for the **history of the current disease**, attention should be focused on the presence of major symptoms of intestinal passage absence, which include stoppage of gas and stool elimination, vomiting and pain.

During the **objective examination** initially inconspicuous symptoms of **alteration of the general condition** such as tachycardia, tachypnea and decreased blood pressure should not be overlooked and underestimated.

### ■ PHYSICAL FINDINGS

Examination of the abdomen usually starts with a **viewing**, which may show apparent bulging of the abdomen, scars after prior surgeries, hernias and possibly also hardening of intestinal loops. During **palpation**, hernias and hernia gates, resistances, points of pain and possibly any circumscribed or diffuse muscle contraction should be sought. The **auscultation findings** are no less important. Instead of usual sounds of intestinal peristalsis, so-called "metallic sounds" can be heard, and the sound of the "falling drop", caused by increased peristalsis above the obstruction. Completely "dead" silence in the abdominal cavity is characteristic for paralytic ileus. **Per rectum** examination may reveal stenosis of the anus, a stenotising tumor in the rectum, resistance in the minor pelvis, or exudate in the Douglas space with an advanced ileus. Empty, dilated and atonic ampulla of the rectum with a weakened sphincter is often characteristic of an obstruction localized in distal parts of the colon.

### 16.5.2 Imaging Methods

**Native radiography** of the **abdomen in the standing position** still remains the primary and basic **examination using imaging methods**. The radiographic scan shows the presence of step-like air-fluid levels characteristic for ileus; these levels reflect the presence of air over the level of liquid material in individual intestine loops. Based on their distribution in the native scan, the place of the obstruction can be accurately assessed. For example, two levels are usually present in the epigastrium and several levels in the middle of the abdomen when the obstruction is found in the small intestine; or in cases where the obstruction is localized in the area of the terminal ileum and cecum, the levels are usually arranged in cascades in the whole abdomen, and dilatation of the small intestine is usually also present. The amount of levels and the dilatation of the small intestine are characteristic also for paralytic ileus. Isolated dilatation of the small or large intestine is usually conditioned by inflammation in the surroundings, by pancreatitis, appendicitis, cholecystitis or diverticulitis.

In addition, any potential presence of pneumoperitoneum should be sought in the scan. Gas in the free abdominal cavity provides evidence of perforation of a hollow organ. The presence of loose gas and a number of levels are signs of advanced AA where stoppage of intestinal passage is also clinically manifested upon peritonitis, or where distension perforation has already occurred in the event of an advanced ileus. Apart from sporadic exceptions, pneumoperitoneum is a clear indication for surgical revision.

In cases where an organic obstruction is found in the left half of the large intestine but also in cases of pseudo obstruction, levels in the colon are localized along the sides of the abdomen, and an increased content of gas can be found in the small intestine. Assessment of the dilatation of the cecum in the native scan is important; if its width reaches more than 12 cm, a high risk of distension perforation is present. In the event of Bauhin's valve insufficiency, the levels also occur in the small intestine.

If the patient is unable to stand, the scan is performed in the supine position using a horizontal beam. Yet, it cannot be used to estimate the height of the obstruction.

Sensitivity of the native abdominal scan in the obstruction diagnostics has been reported as only 66%. Therefore in patients where it is not yet clear, based on the clinical finding and a native abdominal scan, whether a complete obstruction is present, examinations using other imaging methods are also exploited – contrast assessment of the gastrointestinal tract (GIT), sonography or computed tomography (CT). Patients with suspected strangulation and acute mesenteric occlusion are exceptions; they are indicated for urgent surgery. Also, contrast assessment of the GIT should not be used when intestinal perforation is suspected, and a highly reserved approach is necessary in patients with marked dilatation of the cecum.

GIT assessment with the administration of a water solution of a hyperosmolar contrast substance is done in order to obtain closer specification of the localization, origin and completeness of the intestinal obstruction. It is associated with lower risks than the administration of a barium contrast substance. Severely dehydrated patients must be rehydrated before the examination. In vomiting patients and patients under general anesthesia, aspiration of the contrast substance can be prevented by introducing a gastric tube. Without the cooperation of the patient, the performance of contrast examination is too demanding. Examination of the **followed intestinal passage** with oral administration of the water contrast solution or **enteroclysis** is performed if functional ileus or incomplete obstruction is suspected. The aim of the examination is to confirm an obstruction in the gastrointestinal tract and to determine its localization. Where the GIT is passable, the administration of a hyperosmolar contrast substance may provide a therapeutic effect with rapid recovery of intestinal peristalsis.

**Acute irrigography** with the contrast substance administration through the rectum after preparation of the intestine using clysmata is indicated where ileus of the colon is suspected, with an obstruction expected in the left half. The aim of the assessment is to confirm and localize the obstruction in the large intestine, and to exclude pseudo obstruction of the colon. A conservative procedure is to be chosen if no mechanical obstruction of the colon is demonstrated and if perforation of the cecum due to distension is not threatening.

In patients with suspected inflammatory process in the abdominal cavity or retroperitoneum, based on the medical history, clinical findings and native abdominal scan, **sonography** or **CT assessment** of the abdomen is indicated. In the ileus condition, sonography is limited due to the gaseous content in the intestine, but also by the experience of the examiner. CT with an oral contrast substance administration can be used to display distension of intestinal loops, thickening of their walls, any inflammatory and tumorous processes or loose liquid or gas in the abdominal cavity.

**Acute colonoscopy** is indicated for the same reasons as acute irrigography, particularly to exclude pseudo obstruction of the colon. It can be used therapeutically to suck gas out of the intestine. Acute colonoscopy requires an experienced endoscopist, since the examination is difficult and the risk of complications during examination of the unprepared intestine is higher.

Acute examinations pose higher demands on the examiner due to the fact that the patient is not prepared, due to urgency of the examination, the period in which it is done, and the fact that the interpretation of the findings is more difficult.

### 16.5.3   Laboratory Assessments

The results of the basic **laboratory assessments** provide information on the condition of the internal environment, function of organs and condition of coagulation and nutrition. The basic laboratory assessments are performed (blood count, minerals, urea, liver tests, glycemia), which are supplemented as necessary.

The results of all examinations must be evaluated as an integral unit.

## 16.6   Therapy

The therapy of ileus is conservative and surgical. The conservative therapy forms part of the complex treatment of the ileus at the time of determining the diagnosis, preparation for surgery and in the postoperative period. Conservative therapy alone is sufficient only in certain cases of functional ileus. The basic and life-saving therapy of intestinal obstruction is surgery, which must usually be performed as acute. The absolute indications for an urgent surgical procedure are strangulation and mesenteric ischemia. The conservative procedure or postponement of the surgery, respectively, may be chosen only in certain, exceptional cases of mechanical ileus. The decision not to perform urgent surgery of the patient or to postpone the surgery must be based on a qualified conclusion of an erudite surgeon, and it is as serious as the decision to perform the surgery.

### 16.6.1 Conservative Therapy

Essential parts of **conservative therapy** of the ileus are ensuring of venous access by inserting a peripheral or central venous catheter (CVC), elimination of **oral** intake and insertion of a nasogastric tube and a urinary catheter. The basic vital functions must be monitored, preferably in a monitored bed. The balance of liquids and possibly the central venous pressure are also monitored.

Low diuresis is not only the manifestation of hypovolemia, but it may be a sign of renal function disorder within the framework of beginning organ failure. Adaptation of the internal environment: parenteral access is used to compensate for the missing volume of liquids, to correct ionic disbalances and to correct diabetes and other diseases. Properly managed intensive conservative therapy in the event of high-positioned ileus may cover its clinical symptoms completely. In case of organ system failure, the function of the organs must be supported, most commonly that of respiration. An urgent surgery is appropriate only after necessary overall preparation of the patient, however, in the event of a long ineffective preparation the overall condition of the patient with mechanical ileus does not improve.

If paralytic ileus is present, conservative therapy is sufficient to manage the condition. It consists in parenteral nutrition, medicamentous support of intestinal passage using cholinergics, administration of osmotic laxatives, clysmata and the treatment of associated diseases.

### 16.6.2 Surgical Treatment

The conditions of **strangulation, vascular** and **mechanical ileus** are an indication for urgent surgery.

**The main objectives of the surgical treatment** of intestinal obstruction include emptying of the stagnating intestinal content above the obstruction and release thereof. This can be achieved using any of the procedures below or a combination thereof:
- Freeing the intestine from adhesions, derotation of the volvulus, reposition of any incarceration, desinvagination
- Resection of the affected intestinal segment
- Bypassing the obstruction using intestinal bypass
- Establishing an intestinal outlet above the obstruction
- Resection of an irreversibly modified part of the intestine upon vascular supply disorder

Postoperative care depends on the extent of the procedure performed and/or support of failing organ systems.

Decompression of the dilated intestine above the obstruction can be achieved by sucking off the intestinal contents. Peroperative manipulation with filled and dilated intestinal loops requires caution, patience and experience of the operating surgeon. Subsequently, the obstruction of intestinal passage is removed or bypassed, and/or a derivative stoma is established above the obstruction.

In the event of strangulation, the intestine must be loosened by cutting the strangulation band, loosening the hernia gate, derotating in the event of volvulus, and desinvagination upon invagination. When the strangulation has been removed, the vitality of the loosened segment of the intestine should be reviewed. An irreversibly affected segment of the intestine must be resected and continuity of the digestive tract can be reestablished using intestinal anastomosis. In the event that a longer segment of the small intestine is affected and its vitality is unclear, the procedure can be terminated and a "second look" surgery can be planned. In cases of multiple adhesive affection of the small intestine, the disintegration of all adhesions is recommended, since upon incomplete loosening of the adhesions, impairment of intestinal passage may manifest clinically again due to adhesive involvement kept aborally from the treated segment in the postoperative period.

A tumor is the most common cause of ileus of the colon, i.e. colorectal carcinoma localized particularly in the left half of the colon. The obstruction can be resolved in several ways:
- Resection of the intestine in the acute condition with immediate recovery of intestinal continuity ("primary anastomosis")
- Resection of the intestine in the acute condition, establishment of a stoma and blind closure of the aboral segment (Hartmann's operation, with exclusion of anastomosis)
- Establishment of a stoma

Intestinal resection with anastomosis can be done in a single period. The other procedures require surgery in one additional or even two additional periods even if the finding is resectable; this means that the stoma is removed in the first case and intestinal continuity is recovered using anastomosis; or in the second case, the intestine is resected in the second period and the stoma is removed in the third period.

The procedure performed in multiple periods is burdened with high summary morbidity, frequent disturbances of the sequence of necessary operations, and long repeated hospitalizations, and therefore, it has been abandoned.

In terms of extent, a surgical procedure due to intestinal obstruction should meet the criteria of oncological radicality including respective lymphadenectomy as in the event of an elective procedure. A subtotal colectomy with primary ileocolic anastomosis is an alternative to the single-period operative solution of obstructions in the left half of the colon with accumulated intestinal contents in the distended colon. Removal of the colon together with its contents reduces the risk of potential peroperative contamination of the surgical field, and ileocolic anastomosis provides higher safety than colocolic anastomosis. An increase in stool elimination frequency up to relative incontinence with loose stools may be a disadvantage, particularly in elderly patients.

In patients with tumor metastases, limited intestinal resection with anastomosis can be done in locally removable lesions. Ileocolic or colocolic intestinal bypass or derivation of stool using a stoma established above the obstruction is indicated in locally inoperable tumors. In the event of an obstruction caused by a locally advanced rectal carcinoma, it is recommended to establish a derivative stoma. This makes it possible to perform additional examinations and therapeutic irradiation in potentially surgically curable tumors, which should be followed by definitive elective surgical treatment. In patients with advanced cancer stemming from organs in the abdominal cavity where peritoneal carcinosis may already be present, a chronic ileus condition can be palliatively affected by surgery only with difficulty or may not be resolvable at all.

In the event of tumors of the colon an acute ileus condition can be managed in some exceptional cases by recanalization of the tumor using a laser or by establishing a metallic stent. Such a procedure allows for early elective surgery of the patient with a surgically curable tumor or may remain a palliative solution of intestinal obstruction in an advanced colorectal carcinoma not removable by surgery.

The laparoscopic treatment of ileus in the small intestine is possible; however, it is burdened with a high number of conversions. Therefore, when deciding on the management of ileus in the small intestine, it is recommended to perform preoperative selection of patients suitable for laparoscopic operation.

## 16.7 Prognosis

Ileus is a serious acute disease. In spite of all progress in the diagnostics, surgical treatment and intensive care, this condition is burdened with high morbidity and lethality rates. Morbidity and lethality rates depend on the extent of the underlying disease, duration of the obstruction, associated diseases, the age of the patient and also on the promptness and manner of treatment. Every condition of absence or impairment of intestinal passage should be examined by a surgeon who decides on further procedures; whether, how and when the patient is to be operated on.

# 17 PERITONITIS

*17.1 Definition*
*17.2 Pathophysiology of Peritonitis and Sepsis*
*17.3 Peritonitis Classification*
*17.4 Clinical Symptoms*
*17.5 Paraclinical Diagnostics*
*17.6 Indications for Surgical Treatment*
*17.7 Peritonitis Therapy*
*17.8 Prognosis in Patients with Peritonitis*

Inflammation of the peritoneum – peritonitis – has been the most frequent and most serious problem of daily surgery for at least 150 years. A lot has obviously changed during this time in terms of knowledge of pathogenesis of abdominal sepsis, and the capabilities of peritonitis diagnostics and the therapy have improved considerably. Although the basic requirement of therapy, as defined as early as in 1926 by Kirschner, still applies i.e. removal of the focus of any inflammation and contamination from the peritoneal cavity, the problems of peritonitis spread beyond a simple surgical intervention a long time ago. Similarly, timely use of the capacities of modern intensive therapy is just as important for improving the fate of the patient since peritonitis is from the very beginning a general disease, not just limited to the abdominal cavity. The advancements in intensive medicine, which include particularly the support of organ functions (circulation, ventilation, detoxification, nutrition) have meant substantial improvement in the results of surgical treatment. In spite of this, the lethality rate of patients with developed peritonitis is about 30% depending on the inflammation origin.

## 17.1 Definition

**Peritonitis is a localized or diffuse inflammation of the peritoneum, usually caused by bacteria or stimulations of a chemical-toxic nature.** Rapid development of the system disease, sepsis, is possible due to the large resorption area of the peritoneum and close structural and functional relationships of the peritoneal mesothelium to the lymphatic system and thus also to vital organs, particularly the liver, lungs and RES.

## 17.2  Pathophysiology of Peritonitis and Sepsis

Peritoneum is a smooth serous membrane that covers the whole abdominal cavity – viscera as the visceral peritoneum and the wall as the pariteal peritoneum. The area surface of this membrane is roughly equivalent to the body surface and in adults it amounts to about 1.7 m$^2$. Under physiological conditions, the peritoneal cavity contains 50–150 mL of clear yellowish fluid, which allows for the sliding of the surfaces of abdominal cavity organs. It contains less than 3,000 cells in 1 mm$^3$. Out of that, lymphocytes amount to 50%, macrophages to 40%, and the rest consists of eosinophils, mastocysts and mesothelial cells. With the exception of outlets of fallopian tubes, the peritoneal cavity is an enclosed space.

Due to its large surface, the peritoneum works as a membrane that allows for the diffusion of water and electrolytes. Especially in dependence on perfusion the equilibrium between secretion and absorption may be considerably disturbed, and when the peritoneum is irritated, for example, by an inflammatory process, the fluid from the intravascular and interstitial area is transferred rapidly to the free peritoneal cavity. Absorption of large molecules and particularly of cells and bacteria occurs only in the diaphragmatic part of the peritoneum where space exists between mesothelial cells (stomata). This process is active, unidirectional and continues to lymph vessels and further through the thoracic duct to venous blood. Reverse flow is prevented by valves in lymph vessels and by negative intrathoracic pressure in the inspiration.

Vasoactive substances released from peritoneal cells upon chemical, bacterial or traumatic insult provoke vasodilatation and increased permeability of the walls of small venules in the peritoneum, thereby allowing for exudation of large protein molecules, especially fibrin. Since fibrinolytic activity of the mesothelium is considerably suppressed in these situations, fibrin exudation is formed in the affected areas. While fibrin exudation makes it possible that the process is circumscribed and localized, on the other hand, it makes absorption of the bacteria more difficult and provides "fertile ground" for their further persistence in the body. This reaction thus prevents quick development of acute sepsis; however, it leads to a subacute to chronic course with the formation of abscesses. It should be mentioned here, that according to the current views of sepsis, activation of the immune system by parts of bacterial bodies, particularly by endotoxin, is the crucial principle of the system response of the organism. Activation of macrophages by the endotoxin of gram-negative bacteria or "superantigens" of gram-positive bacteria leads to releasing the tumor necrosis factor (TNF) and

# PERITONITIS

interleukins, thereby initiating a cascade of inflammatory acute phase reactions, which includes a number of mediator systems. Mediators affect the permeability of capillaries to a varied extent, as well as peripheral vascular resistance (hyperdynamic circulation), blood coagulability and viscosity, and also directly the function of vital organs. Inflammatory mediators are not regulated by negative feedback but rather on the contrary, increased release of the mediators leads to further intensification of their release. This condition results in the multiple organ dysfunction syndrome (MODS) associated with extremely high lethality if early and successful therapeutic intervention is not granted.

## 17.3 Peritonitis Classification

The term peritonitis is a **summary expression used for a group of diseases non-uniform from the etiological, morphological and clinical point of view**, which makes any classification and comparison of results achieved using various therapeutic procedures difficult.

1. According to the clinical course, peritonitis diseases can be classified as acute and chronic (for example, intra-abdominal abscesses, tuberculous or plastic peritonitis).
2. According to the characteristics of the content in the abdominal cavity, peritonitis can be categorized as serous, fibrinous, hemorrhagic, suppurative, stercoral, biliary and chemical (acute pancreatitis, fresh gastroduodenal perforation, urinous peritonitis).
3. According to localization or spreading of the finding in the abdominal cavity – diffuse peritonitis – spread in all 4 quadrants; circumscribed peritonitis – circumscribed around the source; intra-abdominal abscess (subphrenic, interloop, abscess of Douglas space).
4. According to etiology, peritonitis can be categorized as primary, secondary, tertiary and special types.

### 17.3.1 Primary Peritonitis

Primary peritonitis has no demonstrable intra-abdominal cause. It often develops as hematogenic (pneumococcal peritonitis in children) or lymphogenic ("spontaneous peritonitis" in patients with liver CI and ascites). In women, ascendent infection through the external genital and tube may also occur. A microbiological finding is often monoinfection with gram-positive cocci.

### 17.3.2 Secondary Peritonitis

Secondary peritonitis develops due to the disease of an intra-abdominal organ through perforation or transfer of an infection through an impaired but integral wall. Mixed infection with predominant gram-negative and anaerobic flora is often found upon microbiological examination (*E. coli*, enterococci, *Enterobacteriaceae*, *Klebsiella*, *Proteus*, streptococci, *Bacteroides* and other anaerobes).

The speed and gravity of bacterial contamination are conditioned by **localization of the primary process** (fresh perforation of the gastroduodenal ulcer is primarily aseptic, while bacterial settlement of hollow organs rises aborally), and they increase **with the duration of peritonitis** (or the content is infected secondarily).

The most common sources of secondary peritonitis include perforations of hollow organs – gastroduodenal ulcer, appendicitis, gangrenous cholecystitis, diverticulitis, perforation of the ileus intestine before the obstruction (cecum) or at the place of incarceration, traumatic perforation (of the intestine, stomach, gallbladder, urinary bladder). The passage of the infection through the impaired wall without perforation is typical for perfusion disorders of the intestinal wall upon mesenteric vascular occlusion, long-lasting ileus or toxic megacolon.

### 17.3.3 Tertiary Peritonitis

Tertiary peritonitis develops after surgical or other intervention procedures in the abdominal cavity. Most commonly it includes insufficiency of anastomoses in the GIT, ischemia or injury to the wall of a hollow organ, peroperative contamination with infectious content, etc.

Symptomatology is often modified by the postoperative condition of the patient, and determination of the correct diagnosis is difficult and often delayed. This is why the lethality in this group is the highest. Microbiological findings are similar to those of secondary peritonitis.

### 17.3.4 Special Types of Peritonitis

Special types of peritonitis include tuberculous peritonitis and peritonitis after irradiation (plastic), which are chronic and are often manifested as the picture of the small intestinal ileus.

## 17.4 Clinical Symptoms

Predominant **clinical symptoms** of peritonitis are **local** and **general**. Both may be modified to a various extent by the primary cause and by the place of inflammation origination, but also by the age and general condition of the patient including his/her previous therapy. In general we may say that local symptoms prevail in initial stages of peritonitis, which often allow for diagnostic determination of the initial organ. General symptoms of sepsis and organ dysfunction start to predominate with the prolonged duration of peritonitis. Local findings of advanced peritonitis are then considerably uniform and often make it impossible to determine a more specific organ diagnosis. However, it should be emphasized here that timely indication for the initiation of therapy, which should be intensive, general and surgical, is substantially more important than accurate determination of the source of peritonitis.

The main and characteristic problem in patients with peritoneal inflammation is **pain**. Peritoneal pain is steady, permanent and relatively accurately localized (at least at the beginning of the disease). The pain is carried by spinal nerves – somatic pain. The pain rises upon movement, cough or shaking, and thus the patient typically assumes a **resting** supine **position** with partially bent legs and his/her respiration is superficial. When the position is changed, the pain sometimes irradiates in the shoulder (signs of pneumoperitoneum or subdiaphragmatic abscess – pain carried by the phrenic nerve).

Objective findings include **absent respiratory movements in the abdominal wall, pain in the anterior abdominal wall upon tapping (Plenies sign) and palpation, with the typical defensive contraction of muscles (défense musculaire)**. **Intensification of pain** not only upon compression of the wall but also after rapid release of compression is typical. A number of more or less common symptoms of peritoneal irritation (see acute abdomens in general), which may also be helpful in determining the primary source of the inflammation especially at the beginning of the disease, have been described for the most common causes of peritonitis. Silence is usually found upon auscultation with **absent peristalsis**, and **pain of the anterior wall** is typically **present** upon rectal examination.

The overall finding is dominated by **tachycardia** from the beginning of the inflammation (attention should be paid to its absence in some patients on beta-blockers or with stimulated heart rhythm) and often also signs of **circulatory instability, oliguria, tachypnea, fever** (the difference between rectal and axillary temperature over 0.5 °C is more sensitive than the axillary temperature itself). However, the determination of an early diagnosis of peritonitis cannot wait until all typical signs of peritonitis occur; the treatment must be initiated immediately and indication for surgery cannot be delayed because a certain, even important, symptom is missing. Auxiliary examinations should be used in a targeted mode to confirm the diagnosis and also to exclude some conditions that simulate symptomatology similar to that of peritonitis. Differential diagnostics based on localization of the initial causes is described in Chapter 15; other than surgical diseases that simulate peritonitis, inferior myocardial infarction, spontaneous pneumothorax (in certain cases both may be showing the picture of intense pain in the peritoneum with muscular contraction at the same place and circulatory symptomatology), as well as some serious metabolic disorders (for example, juvenile diabetes decompensation – diabetic pseudoperitonitis) should be excluded.

## 17.5 Paraclinical Diagnostics

**Inflammatory response** (leukocytosis, elevated CRP levels) can be demonstrated in **laboratory findings** from the beginning; however, this may not apply to individual cases. **Liver functions** are **altered** to a varied degree with the development of the system response (rise in transaminases and bilirubin), and pathological findings are present in **acid-base equilibrium** (respiratory alkalosis, metabolic acidosis) and in **blood gases** (both $p_aO_2$ and $p_aCO_2$ decreased). Rising **serum lactate** levels correlate well with the gravity of the general condition. However, none of the findings above is typical only for peritonitis or intra-abdominal sepsis, and therefore, they do not allow for revealing the primary source.

Other than the clinical examination, the dominant position in the diagnostics of peritonitis is that of **ultrasonography (US)**. US is a non-invasive assessment, generally and acutely available, which also allows for monitoring any further development of the finding. The **evidence of free fluid in the abdominal cavity** is decisive in the US finding for acute peritonitis. US sensitivity and specificity in the demonstration of any higher amount of intra-abdominal fluid exceeds 95%. **Targeted puncture** may also be undertaken in diagnostically unclear cases in order to assess the characteristics of the fluid and for biochemical (pancreatitis) and bacteriological assessment (clear vs. turbid ascites). When the course of the disease is subacute or in cases of intra-abdominal sepsis, US assessment can contribute to finding a collection of fluid corresponding to an abscess in the subphrenic area, between intestinal loops, in the area of the appendix or in the Douglas space, but also to demonstrate abscess in parenchymatous organs. In these cases, too, an intervention can be undertaken using the puncture technique and the lesion can be drained under US inspection. Besides the demonstration of fluid the US examination makes it possible to obtain additional information, for example, about the integrity of parenchymatous organs or about the thickness of the gallbladder or appendix wall.

**Native abdominal radiography in the standing position** is a standard method in all cases of unclear abdominal pain. The finding of **free air in the subdiaphragmatic region** provides convincing evidence for acute peritonitis due to perforation of a hollow organ. Most commonly, this finding is demonstrated upon the perforation of the gastroduodenal ulcer; however, it may also accompany the perforation of the appendix with gangrenous appendicitis, of the sigmoid due to diverticulitis or cecum due to distension above any obstruction in the colon. If the patient is unable to stand, the radiography can be done with the patient lying on the left hip, using a horizontal beam, and a crescent of free air is displayed over the convex part of the right lobe of the liver. A **thoracic scan** must always be done to complete radiographic diagnostics. In addition to its undoubtful value for the complex assessment of the patient's general condition, sometimes it may surprisingly change further procedures by providing evidence of spontaneous pneumothorax in a patient with thus far convincing symptomatology of gastroduodenal perforation.

Indication for **CT assessment** is very limited in clinically apparent peritonitis. In cases of justified suspicion of acute pancreatitis (hyperamylasemia, absent pain per rectum), CT assessment is often the only possibility to confirm the diagnosis, and thus to avoid unnecessary diagnostic laparotomy. On the contrary, CT assessment is the "gold standard" in cases of subacute development and suspicion of an intra-abdominal origin of sepsis. It allows for not only demonstrating and localizing lesions of fluid or necrotic tissue in the abdominal cavity and retroperitoneum, but at the same time performing a therapeutic intervention – targeted puncture and drainage using special drains under CT inspection.

Other auxiliary assessments are used only in special and unusual situations and are of no essential importance for deciding on the therapeutic procedure. The only exception is endoscopy when perforation of the gastroduodenal ulcer is suspected. In the event of unclear clinical and radiographic findings endoscopy can be used not only to demonstrate the lesion in the anterior wall, but a new abdominal radiography after endoscopy typically demonstrates free air below the diaphragm (insufflated during endoscopic examination) and the indication for laparotomy becomes apparent.

## 17.6 Indications for Surgical Treatment

It should again be repeated that in the event of peritonitis timely indication for laparotomy is more important than exact organ diagnosis. The basic findings that lead to the indication of laparotomy include in particular:
1. Duration or intensification and spreading of abdominal pain
2. Increasing pain and muscular contraction upon repeated examinations
3. Rising tachycardia and circulatory instability upon adequate intensive therapy
4. Radiological demonstration of free air in the abdominal cavity
5. Sonographic demonstration of a rather large or growing amount of free fluid in the abdominal cavity (with the exception of ascites in liver CI and acute pancreatitis)

Early laparotomy is an essential part of therapy in cases of the most common secondary but also tertiary peritonitis. Any intensive therapy will be unsuccessful without resolving the cause of the sepsis. Only in a part of patients with subacute course and circumscribed inflammatory lesions, the alternative procedure of puncture drainage under CT or US inspection is possible depending on the general condition, localization and cause of the process. The same applies to abscesses in parenchymatous organs, particularly as part of postoperative intra--abdominal sepsis.

Upon the clear diagnosis of rare primary peritonitis (pelveoperitonitis of gynecological origin, patients with liver CI and ascites and patients with chronic peritoneal dialysis), conservative therapy (antibiotics, general therapy) is indicated at the beginning. However, laparotomy is also indicated in these patients if the finding progresses, at least for differential diagnostic reasons to exclude secondary peritonitis.

## 17.7 Peritonitis Therapy

The current **standard** of peritonitis therapy corresponds to the current situation for the possibilities of sepsis therapy. The basic parts of the therapy include the following:
1. Surgical rehabilitation of the septic lesion
2. Antimicrobial therapy – preferentially bactericidal antibiotics and chemotherapeutics (cave: release of a rather large amount of endotoxin from disintegrated bacterial bodies upon the initiation of therapy!)
3. Intensive – medical measures to prevent and treat organ dysfunctions (volume replacement and inotropic support, ventilation support, active detoxification)
4. Immune support in prolonged septic symptomatology
5. Early initiated enteral nutrition to recover the intestinal barrier

Although in individual cases the intensity of applied measures closely depends on the clinical condition of the patient, it is a complex of mutually linked and purposefully complementary therapeutic methods of which none may be left out or underestimated. The therapy should be initiated immediately, during diagnostic tests, and further procedure should be aimed at removal of the septic source in the fastest and most effective way possible.

### 17.7.1 Surgical Treatment and Options

The aim of surgical treatment is to remove the source of the inflammation (suture of the perforated duodenal ulcer, cholecystectomy of the gangrenous gallbladder, appendectomy of the perforated appendix, resection of the affected segment of the intestine, etc.), and therapeutic **effect on the peritoneal inflammation**. Particularly upon diffuse contamination of the abdominal cavity, complete removal of bacteria, fibrin, exudate and/or any pus or stool using simple on-time peroperative lavage usually cannot be achieved by the primary surgery. For cases of severe diffuse purulent and stercoral cases of peritonitis, supplementary surgical measures have been developed – **enclosed continuous lavage of the abdominal cavity, lavage in stages or repeated revisions with lavages upon the open abdomen**. The aim of all these methods and of their numerous modifications is the removal of residual peritoneal contamination and of newly formed exudate, prevention of secretion accumulation in the abdominal cavity, and possibly checking the completeness of, or additional performance of rehabilitation of the primary lesion unless it cannot be achieved during the first surgery. Irrespective of the chosen alternative method, postoperative peritoneal lavage is a method which is demanding for both the patient (for example, repeated general anesthesia for surgical lavages) and the attending personnel (treatment of many drains, immobile patients, etc.). The risks should not be neglected because of possible damage to organ walls by the used drains, bleeding, intestinal fistula and potential contamination from the external environment or an overload of the circulation due to absorption of large amounts of liquid of the lavage solution by the peritoneum. Therefore, the indication for postoperative peritoneal lavage is limited only to the most severe cases – diffuse stercoral and purulent cases of peritonitis and cases where causes and sources of peritonitis cannot be examined completely in the peroperative period. In other cases, thorough **extensive peroperative lavage of all 4 quadrants of the abdominal cavity** is sufficient (10–30 liters of the flushing solution heated to body temperature), and effective drainage of the primary inflammation site and areas of the most common accumulation of intra-abdominal fluid – subphrenic areas and the Douglas space. In localized circumscribed cases of peritonitis and intra-abdominal abscesses, **flushing of the lesion and drainage** in addition to rehabilitation are usually sufficient. The drain(s) can also be used in the postoperative period for intermittent or less commonly continuous lavage of the abscess cavity.

Supplementation of antibiotics to lavage solutions has not proven to be useful (low effectiveness, rise in resistance, local allergization, etc.); of decisive importance is the mechanical function of the lavage. On the contrary, a favorable effect has been reported in the use of some antiseptics; noxytiolin and taurolidine provide, in addition to their bactericidal effect, the ability to bind released endotoxin.

**Enclosed continuous lavage of the abdominal cavity** is usually done by introducing 2 inlet drains and 3–4 outlet drains (subphrenia, paracolic recesses, Douglas space) before closing the laparotomy. A lavage solution (Peridial, Max II, etc.) is instilled permanently to both inlet drains, and brought to collection systems by the outlet drains, while measuring the flushing balance. The amount of 6–24 l of the solution is used for 24 hours based on the operative finding, based on how the lavage works and based on the characteristics of the removed eluate. Enclosed lavage provides the advantage of early food intake, orally or enterally. Repeated anesthesia to remove the peritoneal secretion is not needed, and at the same time, the traumatization of the abdominal cavity organs is reduced, which may limit the formation of intra-abdominal adhesions. The disadvantage of the method is that the drainage of some areas is not effective and abscesses may form in such areas. A certain risk also follows from the use of drains – damage of organ walls by pressure.

The principle of **lavage in stages** is the direct visual control of the situation in the abdominal cavity by repeated surgical revisions in 24–48h intervals. Besides thorough removal of the pathological content from all areas of the peritoneal cavity, it allows for repeated checks and for additional treatment of the primary inflammatory source and/or other intra-abdominal complications. This approach provides the advantage of not having to use any drains, and thus the risk of complications caused by them is not present. The disadvantages include the need of repeated general anesthesia with persisting postoperative intestinal atonia, more common occurrence of specific complications (intestinal fistulae) and the laparotomic wound healing disorders.

The method of **repeated lavages while leaving the abdomen open (laparostomy)** is indicated similar to the lavage in stages, while instead of repeated closures of the laparotomic wound, a temporary closure is performed using a foil with a zip fastener or only by lining the surgical wound with moist abdominal cloths. Compared to the lavage in stages, released intra-abdominal pressure and thus also an improvement of the perfusion of abdominal organs, particularly of the intestine, is the principal benefit. Other advantages and disadvantages are similar. As a rule, definitive closure of the laparostomy is difficult due to retraction of the edges of the fascia; the closure must thus be more commonly resolved by postponed plasty of the abdominal wall in two periods.

### 17.7.2 Complications of Peritonitis Therapy

**Intra-abdominal abscesses** are the most common local **complication** after surgeries due to peritonitis. Typically, they are localized in the lowest areas of the peritoneal cavity in a supine patient (subphrenia, the Douglas space) and in areas inaccessible for drainage and lavage (interloop abscesses). The clinical picture is usually dominated by **persisting symptoms or by recurrently manifested septic organ dysfunctions**, and the abdominal finding is undistinctive in a number of cases. **US and CT assessments** provide indispensable help in the diagnostics of these complications. Both methods also allow for **targeted diagnostic puncture and drainage of the lesion**. When the drainage is effective, surgical intervention is usually not needed. However, the effect of puncture drainage is only temporary in septic cavities with a dense content and tissue shreds, and surgical **revision including the evacuation of the abscess and drainage using a larger drain** must be performed.

## 17.8 Prognosis in Patients with Peritonitis

The **prognosis** in patients with peritonitis is always serious and depends on the inducing cause of the inflammation, general condition of the patient, and timely initiation of adequate therapy. While a mean lethality rate of less than 10% is seen in patients with gastroduodenal ulcer perforation operated within 6 hours from the onset of symptoms, a lethality rate of about 80% is found in patients with developed septic failure of two and more systems, irrespective of the primary source of the sepsis.

Even if the disease of peritonitis is successfully overcome, its carrier is endangered by the consequences in his/her further life. **Adhesions** in the abdominal cavity may be the cause of intestinal obstruction.

# 18  ABDOMINAL TRAUMA

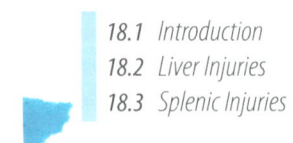

> 18.1  Introduction
> 18.2  Liver Injuries
> 18.3  Splenic Injuries

## 18.1  Introduction

In terms of their characteristics, abdominal injuries belong to an acute abdomen. As for their basic classification, traumas are divided into **closed injuries,** e.g. deceleration upon impact and falls, compression, blows to the abdomen, and **open injuries,** e.g. stabs, cuts, gunshot wounds, and dilacerations, and **iatrogenic injuries,** e.g. those due to invasive examinations or occurring during operations. The result of an injury depends on the nature of the trauma, on the intensity, direction and duration of the acting force, on localization of the injury, on the volume of the content in hollow organs at the time of the injury, and certainly on the condition of the injured person.

Injuries may be isolated, combined or constituent of compound injuries or polytraumas.

**Closed injuries** cause contusion of the abdominal wall, and contusions and ruptures of parenchymatous and hollow organs in the abdomen and in the retroperitoneum.

**Contusions of the abdominal wall** (often with a hematoma in layers of the wall) are painful and cause muscle tension. It is often difficult to distinguish whether only the wall has been affected or whether the muscle tension is caused by peritoneal irritation. Diagnosis involves a medical history, US/CT examination, development during observation.

**Contusions of parenchymatous organs** (liver, pancreas, spleen, kidneys) are indistinctive in terms of symptomatology: in addition to pain of the affected area, the finding of a US/CT examination provides evidence of contusion, confirming contusion lesions in the parenchyma. **Laboratory** assessments usually demonstrate leukocytosis, a rise in CRP values, liver test and bilirubin values for liver contusions, hyperamylasemia for pancreatic contusions, and micro- and macroscopic hematuria for renal contusions.

Injuries caused by falls or impacts where intense deceleration is the primary mechanism of the injury may also cause damage to parenchymatous organs by ruptures of the capsule or parenchyma or by tearing out the organs from their suspensions. As for hollow organs, the suspension is often torn out in such situations (for example, the mesenterium, the mesocolon), especially when there is some content in the lumen of the organ. The rupture of hollow organs is often caused by compression of the abdomen. Rupture poses more of a threat to the fixated and voluminous colon than to the more delicate and movable small intestine or to the stomach with its strong musculature.

**Symptoms** are derived from the affection, i.e. ruptures of suspensions that cause bleeding, the manifestations of which tend to be the major symptoms, and also hemoperitoneum, while ruptures of hollow organs result in the escape of their content into the abdominal cavity and peritonitis.

**Penetrating injuries** are characterized by an injury to the abdominal wall and injury to abdominal viscera. The insidiousness of such an injury follows from the impossibility to estimate whether only the abdominal wall or also the viscera have been injured. Stab and gunshot wounds are the most common mechanisms of a penetrating injury; penetrating injuries are less commonly cut wounds, and exceptionally they may occur due to lacerations or compressions. Consequences of the injuries depend on similar circumstances as those of blunt abdominal injuries, which also influence the **symptoms**. Abdominal wounds as a rule bleed; bleeding originates directly in the wall or blood from the abdomen may flow out through the wound. In the event that no large vessel has been injured, the bleeding may stop spontaneously (illusively!) within a few minutes.

The **diagnostics** are focused more on estimating the localization, scope and gravity of the injury (accurate medical history and description of the injury) and on the preoperative examination and ensuring surgery than on excluding or confirming an intra-abdominal injury because **every penetrating injury must be revised** (diagnostic laparotomy). When the injured person is in generally good condition and shows no signs of circulatory instability, the surgical finding may be specified closer using radiography in the standing position (in the search for pneumoperitoneum), radiography of the chest (hemo- or pneumothorax upon an injury through the diaphragm) and US/CT examination of the abdomen (in the search for any fluid and/or apparent organ lesion).

**Surgical treatment** of abdominal injuries is initiated at the time of the first examination with elimination of oral intake, securing the injured person in the supine position and calm, monitoring of vital functions. In the event of penetrating injuries, the wound should be disinfected and covered; if the viscera are prolapsed, they should not be repositioned and no present foreign bodies should be removed!

The treatment of blunt injuries differs based on the symptoms:
- Injured persons in generally good condition and with stable circulation – the methods above are used to search for any manifestations of internal injuries; where visceral perforation and continued intra-abdominal bleeding can be excluded, the procedure is conservative (resting regimen in bed, monitoring

of vital functions and/or limited oral intake, infusion therapy, repeated checks of the clinical finding, repeated US examinations).
- Injured persons with instable circulation – support of vital functions (O$_2$, infusions, transfusions), US/CT examination of the abdomen; in the event of free fluid – surgery (laparoscopy, laparotomy). Rapid development of hypotension after demonstrable abdominal injury is an indication for urgent laparotomy with no additional examinations.

The manner of surgical treatment depends on the type of injury. The aim of the operation is to stop bleeding, and treat any ruptures and perforations by ligature, suture, resection of injured viscera or their removal, by compression using tamponades, etc.

**Treatment of penetrating injuries** consists in surgical revision. Laparotomy is performed outside the place of injury, and the surgical solution is based on the finding. The extent of surgical procedures ranges from local treatment to organ removal (for example, splenectomy, nephrectomy) or removal of their parts (for example, intestinal resection). Besides the surgical finding, the deliberation regarding the extent of the surgery also takes into account the nature of such injury (contamination in the abdominal cavity, necroses due to gunshot injuries – the zone of molecular commotion).

The **prognosis** is influenced by the extent of the injury, the promptness and quality of its treatment, and any **complications**. The most common complications include late bleeding, vascular thromboses (with subsequent necroses of affected tissues), intra-abdominal and retroperitoneal hematomas, paralytic ileus and infections.

Special attention ought to be paid to **injuries caused by foreign bodies** that have entered the abdomen via natural body openings – by swallowing, or via the rectum, vagina or urethra. Such foreign bodies then cause an obstruction in the gastrointestinal tract manifested by the symptoms of intestinal obstruction or perforation, symptoms of intra-abdominal abscess or peritonitis, and/or they may perforate into another system.

In addition to careful collection of a medical history, radiography and US examinations are also helpful for the diagnostics, since they can be used to find any such foreign body. The treatment is surgical and the operation consists in the extraction of the foreign body, treatment of the affected organ, and treatment of any complications caused by such foreign body.

**Iatrogenic abdominal injuries** include surgical injuries and injuries due to invasive diagnostic and therapeutic procedures. Injuries to other organs and localizations than those to be operated on are considered as **surgical** injuries. They originate in the course of abdominal surgeries when they are, with certain exceptions, also revealed and treated. Their consequence in such cases is normally only unplanned expansion and prolongation of the surgery. If overlooked, they are manifested by bleeding, abscesses or peritonitis.

Other injuries originate during **endoscopic procedures** and also during **transparietal punctures** of abdominal organs. Injuries are caused by perforation of the intestinal wall (duodenum, colon) upon difficult insertion of the endoscope or by perforation upon biopsies and polypectomies. Perforations are either noticed by the endoscopist or they are manifested by increasing pneumoperitoneum or peritonitis.

The solution is usually surgical and consists in resuturing the affected area or resecting the affected intestinal segment.

Injuries due to a puncture normally apply, with certain exceptions, to bleeding from the punctured area – usually the liver.

Their manifestations provide evidence of hemoperitoneum and the treatment is surgical, e.g. resuture or tamponade of the bleeding area.

Note: All invasive medical activities, even if performed **lege artis**, may cause an injury. It is important to know about the possibility of an injury, not to overlook any injury and to ensure adequate treatment!

## 18.2 Liver Injuries

Although the liver is protected relatively well against being injured, injuries to it are the most common among all abdominal organs, with only the spleen being injured more often upon blunt abdominal trauma. The main **mechanism of trauma** in liver injuries in Europe are blunt abdominal injuries (up to 80–90% of all liver injuries), in the US or in South Africa penetrating abdominal injuries (90% and 70%, respectively). Blunt injuries are caused by laceration of the parenchyma or capsule upon intense deceleration or by compression between the ribs and the spine. Penetrating injuries are usually caused by stab or gunshot wounds.

The severity of any injury depends on the nature of anatomic changes and on the extent of liver damage, ranging from a small laceration of the capsule or subcapsular hematoma to extensive rupture of the liver with an injury to hepatic veins or to the inferior vena cava. The gravity of the injury can be expressed using a 6-point classification (Table 18.1).

**Symptoms** of the injury and the clinical picture depend on the extent of liver injury, on its mechanism, and on the nature of other associated injuries. Bleeding in the abdomen accompanied by hypotension up to hemorrhagic shock is the main consequence of severe liver injuries (gr. III and higher), and upon injuries of gr. V and VI, the injured person may bleed to death immediately at the place of the injury.

**Table 18.1** Classification of liver injuries

| Grade | Injury | Characteristics |
|---|---|---|
| I | • Hematoma | • Subcapsular hematoma, less than 10% of liver area |
|  | • Laceration | • A tear in the capsule affecting the parenchyma to the depth of up to 1 cm |
| II | • Hematoma | • Subcapsular hematoma, 10–50% of liver area<br>Intraparenchymatous hematoma with less than 10 cm diameter |
| III | • Hematoma | • Subcapsular hematoma, more than 50% of the area (or progression), subcapsular or intrahepatic hematoma with rupture<br>Intraparenchymatous hematoma larger than 10 cm |
|  | • Laceration | • Tear deeper than 3 cm |
| IV | • Laceration | • Tears in the parenchyma with affection of 25–75% of the parenchyma<br>Single lobe |
| V | • Laceration | • Affection of more than 75% of the parenchyma |
|  | • Vascular affection | • Injury to juxtahepatic veins, retrohepatic segment of the inferior vena cava and hepatic veins |
| VI | • Vascular affection | • Liver avulsion |

**Diagnostics**: Upon a penetrating injury, the finding of wounds on the body leads to the diagnosis of an intra-abdominal and liver injury, while upon the blunt injury hypotension and signs of hemoperitoneum come to the fore.

The combination of a blunt abdominal injury and unconsciousness is difficult in terms of diagnostics, where the presence of a liver injury can be concluded only based on the history (if determinable) and rapidly progressing hypotension.

The scope of examinations differs based on the condition of the injured and the nature of the injury. Injuries associated with penetrating or blunt abdominal injury and signs of hemorrhagic shock – **hemodynamically unstable** – are indicated for **immediate surgical revision with no additional examinations**. Injured persons who are **hemodynamically stable** may be examined, while the finding of fluid around the liver or in the free abdominal cavity by US or CT examination, in connection with information on an abdominal injury from the history, is assessed as a sign of hemoperitoneum. US or CT examination can also be used to directly diagnose an injury to the hepatic capsule, parenchyma or possibly vascular structures. In hemodynamically stable patients, the finding can be confirmed using diagnostic laparoscopy.

The **therapy** of liver injuries is conservative and surgical. In up to 2/3 of liver injuries the bleeding stops spontaneously, particularly in less extensive ones (gr.

# ABDOMINAL TRAUMA

I to III). Conservative therapy consists in a resting regimen in bed, monitoring of vital functions, observance of the development of the physical findings and of the findings upon repeated US or CT examinations. Similarly to spleen injuries, a two-period rupture should always be taken into account.

The purpose of surgical treatment is to achieve provisional and/or definitive stoppage of bleeding with concurrent circulatory resuscitation. Provisional stoppage of bleeding can be achieved by compression of vascular structures, particularly in the hepatoduodenal ligament using the so-called Pringle maneuver, or by compression of the parenchyma through temporary tamponades. Definitive stoppage of bleeding can be achieved by direct ligation of the bleeding vessels or by anatomic or extra-anatomic resection of the liver.

Stabilization is another possibility of treatment, i.e. tightening the liver using a grid, or possibly performing tamponade of bleeding tears of the tissue itself or those caused by foreign material, or by performing tamponade of the bleeding canal in the parenchyma using a catheter with a long balloon in the event of gunshot and stab wounds. Surgical treatment becomes extraordinarily difficult upon extensive dilacerations affecting a substantial part of the parenchyma and upon injuries to hepatic veins.

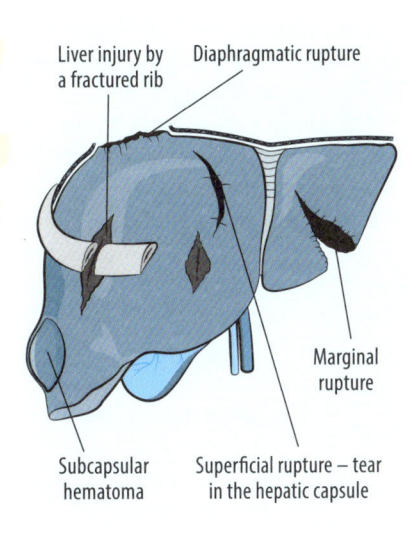

*Fig. 18.1 Liver injury*

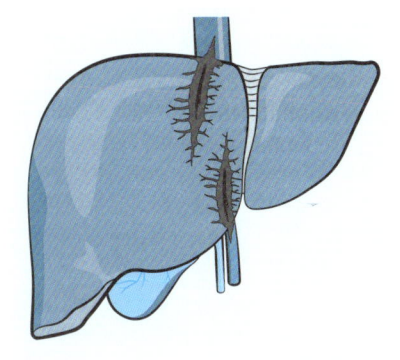

*Fig. 18.2 Deep tear in the hepatic hilum*

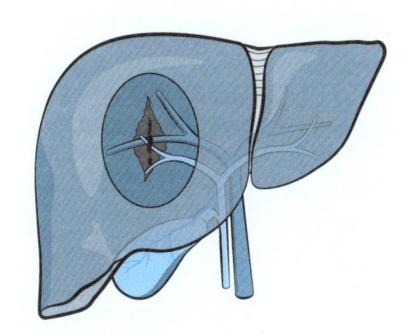

*Fig. 18.3 Central tears in the liver with affection of intrahepatic veins and bile ducts*

**Complications of the therapy** include particularly bleeding in the second period or after the surgery, infections and sepsis, necroses of the parenchyma, liver failure and biliary fistula.

The **prognosis** depends on the manner and extent of the liver injury, on any additional injuries, on the condition of the injured person, and on the time and success of the treatment.

Contusions and subcapsular hematomas usually heal without any later consequences; the prognosis of more severe injuries depends on all the above factors. Based on the mechanism of the injury, blunt liver injuries have up to a 30% mortality rate, and penetrating injuries about 10%.

## 18.3 Splenic Injuries

The issues regarding splenic injuries are explained in Chapter 14.

# 19  GIT HEMORRHAGE

> *19.1* Upper GIT Hemorrhage
> *19.2* Lower GIT Hemorrhage

GIT hemorrhage or bleeding in the GIT is classified as a serious disease. About 80% of all bleeding events stop spontaneously; the remaining 15 to 20% are massive bleedings which may lead to death due to quickly developing hemorrhagic shock, even in a young person. Therefore, every patient with current bleeding in the GIT must be promptly examined, diagnosed, treated and monitored in an intensive care unit (ARU or ICU).

Based on localization, the disease is classified as bleeding in the **upper part** of the GI tract (esophagus, stomach, duodenum) or in the **lower part** of the tract (rectum, colon, small intestine).

Based on the extent of blood loss we distinguish two types of bleeding events: **massive bleeding**, which is always associated with circulatory instability and **hemorrhagic shock**. Patients usually need four or more units of blood through transfusions during the first 12 hours and are at a high risk of death. Less **serious bleeding** events are free of any symptoms of shock.

Bleeding in the GIT is manifested by at least one of the following symptoms:
- **Hematemesis** – vomiting of fresh or darker blood, and sometimes vomit the color of coffee sediment. In most cases, such vomiting indicates bleeding from the esophagus or stomach up to the pylorus. The color and characteristics of the vomit depend on the bleeding intensity and also on the time of contact with HCl in the stomach.
- **Melena** – black, greasy, tarry, strange smelling stool is a symptom of bleeding from the exit part of the stomach or from the duodenum, and exceptionally from the proximal segment of the small intestine. Melena develops upon bacterial degradation of hematin in the intestine.
- **Hematochesis** (often incorrectly called enterorrhagia) – is the excretion of fresh blood and coagula through the rectum. It is usually a symptom of bleeding from the lower part of the GIT; however, it may also come from a source of massive bleeding found in the upper part of the tract, which passes through the intestine too quickly for any melena to develop.

After the clinical examination and determination of bleeding in the GIT, it is necessary to immediately ensure sufficient venous access, determine the blood type, order blood, place the patient in the ICU and monitor his or her circulatory parameters.

**Urgent endoscopy** plays a crucial role in these patients. Today, urgent endoscopy is understood as an examination performed immediately, not later than within 2 hours, in exceptional situations within 6 hours. A patient for urgent endoscopy should be circulatory stable. Patients with consciousness disorder must be intubated before an endoscopy due to the risk of aspiration. An urgent endoscopy should explain the origin and intensity of the bleeding. Based on the finding, the therapy is conservative, endoscopic or surgical.

**Conservative therapy** includes circulatory resuscitation, i.e. supplementation of effective circulatory volume of the bloodstream by administering infusion solutions of crystalloids and plasma expanders, and also blood transfusions and frozen plasma in the case of more severe bleeding. Another measure is oxygen therapy. Parenteral administration of certain hemostyptics (Pamba, Dicynone) is no longer performed. Minor bleeding stops spontaneously and major bleeding, usually from the bleeding vessel, is not affected by this medication.

After such bleeding, peristalsis should be supported to remove the toxic intestinal content. Products administered include lactulose and purgative clysma.

Conservative therapy includes special medications, for example, proton pump blockers upon the peptic ulcer, drugs to reduce portal hypertension (Remestyp), and others.

**Endoscopic therapy** includes the methods of **endoscopic hemostasis**. These methods are being used more and more often and the effect of their use rises with the capacities of departments and with the experience of the examiner. Injection therapy using an endoscopic injector, which is a thin flexible accessory equipped with a telescopic needle at one end and a syringe at the other, is the most common, simplest and least expensive method. The instrument is introduced in the endoscope through the working channel and hemostasis is achieved by application of adrenalin, absolute alcohol, polydocanol (Aethoxysklerol) or in exceptional cases other substances into the bleeding tissue or the bleeding vessel. Other special hemostatic methods include application of a clip on the vessel, bandage of varices, application of tissue adhesives and thermocoagulation methods: monopolar or bipolar electrocoagulation, use of a laser and argon beam coagulation. Endoscopic methods are being used more and more commonly as a definitive solution to bleeding in the GIT because they are effective and the number of bleeding relapses after their application considerably decreases.

Surgical solutions still have their essential place in the therapy of bleeding. Surgery is indicated as **urgent** in cases where intense bleeding that cannot be affected by endoscopy needs to be stopped. An **early elective** surgery is indicated within 24 to 36 hours after successful endoscopic hemostasis where there is a high risk of a bleeding relapse given that relapsed bleeding increases both morbidity and mortality.

In summary, the care of patients with bleeding in the GIT has several goals – to ensure circulation in the patient, to promptly determine the diagnosis and to stop the bleeding and prevent a relapse.

## 19.1 Upper GIT Hemorrhage

**Peptic ulcer** is the cause of about 60% of bleeding events, with duodenal ulcers being the source of bleeding more commonly than gastric ulcers. Any type of ulcer may bleed (solitary, multiple, callous, penetrating, stress, drug-induced).

For the sake of clarity of the diagnosis and to determine the therapy, findings are classified based on the modified **Forrest classification** as follows:
- Group I – Actively bleeding ulcers
  - F Ia – Spurting arterial bleeding
  - F Ib – Non-spurting capillary bleeding
- Group II – Ulcers with signs after bleeding (stigmata)
  - F IIa – Visible vascular stub at the base of the ulcer
  - F IIb – Coagulum firmly attached
  - F IIc – Base of the ulcer having the color of coffee sediment
- Group III – Non-bleeding ulcers
  - F III – Ulcer with no signs of bleeding

**Endoscopic hemostasis** is used for active bleeding classified as F Ia, F Ib, and for findings associated with a high risk of bleeding relapse, i.e. F IIa. The most commonly used methods include injection therapy and vessel clipping; argon beam coagulation and application of tissue adhesives can also be used.

Other findings, when there is no more bleeding, are treated using **conservative** therapy. This therapy includes specific antiulcer medications – particularly proton pump blockers.

An indication for **surgical treatment** is a specific surgical issue. In general, it can be said that all bleeding events are indicated where endoscopic hemostasis has failed. Such operations are **urgent**, i.e. they are undertaken immediately. A relapse of bleeding should be prevented, and that is why findings with a high risk of such relapse are also indicated for surgical treatment. These are **early elective** surgeries, undertaken within 24–36 hours after successful hemostasis. Their indications include stopped bleeding classified as F Ia and some F IIa findings with some other, so called risk factors – advanced age of the patient, complicating diseases (IHD, DM, etc.), ulcer larger than 2 cm, and risk associated with the localization of the ulcer (lesser curvature of the stomach or posterior wall of the duodenal bulb).

At present, we prefer **local operations**, such as injection of the ulcer through gastrotomy or duodenotomy, excision and suture of the bleeding ulcer, and devascularization of the bleeding area. These procedures are simpler and, therefore, they are preferred in patients exhausted from the bleeding. A certain disadvantage of these methods is the possibility of a bleeding relapse. Resection procedures not only stop the bleeding, but they also exert a therapeutic effect on the ulcer disease itself. They are used predominantly in gastric ulcers. Vagotomy combined with injection of the ulcer can also be used for ulcers of the duodenal bulb. Individual types of surgeries are described in greater detail in Section 8.5.

This modern approach to therapy is associated with bleeding relapses of less than 10% and mortality ranging from 5–8%.

**Hemorrhagic or erosive gastropathy** is the cause of an upper GIT hemorrhage in about 30% of cases. It is the diffuse bleeding of the mucosa or bleeding superficial multiple erosions. The etiology is often similar to that of acute ulcers, i.e. reduced mucosal perfusion. It may also be induced by drugs, particularly by non-steroid antirheumatics (NSAID).

The therapy is **conservative** on principle. In addition to antiulcer medications, vasopressin, terlipressin and possibly somatostatin can also be used for extensive bleeding.

**Bleeding from esophageal varices** is in third place in terms of frequency, 5–10%. It is always associated with portal hypertension, usually caused by liver cirrhosis in adults. The patients are always at risk and show high mortality. This severe condition is caused by several co-acting factors – profuse bleeding from varices with rapidly developing hemorrhagic shock, liver failure, coagulopathy, thrombocytopenia. Last but not least, there is a tendency to early relapsing, even if the bleeding has already been stopped.

Therapy is focused on prevention and treatment of the hemorrhagic shock, on the prevention and treatment of liver failure, and on hemostasis. Endoscopic methods are combined with conservative therapy to achieve hemostasis; urgent surgeries are almost never performed due to the high risk of death.

**Endoscopic hemostasis** plays a main role in the therapy. The most commonly applied is **injection therapy** using sclerotizing solutions (polydocanol – Aethoxysklerol) that are administered to varices or their surroundings. Endoscopic ligation of the varices is another option, i.e. strangulation of the bleeding vessel using a rubber ring, or possibly coagulation using an argon beam, laser, or application of synthetic adhesives (histoacrylates).

**Pharmacotherapy** forms an integral part of the conservative therapy. Portal hypertension can be reduced by vasopressin administration. Due to the cardiotoxic effect of vasopressin, a less toxic derivative of vasopressin, terlipressin (Remestyp), is used. Hemostasis can also be achieved using somatostatin, which may substitute for endoscopy when not available.

Therapeutic measures include the use of the three-lumen Sengstaken-Blakemore tube. After insertion in the stomach, one lumen is used to remove blood, one to fill a gastric balloon located at the end, which is upon slight pulling captured in the cardia. Besides fixing the tube in place, the balloon compresses subcardial venous plexuses, which supply the varices with blood. The third lumen is used to fill the oblong esophageal balloon that compresses the varices. The resulting hemostasis is very good but the balloons can only be left filled for 12 to 24 hours at the maximum due to the risk of the development of decubitus, necrosis and potentially perforation. Bleeding relapses occur often (in up to 60% of cases) after the pressure has been removed.

As mentioned above, urgent surgeries are performed in exceptional circumstances when there are no other possibilities. These include various procedures, such as injections of the varices from the transthoracic access, devascularization of the cardioesophageal passage from the abdominal access, or transection of the distal esophagus using the circular stapler from the abdominal access.

An early relapse of the bleeding can also be prevented by elective sclerotization (highly debated), pharmacotherapy (administration of nitrates or trimepranol), elective surgery consisting in the establishment of a portosystemic connection (usually the distal splenorenal shunt according to Warren), and TIPSS (a mini invasive method). However, early bleeding relapses still represent about 40%, and early mortality reaches approximately 60% of these patients. The only definitive solution is a liver transplant. For more details see Section 12.6.

**Mallory-Weiss syndrome** is the cause of about 5% of bleeding events. It is a longitudinal tear in the passage of esophageal and gastric mucosa, which as a rule develops after strenuous vomiting, and sometimes after excessive consumption of alcohol. The therapy is conservative; in the event of a major bleeding endoscopic.

**Tumors** are not a common source of macroscopic bleeding in the upper GIT; however, if they occur, the immediate therapy is usually endoscopic, with subsequent surgical treatment.

**Aorto-enteral fistula** is a rare source of bleeding. The fistula usually develops after vascular replacements, and is most commonly localized in the duodenum. Urgent surgery is always indicated since the only solution is surgical. The mortality rate is high even upon timely surgery and reaches 50%.

Other rare causes of upper tract hemorrhage may include reflux esophagitis, hiatal hernia, angiodysplasia, more severe hemorrhagic diseases, and anticoagulation therapy. Potential complications after endoscopic procedures must not be forgotten.

## 19.2 Lower GIT Hemorrhage

The main symptom of lower GIT bleeding is hematochesis. It occurs less commonly than bleeding in the upper tract, and is only rarely associated with hemorrhagic shock. In spite of this, it is a serious condition.

The diagnostics are based on an urgent endoscopy. Rectoscopy is usually not sufficient, and sigmoidoscopy may reveal about 75% of such sources in the rectosigmoid area. However, **urgent total colonoscopy** is the ideal method. The source may sometimes not be identified since upon heavier bleeding the coagula and often the stool make visibility and the examination procedure quite impossible. The following procedure is then recommended: upper endoscopy to exclude any source in upper GIT; demonstration of bleeding using angiography or a scan after the blood cells have been labeled with the radioisotope $^{99m}$Tc; and total colonoscopy after preparation of the intestine. The source of bleeding in the small intestine can be diagnosed and possibly also treated using enteroscopy (double-balloon enteroscopy).

The most common sources of lower GIT hemorrhage include:
- **Hemorrhoids** – the most common source. The therapy is conservative, endoscopic as well as surgical (see Chapter 9).
- **Polyps** – the maximum occurrence of adenomas is found in the rectosigmoid, but they may be localized anywhere in the colon. The therapy is usually endoscopic, **polypectomy** using the loop, or exceptionally surgical in large, sessile polyps.
- **Tumors** – see Sections 9.4.4 and 9.5.4. The solution is surgical. Exceptionally, in large inoperable tumors, the solution may consist in endoscopic hemostasis or embolization of supply vessels as part of angiography.
- **Diverticula** – are found in elderly patients and usually in the left half of the colon. The therapy for bleeding is usually conservative.

Other rare sources of intestinal bleeding include angiodysplasia, ulcerous colitis, Crohn's disease, infectious colitis, rectal ulcer, any hemorrhagic disease, anticoagulation therapy, conditions after polypectomy, and others.

# 20  MINI-INVASIVE SURGERY

> 20.1 Laparoscopic Cholecystectomy
> 20.2 Laparoscopic Appendectomy
> 20.3 Laparoscopic Inguinal Hernioplasty
> 20.4 Gastroesophageal Reflux Disease and Hiatal Hernias
> 20.5 Laparoscopic Colorectal Procedures
> 20.6 Diagnostic and Therapeutic Thoracoscopy
> 20.7 The Future of Minimally Invasive Therapy

The concept of major operations, particularly abdominal ones, first came into question in the middle of the 20$^{th}$ century. Extensive surgical incisions justified by the need for sufficient access to affected organs or areas are the main characteristics of this surgery built on knowledge from the end of the 19$^{th}$ century on wound healing, anatomy and physiology. The whole chain of known negative consequences, particularly pain with difficulties and slow restitution of gastrointestinal functions, especially motility, represented a challenge for improving the surgeon's access, with ultimate significant benefit for patients.

The post-war developments in medicine followed up with knowledge in the area of diagnostic endoscopy and then through **fiber optics** to serial production of diagnostic **flexible endoscopes**. **Mini-invasive therapeutic procedures** gradually found their way into neurosurgery (**stereotaxis**) and radiology (atrioseptotomy, angioplasty of peripheral and coronary arteries). These were followed by **endoscopic therapeutic procedures** in the oral and aboral parts of the gastrointestinal tract and in bile ducts, as well as transurethral and percutaneous urological procedures and diagnostic and therapeutic arthroscopy. This trend was then continued by the pioneering work of K. Semm in the field of laparoscopic approaches in gynecological surgery.

The first reports of laparoscopic removal of the gallbladder (E. Muhe, 1985) were published in the second half of the 1980s. Only further improvement and use of this method by French surgeons in 1987–1989 (P. Mouret, F. Dubois, J. Perissat) was met with worldwide response. The year of 1990 was the turning point, representing the turbulent development of laparoscopic surgery both in the US and Europe after previous excellent results achieved with gallbladder operations. Only laparoscopic cholecystectomy has influenced the development of surgery in an extraordinary manner. It has definitely turned attention of both doctors and patients to mini-invasive diagnostic and therapeutic techniques. It has become the foundation for rapid introduction of further mini-invasive, predominantly endoscopic, variants of operations in clinical practice. The first laparoscopic cholecystectomy performed by Czech doctors was performed in 1991 in České Budějovice.

Today, approximately 60% of abdominal surgeries in the Czech Republic are performed using the laparoscopic technique. At a number of departments, laparoscopic cholecystectomy represents more than 90% of performed cholecystectomies. In some diagnoses, mini-invasive access is the method of choice. A number of other new operations have been or are being introduced, including in particular:
- Laparoscopic cholecystectomy, appendectomy, inguinal hernioplasty, fundoplication and antireflux surgery, suture of perforated peptic ulcers, choledocholithotomy, splenectomy, intestinal resection, abdominal phase of rectum amputation, enterostomy, adhesiolysis, vagotomy, varicocele surgery, nephrectomy, lymphadenectomy, adrenalectomy, resection of hepatic metastases and cysts, laparoscopic gastric banding and other bariatric procedures and laparoscopic procedures in large vessels
- Gynecological surgeries (of cysts, hysterectomies)
- Thoracoscopic pulmonary resection, bulla suture, pneumonectomy, upper thoracic sympathectomy, truncal vagotomy, esophageal myotomy, pleurodesis, pericardectomy, combined laparoscopic and thoracoscopic total esophagectomy
- Endoscopic surgery of varices in lower limbs, etc.

The listing of surgeries is neither complete nor finite; nevertheless it documents the turbulent development of minimally invasive surgery during the past 20 years.

How do we define mini-invasive surgery and what are the reasons for its introduction? What advantages does it offer? What are its limits and disadvantages?

**Mini-invasive surgery**, perhaps more appropriately called **minimal access surgery** or **maximally sparing surgery**, represents not only new ways of surgical approach, new surgical techniques, technologies and stereotypes, but also a change in the existing concept and philosophy of the field. The basis of the change can be specified using a simple formulation: the maximum comfort for the patient at the price of discomfort and demand for the doctor and economy as well.

The fundamental idea of this line of surgery, or therapy in the broader sense of meaning, is substantial limitation of the burden to the patient, of tissue traumatization and of everything not directly related to the therapeutic procedure on the operated organ. Characteristic features of mini-invasive surgery include reduced surgical load and postoperative pain, and reduction of early as well as late early complications. The time of hospitalization and overall convalescence is shorter, and the patients return sooner to their personal and occupational activities. The final result is lower total financial costs of the therapy. In view of the minimal

## MINI-INVASIVE SURGERY

surgical access, the cosmetic result of the surgery is advantageous, too. The contact of the surgical team with the blood of the patient is also significantly limited, which reduces the possibility of any infection transfer.

Mini-invasive surgery obviously has its own limits and certain disadvantages. These are given by the change in the access and technology, and are often specific for the mini-invasive approach. For example, in laparoscopy it is necessary to establish **capnoperitoneum**, which especially entails the potential risk of cardiopulmonary complications in the peroperative period. In addition, there is the risk of the so-called **trocar injuries,** although fortunately quire rare, which may be very serious. Some surgeries require general anesthesia and intra-abdominal access in contrast to conventional surgery (e.g. inguinal hernia surgery). In the event of intense peroperative bleeding the possibilities of endoscopic techniques are quite limited. Therefore, the possibility of converting to conventional, open surgery should always be taken into account. Specific problems are also the result of the necessity to change the anesthesiological approach, often extending the time of the surgery. And last but not least, the listing of disadvantages includes higher direct costs of the surgery compared to conventional surgery.

Today, laparoscopic and thoracoscopic surgery, similarly to other diagnostic and therapeutic mini-invasive procedures, are quite standard, and they are a routinely used way of access in spite of certain disadvantages; however, they have been used more and more often because of their indisputable benefits.

Endoscopic surgeries are characterized by a number of special features. The surgery is performed in an enclosed area with access limited to several ports. The manipulation area, secured by pulling hooks in conventional surgery, is secured by expanding the abdominal cavity using **insufflated gas** ($CO_2$), by positioning the patient, and only secondarily by pushing away the organs with an instrument or using a special retractor. Gas insufflation is not needed in thoracic surgeries. On the contrary, communication with the external environment helps the lung to collapse and thus to form the space for the surgery. A disadvantage of the endoscopic technique is the impossibility of direct palpation examination of the organs. The mediation of visual perception by the monitor is two-dimensional, which makes spatial orientation more difficult, especially at the beginning. However, the most recent modern instruments are able to work under 3D visualization. Estimating the depth and guiding the instrument accurately to its target require new experience and training. At the beginning, a proper estimate is made more difficult by the image being zoomed 6 to 8 times. Therefore, even tiny bleeding makes a frightening impression with this zoom. Limited visibility of only a certain sector of the surgical field, depending on whether straight or oblique optics are used, means another considerable difference compared to open surgery when the surgical field is perceived as a whole by the surgeon. All these facts increase demands on the coordination of movements, orientation and imagination of the surgeon.

Mini-invasive procedures entail quite specific demands on the instrumentation. An insufflation system is needed for the procedure, and it must meet the following conditions:
- Measurement of intra-abdominal pressure
- Measurement of the current gas flow
- Automatic maintenance of parameters based on the preset maximum cavity pressure of the gas (12–15 mmHg, i.e. 1.6–2.0 kPa
- Optic and acoustic alarms for situations exceeding the preset gas pressure

These parameters are important for maintaining the safety of gas insufflation. Another necessary device is the imaging system, which is composed of the optics, a source of light, a camera and a monitor. Powerful **irrigation and suction systems** are needed to provide a clear view of the surgical field – both these systems are integrated in a single tube. Then there is the **coagulation** set, with the most often used type of **monopolar** coagulation, similarly as at open surgeries. Instruments used for laparoscopic and other mini-invasive surgeries are quite special, including various types of **trocars – ports**.

The most common mini-invasive operations in surgery include laparoscopic cholecystectomy, appendectomy, inguinal hernioplasty, diagnostic laparoscopy, procedures in the area of esophageal hiatus and in the stomach. Other procedures include diagnostic and possibly therapeutic thoracoscopy. Additional procedures are only being introduced in clinical practice and are performed at specialized centers of mini-invasive surgery.

A novelty in the instrumentation techniques of recent years are robotic systems. When such instruments are used, the surgeon works away from the surgical field using a remotely controlled robot and with the help of assistants. Three-dimensional images transmitted and perfect manipulation skills of the surgical instruments provide a great advantage. This technique can be used for safe laparoscopic procedures of the highest difficulty, including surgeries of large vessels. The most common robotic surgery is a urological procedure – radical prostatectomy. A limiting factor of its routine introduction in practice is the extraordinary high purchase price of the instrument as well as very high operating costs.

## 20.1 Laparoscopic Cholecystectomy

Laparoscopic cholecystectomy is among the most common surgeries at departments of surgery both in the Czech Republic and in the world. While in open surgery, cholecystectomy is classified as a moderately difficult procedure, in laparoscopy it is a basic procedure. The principles of surgery remain the same, but the access to the abdominal cavity is different. Indications for surgery – symptomatic cholecystolithiasis – are also identical. The originally determined

criteria of relative contraindications of a laparoscopic procedure (obesity, wrinkled gallbladder, acute cholecystitis, adhesions after previous operations, etc.) are no longer generally recognized. Absolute contraindications for laparoscopic cholecystectomy include:
- Gallbladder carcinoma
- Liver cirrhosis with portal hypertension
- Third trimester of pregnancy
- Cardiac decompensation
- Respiratory insufficiency
- Hemorrhagic diathesis
- Untreated block in bile ducts

The importance of the role played by **ERCP** in the solution and treatment of choledocholithiasis has been rising with the growing number of performed laparoscopic cholecystectomies. ERCP is indicated based on medical history data on a previous icterus, upon laboratory findings of an elevation in obstruction enzymes, and upon sonographic findings of bile duct dilatation over 8–10 mm. If the findings are uncertain, **peroperative cholangiography** can also be performed using laparoscopy through the cystic stub, and in some cases also a procedure in bile ducts – **choledocholithotomy**.

The technique of the surgery consists in establishing capnoperitoneum in the abdominal cavity, in the umbilical area, using a **Veres security needle**, where a 10 mm port is then inserted for the optics. After the basic inspection of the abdominal cavity and gallbladder area, laparoscopic operability is assessed and an additional 2–3 working ports are inserted. The gallbladder is captured using forceps, the liver is elevated by pulling the fundus, and the patient is positioned in a way so that the **Calot's triangle** becomes sufficiently accessible. The cystic duct and cystic artery are then prepared, clipped and cut. Here, it is necessary to keep in mind frequent anatomic varieties of the course of the cystic duct and the bifurcation point of the hepatic and cystic arteries. When the structures above have been cut, the cholecystectomy is completed in the retrograde mode from the bed using an electrocauter with continuous stoppage of bleeding. A security drain is usually inserted in the subhepatic area.

The perioperative and postoperative periods may be accompanied by varied complications of a general character or those specific for the laparoscopic approach. Most commonly they include: bleeding from the bed, bleeding from the cystic artery, gallbladder perforation and injury to extrahepatic bile ducts. During the surgery, these complications may be a reason for converting to an open surgery, as well as an unclear anatomic situation or severe adhesions. Generally, intra-abdominal or early complications may occur in the postoperative period, similar to other surgeries.

An injury to or complete cutting or extraction of magistral bile ducts is the most feared and most widely monitored complication. It may result in **icterus**, biliary collection, or **bilioma,** in the subhepatic area up to **diffuse biliary peritonitis** in the early postoperative period. Chronic biliary obstruction, or **cholestasis,** with subsequent **biliary cirrhosis** may be the final consequence even after reparation (direct suture of the bile duct or possibly biliodigestive anastomosis). Laparoscopic cholecystectomy is burdened with two or three times higher risk of injury to the bile ducts compared to open surgery; however, it does not exceed approx. 0.5%. ERCP is of crucial importance in the diagnostics and therapy of such injuries.

## 20.2  Laparoscopic Appendectomy

While opinions about indications of the laparoscopic approach vary, they come to an agreement on the following, generally presented groups of patients:
- Women with pain in the right lower abdomen and lesser pelvis
- Atypical localization of pain and problems with suspected appendicitis
- Obese patients

The principle of the surgery does not differ from a classic appendectomy. The surgery is initiated by introduction of capnoperitoneum and a port for the optics in the umbilical area. Another port is inserted above the symphysis, and the abdominal cavity is inspected using the instrument, especially lesser pelvis organs in women, the position and changes in the appendix, terminal ileum and mesenterium, adhesions or other pathological changes. Further procedures depend on the findings. In severe inflammatory changes of the appendix, peritonitis, etc., the conversion to open surgery is more appropriate. However, an experienced laparoscopic surgeon can handle even advanced acute appendicitis. In slim adult or pediatric patients, the surgery is usually continued as a so-called assisted laparoscopic appendectomy, when the appendix is pulled out through the umbilical wound using laparoscopic instruments and common appendectomy is completed in front of the abdominal wall. In other cases, classic laparoscopic appendectomy is performed intra-abdominally using an additional port and instrument inserted in the left or right hypogastrium, respectively. The stub of the appendix is usually ligated using a loop; then the tobacco suture is not used. The choice of the method depends, in addition to the intra-abdominal and general findings, also on the experience of the surgeon since, unlike an open appendectomy, a laparoscopic procedure may be technically difficult.

Complications after a laparoscopic appendectomy are rare. The most common are inflammatory complications – early or intra-abdominal. Similar to open surgery, the most feared complication is the **insufficiency of the stub** of the appendix and subsequent stercoral peritonitis. Postoperative ileus as a consequence of the inflammation and adhesions is, compared to classic appendectomies, quite rare. However, it has to be noted that the gravity of an inflammatory finding in a laparoscopic appendectomy is usually not high as follows from indication groups.

## 20.3 Laparoscopic Inguinal Hernioplasty

The indication criteria of this surgery still remain the subject of debates. The following indications can be considered as generally accepted:
- Relapsing inguinal hernia
- Bilateral inguinal hernia

Other indications depend particularly on the experience and habits of the surgical department; conventional and laparoscopic operations are considered equal but each of the ways of access has its pros and cons. General advantages of the mini-invasive procedure support the laparoscopic approach, as well as its operation principle free of tensioning the tissues and a lower number of relapses. A disadvantage is the need for general anesthesia, intra-abdominal access, implantation of foreign material and higher economic costs of the surgery. Out of the number of laparoscopic methods originally used for the treatment of inguinal hernia, the following methods are still used:
- Transabdominal preperitoneal approach – **TAPP**
- Total extraperitoneal approach – **TEP**

TAPP is the most commonly used method of surgery at the majority of departments. The principle of the surgery is based on settling and fixating a grid made of non-absorbable material using the **preperitoneal transabdominal** access, upon prior preparation and inversion or resection of the hernia sac. The procedure of establishing the capnoperitoneum and the port for the optics does not differ from previous surgeries; in addition other ports are inserted in both lower abdominal areas. Subsequently, the peritoneum and the hernia sac are opened and prepared, inguinal structures are identified, the prolene grid is applied and fixated, and the peritoneal defect is closed.

Complications after laparoscopic solution of inguinal hernias are rare. They include the general postoperative complications mentioned above, and complications specific for the laparoscopic approach: trocar injuries; however, in this case also peroperative injuries to large vessels in the area of the iliac vein. Also included are complications similar to those in classic open surgery in the inguinal area: inguinal and scrotal hematoma, hydrocele, testicular atrophy, neuralgia, injury to the urinary bladder. The rate of inguinal hernia relapses after a laparoscopic plasty is slightly higher than after open inguinal plasty using the grid (for example, according to Lichtenstein), as indicated by recent large studies.

## 20.4 Gastroesophageal Reflux Disease and Hiatal Hernias

From the technical point of view, surgeries in the area of the esophageal hiatus are some of the most demanding procedures in laparoscopy. Indications for surgical treatment of gastroesophageal reflux disease and of hiatal hernias, both sliding and paraesophageal, are still the subject of debates among surgeons and gastroenterologists. Due to the marked advantages of mini-invasive approaches, such methods have become the standard solution to these diseases; however, because of their demandingness they are still performed to a limited extent and only at selected departments. Generally accepted indications include:
- Hiatal hernia with reflux and esophagitis
- Paraesophageal and mixed hernias
- Unsuccessful conservative therapy of the gastroesophageal reflux disease
- Reflux complications (stenosis, bleeding, Barrett's esophagus, ulcer, frequent bronchitis, pneumonia)

The principle of surgery is identical to that of an open operation. Most commonly performed is the "360-degree" **Nissen-Rossetti fundoplication**, or turning the cuff of the fundus of the stomach around the loosened abdominal esophagus. If needed, a suture is added, narrowing the esophageal hiatus. Five points of access are usually needed for the laparoscopic solution, which must be placed high enough, including the port for the optics.

Other procedures in the esophagus (myotomy due to achalasia) and in the stomach (vagotomy, suture of the perforated ulcer, gastric banding, etc.) are also performed using a similar access.

A feared complication of procedures in the hiatal area is esophageal perforation with subsequent **mediastinitis** or peritonitis, posing a direct threat to the patient's life. Another risk is injury to the pleura with subsequent pneumothorax. Late complications may include persisting reflux or, on the contrary, dysphagia up to odynophagia when the cuff is too tight.

## 20.5 Laparoscopic Colorectal Procedures

In recent years laparoscopic approaches have also been finding their way into the field of resolving both benign and malignant colorectal diseases. Currently, it is estimated that approximately 15% of these procedures in Western Europe, and also in the Czech Republic, are performed using laparoscopy. Multicentric studies have disproved the initial concerns about insufficient oncological radicality in malignancies as the long-term survival of patients both after laparoscopic and conventional resection of the colon and rectum is comparable. The principle and extent of the laparoscopic procedure remain the same as those of open surgery. In principle, any intestinal procedure can be performed using laparoscopy ranging from ileocecal resection to low rectal resection, including total colectomy. The so-called minilaparotomy has been a point of contradiction, which must be used to remove intestinal resecate and possibly to construct the anastomosis. In left-sided hemicolectomy, however, and even more in right-sided hemicolectomy, the extent of the needed minilaparotomy is almost the size of the common laparotomy, and therefore, the mini-invasive character of the procedure is in such cases disputable. Therefore, the interest of surgeons has been turning to resections of the rectosigmoid and rectum including abdominoperineal amputation where the whole abdominal phase of the surgery can be performed using laparoscopy without any minilaparotomy, since the resecate is removed through the perineal access. The majority of laparoscopic surgeries in the intestine are performed at specialized centers.

## 20.6 Diagnostic and Therapeutic Thoracoscopy

**Video-thoracoscopic** procedures and **video-assisted** procedures in the thoracic cavity and in the mediastinum are performed at departments with sufficient experience in mini-invasive surgery, and also with erudition in thoracic surgery. Separated ventilation of the lungs is a necessary precondition for such procedures, as it allows collapsing the operated lung. Besides the port for the optics, additional two or three ports are inserted, usually of rather large diameter, which can also be used to insert the **endostapler**. No insufflator is needed. Indications for these procedures are relatively wide and, to a considerable extent, they depend on the experience and habits of the given department. Usual indications include:
- Relapsing pleural exudate of unclear etiology
- Acute and chronic pleural empyema
- Malignant exudate (pleurodesis)
- Relapsing spontaneous pneumothorax
- Hyperhidrosis (upper thoracic sympathectomy)
- Non-manageable pain (for example due to pancreatic carcinoma – splanchnicectomy)

Thoracoscopy is used to perform anatomic pulmonary resections using the video-assisted technique (VATS), atypical pulmonary resections, most commonly due to pulmonary bullae and relapsing pneumothorax. A number of procedures are also performed in the mediastinum, pericardium, esophagus, etc. Complications depend on the demanding character of the procedure, the most feared ones being intense bleeding and injury to the esophagus with subsequent purulent mediastinitis.

## 20.7 The Future of Minimally Invasive Therapy

The aforementioned mini-invasive procedures represent only a part of performed operations; a number of other procedures are known in surgery, urology, gynecology and other fields. The present turbulent development indicates that these procedures have been gaining gradually more important place in medicine. The development also brings a number of problems, such as erudition, new technologies, ethical and economic aspects. Some surgeries, for example laparoscopic cholecystectomy, are the first-choice methods, while others provide an equivalent variant of the classic approach, and yet others have not spread in general in spite of large sets of operated persons (colon resection). Other endoscopic surgeries will certainly come in the future, gradually replacing classic surgeries.

The most recent methods introduced in an effort to further reduce the invasiveness of surgical procedures can be mentioned as an example. They include the SILS (single incision laparoscopic surgery) method. The single incision access has been a standard in simple procedures for a number of years – for example, tubal thermocoagulation in sterilization. However, SILS has been gaining ground also in other procedures such as cholecystectomy, appendectomy and others. SILS is a certain alternative for another new method – NOTES (natural orifice transluminal endoscopic surgery), which uses natural body openings and cavities (stomach, rectum, vagina) to access the operated organs. The debate on limited possibilities of hemostasis, bacterial contamination and other aspects has not yet been resolved.

However, the credo of mini-invasive surgery, as well as of conventional surgery, is an unequivocal benefit for the patient.

# 21 VASCULAR SURGERY

> 21.1 Introduction
> 21.2 History of the Discipline
> 21.3 Vascular Replacement and Sutures
> 21.4 Acute Arterial Closures (Outline)
> 21.5 Chronic Arterial Closures
> 21.6 Large Vessel Injuries
> 21.7 Single Large Vessel Affections
> 21.8 Vascular Approaches for Hemodialysis

## 21.1 Introduction

Vascular surgery involves surgical treatment of arterial, venous and lymphatic system diseases. The most common cause of arterial affections is atherosclerosis. The most common venous affections are varicose veins (varices) of the lower limbs which are also the most common reason for venous surgery. In the lymphatic system it is mostly the blockage and impairment of lymph drainage. The treatment is conservative.

Vascular surgery is currently closely intertwined with invasive radiology and both specializations are often involved in the treatment. For the vascular surgeon it is necessary to know in detail the possibilities of current **invasive angiology**. Both fields are quickly converging. Hybrid rooms are being built, which allow combining of surgical and invasive angiological procedures at the same time.

## 21.2 History of the Discipline

In 1912 Alexis Carrel was awarded the Nobel Prize for development the basic procedures in vascular surgery. However, the actual development of vascular surgery came after World War II, when modern surgical procedures were introduced and have been used until now – thrombendarterectomy (Dos Santos, 1947), bypass (Kunlin, 1949), coarctation of the aorta (Crafoord, 1945), resection of abdominal aortic aneurysms (Dubost, 1952), reconstruction of internal carotid artery (Eastcott, Pickering and Rob, 1954).

The main obstacle for the development of vascular surgery was the lack of suitable vascular replacement. The patient's own veins can only be used for reconstruction of smaller vessels. Only the implementation of artificial vascular graft into clinical practice (Voorhees, Jaretzki and Blakemore, 1951) has made it possible for vascular surgery to quickly develop.

Another major breakthrough was the development of invasive radiology. Diagnostics have become much more specific. Besides the classic angiology, CT angiography (with a contrast substance) and magnetic resonance are currently used. Both examinations allow for a three-dimensional reconstruction of vessels. Another improvement is the introduction of stent grafts into clinical practice. This has significantly reduced the proportion of high-risk surgeries in thoracic and abdominal aorta. From among many other options it is necessary to mention the method of subintimal recanalization, which allows clearing long sections of closed arteries with even a small caliber where surgical treatment is less reliable.

## 21.3 Vascular Replacement and Sutures

Venous or arterial grafts and artificial vascular prostheses are used as artificial vascular replacements.

### 21.3.1 Venous Grafts

■ VENOUS AUTOGRAFT

Venous autograft is the patient's own vein, most commonly **great saphenous vein (GSV)**. Other veins (veins of the deep venous system, upper limb veins or internal jugular vein) are used only occasionally. Venous graft is suitable for the reconstruction of vessels with small vascular flow rate, approximately 150 mL/min, especially for the vessels in the lower limbs distally from common femoral artery (CFA) (femoropopliteocrural area), upper limb vessels and carotid arteries. A venous graft can serve as a patch in the artery. Venous grafts are also used almost exclusively for reconstructions of the deep venous system.

Advantages of Venous Grafts
- They are suitable for bypasses on small vessels with low flow, where venous grafts have a significantly higher patency than prostheses (particularly arteries distally from the knee slot)
- Higher resistance against infection
- Reconstruction of the deep venous system

Disadvantages of Venous Grafts
- They are not suitable for reconstructions of large vessels (aortocolic area)
- Not always available (varicose veins, veins used for previous vascular or cardiac surgery)

# VASCULAR SURGERY

## ■ VENOUS ALLOGRAFT

Venous allograft is used when an autologous vein is not available in the same indications. Due to low antigenicity, pharmacological immunosuppression is either not necessary at all, or necessary only in very small doses. However, the venous allograft is subject to faster rebuilding compared to the autograft, and the development of an aneurysm or the rupture of the wall is not exceptional. Therefore, it is used only in case of severe and symptomatic ischemia, as an emergency graft, and in the event of a threat of limb loss when there is no other possible solution.

## ■ ARTERIAL AUTOGRAFT

With regard to the limited availability it is used very rarely. It is possible to use a short segment of internal iliac or radial arteries.

## ■ ARTERIAL ALLOGRAFT

This is used as well very rarely and it is subject to fast degeneration.

### 21.3.2 Vascular Prostheses (Artificial Vascular Replacements)

**The advantages** of vascular prostheses are the following: they do not undergo degeneration, are resistant to pressure, and are always available and suitable for handling. **Their disadvantages** are worse long-term patency with lower flows rates, below 150 mL/min, and a higher risk of infection. All up-to-date prostheses have zero porosity and differences between individual types of prostheses gradually disappear.

There are currently three groups of vascular prostheses available – knitted, woven and molten.

**Knitted prostheses** are used for the reconstruction of vessels distally from the diaphragm – for the aorta and pelvic arteries. If crural arteries are in good condition, the prosthesis can be sewn on popliteal artery above the knee slit. Bypasses in crural arteries using the prosthesis have worse results compared to venous grafts. Knitted prostheses are also suitable for the reconstructions of aortic arch branches.

**Woven prostheses** are somewhat tougher and they are used for aortic replacement from the aortic valve up to the diaphragm.

**Molten prostheses** are expected to maintain a higher long-term patency even at lower flows compared to other types of prostheses, and in the event of emergency they can be used even for the reconstruction of crural arteries. Nevertheless, still the best graft with the best results for the reconstruction of the arteries with lower flow rates is the venous autograft.

Exclusively used **for vascular connection (anastomosis)** of biological grafts or vascular prostheses are **non-absorbable**, usually **monofilament fibers**. The suture most commonly used is a continuous stitch. In young children, where growth of the arteries is expected, it is more appropriate to perform at least a part of anastomosis with individual stitches, which allow extending the anastomosis with the growth of the artery. Individual stitches are also used in microsurgery for anastomosis of very small vessels under 1 mm in diameter.

The polytetrafluorethylen (Teflon) pads can be used under sutures when sclerotic or very fragile blood vessels are sewn to avoid stitch cuts and bleeding from punctures.

### 21.3.3 Constructions and Types of Anastomoses

First, it must be emphasized that the location of an anastomosis is one of the key factors that affect both short-term and long-term patency of the reconstruction. It is important to find the least affected section of the artery.

We distinguish **proximal, distal, end-to-side, end-to-end, and side-to-side** anastomoses (Fig. 21.1).

**A proximal anastomosis** is sewn above and **a distal anastomosis** below the site of the lesion.

**An end-to-side anastomosis** is the most common method of connection. The arteriotomy in the operated artery should be 1/2–1/3 longer than its lumen. The prosthesis which is sewn to the artery should be sidelong arched cut. The venous graft should be cut sidelong and/or longitudinally in the foot.

**An end-to-end anastomosis** is used less commonly, mostly in aneurysms when the vascular replacement is inserted after the opening of the aneurysm, usually intraluminally. Small vessels should be cut sideways or longitudinally on one side so that narrowing of the lumen is avoided after the construction of the anastomosis. It is also suitable to use more sutures to avoid constriction in an anastomosis.

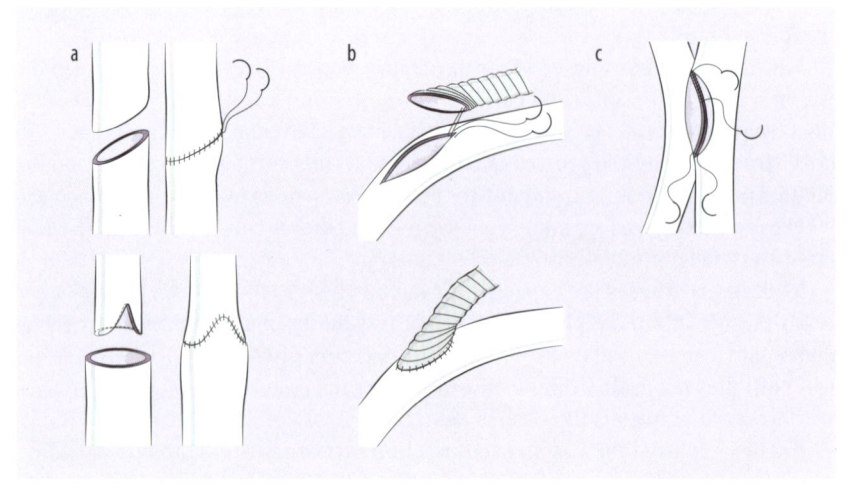

**Fig. 21.1** *Methods of vascular connections: a) Anastomosis "end-to-end"; b) Anastomosis "end-to-side"; c) Anastomosis "side-to-side"*

**A side-to-side anastomosis** is used relatively rarely in vascular surgery compared to cardiac surgery, and the **distal anastomosis** is always concerned. It is used in cases where one graft supplies several arteries (i.e. several distal anastomoses). Besides the end distal anastomosis, the distal anastomosis is also sewn on other arteries located along the graft. The connected vessels or vascular replacements are longitudinally opened and sewn using a continuous suture. In small vessels we use more sutures (2–4) to avoid constriction.

### 21.3.4 Basic Methods of Reconstruction

#### ■ BYPASS (BRIDGING)

Bypass is the most common method of reconstruction. The proximal anastomosis is sewn above and the distal anastomosis below the site of the lesion. It is therefore not necessary to prepare long sections of the vessels (Fig. 21.2a).

The Key Factors of Successful Reconstruction Include:
- Quality inflow (proximal anastomosis may not be sewn below the constriction)
- Quality outflow (circulation below the reconstruction site should be relatively intact)
- Technically perfectly performed anastomoses without stenosis at the site of anastomosis
- Breaking of the graft must be avoided
- Selection of a suitable graft (prosthesis)
- Selection of a suitable place for the anastomosis

#### ■ REPLACEMENT

This method of reconstruction is mostly used in the surgery for aneurysms, and the replacement is laid anatomically. After placing clamps above and below the aneurysm, the aneurysm should be opened longitudinally up to the site where the artery has a normal lumen. The artery should not be interrupted in its entirety, but about one third of the back wall is left intact. **The proximal and distal anastomosis is sewn end-to-end from the lumen of the aneurysm (inclusion technique).**

If the vessel is interrupted in its entirety, then the proximal and distal end of the vascular replacement is sewn to the interrupted blood vessel stumps end-to-end by means of a continuous suture. This type of replacement is sometimes called **interposition** (Fig. 21.2b).

#### ■ PLASTIC

Plastic is mostly used in the event that there is a threat of constriction upon the direct suture of the artery. Instead of the direct suture **a patch** is sewn into the lon-

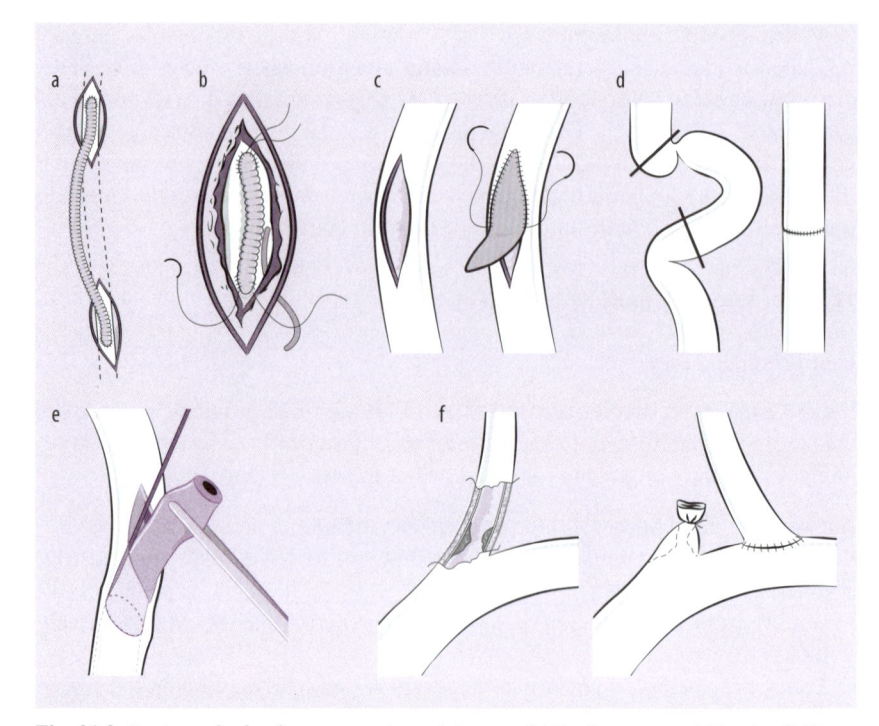

**Fig. 21.2** *Basic methods of reconstruction: a) Bypass; b) Replacement; c) Plastic; d) Shortening; e) Endarterectomy; f) Reimplantation*

gitudinal arteriotomy. A part of the vessel or prosthesis is used for such a patch. Generally, the same replacement is chosen which would be used in the given localization for the reconstruction. It is used either as **a separate reconstruction procedure** or together with another method of reconstruction, most commonly with an **endarterectomy** (Fig. 21.2c).

### ■ ENDARTERECTOMY

Currently, the so-called **open endarterectomy** is almost exclusively used. The affected vessel is opened sideways at the constriction site and the sclerotic plaque is removed from the lumen of the artery. Peripherally (down-stream) the endarterectomy is "taperingly" terminated. In other words, no big step or released endarterium may remain in the lumen of the artery. It could be torn off with the blood flow and a closure of the artery may occur. If endarterium is not stuck firmly it must be fixed with sutures. The artery is then closed either by a primary suture or, if there is the threat of constriction of the artery, a plastic of the artery with a patch is used. Endarterectomy is most commonly performed in reconstructions of carotid artery and common femoral artery (Fig. 21.2d).

# VASCULAR SURGERY

### ■ SHORTENING

If the vessel is too long and wrapped (**kinking**) the redundant part of the artery is resected and stumps are sewn together end-to-end. The elongated internal carotid artery is most often reconstructed in this way (Fig. 21.2e).

### ■ RE-IMPLANTATION

Re-implantation is performed if a short section of the artery is affected at the branching from the main trunk. The affected section of the artery is ligated at its branching, resected and after mobilization the peripheral end is sewn back to the main trunk or to the adjacent unaffected artery. This procedure is used if internal carotid, subclavian, superior mesenteric or renal artery is affected (Fig. 21.2f).

## 21.4 Acute Arterial Closures (Outline)

Acute arterial closures are caused either by **embolism, thrombosis, injury or puncture of the artery** (**iatrogenic cause**). The results of acute ischemia and reperfusion can be general – **myonephropatic-metabolic syndrome**, and local – **compartment syndrome**.

### 21.4.1 Embolism

Embolism is an acute arterial closure caused by **embolus** mostly at the site of the branching of arteries or in a physiological or acquired (stenosis on the basis of atherosclerosis) constriction. The source of emboli is most commonly the left atrium auricle. Inside the auricle, particularly in the case of atrial fibrillation, blood stagnates and forms thrombi which may release and get into the blood stream. Another source of embolism may be myxoma of the left atrium or atherosclerotic masses, especially aneurysms (aorta, subclavian or popliteal arteries). The emboli from aneurysms are often smaller and affect arteries with a smaller diameter. Sometimes a fragmentation of the embolus and multiple small emboli in small peripheral arteries appear, a so-called emboli shower (disperse embolism).

With the embolism a sudden interruption of blood supply to the area occurs perfused by the blocked artery.

The result of an embolism depends on several factors:
- The size of the artery and the perfused area.
- Collateral circulation – worse consequences may paradoxically appear in the event of embolism in healthy circulation. In the atherosclerotic circulation a partial collateral circulation is already developed.
- Embolism in an upper limb usually has less serious consequences than in a lower limb.
  Embolism is commonly localized in arteries of the lower limbs (bifurcation of the aorta, common femoral artery, popliteal artery, branches of crural arte-

ries), arteries of the central nervous system and less often the upper limbs arteries (subclavian, axillary, brachial artery or branching of cubital artery).

### Symptomatology
Sudden, severe pain, feelings of cold, paresthesia up to the loss of sensation or movement. The limb is cold, pale and pulsation under the closure site is missing.

### Diagnostics
The clinical picture is usually sufficient. An ECG often shows atrial fibrillation. Angiography is indicated in the case of a dubious diagnosis; most often it is not necessary.

It has to be emphasized that the symptoms may vary and sometimes they can be milder and less pronounced.

### Treatment
In smaller peripheral embolisms, especially in the upper limb arteries, **thrombolysis** is currently the first choice of therapy. Embolectomy is indicated in embolisms into aortic bifurcation and in the event of failure or contraindication of thrombolysis.

**Embolectomy** is usually performed from a short arteriotomy. A flexible thin catheter with a balloon (**Fogarty catheter**) at the end is used for the embolectomy (Fig. 21.3). Following the insertion of the Fogarty catheter above the site of the embolus the balloon is inflated and pulled back to the site of arteriotomy from where the embolus is removed. The catheter is then inserted repeatedly until no embolic masses are obtained. The whole process is repeated, including the insertion of the catheter in the periphery of the artery, until the embolic masses are removed. Heparin is instilled in the artery proximally and distally and sufficient inflow and outflow are monitored. Each embolus should be examined histologically. The artery is closed by direct sutures; a venous patch is used in arteries with a smaller diameter.

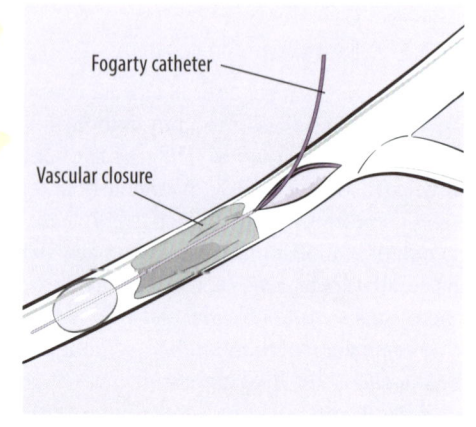

*Fig. 21.3 Embolectomy by the Fogarty catheter*

Each patient should undergo echocardiography before his/her discharge from hospital which should reveal potential thrombi in the left atrium. Anticoagulation therapy is indicated in the event of chronic atrial fibrillation.

## 21.4.2 Arterial Thrombosis

Thrombosis occurs when blood coagulates at the site of impaired intima, especially at the site of atherosclerotic arterial constrictions. However, thrombosis may develop in a relatively intact vessel in cases of hypercoagulation status, shock, and slower flow rate for any reason, etc. There is often a combination of several factors (impairment of intima and hypercoagulation status).

### Symptomatology
The symptoms may be very similar to embolisms, sometimes the onset of problems is slower and the problems are milder. In the event of more detailed medical history it is often found that the patient suffered from the symptoms associated with the impairment of perfusion, mostly in the lower limbs, for a longer period of time.

### Diagnostics
The clinical picture is usually sufficient. Angiography or CT angiography is indicated in the event a thrombosis is suspected.

### Treatment
The first choice method is **thrombolysis**, and sometimes the thrombus can be evacuated and primary **angioplasty, usually with subsequent insertion of a stent**, can be performed. Following the removal of the thrombus the local finding in the arterial circulation is solved according to the standard indications. If the cause of thrombosis was a **hypercoagulation condition, antiaggregation or anticoagulation therapy is indicated.**

## 21.4.3 Compartment Syndrome

Compartment syndrome occurs when the compression of arteries and impairment of circulation develop due to increased tissue pressure in the closed fascial space. This leads to ischemia of the respective muscle groups. Compartment syndrome usually develops following the recovery of perfusion in the ischemic area, e.g. after successful embolectomy or thrombectomy. It mostly occurs in the area of calf muscles, less commonly in the forearm.

### Symptomatology
Muscles of the given area are swollen, painful on palpation, the calf is rigid, the periphery of the limb shows signs of ischemia (it is cold, pale, without palpable peripheral pulsation) with limited movement and sensation of the limb. The clinical picture after recovery of the circulation is usually sufficient for determination of the diagnosis and indication for surgery. If there is any doubt, the pressure in the relevant fascial space can be measured. Normal tissue pressure values range from 0 to 10 mmHg (up to 1.33 kPa). Fasciotomy is indicated if the tissue pressure exceeds 30–40 mmHg (4.0–5.3 kPa).

## Treatment

The treatment initially starts conservatively – elevation of the limb, mannitol. The surgical treatment consists in **fasciotomy**. There are four fascial spaces in the calf – **anterior tibial** (it is affected most often), **lateral fibular, posterior superficial and posterior deep**.

### 21.4.4 Myonephropatic-Metabolic Syndrome (Reperfusion Syndrome)

After restoring blood flow in the lower limbs the patient is threatened by acute egestion of metabolites of anaerobic metabolism from the large mass of muscles. This results in acidosis, hypercalcemia, myoglobinuria, and a shocked lung. Precipitation of myoglobin in the kidneys and renal failure may develop. The treatment includes forced diuresis, adjustment of metabolic acidosis, e.g it is suitable to administer bicarbonate before recovery of the blood flow. Temporary hemodialysis is also often needed.

Reperfusion syndrome regularly follows embolectomy of the aortic bifurcation. In the case of reperfusion of only one limb the metabolic consequences are usually not so serious and the life of the patient is not in danger.

## 21.5 Chronic Arterial Closures

The problems usually begin as intermittent claudications which are characterized by convulsive pain in the muscles of the lower limbs during exercise (walking).

**Localization of pain is connected with the site of impairment of the arterial circulation:**
- Aorta and pelvic circulation – thigh (in case of aortic affection sometimes also the buttocks)
- Superficial femoral artery – calf
- Crural circulation – plantar

The grade of impairment of perfusion is in practice classified according to **Fontain:**
- I. Without problems
- II. Intermittent claudications
  a) Tolerated walking distance > 100 m
  b) Tolerated walking distance < 100 m
- III. Pain at rest
- IV. Trophic defects

Although several factors, such as the overall condition of the patient, concomitant diseases, age, lifestyle, etc., are assessed in the event of a patient's indication for invasive treatment (surgery, percutaneous intravascular interventions), it generally applies that patients in stage II are indicated b. The rapid development of invasive radiology and the outstanding surgical results have made it possible for many patients to move the indication for invasive examination and subsequent intervention to an earlier stage of the disease – IIa.

## 21.6 Large Vessel Injuries

The injuries are divided into **sharp, blunt and deceleration injuries** (Fig. 21.4).

### 21.6.1 Sharp Injuries

- **Injuries of the posterior wall of the artery** not penetrating into the lumen are less serious and usually are not diagnosed. They are completely **healed** or cause an **aneurysm**.
- **Perforating** injuries penetrate into the lumen of the artery and cause external bleeding. In the event of a larger artery it is usually necessary to stop the bleeding surgically. The first aid involves compression. In the case of smaller arteries the bleeding stops by compression and hematoma in soft tissues is

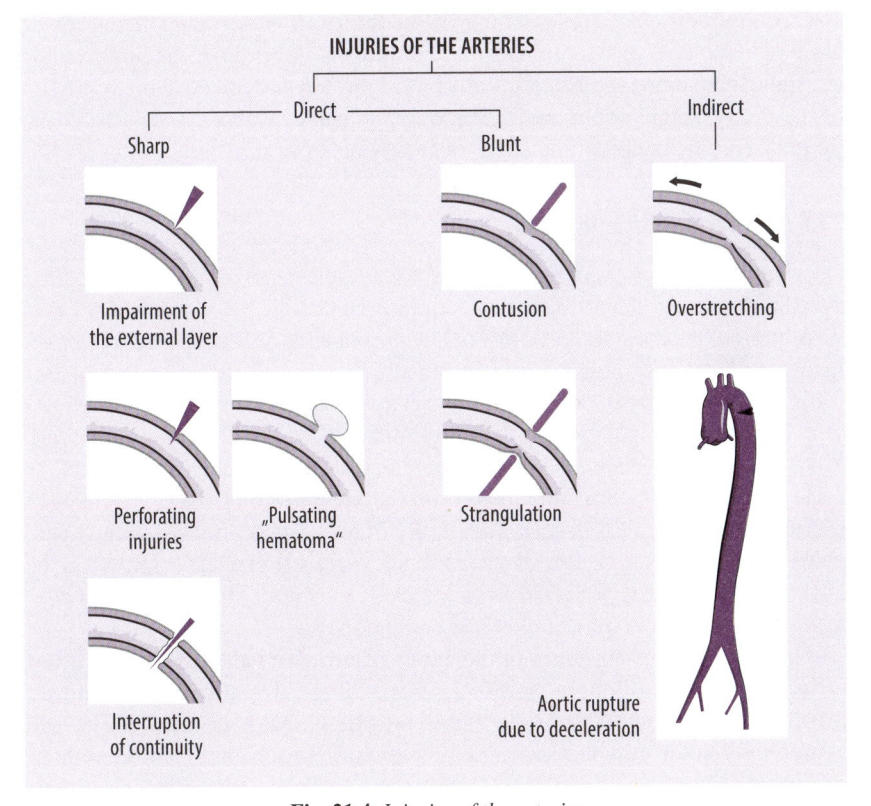

**Fig. 21.4** *Injuries of the arteries*

then absorbed. The artery is usually also healed. Sometimes a communication between the artery and hematoma that is encapsulated may persist and a so-called **false aneurysm** develops. This is indicated for reconstruction – most often surgically. A vein can be injured at the same time and then an **arteriovenous fistula** develops which is indicated for surgery. Invasive radiologists are often able to close the communication using an occluder. If this fails or if the finding is not suitable for implantation of the occluder, surgical closure of the a-v fistula is indicated.
- The **full arteriotomy** causes bleeding but also ischemia of the perfused area. Smaller arteries can constrict and bleeding from them can stop. In larger arteries surgical revision and reconstruction are indicated – mostly interposition of a graft (vein or prosthesis based on the lumen of the artery). Sometimes, especially in younger individuals, the direct suture of the stumps end-to-end is possible.

### 21.6.2 Blunt Injuries

These may occur directly by compression, strangulation or contusion of the artery, or indirectly by overstretching of the artery in the event of luxations or fractures. The typical symptom of these injuries is ischemia of the limbs below the site of the injury. A ruffled intima and/or thrombosis can develop at the site of the injury. Angiography or CT angiography can contribute to the diagnosis. Surgical reconstruction of the artery is mostly necessary.

### 21.6.3 Deceleration Injuries

Deceleration injuries occur upon a sudden, intense change of movement (falling from heights, car accident). The most serious deceleration injury occurs in the aortic isthmus of the thoracic aorta, just below the branching of the subclavian artery. In the event of aortic interruption most patients die at the place of the accident. Because there is rigid tissue around the aorta at this area, the bleeding can sometimes stop. Exceptionally, patients are healed spontaneously, or an aneurysm develops. More often, more bleeding occurs within hours or days, which is usually fatal.

The **diagnosis** is determined based on the knowledge of injury mechanism and the clinical status. A deceleration injury of the aorta is often associated with pulmonary contusion. X-rays of the chest show pleural exudate (usually on the left). Arterial blood is collected from the chest puncture. The diagnosis is confirmed by CT angiography or classical angiography.

**The treatment** is currently in the hands of invasive radiologists who insert an intraluminal stent-graft in the affected aorta. Surgical treatment which mostly involves replacement of the aorta with a prosthesis that is inserted end-to-end is used only in the case that the patient is found to be unsuitable for stent-graft implantation.

The usual rule is that the bleeding artery can be ligated distally below the knee or elbow; of course, with regard to the extent of the injury and the status of the vascular circulation as a whole. Injuries to the proximal arteries, above the knee or elbow, are to be reconstructed and preserved.

## 21.7 Individual Large Vessel Affections

### 21.7.1 Aortic Arch Branches

The most common cause of affection is atherosclerosis which causes constriction, closures or aneurysm of arteries. Non-specific arteritis can occur rarely.

Based on the surgical approach the affections are classified into **central (intrathoracic)** if the aortic arch branches are affected at their branching up to the edge of the breast-bone or clavicle, and **peripheral** if the vessels on the chest are affected.

■ CENTRAL (INTRATHORACAL) AFFECTION – SYMPTOMATOLOGY

**The steal syndromes** – the most common is the **subclavian steal syndrome** which occurs in the central affection of the subclavian artery or brachiocephalic trunk. Flow is reversed in the vertebral artery which becomes the main source of blood supply to the upper limb and derives blood from the vertebrobasillary drainage area to the arm. Resulting to decrease ("steal") of the blood supply to the cerebral circulation manifests with symptoms of vertebrobasillary insufficiency, which worsen especially when arm is working.

**Ischemic problems in the upper limbs** are manifested at work, especially if they are elevated. Tiredness, claudication in the upper limbs and the feeling of cold in the acral parts are the main symptoms.

Other symptoms can include minor **embolisms** (especially from aneurysms) to the brain which can result in **transitory ischemic attack (TIA) or cerebrovascular accident** (CVA), or to the upper limbs where they can cause ischemic changes, especially in the acral parts. These can lead to trophic defects in the fingers.

Diagnostics
Clinical picture, pressure difference in the upper limbs, ultrasound (suitable for peripheral affections), CT angiography or standard angiography.

Indications for surgery:
- Neurological symptomatic affections
- Steal syndrome
- Significant ischemia of the upper limb
- Asymptomatic affection only in the case of serious affection of at least two main trunks

## Methods of Reconstruction

Commonly **an extracranial** solution is possible – implantation of the subclavian to the internal carotid artery and vice versa. If direct connection of the arteries is not possible the carotid-subclavian bypass is another possibility. A prosthesis is preferred due to the risk of breaking the venous graft.

**Intrathoracic procedures** are performed from the middle sternotomy and the method of reconstruction is almost always a bypass. The central anastomosis is placed into the aorta ascendens and the peripheral anastomosis into the respective artery (brachiocephalic, common carotid, subclavian artery) behind the lesion site. Since there are usually two arteries reconstructed, the branching (bifurcation) prosthesis is used.

### PERIPHERAL AFFECTION – SYMPTOMATOLOGY

Neurological symptoms in terms of TIA or cerebrovascular accident are mostly associated with the affection of the carotic circulation. Small and often repeated embolisms are mostly involved in TIA. Closure of the carotid artery is often associated with a cerebrovascular accident. If the vertebral arteries are affected there can be signs of vertebrobasillary insufficiency (dizziness, insecure gait, nausea, etc.).

The above symptoms apply only generally. Various symptomatologies can develop in case of the affection of head vessels and these depend on many factors (variability of head vessel anatomy, collateral circulation, localization of embolisms, etc.). For example, closure of the carotid artery may be clinically silent or may be manifested only as TIA. On the contrary, sometimes a relatively small embolism can cause a large cerebrovascular accident.

### Diagnostics
- Clinical symptoms
- Ultrasonography (mainly carotid arteries in the neck are well accessible)
- Angiography, CT angiography or MRI

### Indications for Surgery
*Carotid Arteries*
- Significant asymptomatic stenoses (> 50%, rather 70%)
- Significant symptomatic stenoses
- Acute closure of the carotid artery within 4 hours after initial symptoms

*Vertebral Arteries*
- Significant symptomatic stenoses

### Methods of Reconstruction
*Carotid Artery*
The affection of branching (bifurcation) of the common carotid artery to the internal and external carotid artery is by far the most common. The surgical

intervention consists in an **endarterectomy** of the bifurcation and the common, internal and external carotid artery. The arteriotomy is closed by direct suture, and in the event the artery is thin and the direct suture could cause constriction of the artery a venous or prosthetic patch is used to close the arteriotomy (Fig. 21.5).

Exceptionally, a part of the artery **must be replaced**. In such event the **venous graft** is usually inserted from the great saphenous vein with end-to-end anastomoses.

If the internal carotid artery **is extended and cranked (kinking) the resection and suture of the stumps end-to-end** is performed.

*Vertebral Artery*

The vertebral artery is often affected at the branching from the subclavian artery. An **endarterectomy is performed** if it is **constricted**. In the event of elongation and kinking of the **vertebral artery, the subclavian artery is rotated** so that the branching of the vertebral artery is shifted from dorsocranial to ventrolateral periphery. If the elongation is too large it is possible to **interrupt** the vertebral artery, **perform a resection and re-implant it into the subclavian artery**.

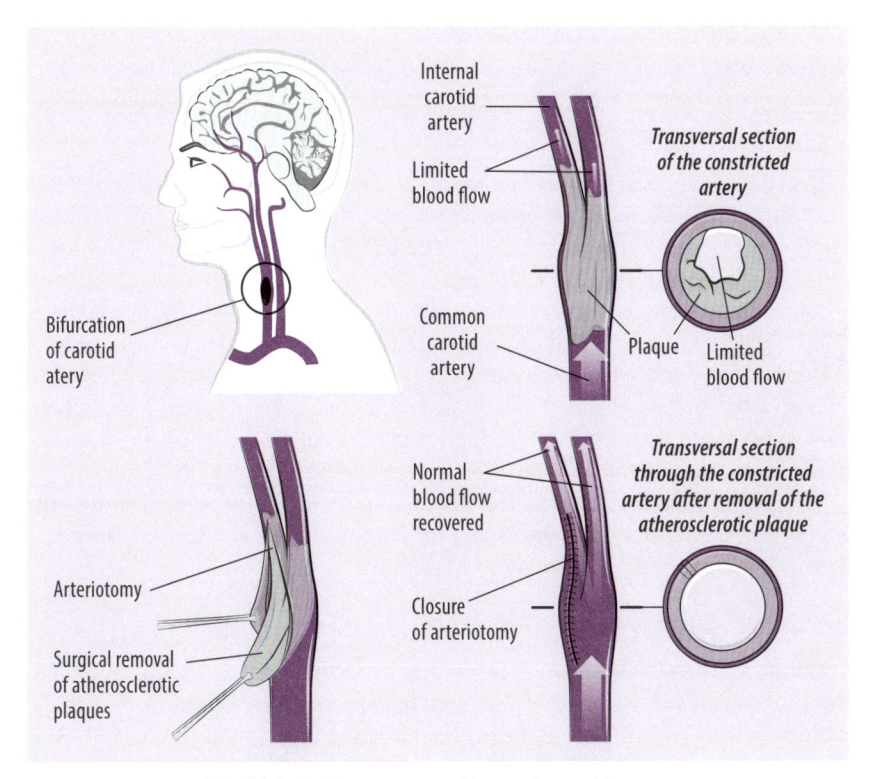

Fig. 21.5 *Endarterectomy of internal carotid artery*

## 21.7.2 Arteries Supplying the Upper Limbs

### ACUTE ARTERIAL CLOSURES

Acute arterial closures of the upper limb arteries are almost always caused by an embolism. The clinical impact is often less significant compared to acute arterial closures in the lower limbs. The origin of embolism is most often in the heart, mostly in the left atrium upon atrial fibrillation. Another less common cause of embolism is an aneurysm of the subclavian or axillary artery. In such events it is mostly small, multiple embolisms that close small arterioles in the fingers.

#### Symptomatology
Acute arterial closure of larger trunks is manifested by sudden and severe pain in the limb below the site of the closure. The limb is pale, cold, with impaired sensation and sometimes with limited movement. Pulsation is not palpable below the site of closure. Despite severe pain the limb is not at danger.

Small embolisms in fingers are manifested by cold and pain and there may be livid spots in fingers sometimes also with small necroses.

#### Diagnostics
The clinical picture and symptoms are usually sufficient for the diagnosis, angiography is not usually necessary. However, secondly the cause of the embolism must be investigated – echocardiography, or angiography, CT angiography or MRI.

#### Treatment
Heparin should be administered immediately after the determination of the diagnosis. **Fibrinolysis** is usually the method of choice. **Surgical therapy – an embolectomy** is performed either in the case of failure of the conservative therapy or in the event that the embolism is localized proximally with significant symptomatology.

An embolectomy is mostly performed with a short incision in the cubital hole. The cubital artery is prepared up to the branching to the radial and ulnar artery so a Fogarty catheter can be inserted proximally via the brachial artery up to the subclavian artery and peripherally to both arteries (radial and ulnar artery). Exceptionally an approach from the brachial artery can be used. A successful embolectomy is confirmed by palpable pulsation on the wrist in the radial and ulnar artery.

Following a successful embolectomy it is important to solve the cause of the embolism, e.g. resection of the aneurysm of the subclavian artery or cardioversion and anticoagulation upon atrial fibrillation.

### CHRONIC AFFECTION OF THE ARTERIES SUPPLYING THE UPPER LIMBS

Atherosclerosis which causes **constriction or closure** of the arteries of the upper limbs occurs incomparably less often than in the lower limbs. In view of the affluent collateral circulation the problems in the upper limbs are usually less dramatic. Therefore, surgical reconstructions of the arteries in the upper limbs are very rare. Moreover, advances in invasive angiology make it possible to solve most stenoses by percutaneous dilation and insertion of a stent.

Rarely an **aneurysm of the subclavian artery** or other upper limb arteries appears. The most common symptom is small repeated peripheral embolisms. Most aneurysms are solved by invasive radiologists using percutaneous interventions. The surgeon performs occlusion of the aneurysm and bypass only occasionally.

We have to note here that if the **subclavian artery is to be ligated**, it can be done without any major risks. The ligation usually does not cause serious symptomatology and there is practically no risk of the loss of a limb. If there are any symptoms of ischemia of the limb (especially in exercise), the reconstruction of the artery can be performed and it usually consists in bypass above and below the site of the lesion with both anastomoses end-to-end. A vein or prosthesis can be used as a graft. A venous graft should be used for rare reconstructions of the brachial artery. Ligation of one of the forearm arteries usually causes no symptoms or quite mild symptoms which require no surgical intervention.

## ■ THORACIC OUTLET SYNDROME – TOS

TOS is relatively common and is characterized by compression of plexus brachiocephalicus and subclavian vessels either between the scalenus anterior and medius or between the clavicle and the first rib, less often between the pectoralis minor and the first rib. The causes may include an abnormal cervical rib or elongated processus transversus of the $7^{th}$ cervical vertebra. Irritation of the brachial plexus usually appears which is manifested by pain, paresthesias, impairment of sensitivity, etc. If there is the compression of the subclavian artery it is manifested by ischemic affection of the upper limb, especially upon work with the elevated limb. Claudications (muscle pain) are often associated with pallor of the fingers, cold, sensation impairment and reactive hyperemia after the limb is hung down. The compression can also be only intermittent when the head is rotated. The compression of the subclavian artery may also cause an aneurysm of the artery. The most common symptom is a peripheral embolism.

### Diagnostics
A high emphasis is put on the medical history and physical examination (extinction of peripheral pulsation during rotation of the head).

X-ray of the chest with the first rib visible, or constriction in between the collarbone and the first rib. The course of the arteries, location of the affection, including the aneurysm, is best displayed by angiography, CT angiography, and/or MRI.

### Indications for Surgery
If the symptomatology is not significant, a conservative approach is preferred (physiotherapy, physical therapy, adjustment of posture, analgesics, anti-inflammatory medication). Surgical therapy is indicated in the case of significant symptomatology and detected TOS. The surgical procedure consists in the resection of

the first rib by transaxillary approach. In the case of an aneurysm of the subclavian artery, the procedure consists in its exclusion and reconstruction of the artery.

### 21.7.3 Abdominal Aorta and Lower Limbs Supplying Arteries
### Acute Arterial Closures

#### ■ CLOSURE OF THE BIFURCATION OF THE ABDOMINAL AORTA

The closure of the bifurcation of the abdominal aorta is usually caused by an embolism; thrombosis is less common. The source of embolisms (as well as in cases of closures in other levels of the lower limbs arteries) is usually thrombi in the left atrium auricle during atrial fibrillation. This is the most serious acute arterial closure that endangers the patient not only by ischemia of both limbs but, due to metabolic consequences, the patient's life is also at risk. A saddle-shaped embolus usually sits in the aortic branching and its partial breakup may occur with subsequent embolization in the periphery of the limbs ("a shower of emboli").

#### Symptomatology
The clinical picture is dramatic. Acute, intense pain in both lower limbs is typical; it may later disappear with the progression of ischemia of the nerves. Impairment of sensation and mobility develops which can eventually result in paraparesis or paraplegia of both limbs. The limbs are pale, cold, immobile and later cyanotic and marbled.

#### Diagnostics
The diagnosis is based on the symptoms. The lower limbs are apparently ischemic, cold in the peripheral parts without palpable pulsation in the femoral arteries. ECG quite often shows atrial fibrillation.

Acute dissection of the thoracic aorta must be diagnostically differentiated. However, it is characterized also by back or chest pain and the signs of ischemia of the lower limbs are completely symmetrical and serious, and the general condition is often altered. In acute spinal lesions the symptoms of ischemia of the lower limbs are missing.

#### Treatment
The most effective manner of therapy is an embolectomy using the Fogarty catheter from both common femoral arteries which are prepared from a short incision in the groin.

#### ■ ACUTE CLOSURE OF THE PELVIC ARTERIES

Symptomatology is very similar to the closure of an aortic bifurcation but the difference is that only one limb is affected. If the flow in the internal iliac artery is preserved the ischemic changes in the respective lower limb can be less dramatic. Nevertheless, the blood flow must be restored as soon as possible.

# VASCULAR SURGERY

The diagnostic and therapeutic procedure is the same as in acute closure of the aortic bifurcation. The difference is that usually a unilateral affection is concerned and the general consequences for the body are less serious.

### ■ ACUTE CLOSURE OF THE COMMON FEMORAL ARTERY

Embolism into the bifurcation of the common femoral artery is the most common location of an embolism and it closes the branches of the superficial and deep femoral artery. Ischemic symptoms (pain, impairment of sensation and movement, color changes, cold) reach mainly to the upper third of the crus and they are most distinctive in the acral parts. The limb is often colder up to the knee.

#### Diagnostics
Pulsation in the common femoral artery below the ligament may be palpable, even stronger than in the other side. A thrombus which reaches up to the first major branch regularly develops above the embolus. If the thrombus continues above the ligament the pulsation in the groin does not have to be palpable. Peripheral pulsation (popliteal, posterior tibial and dorsal pedis artery) is usually not palpable. If the collateral circulation is well developed it can be weakly palpable.

#### Treatment
Surgical embolectomy from the femoral artery is very effective. Thrombolysis is the method of choice. General metabolic symptoms are usually not imminent or are weak. The **compartment syndrome**, which sometimes requires surgical fasciotomy, can develop.

### ■ ACUTE CLOSURE OF THE POPLITEAL ARTERY AND CRURAL CIRCULATION

#### Symptomatology
The symptoms are identical as in the event of embolism in higher levels and they are localized more peripherally. In the popliteal artery they are localized up to the half of the crus at the maximum; in crural arteries up to the tarsus.

#### Diagnostics
The diagnosis is based on the symptoms and clinical picture. Pulsation is palpable on the popliteal artery and it is missing distally.

#### Treatment
**Thrombolysis** is indicated in the event of peripheral closures. **Surgical therapy is indicated in the event of unsuccessful thrombolysis.** The femoral artery is usually used to approach the popliteal artery. In the case of failure, the proximal part of the popliteal artery above the knee must be prepared. In the case of embolism in the crural circulation, the distal part of the popliteal artery should be prepared in the crus up to the branching of the crural arteries. The Fogarty catheter should be inserted selectively to all crural arteries. It is also possible to prepare and open the posterior tibial artery behind the internal ankle and exceptionally even the dorsal pedis artery in the crus and to perform a retrograde embolectomy.

# Affections of the Abdominal Aorta

## ABDOMINAL AORTA ANEURYSM

The subrenal part of the abdominal aorta is one of the most common sites of aneurysms. The most frequent cause is atherosclerosis. This occurs mostly in elderly patients above 65 years of age and more often in males. Proximally, it starts immediately below the renal arteries and only exceptionally above them, and distally it reaches up to the bifurcation. The pelvic arteries are also relatively often affected.

### Symptomatology
There are often no symptoms or only nonspecific problems that are caused by compression of the surrounding organs (loss of appetite, meteorism, nausea, feeling of pressure in the abdomen, back pain, etc.).

### Diagnostics
A pulsating resistance in the epigastrium is often present upon the palpation examination of the abdomen. The diagnosis is confirmed by an ultrasound, angiography, CT with contrast or MRI.

Prior to invasive surgery, all patients should undergo cardiological examination, including echocardiography, or coronarography or CT of the heart with contrast medium and ultrasound of the carotid arteries.

### Indications for Surgery

*Asymptomatic Aneurysms*
Because of the risk of rupture each aneurysm is indicated for invasive surgery. The patient's general condition, accompanying diseases and the size and symptoms of the aneurysm must be evaluated. The indication must be carefully considered in the elderly and at risk patients with small asymptomatic aneurysms (between 4 and 5 cm). On the other hand, large and especially symptomatic aneurysms are unambiguously indicated for reconstruction (Fig. 21.6).

*Symptomatic Aneurysms*
Aneurysms with symptoms of compression of the abdominal organs are practically always indicated for surgery.

*Bleeding Aneurysms*
The most serious complication that directly threatens the patient's life is the rupture of an aneurysm. It is sometimes manifested as a serious condition with hemodynamic responses – hypotension, alteration of the general condition that can result in shock and death. Surgery is urgent from vital indications.

Sometimes the first symptom may be severe pain in the lumbar area with relatively small general response. Besides the aneurysm, we can see retroperitoneal hematoma during the examination (CT, ultrasound). In such event surgery is also

## VASCULAR SURGERY

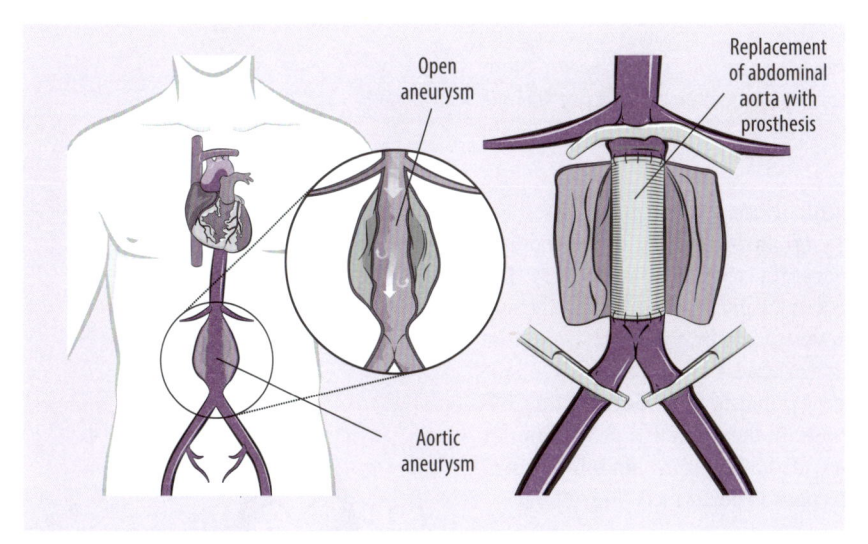

**Fig. 21.6** *Abdominal aorta aneurysm. Replacement of abdominal aorta with prosthesis*

urgently indicated since the aneurysm is already with the rupture covered by coagula. Bleeding may be temporarily stopped but the risk of rupture and repeated bleeding is extremely high.

### Treatment
The first choice method is currently the insertion of an intraluminal stent-graft, most often from the common femoral artery. The surgical solution is in place only in the event that an anatomical finding is not suitable for implantation of the stent-graft.

The surgical procedure consists in the replacement of the affected section of the abdominal aorta by a vascular graft. If the aneurysm extends to the pelvic arteries an aortoiliac (or biiliac in case of the affection of both common pelvic arteries) bypass is performed. If the external pelvic arteries are also affected, an aortofemoral (bifemoral) bypass is performed.

The approach to the aorta is achieved from a medial laparotomy from the xiphoid process to the half distance between the symphysis and navel. If pelvic arteries must be prepared, it is possible to extend the section distally.

### ■ CLOSURE OF THE ABDOMINAL AORTA (LERICH SYNDROME)
**Lerich syndrome** is a chronic closure of the distal aorta or its bifurcation.

### Clinical Picture
Claudications in the buttocks and thighs and erectile dysfunction. Claudications are not so marked and they are usually graded as IIa according to Fontain. The disease is sometimes manifested after 40 years of age but it is usual in the 5$^{th}$ or 6$^{th}$ decade of life. The limbs may be colder. If there is a chronic isolated aortic bifurcation

closure without any major impairment of the limb arteries on other levels, no trophic changes or serious symptoms of chronic ischemia are expressed.

### Indications for Surgery

Symptomatic closure of the abdominal aorta is indicated for surgery. The patient's general condition, age and severity of the symptoms must be considered for indication. The surgery consists in an **aortobiiliac bypass**. In the event that pelvic arteries are also affected an **aortobifemoral bypass** is performed (Fig. 21.7).

## Affection of Pelvic Circulation

### Symptomatology

In the case of isolated impairment of the pelvic circulation, the symptomatology is usually not dramatic and indications follow the general rules described above. Affection of the pelvic circulation can very often be solved intravascularly by percutaneous dilation and insertion of a stent. Surgery depends on the site of the affection. In the case of affection in the branching of the common iliac artery a unilateral or bilateral aortofemoral bypass is appropriate. An iliofemorral bypass is performed in the case of affection of the external iliac artery. The access to the pelvic artery is performed by a transversal section that starts proximally below the rib arch at the level of the anterior axillary line, extends distally about 4 cm above the inguinal ligament and ends by a sheath of the direct oblique muscle. The pelvic artery should be prepared extraperitoneally. The surgery is relatively simple and since the abdominal cavity is not opened it is well tolerated by patients.

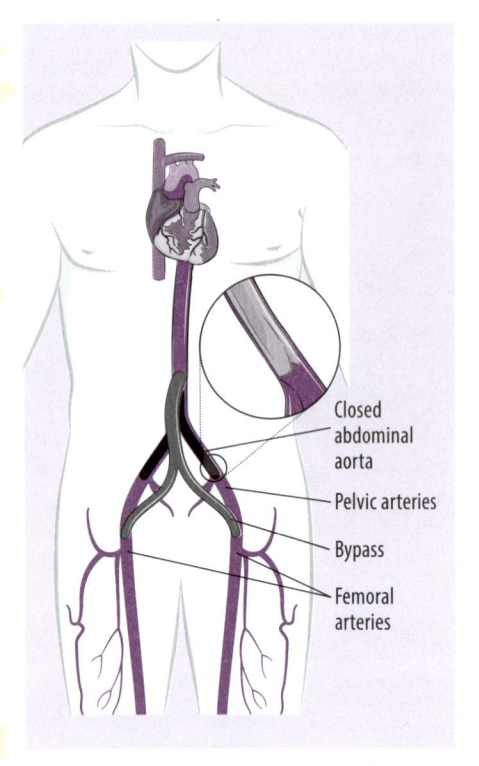

*Fig. 21.7 Aortobifemoral bypass – diagram*

## Affections of the Common Femoral Artery

### Symptomatology

The extent of the problems can be relatively variable and depends on many factors:
- Severity of arterial affection (stenosis and its grade, closure)

- Whether the stenosis also affects the branches of both arteries (superficial and profunda femoral artery), if both arteries are closed or significantly affected, the problems are mostly significant
- How the collateral circulation is developed
- The extent of affection of other arteries of the respective limb

Diagnostics and indications for surgery follow the general rules. In this location the surgical procedure is more common compared to percutaneous intravascular intervention. The surgical procedure mostly consists in **endarterectomy of the common femoral artery**, or the branching of both branches. The arteriotomy is closed directly or by using a patch – it is possible to use a venous or a prosthetic patch (Fig. 21.8).

## Reconstruction of the Profunda Femoral Artery

The profunda femoral artery can sometimes provide sufficient blood supply to the lower limbs even when the superficial femoral artery is closed. This works as natural collateral. It is usually less affected by atherosclerosis, especially in the medial and peripheral parts. The branching from the common femoral artery is most often affected. The methods of reconstruction depend on the site of affection.

**Endarterectomy** of the branching of the profunda femoral artery. The arteriotomy should be performed from the common femoral artery to the profunda femoral artery based on the extent of the affection. The sclerotic plaques should be removed under direct visual control. The arteriotomy should be closed directly or more often using a venous graft in the case of an isolated reconstruction.

In an aortofemoral or ileofemoral bypass it is possible **to sew the distal anastomosis of the bypass above the branching of the profunda femoral artery** or more peripherally to a healthy (or endarterectomized) part of the profunda femoral artery.

In the case of an affection of the longer part of the profunda femoral artery the bypass should be performed from the common femoral artery to the peripheral part of the profunda femoral artery, at best using a vein, but a prosthesis can also be used.

## Affection of the Superficial Femoral Artery

This is a relatively commonly affected area. Symptomatology can again be very variable. Diagnostics and indications for surgery follow the general rules. The superficial femoral artery is usually very suitable for percutaneous intervention, often repeatedly. If it is not possible to perform a percutanenous procedure, a **femoropopliteal bypass** is indicated (Fig. 21.9). If the popliteal artery is not affected, a so-called **proximal femoropopliteal bypass** is performed by placing the distal anastomosis in the proximal part of the popliteal artery. If the crural circulation is

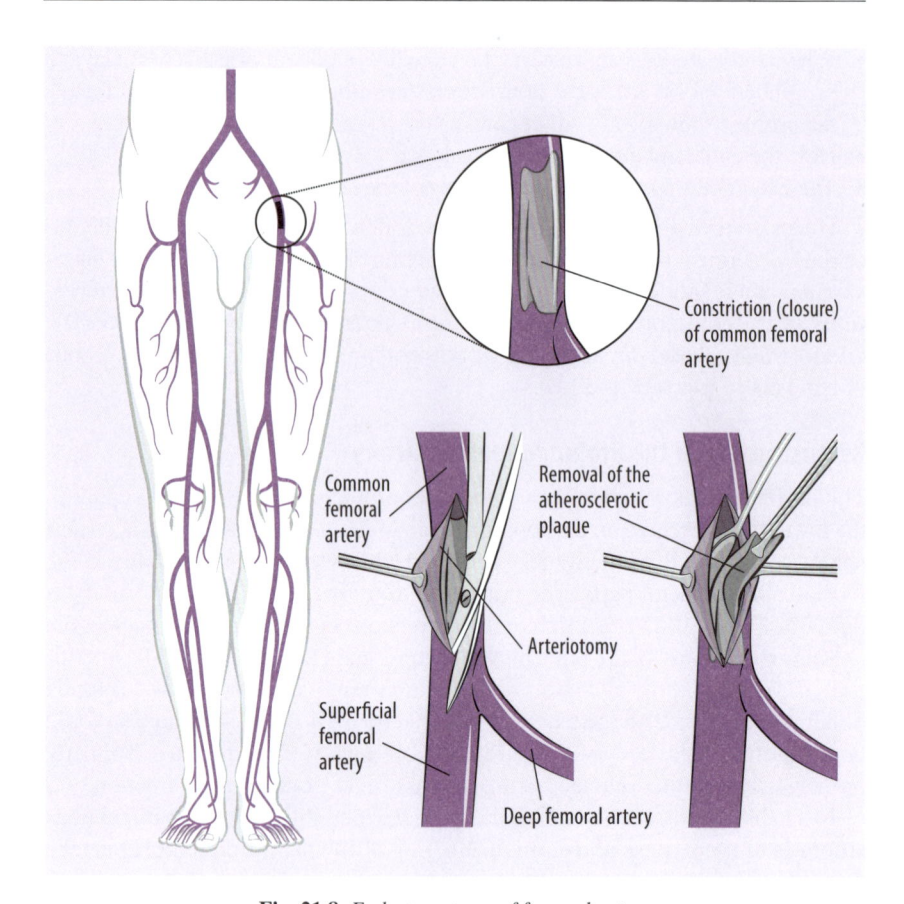

**Fig. 21.8** *Endarterectomy of femoral artery*

intact, it is possible to use either **the vein (great saphenous vein) or an artificial prosthesis** as a graft. Long-term patency of both grafts is similar. If the great saphenous vein is of good quality a venous graft is preferred since a higher and longer patency is expected. Moreover, a venous graft is more resistant to infection compared to a prosthesis. The prosthesis also has certain advantages – the surgery is faster and technically less demanding and the venous graft remains preserved for potential future reconstructions (vascular, aortocoronary bypass). In the case of affection of the crural circulation (closures or significant stenoses of the crural arteries) the outflow from the bypass is limited. The quality of the outflow circulation is reflected in the blood flow through the bypass, and therefore it is one of the basic factors of the short-term and long-term reconstructions. This is the reason why the venous graft is preferred in these cases because it retains high patency with lower flow rates.

If the proximal part of the popliteal artery is affected, a so-called distal femoropopliteal bypass should be performed when the peripheral anastomosis is below the knee. A venous graft is preferred in this case. The prosthesis is used only in emergency situations, in the event of severe symptomatology or if the limb is threatened.

The access to the **common femoral artery** is by transversal section below the inguinal ligament. **The proximal part of the popliteal artery** should be prepared from the transversal section on the internal side of the distal part of the thigh along with the anterior edge of the sartorius muscle in the sulcus femoris medialis up to the medial condylus of the femoral artery. The distal part of the popliteal artery should be prepared from the transversal section below the knee from the medial condylus of the shin-bone distally, evenly with posteromedial margin.

## Affection of the Popliteal Artery

The popliteal artery is often affected by constrictions, closures or aneurysms. In the case of constrictions or closures of the popliteal artery the indication for surgery should follow the general rules. Given that the patency of the reconstructions in the femoropopliteal area is worse than in the reconstructions of the aorta and pelvic circulation, patients with significant symptomatology, i.e. usually at stage III and IV according to Fontaine, are indicated for surgery. Generally speaking, the more peripherally the distal anastomosis must be placed the worse are the results of the reconstructions and the indications are postponed to later stages of the disease with pronounced symptoms or if the limb is threatened. In the event the poplitea is affected together with the superficial femoral artery,

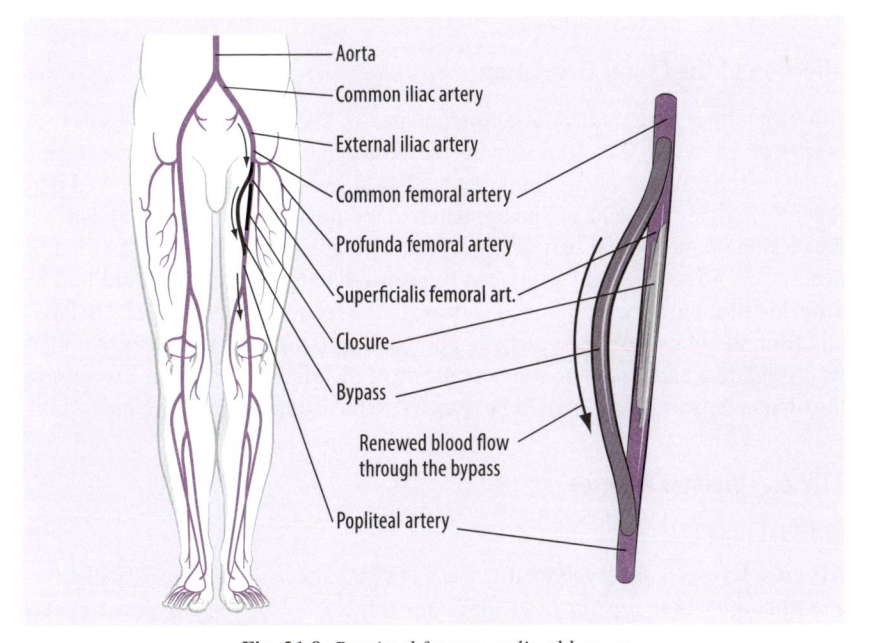

Fig. 21.9 *Proximal femoropopliteal bypass*

a **femoropopliteal distal bypass** is usually indicated; in the event the whole part of the popliteal artery is affected, the **distal anastomosis is placed on one of the crural arteries**. If only the popliteal artery is affected it is possible to perform a **popliteopopliteal bypass**. The proximal anastomosis should be placed on the proximal part of the popliteal artery (or the distal part of the superficial femoral artery) and the distal anastomosis is placed on the distal part of the popliteal artery. A venous graft is chosen as a replacement.

### ANEURYSM OF THE POPLITEAL ARTERY

An aneurysm of the popliteal artery occurs mostly on the basis of atherosclerosis.

### Symptomatology

It may be asymptomatic for a long period of time and the first symptoms are usually small peripheral embolisms or thrombosis of the aneurysm. Therefore, each aneurysm of the popliteal artery is indicated for surgery.

The surgery consists in the **exclusion of the aneurysm**. The popliteal artery is ligated below and above the aneurysm and a **short bypass** is performed. The use of the inclusion technique is another possible reconstruction. The aneurysm is prepared from the sigmoid section in the popliteal hole and after placing staples on unaffected sections of the popliteal artery above and below the aneurysm, it is opened sideways and the replacement from the **lumen of the aneurysm with the anastomoses** is sewn in **end-to-end**.

## Affection of the Crural Circulation

Atherosclerosis is again the most common cause. The reconstruction in this area is performed mostly as a limb-saving procedure in the case of serious ischemia of the peripheral part of the limb. Patency of at least one crural artery is a prerequisite for this procedure. The approach to the **posterior tibial artery** is from the section on the medial part of the crus along the posterior edge of the tibia. If needed, the posterior tibial artery can be prepared behind the internal ankle. The **anterior tibial artery** is approached through the section placed about 2 cm laterally from the tibia. The most difficult approach is to the **fibular artery**. An incision should be performed on the lateral side of the medial part of the crus above the fibula whose segment should be resected to the extent of approximately 8 cm.

### 21.7.4 Visceral Arteries

### RENAL ARTERIES

**Atherosclerosis** is involved in affections of renal arteries in about 70% of cases and **fibromuscular dysplasia** in approximately 25%. Vasorenal hypertenison is the most serious consequence of constrictions and closures of the renal arteries.

# VASCULAR SURGERY

The therapy of renal arteries currently belongs to invasive radiology. The most common form of surgical reconstruction is an **aortorenal bypass**. The prosthesis is mostly used as a replacement.

### ■ ARTERIES SUPPLYING INTESTINES

In this area we should keep in mind the acute closure of the **superior mesenteric artery**, a serious condition that results in intestinal gangrene, metabolic dysbalance and death. Complete interruption of the blood supply in the superior mesenteric artery is often within hours followed by secondary stagnation thrombosis of mesenterial veins. The intestine is then edematous, livid, and perfused from hemorrhage.

#### Etiology
Acute closure is caused either by embolism (usually originating in the left atrium upon chronic atrial fibrillation) or thrombosis on the basis of atherosclerosis.

#### Symptomatology
The first symptom is severe and sudden pain, diffuse or localized in the epigastrium. This is followed by abdominal cramps and hyperperistalsis sometimes with diarrhea, often with blood. In the next phase paralytic ileus develops and abdominal pain may be reduced. However, the general condition is deteriorated and signs of peritoneal irritation appear followed by metabolic disruption, shock and death.

#### Diagnostics
The discrepancy between the problems of the patient – severe abdominal pain and a serious general condition – and a weak physical finding is typical for acute closure of the **superior mesenteric artery**. The signs of peritonitis appear relatively late when the intestine is already necrotic. The hope for saving the intestine consists only in early intervention. The diagnosis should be confirmed by angiography, CT angiography, or explorative laparotomy.

#### Treatment
Surgical treatment **is clearly indicated**. As far as the **embolism** is concerned, the **embolectomy** is performed using a Fogarty catheter. In the case of **thrombosis** the simplest solution is an **aortomesenteric bypass**, usually with prosthesis but a venous graft from the great saphenous vein can also be used. The diagnosis is mostly confirmed late when the intestine is irreversibly impaired and there is no chance to save it. Therefore, it is vitally indicated to perform an **intestinal resection**.

## 21.7.5 Large Vein Affections

The main symptom of closure of the large veins is the impairment of drainage of the respective area. The tissues are swollen and cyanotic. **Cave**: the tissues are pale and they are not swollen in arterial closures.

## Closure of the Superior Vena Cava

The cause can be compression from the surrounding tissues, thrombosis, hypercoagulation status, fibrotising mediastinitis, etc.

Symptomatology
The venous blood is congested in the upper limbs and head and the tissues are cyanotic and perfused. In a chronic slow closure collateral circulation develops and the symptoms do not have to be manifested.

Diagnostics
Medical history, clinical picture, echocardiography, angiography, CT angiography, MRI.

Treatment
The treatment is usually conservative and it consists in long-term anticoagulation. Surgical treatment is indicated only in the event of markedly limiting difficulties. Possibilities of surgical reconstruction:
- Connection of the azygos vein to the inferior vena cava
- Replacement of the superior vena cava at best by venous graft that is created by a longitudinal suture of the great saphenous vein; an artificial prosthesis can also be used.
- A bypass bridging the closed part of the superior vena cava
- Closure of the subclavian vein

This usually does not cause major problems and sometimes edemas of the upper limbs occur. An acute closure, most often associated with cannulation of the subclavian vein, results in temporary edemas of the affected limb.

**The treatment is conservative.** In acute closures the therapy is initiated with low-molecular heparin and continues with anticoagulation medication for 3 to 6 months.

In a chronic closure and problems oral anticoagulation medication is recommended. Anticoagulation therapy can be discontinued in the event the problems disappear.

## Inferior Vena Cava

The closure of the inferior vena cava is caused by compression from the surrounding tissues, hypercoagulation status or insertion of intracaval filters. Ingrowth of the tumor from the kidney that expands into the superior vena cava via the renal vein and can reach the right atrium can be involved in the closure of the inferior vena cava.

Symptomatology
The problems are very heterogeneous, from mild venous congestion in the lower limbs to extensive edemas and severe postthrombotic syndrome.

# VASCULAR SURGERY

### Diagnostics
Clinical picture, angiography, CT angiography, MRI, or abdominal ultrasound.

### Treatment
The **treatment** is **usually conservative** – anticoagulation, elastic bandage of the lower limbs, elevation of the lower limbs at rest (in sitting position or while sleeping), venotonics. In the case of severe problems it is possible to try to perform a recanalization percutaneously and to insert a stent.

If the thrombus or tumor from the renal vein with primary renal cancer grows into the inferior vena cava, surgical treatment is indicated. This consists in nephrectomy and removal of thrombi or tumor masses from the inferior vena cava, or from the right atrium. In addition, extracorporeal circulation must be established, the patient must be cooled down and the procedure must be performed with circulatory arrest.

**Intracaval filters** should be inserted in the case of repeated (successive) pulmonary embolisms. Currently, the procedure is not performed by a surgeon but by an invasive radiologist who inserts a filter percutaneously by cannulation of some of the large veins, mostly the internal jugular vein.

## Pelvic Vein Affections

### ■ CHRONIC CLOSURE

As with the closure of the inferior vena cava the severity of symptoms is relatively variable. From mild edemas to severe postthrombotic syndrome with extensive edemas which reach up to hypogastrium, with extended subcutaneous veins, skin induration, which may be eczematous, hemosiderin pigmented and with trophic defects and ulcers.

**The diagnosis** is mostly apparent from the clinical picture. The treatment consists **in the administration of anticoagulants**, elastic bandages, elevation of the lower limbs and local care of trophic defects. Venotonics can be used as supportive pharmacological therapy but their effects are not very significant. It is possible to try to make the closure patent percutaneously and to insert a stent.

**Surgical therapy** is indicated rarely and the results are not convincing. In the event of the closure of the pelvic vein on the one side and with the pelvic circulation patent on the other side a **crossed femorofemoral bypass** is performed using the great saphenous vein that drains venous blood from the affected side.

### ■ ACUTE ILEOFEMORAL THROMBOSIS

Acute ileofemoral thrombosis (thrombosis of the external and common pelvic vein) originates secondarily in patients confined to bed for a long period of time, in the event of compression by an external expansive process in the small pelvis, after delivery and in the case of fractures of the femoral neck or pelvis.

Ileofemoral thrombosis appears when a thrombus grows from the internal iliac vein or from the deep veins of the crus and thigh. Exceptionally, even in thrombosis of the superficial veins of the crus and thigh that spreads into the deep system through shunts between the deep and superficial venous system or through the ostium of the great saphen vein or parva into the deep veins. Hypercoagulation status is often present.

**Symptomatology** depends on the speed of the closure of the pelvic venous circulation. Gradually a feeling of tension in the limb and edema of the limb occur. However, the limb is warm. Sometimes subfebrile conditions are generally present. Edema increases, the limb starts to be livid, and in the event of a complete closure, massive edema, cyanosis and a picture of **phlegmasia coerulea dolens** appear that may eventually lead to venous gangrene. With enormous compression the pulsation in the periphery of the limb, sensitivity and movement disappear.

**The diagnostics** are based on the clinical picture. The imaging method of choice is phlebography and/or CT with a contrast substance.

Treatment
In the case of a less serious finding, heparin is administered or thrombolysis may be applied. A surgical thrombectomy of pelvic veins is indicated rarely – in the case of extensive findings or in contraindication of thrombolysis (after a previous surgery in the small pelvis, fractures, etc.). It is usually most successful in the early phase of thrombosis. After 4–5 days the chance for success of the surgical treatment is already small.

## Affection of the Deep Venous Circulation of the Thigh and Crus

### CHRONIC CLOSURES

The clinical picture is relatively variable and depends on the extent of the closures and the collateral circulation. Significant overpressure in the deep venous system results in the insufficiency of the shunts between the deep and superficial venous systems, swelling of the limb and postthrombotic syndrome with subcutaneous induration, dilatation of superficial veins and trophic defects (crural ulcers).

Anticoagulants and venotonics should be administered systemically; locally elastic bandages, treatment of trophic defects, and elevation of the limb. In the case of insufficiency of the venous shunts surgical removal is indicated.

### ACUTE PHLEBOTHROMBOSIS

**Acute phlebothrombosis** of deep veins in the thigh and crus is characterized by pain and edema below the site of phlebothrombosis. In the case of phlebothrombosis of the crural veins the calf is painful after palpation; dorsal flexion in the ankle is accompanied by pain and feelings of tension in the calf.

VASCULAR SURGERY

The treatment is conservative. Anticoagulation therapy, rest, elevation of the limb and elastic bandages are mostly sufficient.

## VARICOSE VEINS IN THE LOWER LIMBS

Varicose veins in the lower limbs are the most common venous disease. They are characterized by the extension of the superficial veins. The trunk or drainage area of the great saphenous vein, the small saphenous vein or any other superficial vein may be affected. Insufficiency of the valves, congestion of blood and later insufficiency of the shunts within the deep venous system appear.

The most significant cause of varicose vein formation is hereditary predisposition and constitutional inferiority of the venous wall. Besides predisposition there are many other factors that contribute to the development of varicose veins – prolonged standing, heavy physical work, especially lifting heavy objects, conditions increasing abdominal pressure, difficulties with defecation, pregnancy, strangulation of the limb with garters and others. Varicose veins occur more often in women.

**The clinical picture** may be considerably variable and it depends on the extent of affection; symptoms and problems are variable and individual.

The superficial small and so-called **spider varices** usually cause no problems but are a cosmetic issue. Larger and **trunk varices** either do not cause any problems or result in the feeling of fullness, bluntness and edemas of the limbs, especially in the case of prolonged standing. The skin may be pigmented, induration is painful in case of insufficiency of the shunts, and crural ulcers may even appear. Because blood stagnates in the varicose veins they are vulnerable to small thromboses and inflammation (**superficial thrombophlebitis**).

### Diagnostics
A clinical examination is usually sufficient for the diagnosis.

### Treatment
The most important element of the conservative therapy is **elastic bandages**, especially with exercise and prolonged standing. **Anticoagulation therapy** is appropriate in cases of the insufficiency of the shunts and phlebothrombosis. In the event of phlebitis, **antibiotics** are administered and **venotonics** are also administered as supportive therapy.

Effective therapy of spider and small varices is **sclerotherapy** which consists in the instillation of a small volume of concentrated alcohol in the varicose vein. This results in varicose vein thrombosis and later in its transformation into a fibrous tissue and varicose vein disappearance.

### Surgical Treatment
In the event of **trunk varices** the therapy is based on **stripping** (removal) mostly of the great saphenous vein, or the small saphenous vein. Varicose veins which

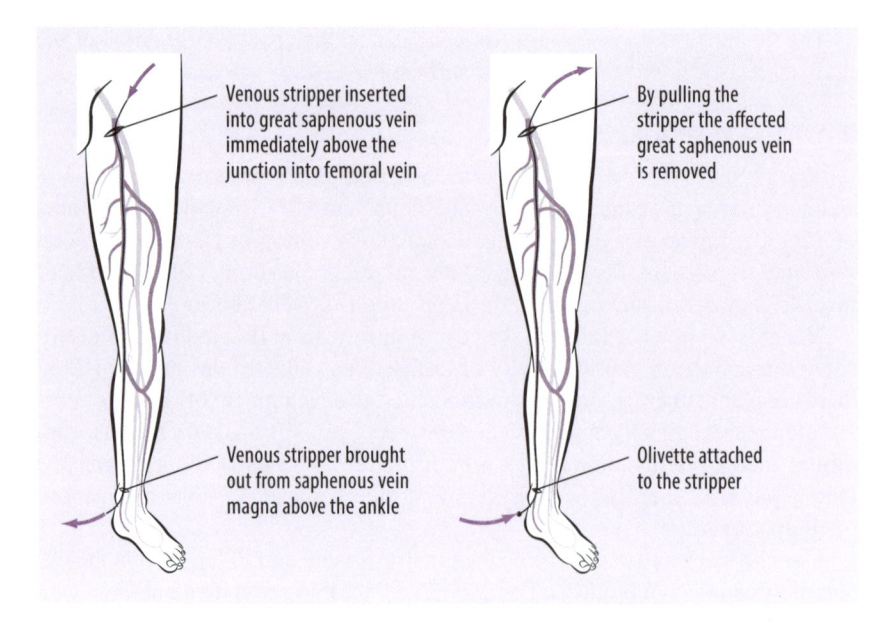

*Fig. 21.10 Varicose veins in the lower limbs, stripping*

are located outside the trunk of the great saphenous vein or parva are removed surgically through small incisions. The vein is prepared and pulled out using either forceps or the so-called Smetana's knife that has a toothed blade onto which the varicose vein is reeled in and pulled out.

There are also less invasive methods that can be used for removal of varicose veins: the veins are "stopped" by laser or radiosurgical procedures and they gradually change into fibrous tissue.

Elastic bandages on the limb or compressive stockings are necessary in the postoperative phase (Fig. 21.10).

## 21.8 Vascular Approaches for Hemodialysis

For patients with renal failure who are included in a chronic dialysis program, and repeatedly, usually several times a week, undergo dialysis, it is necessary to ensure reliable access to a repeated connection to the hemodialysis machine.

Cannulation of the large veins (jugular, subclavian, femoral) is sufficient for temporary hemodialysis. However, it does not fulfill the requirements for chronic dialysis. Therefore, **arteriovenous fistulas, so-called shunts,** are performed. The purpose of the shunts is dilation of the peripheral vein and hardening of their

## VASCULAR SURGERY

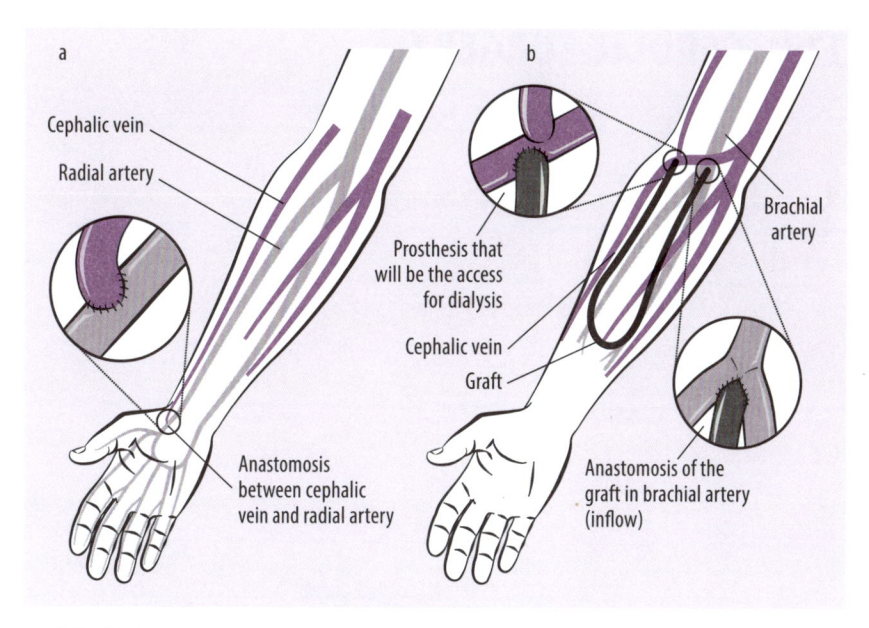

**Fig. 21.11** *Types of shunts: a) Radiocephalic shunt; b) Shunt using a vascular graft*

wall, the so-called **arterialisation of the vein**. Then, by means of a percutaneous puncture, the arterialized vein enables easy and repeated connection (sometimes for several years) to the hemodialysis machine.

The ideal blood flow rate through the shunt is approximately 300 mL/min. Arteriolisation of the vein and the possibility of its use for repeated puncture for dialysis is a process lasting about 1–3 months. The shunts are therefore performed in advance.

Types of shunts:
- Mostly a so-called **radiocephalic shunt in the foveola radialis** is created between the tendons of the extensor pollicis brevis and longus. Dilated cephalic vein in the forearm should be used for punctures (Fig. 21.11)
- A shunt between the **radial artery and cephalic vein** above the wrist
- Radiocephalic shunt in the upper part of the forearm
- Brachiocephalic shunt above the cubital hole
- Shunts in the lower limb between the great saphenous vein and the peripheral arteries are used very rarely
- Exceptionally artificial prostheses or venous allografts are used for the construction of the shunts.

# 22 CARDIAC SURGERY

22.1 Introduction
22.2 Cardiac Surgery in History and Present Days
22.3 Principle of Extracorporeal Circulation
22.4 Preoperative Examinations
22.5 Surgical Approaches in Cardiac Surgery
22.6 Coronary Artery Disease
22.7 Valvular Defects
22.8 Aneurysm of the Thoracic Aorta
22.9 Aortic Dissection
22.10 Cardiac Tumors
22.11 Surgical Treatment of Arrhythmias
22.12 Mini-invasive Procedures in Cardiac Surgery
22.13 Heart Transplantation, Mechanical Cardiac Supports
22.14 Heart Injuries
22.15 Congenital Cardiac Defects

## 22.1 Introduction

Cardiac surgery is a field of surgery that is focused on surgical treatment of acquired and congenital cardiac diseases. The most common cardiac surgery is aortocoronary bypass (ACB) which is performed in the case of affection of coronary arteries in patients with coronary artery disease (CAD); this represents 50 to 70% of all cardiosurgical procedures. Another class of diseases is the affection of cardiac valves, which involves about 20 to 30% of cardiosurgical procedures. Each year approximately 7,000 ACBs, 300 valvular procedures and 50 to 60 cardiac transplantations are performed in the Czech Republic. Cardiac surgery also focuses on diseases of the thoracic aorta (aneurysm, dissections), cardiac arrhythmias, most commonly atrial fibrillation (AF) and congenital heart defects.

## 22.2 Cardiac Surgery in History and Present Days

The history of cardiac surgeries dates back to the 19th century. As early as in 1893 Dr. Williams in Chicago and in 1896 Dr. Rehn in Frankfurt successfully treated a stab wound to the heart. For cardiac surgery, the first 50 years of the 20th century was a period of prospecting and the surgical results were burdened by high mortality.

With the introduction of extracorporeal circulation (EC) into the clinical practice in the early 1950s, cardiac surgery experienced rapid development. In the 1950s, surgeons learned how to use the EC machine, many technical innovations were introduced, and particularly patients with congenital heart defects were operated on.

A turbulent development in cardiac surgery started in the 1960s. In the late years of this decade the number of surgeries soared and ACBs and replacements of heart valves were performed routinely.

In the 1970s and 1980s surgical procedures standardized and the number of cardiosurgeries increased. Since the second half of the 1990s, due to the development of invasive cardiology, the number of cardiosurgeries no longer increased, and after 2000 it even started to decrease. This makes cardiosurgeons reduce the invasivity of surgeries and develop mini-invasive approaches.

The development of cardiac surgery in Czechoslovakia and later in the Czech Republic does not fall behind the world. As early as in 1947, Professor Bedrna in Hradec Králové successfully operated on the patent arterial duct and in 1951, as the first in the Czechoslovakia, dislocated mitral stenosis, and thus laid the foundations of cardiac surgery in the former Czechoslovakia. Further development was then taken over by his disciple, Professor Procházka in Hradec Králové. Another site with a long-term tradition is located in Brno where the first surgery was performed in 1953. In Prague a long-term tradition is that of the 1st Clinic of Surgery of the General Faculty Hospital, where Professor Lichtenberg performed the first ACB in Bohemia in 1970, and the IKEM (the Institute of Clinical and Experimental Medicine). The systematic program of coronary revascularization was initiated there in 1971 under the leadership of Professor Hejhal. Also worth mentioning is the date of the first heart transplant, performed at IKEM in 1984 by a team led by Professor Kočandrle and Professor Firt. The heart transplant has gradually become a routine therapeutic method which, in addition to IKEM, is also performed at the Center of Cardiovascular and Transplant Surgery in Brno.

Surgeries of congenital heart defects have gradually been concentrated at the Faculty Hospital in Motol where a Pediatric Cardiocenter of world parameters was established. Significant contribution to the development of cardiac surgery was provided by the first head of the Department of Pediatric Surgery Professor Kafka and also by Professor Stark, who spent most of his professional life in London and achieved world fame. Despite being behind the Iron Curtain, he co-operated, to the great benefit of the Czech pediatric cardiac surgery, with the Motol Center, and also participated in the education of many Czech cardiac surgeons and cardiologists. On the domestic scene, the greatest influence on the extremely successful pediatric cardiac surgery was that of Professor Hučín who worked as the head of the Department for many years. In the 1990s new cardiac surgery departments were established, and there are currently 13 cardiocenters in the Czech Republic (12 for adults and 1 for pediatric patients); their need is thus fully satisfied.

The unprecedented development of cardiac surgery is supported by the fact that in the year 1990 there were about 100 surgeries per 1 million inhabitants in Bohemia and Moravia per year. After 12 years there was a tenfold increase, and in the year 2002 there were 1,000 surgeries per 1 million inhabitants per year. In the subsequent years there was a slight decline, which stopped however, and now the situation is relatively stable with approximately 900 cardiac operations per 1 million inhabitants per year. As far as cardiac surgery is concerned, the Czech Republic belongs among the most advanced countries in Europe and worldwide in both the number and the spectrum of procedures.

## 22.3 Principle of Extracorporeal Circulation

Most cardiac surgery procedures require the use of a machine for extracorporeal circulation. An exception is the surgical treatment of CAD when ACB is created which can be performed by both methods – with or without the use of the EC machine (Fig. 22.1).

The EC machine substitutes the function of the heart and lungs during a cardiosurgical procedure. It therefore ensures **blood circulation and oxygenation, replacement of carbon dioxide ($CO_2$) and maintaining the acid-base balance**.

Venous, i.e. deoxidized blood is drained away from the **right atrium** to the **venous reservoir**. From the reservoir it is conveyed by the **rotation pump** into the **heat exchanger** where it can be cooled down and the body temperature of the patient can thus be reduced (hypothermia), and then again heated up to the normal values. However, the patient often need not be cooled down and the surgery is performed at a normal temperature around 36 °C (normothermia).

The blood that is still deoxidized flows from the heat exchanger through the **membrane (capillary) oxygenator** where $CO_2$ is removed and the blood is oxidized. After its passage through the oxygenator the deoxidized blood flows to the cannula which is inserted into the **aorta ascendens**. In certain events (aneurysms or dissections of the thoracic aorta, some surgeries and mini-invasive surgeries) the arterial cannula is inserted into femoral or subclavian artery. Prior to the insertion of cannulas into the heart and initiation of the extracorporeal circulation, **heparin** must be administered intravenously to avoid blood clotting in the machine.

After termination of the EC and removal of the cannulas, the effect of heparin is finished by protamin administration.

The EC must provide sufficient perfusion for the whole body during the cardiac arrest. **The flow rate of 2.4 to 3.0 L/m² of the body surface per minute is considered sufficient during normothermia**. Adequacy of the perfusion is continually monitored in many ways. The most important indicators include saturation of venous and arterial blood with oxygen, acid-base balance values, blood lactate, $p_aO_2$ and $p_aCO_2$, blood minerals, diuresis and circulatory stability.

During the cardiosurgical procedure, it is necessary to induce cardiac arrest. The so-called **cardioplegic solution** is used for this. Composition of the solu-

CARDIAC SURGERY

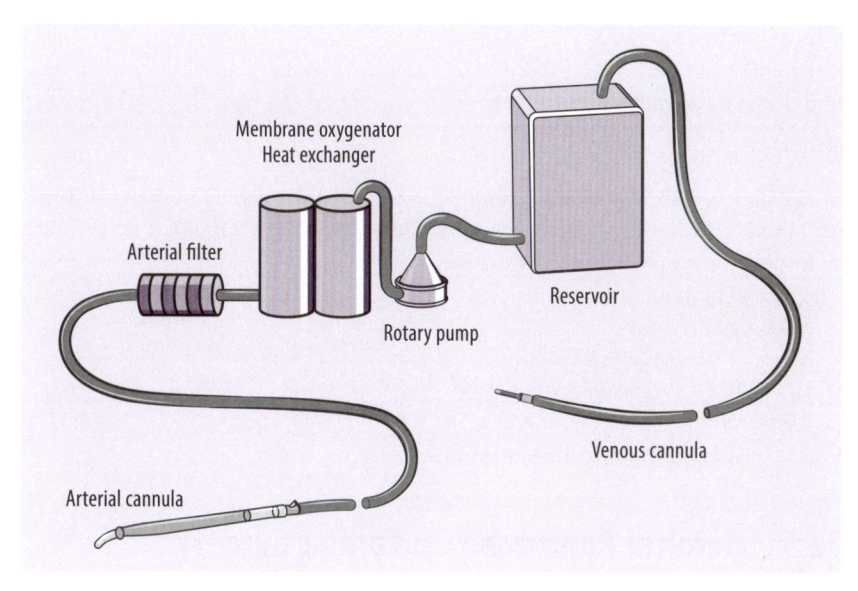

**Fig. 22.1** *Extracorporeal circulation components*

tions, their temperature and method of administration can be in individual cases different and the most often used is a hyperkalemic cold solution which causes cardiac arrest in the diastole. During the cardiac arrest the myocardial energy requirements are reduced to the minimum, nevertheless the metabolism still works, and therefore, there is a need to reduce cardiac arrest to the necessary minimum. Most cardiosurgical procedures can be performed within two or a maximum of three hours of cardiac arrest.

## 22.4 Preoperative Examinations

Summary of standard examinations performed before the aortocoronary bypass and cardiac valve surgeries:

■ AORTOCORONARY BYPASS
- Blood count + Differential blood count
- Biochemistry – glycemia, N, K, Cl, urea, creatinine, bilirubin, ALT, AST, GMT, total protein, albumin, CRP
- Hemocoagulation examination – Quick test, APTT, fibrinogen, antithrombin III
- Urine – chemically + sediment
- Serology – markers of viral hepatitides
- Spirometry
- Ultrasound examination of the carotid arteries
- X-ray of the heart + lungs

- Echocardiography
- ECG
- Selective coronarography

### ■ VALVULAR SURGERY

In valvular surgeries the same examinations are performed as in the aortocoronary bypass. Moreover, a latent infection focus cannot be excluded, and therefore additional examinations are performed:
- Dental examination
- ETN examination
- X-ray of the paranasal cavities
- Smear from the nose and throat
- Bacteriological examination of urine
- Gynecological examination in women

## 22.5 Surgical Approaches in Cardiac Surgery

The **medial sternotomy** is by far the most common access to the heart in all cardiac surgeries, pericardial procedures and procedures in aorta ascendens and aortic arch (Fig. 22.2).

The skin cut reaches from the jugulum to the xiphoid. Electrocoagulation is used to cut the subcutis and soft tissues up to the periosteum. The sternum is broken by an electric saw. Below the sternum there is the visible pericardium where the heart is embedded. Below the upper third of the sternum there is the thymus, in older people its remainders and fat tissue. After opening the pericardium the heart can be freely approached.

Other approaches to the heart (right or left thoracotomy and their alternatives) are used only in the event of special indications (Fig. 22.3).

## 22.6 Coronary Artery Disease

CAD is caused by affection of the coronary circulation, mostly on the basis of atherosclerosis that causes constriction or closure of coronary arteries and consequently ischemia of the heart muscle (myocardium). Less commonly the flow through the myocardium may be reduced due to a spasm of the coronary arteries.

CAD is the most common cause of death of the population in the industrialized world. Approximately 50% of deaths are associated with CAD.

The supply of blood to the myocardium is provided by the left and right coronary arteries. After a short segment the trunk of the coronary artery (**ACS**) branches to ramus interventricularis anterior (**RIA**) which supplies the anterior wall of the left ventricle and the interventricular septum, and ramus circumflexus (**RC**) which supplies especially the lateral wall of the left ventricle and takes part

CARDIAC SURGERY

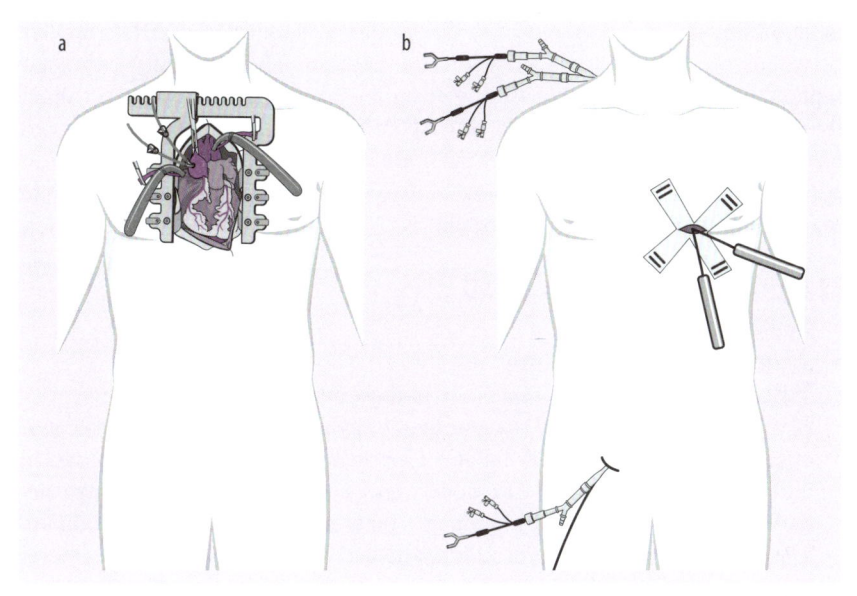

**Fig. 22.2** *Surgical procedure; a) Medial sternotomy; b) Mini-invasive approach*

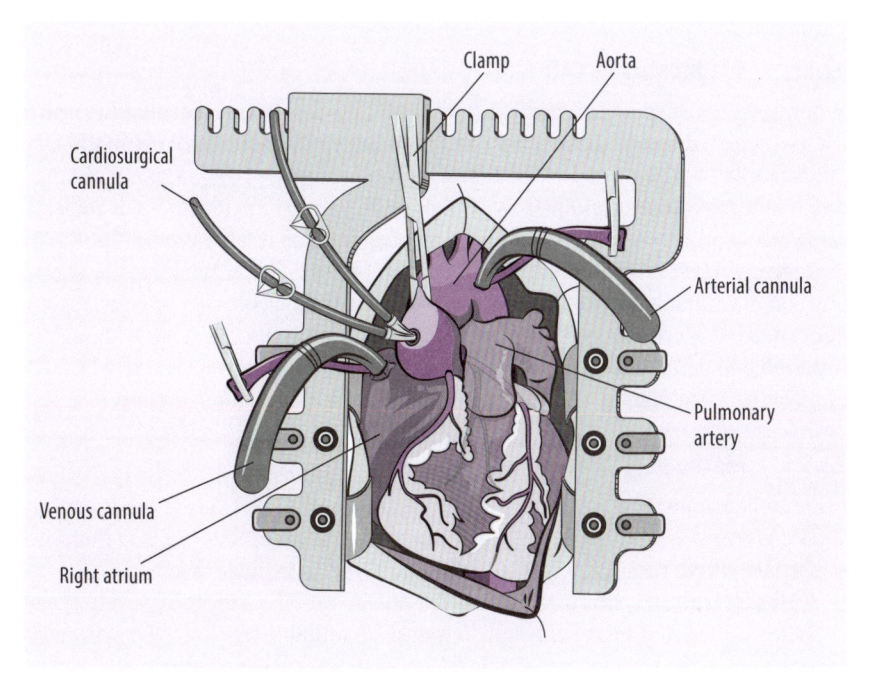

**Fig. 22.3** *Scheme of cannulation for cardiac surgery*

in supplying the papillary muscles. The right coronary artery (**ACD**) supplies especially the right ventricle and takes part in the supply of the interventricular septum, papillary muscles and the lower cardiac wall. Therefore we speak about the **three-artery system RIA, RC and ACD**. The optimal therapy is determined based on the extent of affection of the coronary arteries. Proximal affection of coronary arteries threatens larger area of myocardium with the worst situation in the event of affection of the ACS trunk.

### 22.6.1 Clinical Symptoms of CAD

- Angina pectoris
- Symptoms of **cardiac failure**
- **Without any symptoms** (especially in diabetic patients)
- **Myocardial infarction** (MI) may be the first symptom; it can be fatal – because of malign arrhythmia, cardiac failure or mechanical complication. MI occurs in the event of acute closure of the coronary artery and is characterized by **myocardial necrosis**. The extent of MI depends on the mass of affected myocardium. The extent of the part of myocardium affected by necrosis depends on several factors – the size of the affected coronary artery and the size of myocardium that is supplied by this artery, collateral circulation, time factors, the speed of recanalization of the closed artery and many others.

### 22.6.2 Diagnostics of CAD

When CAD is suspected (medical history, ECG) a **selective coronarography** (**SCG**), which displays the anatomy and pathology of the coronary circulation, is indicated. It is currently possible to display the anatomy of the coronary circulation by means of **CT angiography (CT AG)**. In view of the fact that the contrast substance is administered intravenously, the examination is less invasive. Its disadvantage is a lower resolution capability than in the event of conventional angiography and the inability to immediately intervene in affected coronary arteries, e.g. to perform a balloon dilation of the constricted artery or to insert a stent. Although it is possible to perform CT AG also as a diagnostic test, it is nowadays mostly used as a control examination that evaluates patency of bypasses after surgery.

### 22.6.3 Methods of Therapy of CAD

Prior to determination of the optimum approach SCG or CT AG examination should always be performed. Basically, there are three methods of CAD therapy:
- **Conservative therapy** – i.e. medicines and regimen measures
- **Catheterization** – this therapy is a domain of invasive cardiology; a thin catheter is inserted either through femoral or radial artery into the coronary artery up to the affected site that is treated – mostly using a balloon and a stent
- **Surgical treatment**

# CARDIAC SURGERY

## ■ SURGICAL TREATMENT

The surgical treatment of CAD is a **coronary bypass**. The principle of revascularization surgery is the bridging (bypass) of the closure or stenosis of the coronary artery (using venous or arterial grafts). This leads to the recovery of the arterial blood supply to the ischemic area of the myocardium.

As a venous graft we use almost exclusively great saphenous vein (**GSV**, Fig. 22.6). As an arterial graft we use internal thoracic artery (**ITA**), previously known as the internal mammary artery (**IMA**), usually left (**LIMA**), less often right (**RIMA**) and radial artery (**AR**). Other arterial grafts (right gastroepiploic artery, ulnar artery, inferior epigastric artery) are used only exceptionally.

A 10-year patency of venous grafts is approximately 50 to 60%, a 10-year patency of IMA and AR is about 90% and 70%, respectively.

The **advantage of the venous graft** compared to the VSM is easy handling. **The disadvantage** is its worse long-term patency and the need to perform central anastomosis to the aorta (Fig. 22.4).

The **advantage of IMA** is its high long-term patency, resistance against atherosclerosis and spasms and the possibility to use it as a graft *in situ*. IMA is the branch of subclavian artery. During the collection IMA is not separated from subclavian artery and the inflow to the graft remains natural. Only its peripheral end is interrupted approximately at the 6th rib and the graft is then sewn to the

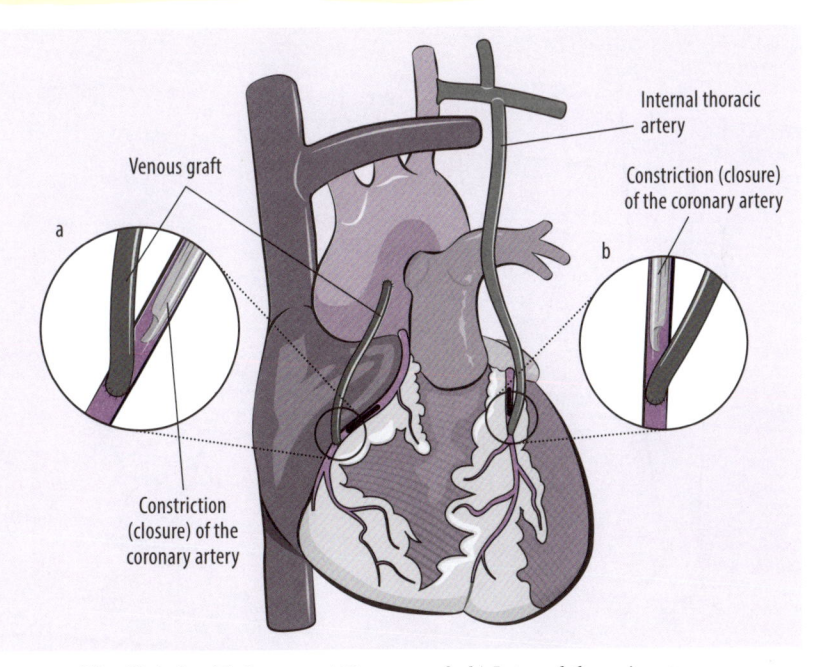

**Fig. 22.4** *Double bypass; a) Venous graft; b) Internal thoracic artery*

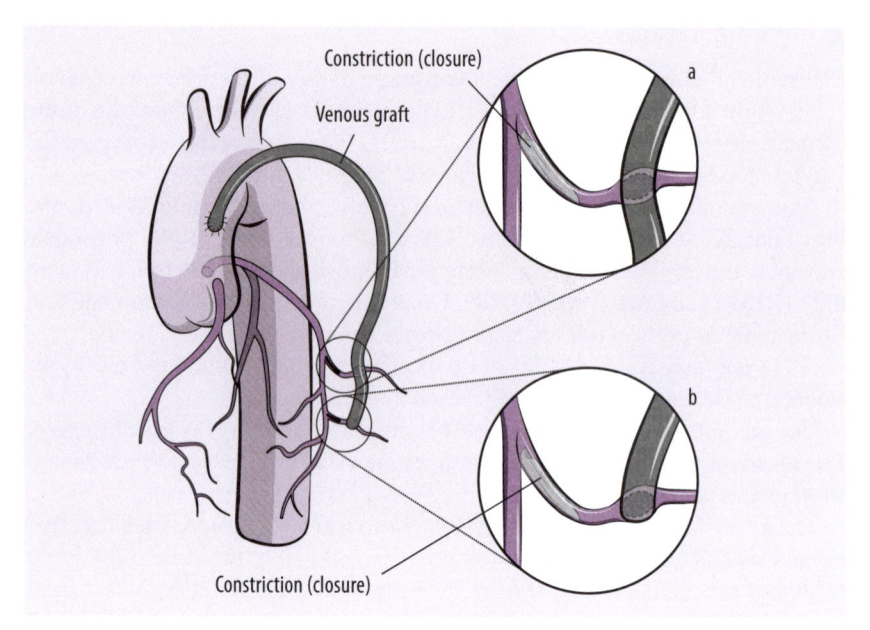

**Fig. 22.5** *Double venous bypass; a) Anastomosis "side-to-side"; b) Anastomosis "end-to-side"*

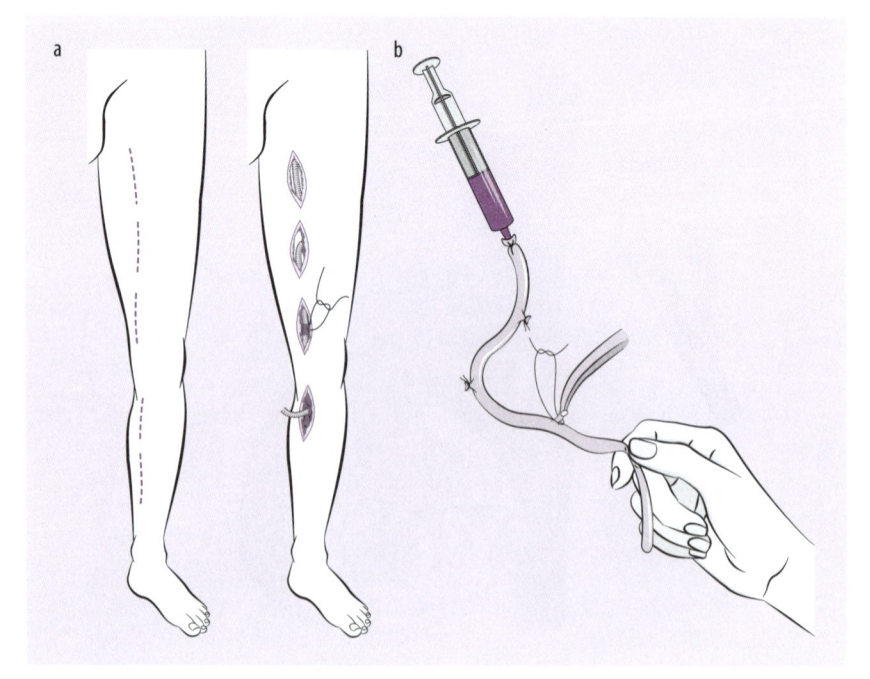

**Fig. 22.6** *Collection of venous graft (vena saphena magna); a) Skin incision; b) Check of graft tightness*

coronary artery below the site of the lesion. Only peripheral anastomosis is thus performed. **The disadvantage** is that after the collection of IMA perfusion of the sternum is reduced, and particularly after the collection of both IMA there is a higher risk of early complications.

The patency of the **AR** is higher than in the event of venous grafts and worse than in the event of IMA. **The advantage** is also relatively easy collection. **The disadvantage** is that the AR cannot be used as a graft *in situ* and it is necessary to perform a central anastomosis – mostly to the IMA, or to the aorta or a venous graft. The disadvantage compared to the IMA is also a smaller resistance against atherosclerosis and a higher predisposition to spasms.

**The most common manner of revascularization is a bypass using the LIMA to the RIA. A venous graft is used for other coronary arteries.** In recent years, arterial grafts are used even more often, at best, both IMAs or even the AR.

With one graft it is possible to revascularize only one coronary artery in which case the anastomosis should be performed by the end of the graft to the side of the coronary artery (end-to-end). If one graft is used for several coronary arteries, the anastomosis to the last artery is end-to-side, and the graft should be sewn to other arteries with its side to the side of the coronary artery (anastomosis side-to-side; Figure 22.5).

The surgery is mostly performed from the medial sternotomy with the use of the EC and during the cardiac arrest. Recently, with the development of surgical techniques and various stabilizers, more and more surgeries are performed **without the EC on the beating heart, by means of the so-called off-pump technique.** This manner of revascularization is more challenging for the surgical technique but less burdensome for the patient.

If only one bypass in the RIA is to be performed, it is possible to do it from the small left anterolateral thoracotomy. The length of the skin section is about 5 cm and the surgery is most often called **MIDCAB** (Minimally Invasive Direct Coronary Artery Bypass).

### 22.6.4 Mechanical Complications of Myocardial Infarction

The **acute** mechanical complications of myocardial infarction include the **interventricular septum defect, rupture of the free cardiac wall** (almost exclusively left ventricle) and **acute insufficiency of the mitral valve** that occurs on the basis of the rupture or loss of contractility of the papillary muscle, or in acute change of geometry and impairment of contractility of the left ventricular myocardium (Fig. 22.7).

They always occur on the basis of the acute extensive **transmural MI**, usually **2–10 days after MI**. It is typical that after transient stabilization a sudden intense worsening of the condition and circulatory instability occurs. The treatment is entirely surgical. Mortality is in the range of several tens of percent, and only

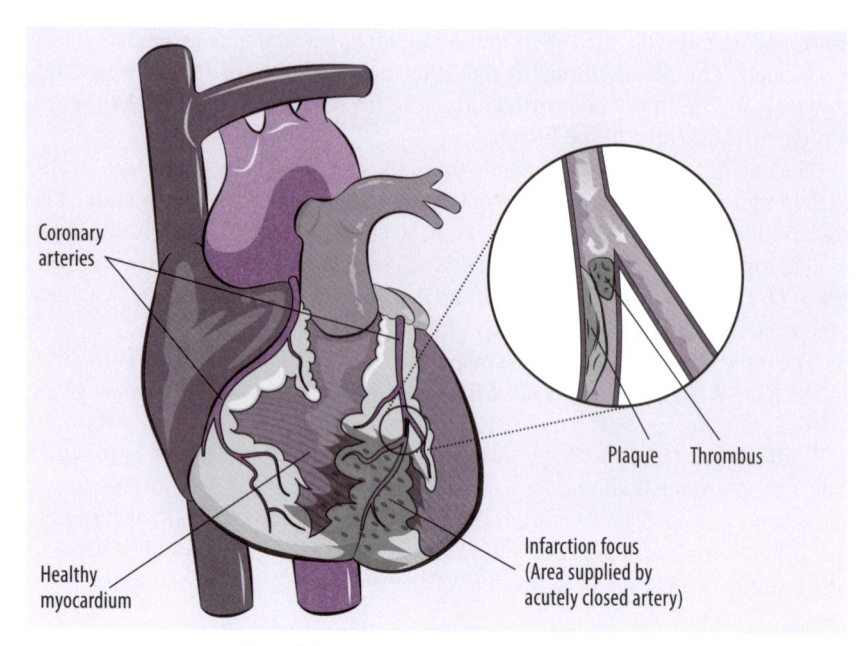

**Fig. 22.7** *Transmural myocardial infarction*

a small number of patients survive without surgical treatment. Most patients die within several hours or days.

**Late** mechanical complications of myocardial infarction include **a true and false aneurysm of the left ventricle**. A false aneurysm is almost always indicated for surgery because there is a risk of rupture and tamponade. A true aneurysm of the left ventricle is indicated for surgery if it is symptomatic and the symptoms cannot be managed conservatively or as an adjuvant procedure during a coronary bypass. The symptoms of aneurysms include dyspnoea, embolism and arrhythmias.

## 22.7 Valvular Defects

### 22.7.1 Aortic Valve

■ AORTIC VALVE STENOSIS

Aortic valve stenosis is often asymptomatic for a long period of time. Following the occurrence of problems the expected survival without surgical treatment is approximately 2 to 4 years.

Symptoms
- Dyspnoea
- Angina pectoris

CARDIAC SURGERY

- Syncope
- Sudden death

Etiology
- Degenerative – the disease of a higher age, mostly above 70 years of age, the valve is severely calcificated, immobile, sometimes associated with insufficiency. Etiology is similar to atherosclerosis.
- The bicuspid valve – the degeneration appears earlier than in the event of a normal tricuspid valve, most often around 60 years of age, but it is very individual. Mostly combined with insufficiency, sometimes with the predominance of insufficiency, sometimes with stenosis.
- Rheumatic – the significant defect occurs mostly between 50 and 60 years of age, currently less common, mostly associated with the mitral defect, often combined with insufficiency, initially fibrotic changes in the cusps, later with calcifications.
- Congenital – at adult age less common – mostly the unicuspid valve
- Other causes of stenosis are rare.

**Stenosis results in a pressure overload** that leads to hypertrophy of the left ventricle and diastolic dysfunction (impairment of relaxation). Systolic function remains preserved for a long time, ejection fraction (EF) is normal or supranormal. Reduction of EF occurs during the very latest phase.

Indication for Surgery
- Presence of symptoms – dyspnoea, angina pectoris, syncope
- Mean gradient above 50 mmHg (6.67 kPa)
- Area of the orifice below 0.8 $cm^2/m^2$

Contraindication
- **Cardial** – since immediately after surgery there appears to be a reduction of the gradient and a release the obstacle for emptying the heart they are exceptional from the cardial point of view and only relative – a terminal stage of cardiac failure if there is practically no functional myocardium left.
- **Non-cardial** – severe organ dysfunction (lungs, liver, kidney), another serious disease which markedly reduces life prognosis (malignancy), serious neurological affection.

After the surgery improvement appears in the function of the left ventricle and the overall prognosis.

### AORTIC VALVE INSUFFICIENCY

It can be without any symptoms for a long period of time.

Symptoms
- Dyspnoea
- Reduced tolerance of exercise

## Etiology
- Bicuspid valve
- Annuloaortic ectasia
- Fibrotic changes of the cusps
- Rheumatic defect (associated with stenosis)
- Degenerative defect (usually with predominance of stenosis)
- Infectious endocarditis (IE) –acute insufficiency may appear during the perforation of the cusps
- Dissection of the ascendent aorta – acute condition

## Consequences of Insufficiency
- Volume overload of the left ventricle
- Dilation of the left ventricle
- Reduction of the peripheral resistance
- Decrease of the diastolic pressure, increase in the systolic-diastolic difference
- Reduction of EF that is initially not high due to the reduced peripheral resistance; progression of the defect and reduction of EF appears with the increase in the dilation of the left ventricle.

## The Result of Acute Insufficiency (in Dissection of Ascending Aorta or IE)
- Acute volume left ventricle overload quickly progressing into cardiac failure

## Indication for Surgery
- Presence of symptoms
- Dilation of the left ventricle
- Significant insufficiency

## Contraindication
**Cardial** – not absolute
- Decrease of EF below 25%
- Diameter of the left ventricle – end-diastolic diameter of the left ventricle above 85 mm
- Cardiac failure

**Non-cardial**
- Severe organ dysfunction (lungs, liver, kidneys)
- Other serious disease that significantly reduces the life prognosis
- Serious neurological disease

In the event of a serious decrease of EF, the postoperative course is difficult, the LV function may not improve and the life prognosis remains worsened.

### SURGICAL TREATMENT
**Stenosis** – practically always a replacement
**Insufficiency** – mostly a replacement. In the event of annuloaortic ectasia, dissection of the ascendent aorta and IE, reconstruction of the valve may be possible.

## CARDIAC SURGERY

### 22.7.2 Mitral Valve

#### MITRAL VALVE STENOSIS

Currently, mitral valve stenosis is not very common (Fig. 22.8).

**Etiology**
- Mostly rheumatic. Commissural adhesions of, shortening of the heart strings, calcification, especially in the annulus. It is usually associated with some insufficiency.
- Carcinoid
- Myxoma
- IE

**Pathophysiology**
- Stasis of blood in the left atrium
- Increased blood pressure in the left atrium – propagation to the lungs – postcapillary pulmonary hypertension
- Dilation of the left atrium causes atrial fibrillation; thrombi which often embolize into the systemic circulation can develop in the auricle
- Low cardiac output per minute at rest and exercise
- Tachycardia – shortening of the diastolic filling
- In the event of clear stenosis – reduced filling of the left ventricle which is small and the systolic function is preserved
- Hypertrophy and dilation of the right ventricle, dilation of the annulus of the tricuspid valve, insufficiency of the tricuspid valve (tricuspidisation of the defect)

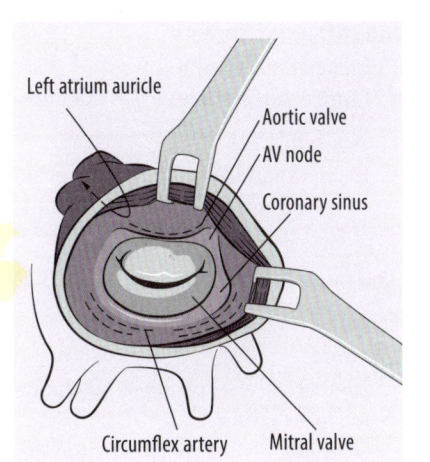

**Fig. 22.8** *Mitral valve and adjacent structures scheme. Left side view*

**Clinical Picture**
- Increased dyspnoea during exercise and later at rest
- Cough during exercise (overperfusion of the lungs)
- Inability to increase cardiac output per minute
- Tiredness and general inefficiency
- Asthenic habitus
- Facies mitralis (lip cyanosis, red face, subicterus)
- Diastolic murmur (presystolic)

**Diagnosis**
- Clinical picture
- ECG (P mitrale)
- X-ray – increased left atrium
- Echocardiography – masterful diagnostic method

### Indication for Surgery
- Presence of symptoms
- Orifice surface below 1.5 cm² (stricter criterion 1.0 cm²)

### Contraindication
- Exceptional from the cardiac point of view

## ■ MITRAL INSUFFICIENCY

The most commonly operated cardiac defect after aortic stenosis (Fig. 22.9).

### Etiology
**Chronic**
- Degenerative – prolapse of the cusp (most commonly posterior, rupture of the heart string)
- Ischemic – dysfunction of the papillary muscles, changed geometry of the left ventricle (impaired kinetics, dilation of the left ventricle in the event of dysfunction)
- Rheumatic

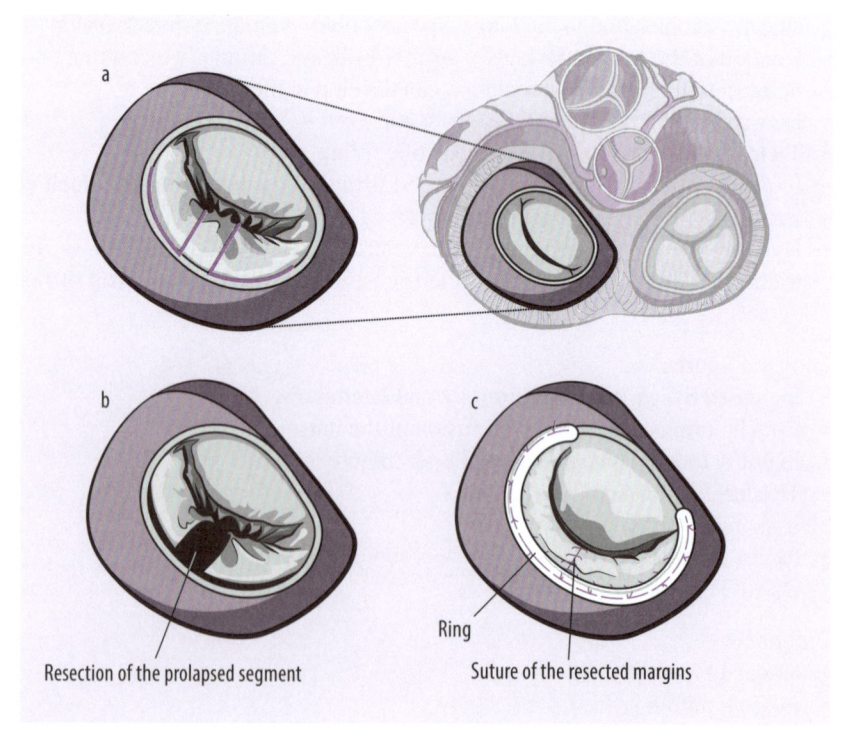

**Fig. 22.9** *Mitral valve insufficiency; a) Posterior cusp prolapse in the P2 area; b) Reconstruction; c) Annulus*

### Acute
- Idiopathic rupture of the heart string
- Post-infarction rupture (insufficiency) of the papillary muscle or heart string
- Perforation of the cusp in bacterial endocarditis

### Pathophysiology
- Regurgitation of blood from the left ventricle into the left atrium (volume overload of the left ventricle and left atrium)
- Dilation and hypertrophy of the left ventricle
- Dilation of the left atrium
- Development of left cardiac failure
- Decrease of LVEF indicates an advanced defect
- In case of acute insufficiency the fast development of pulmonary edema

### Clinical Picture
- Dyspnoea at exercise (later at rest)
- Systolic murmur with the maximum above the apex cordis

### Diagnosis
- Clinical picture
- ECG – hypertrophy of the left ventricle
- X-ray – increased left ventricle and left atrium
- Echocardiography – masterful diagnostic method
- Ventriculography – often inaccurate

### Indication for Surgery
- Acute MR
- Congestive heart failure
- Cardiogenic shock
- Acute endocarditis
- NYHA III, IV
- NYHA I, II with the signs of worsening of the left ventricle:
  - LVEF below 60%
  - End-diastolic diameter of the left ventricle above 40 mm
  - End-diastolic of the left ventricle above 70 mm

### Contraindication
- Markedly worsened left ventricular function
- EF below 20% (25%)
- End-diastolic diameter of the left ventricle above 80 mm

### SURGICAL TREATMENT
- **Stenosis** – practically always a replacement
- **Insufficiency** – in 90% of cases the reconstruction of the valve is possible

### 22.7.3 Tricuspid Valve

**Stenosis** is rare – carcinoid, rheumatic affection, endocarditis, congenital defect, **insufficiency** is much more common.

Etiology
- Primary – only rarely
  - Endocarditis
  - Rupture of the heart string
- Secondary
  - Post-capillary pulmonary hypertension, dilation of the right ventricle and annulus of the tricuspid valve and its insufficiency develop in the case of advanced mitral and less often an aortic defect

Pathophysiology
- Increased filling right-side pressures and venous congestion
- Worsened function of the right ventricle

Clinical Picture
- Edemas of the lower limbs
- Ascites
- Congestion in the liver that is increased, worsened liver function with gradual fibrosis

Diagnosis
- Clinical picture
- Echocardiography

Indication for Surgery

Most often as an **adjuvant procedure** in the surgery of the mitral (less often aortic) valve with significant insufficiency and/or dilation of the annulus above 40 mm (21 mm/m$^2$ of BSA).

As a **separate procedure** it is rarely performed.
- Infectious endocarditis not responding to conservative therapy
- Significant stenosis
- Severe, significantly symptomatic insufficiency, conservatively unmanageable

Treatment
1. **Insufficiency** – almost always reconstruction with the preservation of the valve
   - Reduction of the annulus using the ring
   - In the case of IE removal of vegetation and plastic using the pericardium
   - In the case of prolapse of the heart string
2. **Stenosis** – almost always replacement with an artificial valve

## 22.7.4 Valvular Replacements

- Artificial grafts
  - Mechanical
  - Biological
- Homograft
- Autograft
- Ring

There is no ideal valvular replacement and each has its advantages and disadvantages. Therefore, it is necessary to select the valve individually with a view to its specific properties and always after agreement with the patient.

**Mechanical valves** (Fig. 22.10) are usually indicated in younger patients up to approximately 65 years of age due to their resistance to mechanical damage and durability. Their biggest disadvantage is the risk of valvular thrombosis, and therefore life-long anticoagulation is necessary. **In aortic replacement** the values of the Quick test should be maintained between 2.0 and 3.0 INR and **in the mitral replacement** between 2.5 and 3.5 INR.

The biggest disadvantage **of biological valves** is their limited lifespan. Although they are practically biologically inert, they gradually degenerate. The younger the body is the faster the whole process is. In the event of a patient over 70 years of age there exists a 70% probability that the valve will remain functional for 20 years. In the event of a 20-year-old patient there exists a 50% probability that the lifespan of the valve is ten years and only 10% of biological valves remain functional for 20 years. The big advantage of biological valves is that no anticoagulation (warfarin) is needed. Antiaggregation is sufficient – usually 100 mg of Anopyrin daily. Therefore, biological valves are indicated in patients above 65 years of age in whom anticoagulation is not indicated for other reasons (e.g. chronic atrial fibrillation), and in patients who have anticoagulation contraindicated for whatever reason.

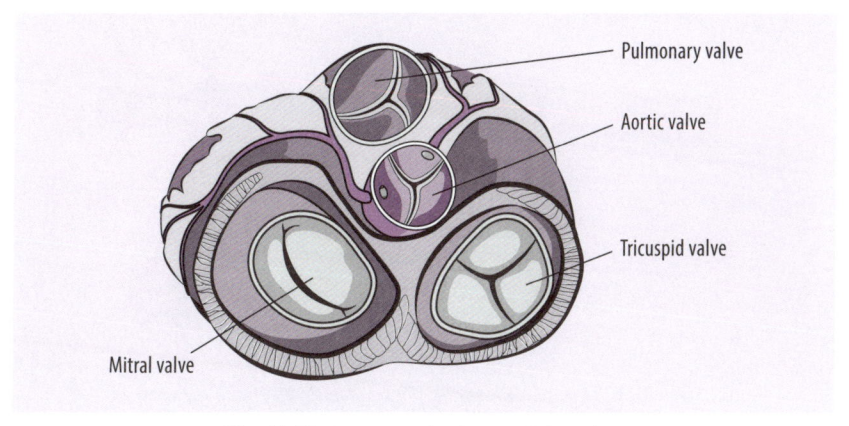

*Fig. 22.10 Anatomical relation of the valves*

Due to increased susceptibility to infection compared with a healthy native valve antibiotic therapy is necessary in the event of both types of artificial valves during intercurrent infections or instrumental interventions (pulling of teeth, catheterization, surgery with the risk bacteremia, etc.).

**Homografts** are human valves collected from dead donors. **An autograft** is the replacement of the valve with one's own valve – exclusively the pulmonary valve that is removed and used in the same patient for the replacement of the aortic valve. The removed pulmonary valve is replaced with a homograft or biological valvular replacement.

The advantage of homografts and autografts is in their outstanding rheological properties; no anticoagulation and antiaggregation are needed and they are very resistant to infection. Their disadvantages are a more complicated surgical procedure and limited durability which is similar to biological valves.

They are used relatively rarely and have special indications:
- Younger patients
- Fertile women
- Contraindications for anticoagulation or antiaggregation therapy
- High risk of infection

The **rings** are used for reconstructions of the mitral or tricuspid valve, separately or as an adjunctive reconstruction of cusps or saving valvular apparatus (Fig. 22.11).

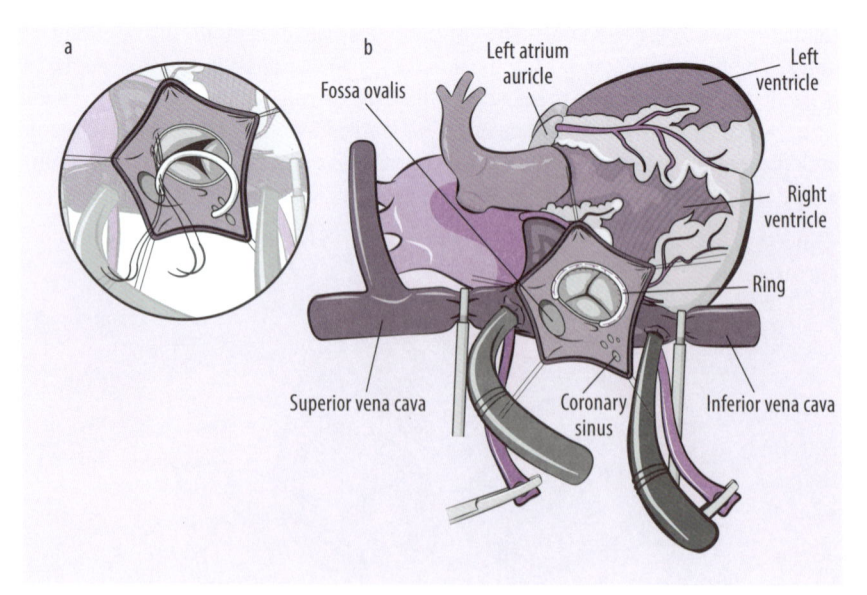

**Fig. 22.11** *Scheme – Plastic of the tricuspid valve with the ring*

## 22.8 Aneurysm of the Thoracic Aorta

Aneurysm means that the artery is extended at a certain part and its wall is weakened. In addition, according to Laplace's law, the pressure of liquid to the hollow body is indirectly proportional to the radius. Hence – the bigger the radius of the vessel is, the higher the pressure on its wall is. A combination of a weakened vascular wall and increased intraluminal pressure to the vascular wall increases the risk of a rupture of the aneurysm. In the case of the aorta it is a serious and life threatening condition.

The development of an aortic aneurysm may be the result of many risk factors. The most common include atherosclerosis, connective tissue affections (e.g. Marfan syndrome, Ehlers-Danlos syndrome, etc.), cystic medial necrosis and high blood pressure.

Aneurysm is asymptomatic for a long time and the first symptom may be the rupture. An aneurysm can be manifested by dyspnoea, wheezing, swallowing problems, hoarseness in case of compression of the recurrent nerve, and pain (behind the chest bone or back pain). The problems result from the compression of surrounding structures.

Aneurysm is usually obvious in an X-ray of the chest. The diagnosis should be confirmed by computed tomography (CT), magnetic resonance imaging (MRI) or echocardiography.

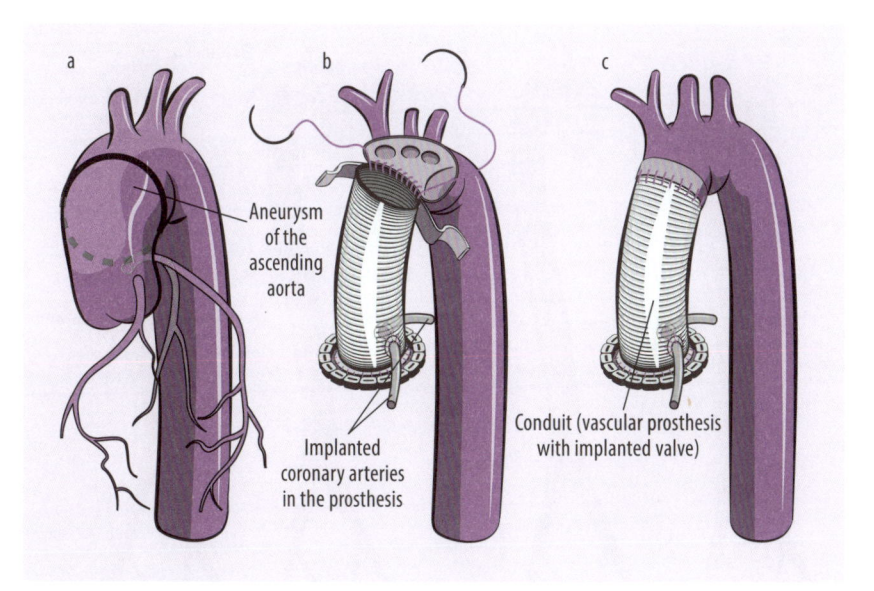

**Fig. 22.12** *Replacement of the aortic valve and ascending aorta by conduit with implantation of coronary arteries according to Bentall*

The indication for invasive surgery includes **symptomatic aneurysms larger than 5 cm.** In the case of affection of the ascendent aorta or aortic arch surgical treatment is needed, which consists in the replacement of the affected section **by a vascular prosthesis**. Sometimes an annuloaortic ectasia may appear when the aortic valve is also affected in addition to the aortic root. Then the surgery also involves the procedure in the aortic valve which consists in either the replacement and sewing of the coronary arteries into the prosthesis (so-called Bentall operation – Fig. 22.12) or the so-called conserving operation when the patient's own aortic valve is left and sewn into the prosthesis (procedure according to David).

In the case of the **affection of the descendent aorta, the surgery is usually not performed but the so-called stent graft is inserted from femoralis artery into the lumen of the thoracic aorta.** The stent graft is a tube made of metal spirals coated with special impermeable fabric that covers the aneurysm.

## 22.9    Aortic Dissection

The dissection occurs when the intima is slightly torn and the blood flows into the vascular wall that is longitudinally split, sometimes up to tens of centimeters. The blood flows both in the original lumen of the vessel (**true lumen**), as well as in the wall of the vessel (**false lumen**).

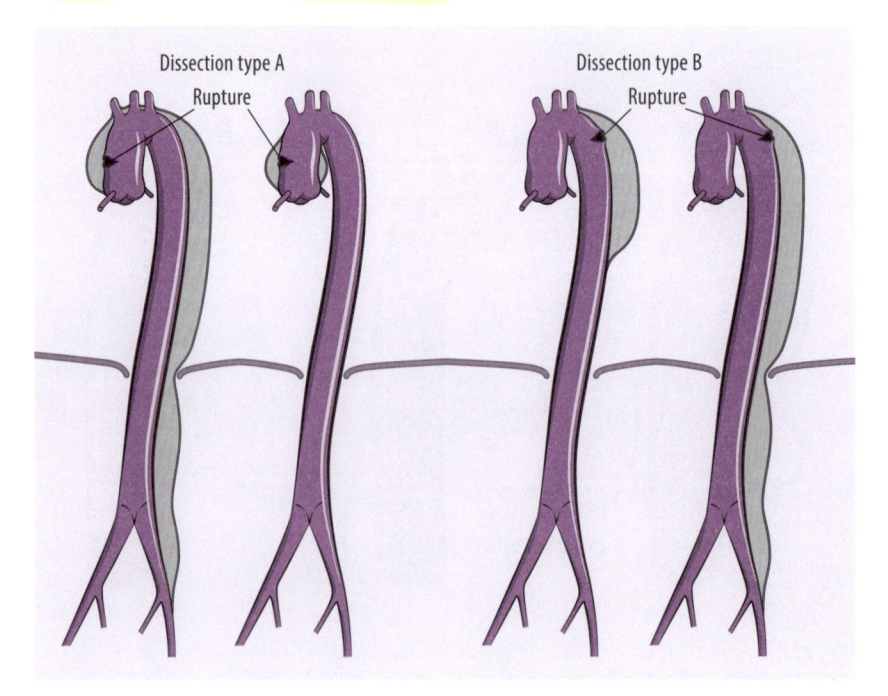

**Fig. 22.13** *Dissection – scheme type A and B*

The biggest risk of dissection is the rupture of the aorta and massive bleeding. There is at the same time the danger of impairment of vital organs (brain, spinal cord, liver, kidneys, and limbs). It is an acute, life-threatening condition.

The symptoms usually include acute back pain, or the signs of worsening of perfusion of the affected organs, including neurological symptoms or acute ischemia of the lower limbs. We distinguish two types of dissection based on the site of their occurrence (Fig. 22.13).

In the event of **dissection type A** the ascendent aorta is always affected. The dissection can but does not have to spread further to the descendent thoracic aorta. The ascendent aorta is connected to the pericardial sac and hence in the case of a rupture the cardiac tamponade can develop with a high risk of death. Therefore, urgent surgery is needed that consists in the replacement of the ascendent aorta with the prosthesis and in the procedure in the aortic valve (replacement or plastic), mostly with the implantation of coronary arteries into the prosthesis.

In the event of **dissection type B** only the descendent thoracic aorta is affected. The aorta is encapsulated by the pleura and the risk of rupture is smaller. This form is usually (in 70 to 80% of cases) treated conservatively – rest and pharmacological correction of blood pressure when the systolic pressure is maintained at about 100 mmHg (13.3 kPa).

In the event of the risk of rupture, symptoms of the spreading of the dissection, invasive therapy is initiated which consists in the implantation of a stent graft.

## 22.10 Cardiac Tumors

Cardiac tumors are rare. **The primary tumors** are usually **benign,** and the most common tumor is **myxoma**. They are mostly located in the left atrium and lay on the septum. Less commonly they occur in the right atrium, rarely in the ventricles, or they are multiple. They often reach the mitral valve and the problems are similar to those of a mitral defect. They are fragile and friable tumors and the first symptom is sometimes embolism. Treatment consists in surgical removal of the tumor.

**Primary malign tumors** are extremely rare, most often angio- or myxosarcoma. More often, although still very rarely, **malign tumors spread** into the heart. Prognosis of malign tumors is very poor even when they are completely removed.

## 22.11 Surgical Treatment of Arrhythmias

The surgical treatment of arrhythmias is almost always related to atrial fibrillation (AF). Primary AF is usually treated conservatively, or by means of catheterization. Surgical treatment is intended only for a very small group of patients in whom the above-mentioned treatment methods are not effective.

The surgical treatment is mostly performed as an adjunctive therapy in secondary AF that is associated with another valvular defect (mostly mitral), or in

CAD. The principle of the operation (so called MAZE procedure) is the creation of scars in the atriums which prevent pathological circulation of electric impulses. To create the scars, other sources of energy may be used – cryodestruction, ultrasound, radiofrequency, etc.

## 22.12 Mini-invasive Procedures in Cardiac Surgery

Mini-invasive procedures have become a routine part of general surgery, gynecology, urology and other surgical fields. With regard to the complexity of cardio surgical procedures only the technological developments in recent years have made implementing these procedures in this field possible. The minimally invasive procedures reduce the surgical burden and enable earlier physiotherapy and return to a normal life.

In the event of a conventional approach the chest bone must be cut and then heals for about 6 weeks. In the minimally invasive procedures the heart is accessed **through the small thoracotomy and intervertebral space**. Not only the size of the surgical wound but also the fact that the body "needs no healing" of the cut bone contributes to a smaller burden on the whole organism. The cosmetic effect is also significant. The scar below the left or right nipple (breast) is only 5 to 8 cm. Small scars after drains which are quite common even in the classical surgeries are almost invisible after several months.

This approach can be used in bypasses in CAD, valvular surgery, surgery of some congenital defects, tumors or arrhythmias.

The most common mini-invasive procedure in the heart is a single bypass that is usually used for bridging the RIA. The access is approximately a 5 cm long left anterolateral thoracotomy in the fifth intercostal space. First, the LIMA is prepared and it is then sewn to the RIA behind the site of affection.

The procedure is performed without cardiac arrest and the need for connection of the patient to the EC is eliminated. In the event of affection of other coronary arteries this surgery can in some events be combined with the catheterization therapy of other coronary arteries. Since the surgical burden is markedly lower compared to the conventional approach, it is indicated especially in elderly and risky patients in whom the reduction of the surgical burden is important.

The other group of mini-invasive cardiosurgeries is the so-called **video-assisted surgery (VATS)** of the cardiac valves and some congenital defects. Using an optic device the picture from the surgical field is transferred to the monitor based on which the surgeon performs the procedure using special tools. The access is a small 5 to 7 cm long right anterolateral thoracotomy below the nipple. The EC is connected to the vessels in the groin. This technique can be used for the treatment of the replacement of the mitral and tricuspid valve, for some congenital cardiac defects, especially atrium septum defects, for removal of some tumors or surgical treatment of atrial fibrillation.

# CARDIAC SURGERY

## 22.13 Heart Transplantation, Mechanical Cardiac Supports

Heart transplantation is currently a routine surgical procedure and there are about 60 cardiac transplantations performed in the Czech Republic every year. Patients with end-stage heart failure, refractory to medical therapy and those in whom another manner of surgical treatment or catheterization is not possible are indicated for heart transplantation. The anticipated life prognosis should be less than 1 or 2 years, an EF of 20% and less.

The most common diagnosis is dilated cardiomyopathy and coronary artery disease, rarely also congenital heart defects or affections of the heart valves.

Contraindications of transplantation are particularly active infection, malignancy, high pulmonary vascular resistance, multiple organ failure, decompensated diabetes mellitus, active phase of gastroduodenal ulcer disease, non-cooperation of the patient and failure to adhere to the treatment.

A brain death must be confirmed in a donor.

In the Czech Republic the so-called principle of **anticipated agreement** with organ donation applies. In other words, if the donor does not at any time in his/her life express a disagreement with the donation of his/her organs it is possible to take organs from him/her.

The heart is stopped with cold and highly concentrated potassium solution and after collection it is placed into the ice solution. The maximum time of cold ischemia, i.e. the time before the heart is sewn to the recipient and the blood circulation is restored, is about 5 to 6 hours. The optimal time is up to 3 hours.

The recipient's heart is completely extracted and only a part of the left atrium, where the pulmonary veins come into and the stumps of inferior vena cava, aorta and pulmonary artery are preserved. The donor's heart is then sewn to them.

All patients after heart transplantation must use immunosuppressive therapy. The hospitalization mortality is approximately 10%; the five-year survival rate is about 70%.

## 22.14 Heart Injuries

Serious heart injuries are associated with significant pre-hospitalization mortality reaching up to 80–90%.

### 22.14.1 Blunt Injuries

The most common cause of blunt heart injuries is **deceleration** which means that the heart is cast against the chest wall or compressed between the chest bone and spine. The blunt injury may be caused by a forceful strike to the chest. The extent of the injury depends on many factors; the most important is the degree of deceleration, strength of impact and the phase of the cardiac cycle at the moment of injury.

Blunt injuries cause various heart injuries – **myocardial contusion** that can lead to necrosis, similar to myocardial infarction, **cardiac rupture with tamponade** that usually causes sudden death, **ventricular septum defect, valvular or coronary artery injuries, impairment of the conduction heart apparatus and pericardial injuries**, etc.

The **symptomatology** is quite varied and depends on the character of the injury.

### 22.14.2 Heart Contusion

Symptomatology
A **small contusion** is not necessarily accompanied by any symptoms. In the case of a **major contusion** patients often have chest pain, arrhythmias, or the symptoms of cardiac failure. Sometimes, there is pericardial exudate, usually hemorrhagic. Larger exudate may result in cardiac tamponade.

Diagnosis
Determination of the diagnosis is not easy because there is no unambiguous diagnostic test available. ECG can show sinus tachycardia or another arrhythmia and the changes of ST-T segment are relatively common. ECG changes may develop either during the first 24 hours or not at all. Therefore, if they occur at this time, no further ECG monitoring is needed. Echocardiography is the basic examination of the heart that can reveal structural changes of valves, abnormal myocardial kinetics, functions of the left and right ventricles, or exudate. Myocardial affection is indicated by the elevation of cardiac enzymes (CK-MB, troponin I or T).

Treatment
The treatment depends on the clinical condition and the extent of injury. In the event of only a **myocardial contusion**, bed rest, monitoring and treatment of arrhythmias or cardiac failure are prescribed. In the event of **structural changes** (injury of valves, cardiac vessels, ventricular septum defect, rupture of the heart, etc.), surgical treatment is usually indicated.

### 22.14.3 Penetrating Heart Injuries

The cause of the penetrating cardiac injury is mostly **stab wounds**, less commonly **gunshot** wounds. Usually the right ventricle, the apex of the left ventricle, or the right atrium is injured. Also coronary arteries, valves and the conduction system may be injured or an interventricular septum defect may be created. The injury may result in pericardial bleeding and cardiac tamponade, arrhythmia or myocardial ischemia.

# CARDIAC SURGERY

### Diagnosis
The diagnosis depends on the character of the injury and the clinical picture. The examination methods include X-ray of the chest, echocardiography or coronarography or contrast CT. In the event of a hemodynamic collapse urgent surgical revision is necessary.

### Treatment
The treatment depends on the character of the injury and the overall condition of the patient. A small injury can be treated conservatively and surgical revision is usually needed. **If a stabbing object remains in the patient's chest, it is removed after the surgical revision, never earlier!** The access is usually median sternotomy or thoracotomy, according to the location of the stab wound or object. Patients are usually young and healthy people who tolerate cardiac procedures well. Suture of the heart is not too technically difficult and consists in several single sutures with Teflon pads.

### 22.14.4 Injuries of the Ascendent Aorta (Intrapericardial Section)

This is a relatively rare localization of injury. The aorta ascendens is more often injured at the site of the isthmus (see section 21.6).

A **blunt contusion of the wall** usually does not require surgical revision, only periodic check-ups (echocardiography, contrast CT). In the event of an aneurysm of the ascendent aorta or injury to the intima and aortic dissection surgical treatment is indicated usually consisting in the replacement of the affected part of the aorta.

A **penetrating injury** is associated with bleeding. Massive bleeding is quickly followed by cardiac tamponade, which without an immediately revision leads to early death. In the event of a smaller injury the bleeding can sometimes be stopped, especially when the blood pressure is reduced. In both cases immediate surgical revision is indicated. An echocardiographic examination can be performed in the operating room. A small wound can be treated with a direct suture. In the event of a larger injury replacement of the affected part of the ascendent aorta is necessary.

## 22.15 Congenital Cardiac Defects

There is a wide range of congenital heart defects. The most common ones are described below.

### 22.15.1 Patent Ductus Arteriosus

Ductus arteriosus (ductus Botalli) is a residue of the fetal circulation ensuring the vascular connection between the left pulmonary artery branch and the aortic isthmus. It usually closes during the first days or weeks after the birth.

If it remains open, a left-right shunt appears (from the aorta to the pulmonary artery). The symptoms and problems depend on the size of the shunt. A broad duct with a large left-right shunt can be the cause of cardiac failure in infants and requires acute intervention.

The closure of the ductus Botalli in children above 10 kg is mostly performed by catheterization and in children of less than 10 kg by surgical therapy. The surgical access is the left thoracotomy in the 4$^{th}$ intercostal space and the principle is the interruption of the duct and closure of the stumps of the duct with suture.

### 22.15.2 Aortic Coarctation

The aortic coarctation is a constriction of the aorta usually below the branching of the left subclavian artery at the isthmus, at the site of the original ostium of the arterial duct. The coarctation causes an obstacle in blood flow, which results in higher blood pressure before the coarctation than in the part below it (pressure gradient). If the coarctation is tight, it is a critical defect requiring an urgent solution.

#### Indication for Surgery

If it is not urgently necessary to operate on the coarctation due to the tight stenosis and imminent cardiac failure in a newborn or infant age, the operation is performed electively at pre-school age.

The access is the left thoracotomy in the 4$^{th}$ intercostal space. More often a resection of the constricted aorta and suture of both ends of the aorta end-to-end is performed. The other surgical possibilities include extension of the coarctation using the lobe plastic from the interrupted and tilted left subclavian artery (the supply to the upper limb is often not interrupted). In the event of the affection of the long segment of the aorta and inability to pull the aortic ends together after the resection, the resected part is replaced by a vascular prosthesis. Another possibility is the extension of the constricted site using a patch from the vascular prosthesis. The risk of this surgery in the long-term perspective is pseudoaneurysm.

### 22.15.3 Atrium Septum Defect

An atrium septum defect is most often located at the fossa ovalis and it is called an **ostium secundum type defect (type II defect)** (Fig. 22.14).

An atrium septum defect located at the site of the entry of the superior vena cava that is usually associated with abnormal return of the right-side pulmonary veins to the superior vena cava is called a **defect sinus venosus superior**. The defect located at the entry of the inferior vena cava is called a **defect sinus venosus inferior**.

It is recommended to perform the closure of the defect at the pre-school age. Most of the defects of type II are currently closed by means of catheterization with the so-called Amplatzer occluder. If the defect cannot be closed, using the catheterization procedure surgical therapy is necessary. This consists in the closure of the defect either by direct suture (small defects in small children) or pericardial patch (larger defects and older children). The use of the patch is almost always recommended in adulthood.

### 22.15.4 Atrioventricular Septum Defect

The atrioventricular (AV) septum defect has a high morphological variability. A certain degree of communication between atriums and ventricles is characteristic, and atrioventricular valves are usually also affected.

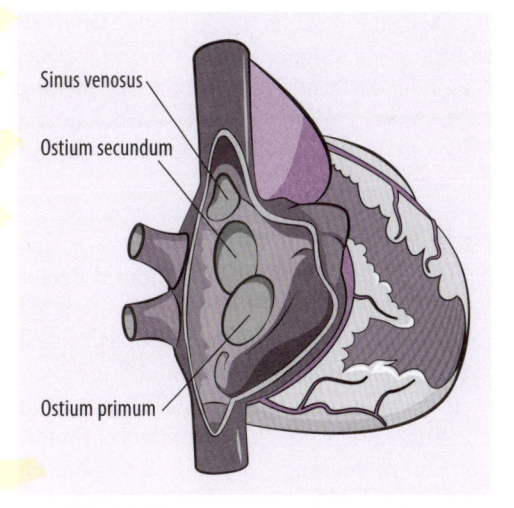

**Fig. 22.14** *Atrium septum defect, scheme*

There are three forms:
- The **incomplete form** of an AV septum defect (incomplete AV canal, atrium septum defect of the ostium primum type) includes an atrium defect (type primum), two separated AV entries with valves, usually the cleft of the anterior cusp of the mitral valve; a ventricular defect is not present.
- The **transient form** is characterized either by the common AV entry without a ventricular defect or AV entries are separated but a ventricular defect is apparent.
- The **complete form** of an AV septum defect includes one AV entry with one common valve and an extensive defect on the level of atriums and ventricles.

The treatment includes surgical correction that consists in the closure of ventricular and atrium septum defects with patches, reconstruction of the common AV valve or the cleft of the mitral valve so that the competence of the valves is ensured.

Surgery of the complete form of the AV septum defect should be performed during the first 6 months of life and the incomplete form should usually be performed at the age of about 3.

### 22.15.5 Ventricular Septum Defect

A ventricular septum defect enables pathological communication between ventricles. It can be either solitary or multiple, of various sizes and locations. It is the most common congenital cardiac defect with a prevalence of about 40%. The indication for surgery depends on the size and location of the ventricular defect. Small defects can be left without any therapy and many of them spontaneously close during childhood. Large defects must be operated on during infancy. The principle of such surgery is the closure of the defect using an artificial patch.

### 22.15.6 Tetralogy of Fallot

The tetralogy of Fallot is a combined defect that consists of a large subaortic ventricular septum defect, dextroposition of the aorta, infundibular stenosis of the pulmonary artery and hypertrophy of the right ventricle. The typical clinical symptom of the defect is a central cyanosis.

In the past, various shunt surgeries between the systemic and pulmonary circulation were performed in order to bring mixed blood from the systemic circulation to the lungs (it was first proposed by Blalock and Taussig and called a subclaviopulmonal shunt). Today, the defect is primarily solved by a radical correction that consists in the closure of the ventricular septum defect with an artificial patch, release of the pulmonary stenosis and extension of the outflow tract of the right ventricle by the patch.

### 22.15.7 Transposition of the Great Arteries

Transposition may be corrected or uncorrected.

In the event of **corrected transposition** the ventricles are inverted in the following sequence of cardiac sections – the mitral valve is behind the right ventricle, the left ventricle is behind the mitral valve and the pulmonary artery stems from the left ventricle and brings blood to the lungs. Behind the left atrium there is the tricuspid valve and behind it there is the right ventricle; the aorta stems from the ventricle and takes blood to the whole body. The configuration shows that the main difference from the normal condition is that the **right ventricle works as the systemic one**. Its muscle is weaker than in the left ventricle and hence the right ventricle may dilate over the years. The life prognosis is worse than in the common population. The corrected transposition does not primarily require surgery and the reasons for surgical intervention are associated cardiac defects which occur in up to 70% of cases.

**Uncorrected transposition** is a serious cyanotic defect that requires surgical solution in the first months of life. The sequence of cardiac sections is as follows: the tricuspid valve and the right ventricle are behind the right atrium, the aorta stems from the right ventricle, the mitral valve and the left ventricle are behind the left atrium, the pulmonary artery stems from the left ventricle. The small and large circulations are therefore separated and survival is possible only in the event of ventricular or atrium defects or an open arterial duct, i.e. when the mixing of blood is ensured. Various methods of surgical correction have been proposed over the years. Currently, the method of choice is the so-called radical anatomical correction (arterial switch) which is performed in the first 3 weeks of life, before the left ventricle "weans" to a pressure systemic load. The principle of surgery consists in the replacement of the aorta and the pulmonary artery and re-implantation of coronary arteries.

### 22.15.8 Congenital Stenosis of the Aortic Valve

This includes a wide spectrum of defects at various levels of the outflow tract. According to the location of stenosis they are divided to **subvalvular, valvular** and **supravalvular**.

There are more indications for surgery and the decisive parameter is the pressure gradient in front of and behind the obstacle. A gradient of more than 60 mmHg (8 kPa) is considered significant.

In a **subvalvular** stenosis a resection of the fibrous membrane or hypertrophic muscle is performed. **The valvular** stenosis in infants and very small children is solved, if possible, by a balloon valvuloplasty, or surgical valvulotomy. If the plastic is not possible the valve must be replaced. In small children, one of the possibilities of the replacement is the so-called Ross operation, an autotransplantation of the patient's own pulmonary valve into the aortic position. Instead of the collected pulmonary valve a homograft from a dead donor is mostly used.

A **supravalvular** stenosis is performed by the extension of the aorta with an artificial patch, exceptionally with a replacement.

### 22.15.9 Isolated Stenosis of the Pulmonary Valve

This belongs among the most common congenital defects and the stricture is mainly located in the valve (**valvular**); however it may also be located on the trunk of the pulmonary artery (supravalvular). The primary **subvalvular stenosis** is rare in the outflow tract of the right ventricle and it usually occurs within the complex defects (e.g. tetralogy of Fallot) and is treated within the therapy of these defects.

The indication for urgent surgery is the condition of the pressure in the right ventricle exceeding the pressure in the left ventricle. The elective procedure is performed at around 2 years of age if there is a pressure gradient of 50 mmHg (6.7 kPa) and more. A plastic, balloon or surgical, of the valve or pulmonary artery is performed.

# 23 NEUROSURGERY

> 23.1 Craniocerebral Injuries
> 23.2 Spine and Spinal Cord Injuries
> 23.3 Peripheral Nerve Injuries
> 23.4 Degenerative Spinal Disorders
> 23.5 Constriction Syndromes
> 23.6 CNS Congenital Anomalies and Hydrocephalus
> 23.7 Infectious Diseases of the CNS
> 23.8 Vascular Brain Diseases
> 23.9 Brain Tumors
> 23.10 Surgical Treatment of Epilepsy

## 23.1 Craniocerebral Injuries

### 23.1.1 Injuries of the Soft Skull Covers

Injuries of the soft skull covers are often associated with severe bleeding from a well perfused scalp; also common is a hematoma. The wound is treated with suture, compression, or puncture of the subcutaneous or subgaleal hematoma in the second phase.

### 23.1.2 Skull Fractures

**Linear fractures** of the skull affect the cranial dome, the area of the supraorbital bones and the temporal area. At the site where it crosses the meningeal artery there is an increased risk of post-injury bleeding. The fracture itself is not an indication for invasive therapy, the therapy is conservative. **Diastatic fractures** continue to cranial commissures and cause dilatation. They can be found in younger patients. In **depressed fractures** the bone fragments are shifted into the intracranial space. A small shift is not an indication for surgery; the criterion is a shift by 8–10 mm or by more than the width of the bone intracranially. **Fragmentation fractures** are a part of serious craniocerebral injuries including multiple fracture lines converging at the site of a stroke. **Basal skull fractures** are complicated injuries and they develop as a result of transferred injury power to the skull base structures; sometimes they are caused by continuation of skull dome fractures. Diagnostics are carried out with the help of CT examination, detection of the fracture and pneumocephalus findings in the event of disruption of the dura mater. The clinical picture often includes **periorbital ecchymosis** or **retroauricular ecchymosis, rhinorrhea or otorrhea**. Administration of antibiotics is indicated in all patients in whom a basal skull fracture is suspected. In some cases it is healed conservatively and in the case of persistent symptoms of intracranial communication a corresponding plastic of the dura mater defects with the reconstruction of the affected bones is necessary. The occurrence of late post-injury meningitides is also a risk. Other potential complications depend on the location – affection of hearing, facial nerve, injuries of the optical nerves, hypophysis, carotid-cavernous fistulas and others.

### 23.1.3 Brain Injuries

Brain injuries caused at the moment of injury are called primary injuries (impact injuries) and they are classified based on the location and severity to **brain commotion, brain contusion and laceration, and diffusion axonal impairment**. This instant brain injury that occurs at the moment of an accident can be complicated by changes which develop following the injury, such as intracranial hemorrhage, cerebral edema, hypoxia and ischemia. The aim of the therapy is to avoid the development of secondary brain injuries. The intracranial space

■ Table 23.1 Glasgow coma scale Table

| | | |
|---|---|---|
| Opening of the eyes | • Spontaneous | 4 |
| | • After verbal stimulus | 3 |
| | • On pain | 2 |
| | • None | 1 |
| Verbal answer | • Oriented | 5 |
| | • Confused, disoriented | 4 |
| | • Only words (not pertinent) | 3 |
| | • Only sounds (inarticulate) | 2 |
| | • None | 1 |
| Best motor response | • Movement after a verbal order | 6 |
| | • Targeted flexion to pain | 5 |
| | • Non-targeted flexion to pain | 4 |
| | • Abnormal flexion (a sign of decortication) | 3 |
| | • Abnormal extension (a sign of decerebration) | 2 |
| | • None | 1 |

■ Table 23.2  Glasgow Outcome Scale

| Grade | Patient's condition |
|---|---|
| 1 | Without problems, mild affection possible, patients are able to perform their original job |
| 2 | Severe affection, the ability to take care of him/herself is preserved |
| 3 | Patients are dependent on the help of others |
| 4 | Apallic syndrome, coma vigile, basic vital functions are preserved, without any contact with the environment |
| 5 | Death |

consists of three basic compartments – the brain tissue with approximately 80% of liquor[liquid?] and vascular circulation. The present compensation mechanisms are limited and allow only small changes in the given proportions. The reserve intracranial volume is reported to be 70–100 mL. For brain perfusion it is necessary to maintain brain perfusion at the CPP level of at least 50 mmHg, i.e. 6,7 kPa (CPP = MAP–ICP). The increasing **intracranial hypertension** is clinically associated with headache, sedation up to the loss of consciousness, conus symptoms and potentially death.

In neurotraumatology the globally established scales are used to evaluate consciousness impairments – the **Glasgow coma scale** (Tab. 23.1) and for assessment of the result the **Glasgow outcome scale** (Tab. 23.2).

### ▨ PRIMARY BRAIN INJURIES

The mildest type of brain injury is **brain commotion**. It is a short, reversible condition including functional changes without any anatomical correlate during the examination with imaging methods. The clinical picture involves short-term consciousness impairment, amnesia, sometimes accompanied by headache and vegetative symptoms – nausea and vomiting. The treatment is conservative and a short-term observation to exclude post-injury complications is appropriate. **Brain contusion** is a more serious grade of injury with focal changes in the brain tissue. An excellent diagnostic method is the CT examination. In the first phase, the focus is often hypotense with a gradual perfusion of the contused tissue associated with expansive progression. Clinical symptoms depend on the size and location of the contusion. In patients with a small contusion outside the eloquent cortex the clinical picture may be practically silent even without any neurological deficit and consciousness impairment (as with the laceration and penetrating brain injuries). The penetrating injuries can be gunshots or caused by sharp objects. The risks include the development of brain edema and in the event of an open injury especially infectious complications.

**Diffusion axonal injury** occurs in the event of acceleration-deceleration and rotation injuries of the head. It is based on the interruption of axons in the white matter, and an acute CT examination does not always prove traumatic changes. The MRI examination is more sensitive and it may demonstrate small petechial bleedings in the white mater, corpus callosum, periventriculary, and in capsula interna. The clinical picture is serious with consciousness impairment of different severity; an increase of intracranial hypertension occurs in the event of the development of brain edema; and there may concurrently appear primary or secondary affection of the brain stem. The prognosis depends on the extent of affection; in some patients the condition progresses to coma vigile, some patients die and some survive with different degrees of impairment.

**Epidural hematoma** (Fig 23.1) occurs when gradual bleeding develops in the area between the dura mater and a bone. The dura mater is further separated from the bone and hematoma also increases due to bleeding from diploic vessels. The most common location of epidural hematoma is the temporal area, the bone is relatively thin and it is a common site where the injury occurs and the fracture crosses the course of the meningeal artery. Besides the arterial source from meningeal artery, a potential source of bleeding is also the injury of sinus at convexities or in the area above the posterior hole. Venous bleeding progresses more slowly and the development of symptoms is delayed from the injury, and therefore can be insidious. Epidural bleeding may also occur without any fracture or bleeding

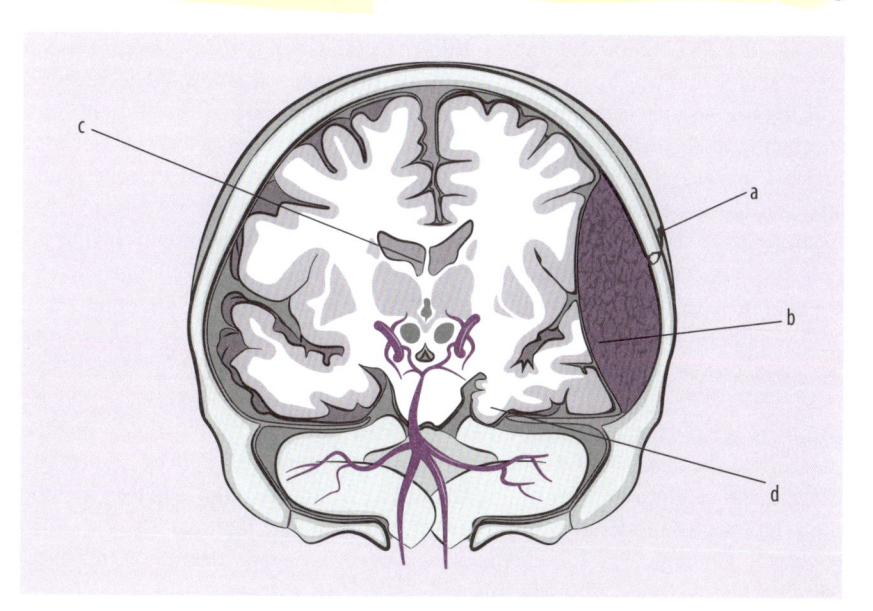

**Fig. 23.1** *Epidural hematoma: a) Fracture of the skull, impairment of middle meningeal artery; b) Epidural hematoma; c) Displacement of chambers and mid-line structures; d) Herniation, temporal conus*

from strongly vascularized diploe in wide fractures in young patients. The clinical symptoms include gradual worsening of consciousness, contralateral hemiparesis, development of anisocoria in about 60% of patients, in 85% at the site of bleeding. Diagnostics include acute CT examination with the finding of hypodense lenticular expansion with the compression of brain tissue. Acute epidural hematoma is a life-threatening condition for the patient and is indicated for urgent surgery. The hematoma is removed via a craniotomy from the dura mater and the source of bleeding is stopped. When surgery is performed early the prognosis is good and most patients are without any consequences. In small hematomas the clinical picture after injury may sometimes be silent; some hematomas may also develop subacutely.

**Subdural hematoma** is the bleeding between the dura mater and the arachnoidea. We distinguish **acute** subdural and **chronic** subdural hematoma as two completely different units.

**Acute subdural hematoma** occurs in severe craniocerebral injuries and it usually develops within several hours. It covers a large part of the cerebral hemisphere and it is coagulated and mostly associated with another injury – brain contusion, edema. The source of bleeding is the bridging veins or superficial vessels on the brain. Consciousness disorder, anisocoria and hemiparesis dominate in the clinical picture. The diagnostics require the performance of a CT examination; acute subdural hematoma is displayed as a hyperdense crescent formation that margins a large part of the hemisphere. The hematoma is largely coagulated and surgery requires an extensive craniotomy, removal of the hematoma, stopping the bleeding and usually external decompression is needed with a plastic of the mater and removal of the bone. The prognosis is serious, morbidity and mortality is 50–80%.

**Chronic subdural hematoma** is a special and etiologically different unit. It affects elderly people above 60 years of age who have brain atrophy. Some patients are alcoholics with a chronic hepatic lesion and impairment of blood coagulation. The source of bleeding is the bridging veins that are stretched during the movement of the brain. The injury may be small and often repeated and the patient does not consider it as significant, and sometimes it is not at all registered by the patient. The non-injury subdural hematoma affects patients with blood disorders, coagulation impairment and those on anticoagulation therapy. It may occur during infectious diseases, tumor affection of arachnoids and in chronic bronchial obstruction with cough. When perfused with blood the hematoma is encapsulated and then again appears bleeding from the wall of the case from newly created vessels and the increase of the subdural hematoma due to the reduced absorption. The clinical symptoms develop slowly, even for several months, and they include the symptoms of intracranial hypertension, headache and hemiparesis often with psychotic changes. The CT examination can reveal a hypodense extracerebral formation, sometimes with septums with brain compression.

The treatment consists in emptying the hematoma from a hole with or without external drainage. Exceptionally, a craniotomy and removal of the hematoma with its case are needed in the event of the recurrent process and if the septa are developed. The prognosis is good.

## 23.2 Spine and Spinal Cord Injuries

Spinal injuries represent about 5% of all injuries and they are dangerous especially due to the possibility of impairment of nervous structures, i.e. spinal cord and neural roots branching. The spinal cord of an adult ends at L1-L2. A spinal cord injury occurs most often concurrently with a spinal injury, less commonly the spinal cord may be damaged even when the spine is obviously unimpaired. The impairment of the cervical spine (approximately in 40% of cases) appears most frequently in the C5-C6 segment. This is followed by injuries of the thoracic spine and the least common is the lumbar spine injury. Nervous tissue impairment is caused either by the direct shift of vertebral bodies or fragments of vertebral bodies or arches. Most spine injuries are caused by traffic accidents and sport activities (especially jumps into shallow water, which are unfortunately still a quite common seasonal phenomenon). Injuries affect mostly younger individuals and may result in severe irreversible consequences.

### CLINICAL PICTURE

The clinical picture is diverse and ranges from a zero finding up to paralysis of all limbs, including respiratory insufficiency (in the case of high spinal cord injuries). When a spinal injury is suspected it is important not to underestimate the risk of possible damage even upon a negative neurological finding. The patients report pain in different spinal segments, sometimes with subcutaneous hematomas and sometimes there may be an apparent defect on palpation between spinous processes. Symptoms of the major lesions vary from sensation and motor disorders in individual segments with the typical level of sensation on the body, etc. For the evaluation of the level of impairment it is important to know at least the basic dermatome, e.g. C4 shoulder, C6 pollex, C8 little finger, Th4 nipples, Th10 navel, L5 hallux, S1 little toe, S4-S5 perianogenital area. The basic graphic examinations include X-ray (AP and lateral projections). The summation of the lower part of the cervical spine with the shoulders is problematic (just the injury of the C5-C6 segment is quite common!). When a spinal injury is suspected it is necessary to add a CT examination for the parts of the spine otherwise not displayed. CT examination is widely available and fast, however, its disadvantage is the worse resolution of soft tissues. Therefore, an MRI examination is already a standard examination to complete the overall examination of spinal injuries.

### TYPES OF SPINAL CORD INJURIES

1. Commotion of the spinal cord that is similar to brain commotion, good prognosis

2. Incomplete syndromes of spinal cord impairments (central cord syndrome, anterior cord syndrome, posterior cord syndrome, Brown-Séquard syndrome)
3. Incomplete cord interruption syndrome

Classification of the spinal injury types is relatively complex, and today we mostly use the Aebi and Nazarian classification in which injuries are divided into type A, B, C and groups 1, 2, 3.

When assessing the therapy we use the so-called Frankel scale with A, B, C, D and E points – from point A which means a completely expressed lesion to point E which indicates a normal function. The therapy can be divided into conservative and surgical. First aid is very important. The principle is that all patients with suspected spinal and spinal cord injury should be treated as if they were diagnosed with unstable spinal trauma, i.e. to fix the cervical spine with a secure collar and to ensure cautious transport. Further medical care consists in providing oxygenation, stabilization of blood pressure, pulse, administration of methylprednisolon (best within 3 hours from injury) at the dose of 30 mg/kg in a bolus and then 5.4 mg/kg per hour continually for 23 (or 47) hours from the injury. In the event the compression of the spinal cord is clearly diagnosed (X-ray, CT or MRI) acute surgery with decompression and stabilization of the impaired part of the spine is needed. In older spinal injuries with transversal spinal cord lesion the neurological functions will not improve after surgery but stabilization of the spine enables physiotherapy and improves handling with such patients.

In principle, the surgical techniques consist in decompression of the impaired nervous tissue, reposition, as needed and subsequent stabilization of the spine. The cervical spine is mostly operated on from an anterior approach and various splints, screws, autografts from the pelvis are used for the fixation. Surgical approaches in the thoracic and lumbar spine are mostly from behind, i.e. the so-called transpedicular stabilization using screws and rods. However, the procedures are combined and some types of injury can be treated with percutaneous vertebroplastic, or kypho- or stentoplastic.

Treatment of patients is very difficult. In immobile patients it is necessary to avoid pressure sores and chronic infections, to train automatic reflex urinary bladder emptying, and to perform active physiotherapy of limbs to prevent contractures. Also important is psychotherapy. The system of spinal units in the Czech Republic has been gradually extended.

## 23.3 Peripheral Nerve Injuries

Injuries of the peripheral nerves occur most commonly in the wrist and forearm regions. If not properly and early treated they may result in irreversible nerve impairment. Iatrogenic impairment may typically occur during osteosyntheses of the upper limb bones. The diagnosis of impairment is based on the subjective problems of the patient (tingling, impairment of sensitivity) and objective motor disorders.

Objectification is possible with EMG (electromyography). Clinical symptoms of nerve impairment are typical. Impairment of the **median nerve** is common in the volar part of the forearm and the patient complains about the impairment of sensation in the I.–IV. fingers (in the ring-finger the sensation impairment is isolated to the radial edge), volar opposition of the thumb is reduced and thenar hypotrophy may appear. Impairment of the **ulnar nerve** occurs mostly in the elbow and is clinically manifested by impairment of sensation in the little finger and ulnar edge of the ring-finger, with paresis of adduction of the thumb and there may be semiflexion of the IV. and V. finger (a claw hand). The **radial nerve** (fractures of the humerus, osteosyntheses) is injured less commonly with the clinical symptoms of paresis of the extension of the wrist and thumb. In the lower limbs nerve impairments are rare. Most of them are in the **peroneal nerve** behind the fibular head where it is located just below the skin and an injury may occur following a small cut wound. Sometimes a so-called pressure paresis occurs which is manifested by the paresis of dorsal flexion of the hallux. Nerve impairment therapy consists either in the release of the nerve, in the event of the compression of the surrounding tissue only (scar, splint), or in a nerve suture, if the continuity of the nerve is impaired. Microsurgical nerve suturing should be performed as soon as possible. The nerve must be prepared and both ends must be sewn together using an epineuro-perineural suture. The suture may not be stretched (which could cause tissue ischemia and worsen the chances to regenerate the nerve). In the event of irreversible damage to the nerves, the missing part is bridged using nerve grafts, mostly taken from the sural nerve. The treatment of the nerve without microscopic techniques outside specialized departments is currently **non lege artis**! Physiotherapy which is no less important usually follows the surgery. The patient must be informed that the function of the nerve is recovered after several months and physiotherapy of the limb must be performed over this time (Fig 23.2).

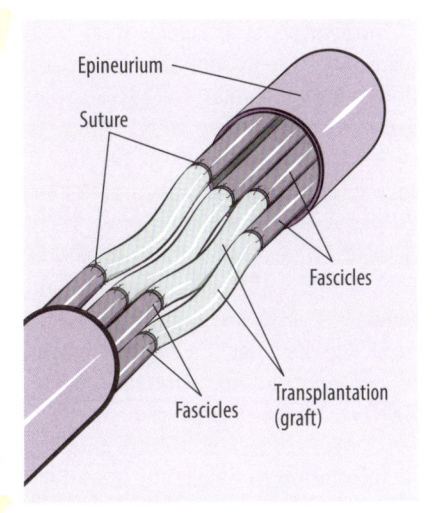

*Fig. 23.2 Microsuture of the peripheral nerve (interfascicular suture)*

## 23.4 Degenerative Spinal Disorders

Spinal pain (cervical, lumbar) is one of the most common diseases of the productive population in developed countries. It is called an epidemic of back pain. The explanation consists most probably in the combination of improper lifestyle, lack of movement, obesity, psychic factors, etc.

Lumbar spine disease is more common compared to cervical spine diseases. Clinically, it is manifested first by pain in the lumbosacral area, and irritation in one or both legs may follow. The patient is not able to bend down and he turns round with the whole body. The most common are radicular irritations S1 (pain shooting from behind to the leg, from the bottom through the foot and ends in the little finger, the patient has a problem stand on tip-toe), L5 (the pain shoots along the external side of the leg over the instep up to the hallux; standing on the heel is reduced), less often L4 (pain shoots from the front to the leg, extension in the knee is reduced). The basic examinations include X-ray, best in AP projection and dynamic lateral images, CT or preferably MRI. The dynamic MRI images are needed to document the shift of vertebral bodies (spondylolisthesis). Sometimes, it is appropriate to supplement electrophysiological examination (electromyography, EMG) that may detect a radicular lesion. The most common pathological finding in younger patients with back pain and irritation to the lower limbs is **protrusion or herniation** (prolapse) **of the intervertebral disk** (Fig. 23.3). In 90% of cases the prolapse is located in L4–L5 or L5–S1 segments, less commonly higher, usually at one level but it can be present in several segments. If the prolapse is located medially or paramedially it may irritate several radices and manifest with mixed symptoms; if it is located foraminally or extraforaminally (i.e. along with the canal which the individual radices pass through) it irritates only this particular radix. In some patients the problems are caused generally by constriction of the spinal canal – **stenosis of the spinal canal**. The symptoms are usually mixed and include pain in both lower limbs, gait impairment, and pseudoclaudication. An extreme form of problems is the so-called **caudal syndrome** (cauda equina syndrome). This is a combination of symptoms, such as LS pain, radicular pain, gait impairment, but especially perianogential hypesthesia with neurogenic impairment of urination, defecation and sexual functions. It is a significant compression of caudal radices, including S2–S4, mostly caused by acute prolapse of the disk. Cauda equina syndrome is a clear indication for examination of the patient and absolute indication for surgery in the case of a corresponding graphical finding. In the event of a prolonged compression of the nerve roots, they may be irreversibly damaged. The

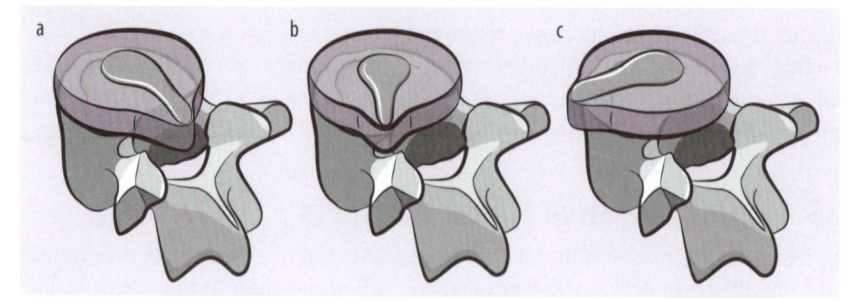

**Fig. 23.3** *Location of prolapse of the intervertebral disc: a) lateral; b) foraminal; c) extraforaminal*

so-called **spondylolisthesis** is another type of disease. Spondylolisthesis is the displacement of adjacent vertebral bodies in the sagittal plane. The displacement can be stable, but usually is instable. The size of the displacement is indicated by a scale from I. to IV., where grade I is displacement up to 25% of the vertebral body. This type of disease requires dynamic lateral X-ray images. The so-called Back Surgery Syndrome (FBSS) is a separate unit. This is a condition that occurs after previous spinal injuries (one or more) with persisting problems. The cause of the problems is usually peridural fibrosis, recurrent disk prolapses, arachnoiditis, but may also be a purpose-built over structure.

The therapy of **lumbar spine** pain should consist in the use of all possibilities of conservative therapy, i.e. analgesics, myorelaxants, lifestyle changes and body weight reduction. If all these methods fail, or in the event of a clear clinical worsening of the patient's condition and corresponding graphical finding, surgery should be used. The correct indication for surgery is most important. Otherwise re-operations may follow, which do not provide the expected effect. The truth is that patients often request surgery rather than work more intensively on changes to their improper lifestyle.

In the majority of cases the surgery is performed from a posterior spinal approach and consists in the release of the dural pouch and roots. In the event of disk prolapse it is sufficient to remove sequesters that compress the nerve tissue; in the event of stenosis of the spinal canal decompression is performed of the canal to various extents (partial hemilaminectomy, hemilaminectomy, bilateral laminectomy, sometimes also in several segments). In the event of spinal instability the decompression of the instable and mostly constricted segment is performed, and if needed the reposition of displaced vertebral bodies and transpedicular screw fixation. A similar approach is used in FBSS. In the last ten years spinal surgery has seen a great development of so-called minimally invasive techniques. Disk prolapses are operated from centimeter cuts using endoscopic techniques, transpedicular stabilizations are performed percutaneously, and there are also other techniques used such as artificial disc replacements (arthroplasty), the so-called dynamic stabilizations (e.g. interspinal implants), and many other techniques. The disadvantage is the higher price of these technologies.

In the **cervical area** it is more often **osteochondrosis** with osteophytes which compress the spinal cord and nerve roots in the foramens than pure disk prolapses. The problems are manifested as cervical pain, irritation in the upper limbs, and impairment of gait in the event of more severe findings. The examination is similar to that of the lumbar spine, i.e. X-ray, MRI, CT or electrophysiological examination. Patients with the signs of myelopathy and graphical finding of compression of the nerve structures should undergo prophylactic surgery.

The surgical approach to the cervical spine is mostly from the anterior side, i.e. an anterior microdiscectomy is performed when the so-called cage (inlay, replacement, graft) is inserted in the drilled space and the segment is fixed with a splint. Arthroplastics of the cervical spine have better results than those in the lumbar spine. In indicated cases the posterior approach is taken (foraminotomy, laminotomy). Minimally invasive procedures are performed as well. Thoracic spine surgery represents a minimum part of spinal surgeries. More often anterior or posterolateral approaches are used so as to avoid handling spinal cord during the procedure.

## 23.5 Constriction Syndromes

These are chronic neuropathies which are caused by nerve compression at typical sites. The most common constriction syndrome is the so-called **carpal tunnel syndrome** (CTS), then **ulnar sulcus syndrome** (USS), and less common is Guyon's canal syndrome and others. Clinical symptoms usually start with painful tingling sensation in the area of the respective nerve and gradually motor impairments and muscle atrophy develop. Paresthesias of the I.–III. fingers are typical for CTS and the patient often wakes up at night with pain in his/her hands that recedes after shaking the limbs. The problems are more common in females in middle age and above (hormonal involvement). The diagnosis of the constriction syndromes is confirmed by EMG and sometimes a cervical spine etiology of problems must be differentiated. The therapy is either conservative (analgesics, immobilization of the limb) or surgical. The surgery consists in the release of the respective nerve (e.g. in CTS ligamentum the carpi transversum should be cut) under either local or regional anesthesia.

## 23.6 CNS Congenital Anomalies and Hydrocephalus

### 23.6.1 Cervico-Cranial Anomalies

- **Platybasia** – abnormal basal angle, without clinical significance, the name is used in anthropology.
- **Basal invagination** – migration of bone structures of foramen magnum and the upper cervical spine to the posterior hole.
- **Basal impression** – secondary basal invagination – result of bone structure impairment – osteogenesis imperfecta, Hurler syndrome, etc.

■ DANDY-WALKER COMPLEX

This complex is the manifestation of developmental anomalies of the posterior hole structures. It involves the Dandy-Walker malformation and the Dandy-Walker variant.

**The Dandy-Walker malformation** occurs during embryonic development between the 5th and 8th week by impairment of the rostral rhombencephalon. It is characterized by a different grade of hypoplasia of the cerebellar vermis and medial structures of cerebellar hemispheres. The IV. chamber is wide, with expansive symptoms and the tentorium is elevated. In 80 to 90% of cases it is associated with hydrocephalus and in 30% with agenesis of corpus callosum.

**The Dandy-Walker variant** is a mild form of the same malformation with the preservation of cerebellar vermis and without the elevation of tentorium. Other authors report an arachnoid cyst of the IV. ventricle ceiling that does not communicate with the IV. chamber. The treatment of patients with hydrocephalus requires shunt surgery with the insertion of drains into the posterior ventricle or cyst in the posterior hole or a combination of both shunts. Morbidity is approximately 15% and the revision of the shunts is more common than in the simple shunt due to hydrocephalus. Patients with other anomalies are reported to have their IQ reduced. The reduction itself of the structures in the posterior hole is not a prognostic factor and does not indicate the extent of the impairment of intellect.

## CHIARI MALFORMATION

Abnormality of the cervicocranial junction is associated with downward displacement of the posterior brain structures caudally through the foramen magnum. The pathologist Hans Chiari published his first clinical series in 1986 and later he set the classification to 4 types. We currently use the following classification: Chiari type I – caudal displacement of cerebellar tonsils through the foramen magnum; Chiari type II – displacement of cerebellar vermis, the medulla oblongata and the IV. chamber through the foramen magnum, associated with meningomyelocele.

**Etiology** is unclear and it is associated with the impairment of organogenesis of the brain, ventricular system and liquor circulation. Risk factors include genetic impacts, impairments of folic acid metabolism and other teratogenic influences.

**Epidemiology** – there are two groups – young adults and children around 7 years of age. There is high incidence of Chiari type II in neural tube defects associated with hydrocephalus.

**Clinical picture** – the most common symptom is a headache in the suboccipital area, cerebellar symptoms, bulbar symptoms, affection of the long nerve lines, weakness of the limbs, spasticity in the lower limbs, sensation impairment and sphincter disorders.

**Diagnostics** – MRI examination with the assessment of tonsillar position. The displacement by 5 mm below the foramen magnum is evaluated as pathological (pathognomonic for Chiari type I). A dynamic MRI examination can detect impairment of liquor circulation in the occipital foramen or impairment of patency. An important finding is syringomyelia, which affects mostly the cervical area but the cervical area up to the spinal conus (holosyrings) can also be affected.

**Treatment** – observation is possible in asymptomatic findings and mild forms of affliction which are stable for a long time. Surgical therapy is necessary in the event of worsening. The objective of the surgery is decompression in the area of the cervicocranial junction with the release of the foramen magnum structures.

## ARACHNOID CYSTS

Arachnoid cysts are benign, congenital non-tumorous expansions which can be found mostly extraaxially and intra-arachnoidally and contain clear fluid which due to its biochemical composition corresponds to cerebrospinal fluid.

**Incidence** is low, 1% of the total number of intracranial expansions, 3% in children. 75% of the total number of diagnosed arachnoid cysts are diagnosed in children. They occur three times more often in boys. Histopathologically they consist of one or several layers of flat arachnoidal cells in the collagen membrane with vascularization and numerous collagen fibers. Cysts may be multilobar, septum, and may communicate with adjacent cisternas. The glial or epithelial layers are not present in the wall. They are often connected with bone structures which may be gibbous by their pressure.

**Etiology** of the cysts is controversial. Starkman's theory is based on the assumption of the congenital development by doubling the arachnoid membrane, proliferation of arachnoid cells which form the cavity and subsequent filling with liquor by several possible mechanisms. The intra-arachnoid localization of the cyst is confirmed by the histological finding of doubling the arachnoid membrane at the edge of the cysts. The second theory is Robins' anticipated hypoplasia or aplasia of the temporal lobe. However, it does not explain the development of cysts in another location, and further the expansion of brain and reduction or disappearance of the cyst following draining. The cysts in the sellar area are possibly the projection of the Lillequist membrane that separates the chiasmatic cistern from the interpeduncular cistern. Cysts in the posterior hole probably occur as a result of the closure of the Luschk and Magendie foramina. Arachnoid cysts are often located supratentorialy (60%), most commonly in the area of a sylvian fissure, in the temporal area, interhemispherally and on the convexity, in the sellar area and intraventricularly. The infratentorial location can be found in 40% of arachnoid cysts – in the area of the cerebellar vermis, pontocerebellar angle, in the IV. chamber and above cerebellar hemispheres and in the cistern magna. Cysts in the area of the corpora quadrigemina may reach supratentorially and infratentorially.

**Clinical picture** – some cysts remain asymptomatic. Cysts with expansion are manifested by the symptoms of increased intracranial pressure and focal symptoms, asymmetry of the calva and epileptic seizures. Cysts in the middle line may be manifested by endocrine symptoms and like cysts in the posterior hole they cause hydrocephalus in the event of liquor circulation disorder. Growth of the cyst can be explained by active secretion from the wall, unilateral liquor flow through the valve mechanism, active osmosis through the wall of the cyst and pulsation liquor waves. Sometimes the cyst may be manifested by acute hemorrhage into the cyst or coincidence with a subdural hematoma.

**Diagnostics** – in view of the availability of CT examination the rate of finding asymptomatic cysts is increasing. An MRI examination is appropriate to document septation and relationship to cisternas. The dynamic MRI also displays the liquor flow. Administration of a contrast substance does not cause any saturation of the wall and there are no calcifications and edema around the cyst. According to the size and relation with the surrounding area we distinguish three sizes of the most common sylvian cysts. Type I are asymptomatic small cysts, type II are cysts with little expansive behavior and type III are cysts with displacement of the medial line and changes of the surrounding brain tissue with bone pressure changes.

**Therapy** – asymptomatic cysts are not indicated for surgery. The cyst can be drained from the hole but this procedure is associated with a high rate of relapses. Craniotomy and resection of the cyst wall with fenestration into the basal cistern is a procedure with a higher surgical risk. The most common method involves a shunt of the cyst using a high-pressure or programmable valve. The latest and in many cases the most appropriate procedure is an endoscopic fenestration of the cyst into the chamber or arachnoid areas. Nevertheless, sometimes shunt surgery is needed in the second phase.

## HYDROCEPHALUS

Hydrocephalus is a pathological condition of abnormal accumulation of cerebrospinal fluid which causes extension of the ventricular system (ventriculomegaly) on the basis of the disproportion between formation and absorption of the cerebrospinal fluid, accompanied by increased intracranial pressure. There are a number of causes that take part in the pathophysiology of hydrocephalus. Congenital hydrocephalus on the basis of stenosis of the cerebral aqueduct, congenital anomalies of the posterior hole – Chiari malformations, Dandy-Walker syndrome, myelomeningocele and other congenital disorders are manifested mostly in childhood. In adulthood hydrocephalus is mostly acquired, post-inflammation, post-hemorrhage, post-injury or neoplasm. From the viewpoint of circulation of cerebrospinal fluid and imaging methods we distinguish hydrocephalus obstructive and communicating (in the communicating hydrocephalus the obstruction is at the level of arachnoid granulations).

**Clinical symptoms** include headache, vomiting, paresis of n. VI, gait and behavioral disorders. The complementary examinations can detect congestion in the fundus oculi. For the diagnostics of hydrocephalus we use imaging methods; CT examination shows an extended ventricular system, periventricular hypodensities in transition of the cerebrospinal fluid, and expansion with obstruction. The MRI can provide more detailed imaging of the causes of obstruction (i.e. higher yield for the posterior hole processes, congenital defects, septations, brain-stem tumor, etc.) and enables a dynamic examination displaying the cerebrospinal fluid flow.

**Therapy** of an active hydrocephalus with the symptoms of intracranial hypertension consists in extracranial drainage of the cerebrospinal fluid or recovery of the circulation by means of removal of or bypassing the obstacle. A number of shunt systems are used with the use of non-programmable valves, programmable valves in which the opening pressure can be used as needed, or with components which prevent overdrainage (the so-called antisiphon devices).

The most common type of drainage is the ventriculoperitoneal shunt (95%). The ventricular catheter is inserted from the hole into the lateral ventricle, the valve is placed subcutaneously retroauricularly and the distal hose is inserted into the peritoneal cavity. In the event of a ventriculoatrial shunt the distal hose is inserted in the area of the cardiac atrium under X-ray or ECG guidance. In lumboperitoneal drainage the hose is inserted into the lumbal subarachnoid space and then through the valve in subcutis into the peritoneum. It can be used only in a communicating hydrocephalus and in a rare clinical units called pseudotumor cerebri.

Neuroendoscopy is the treatment method largely used in recent years in the event of the obstructive form of hydrocephalus. The principle of this method is making the liquor passages patent by means of removal of the obstacle – cyst in the III. ventricle, cyst in the foramen interventricularly, septation and cysts of lateral ventricles, plastic of the liquor duct. The endoscopic method can also be used to remove some types of tumors in the ventricle or in the cranial base. However, the neuroendoscopic technique is used more often to perform ventriculostomy of the III. chamber. Through the hole in the anterior area the neuroendoscopic device is inserted through the lateral ventricle, the foramen of Monro into the III. ventricle and a communication is created from the anterior part of the base of the III. ventricle to the basal cisterns. The circulation of cerebrospinal liquid and patency of fenestration can be verified later by means of a dynamic MRI examination.

**Normotensive hydrocephalus** is a completely specific unit. In some patients it may develop as a secondary hydrocephalus following subarachnoid hemorrhage, trauma or meningitis. The idiopathic form is typical when the persistent classic triad symptoms develop mostly in patients above 60 years of age. First, gait **disorders**, with a broader basis, with small steps, followed by memory **impairment**, bradypsychic symptoms, and continence **disorders**. Measurement of blood pressure during the puncture does not show hypertension, and during prolonged monitoring the periods of pressure increase; the so-called B waves are recorded. The lumbar infusion test is useful in the diagnostics with the instillation of Ringer's solution using the linear dosing device and measurement of the liquor resistance. In indicated patients the method of therapy is a ventriculoperitoneal shunt.

## 23.7 Infectious Diseases of the CNS

Infectious disease of the central nervous system is a serious condition which in its consequence may be life-threatening for the patient. In developed countries these diseases occur significantly less than in developing countries. Acute neurosurgical solutions are indicated for patients with subdural empyema, epidural empyema and brain abscess. Another group includes postoperative inflammations – osteomyelitis of the bone lobe after surgery and infectious complications of shunt surgeries and shunt surgeries due to post-inflammatory hydrocephalus (see section Hydrocephalus in section 23.6.1).

## 23.7.1 Epidural Abscess and Subdural Empyema

These diseases occur as a complication of inflammations in paranasal cavities, the mastoid area, orbit, after scalp infections and skull osteomyelitis, after injuries of the cranial base with intracranial communication and after procedures in the cranial base. Hematogenic infection is rare and it is present in subdural empyema.

**Diagnostics** – CT or MRI examinations may display a hypodense or hypotense focus. The CT examination is sometimes insufficient and may detect only highlighting of the brain meninges following the administration of the contrast substance and brain edema.

**Therapy** is surgical, removal of pus, inflammatory tissue, and temporary drainage of the focus. Treatment of the primary inflammatory focus is always necessary.

## 23.7.2 Brain Abscess

Brain abscess affects mostly younger age groups, more often males. The incidence in developed countries is relatively low and brain abscess represents 2–5% of all intracranial expansive processes. Etiology is diverse. It is often a complication of inflammations in parameningeal spaces with direct transmission (frontal or ethmoidal sinusitis, otogenic infections), hematogenic transmission in cyanotic cardiac defects, pulmonary arteriovenous malformations, secondarily following post-injury conditions or surgeries in the area of the cranial base. More commonly it occurs in patients with immunodeficiency.

**Clinical symptoms** – fever, meningeal irritation and generally the symptoms of inflammation are present in only 40–50% of patients. In 70–80% of cases the abscess is manifested by neurological symptoms, by headache in the case of increased intracranial pressure, vomiting or epileptic seizures in up to 1/3 of patients.

**Diagnostics** – for abscess identification the MRI examination is more appropriate compared to the CT examination; it is more sensitive and better displays the phases of abscess development and the multilocular character.

Brain abscess is an intraparenchymatous inflammatory process that develops in 4 stages. The inflammation is displayed first – the focal stage of early cerebritis at around the 3$^{rd}$ day of infection, after 1 week the last phase of cerebritis occurs highlighting the necrotic central area with expansive behavior. The center of the focus is hypodense in the CT examination and hypotense in the MRI image and saturation appears. At around day 10 a delimitation of the inflammatory focus develops by formation of the necrotic center and abscess case with marked saturation of the case following the administration of a contrast substance – the early capsular phase. At around day 14 after the first signs of infection – the late capsular phase – the case is already formed by the glial tissue with smaller signs of saturation, and the periphery of the focus is created by the cerebritis zone externally from the case.

**Therapy** – conservative therapy with the administration of antibiotics is appropriate only in small, multilocular foci. Most abscesses are operated on by means of puncture and drainage of the abscess cavity or removal of the focus from craniotomy. From the viewpoint of bacteriology the most often identified are *Staphylococcus aureus*, *Streptococcus pneumoniae*, *Haemophilus influenzae*, *Neisseria*, *E. coli* and others. Mycotic infection is less common and it may be *Candida species*, *Nocardiae*, or *Aspergillus*. Parasitary infections are rare and they mostly appear in developing countries (cysticercosis, toxoplasmosis, amoebic infections, *Echinococcus*).

**Prognosis** – in early treated patients good despite the fact that it is a life-threatening condition. Mortality currently does not exceed 5–15%.

### 23.7.3 Cranial Osteomyelitis

It is rare in developed countries and may occur after penetrating injuries, more often as a complication of neurosurgical procedures – osteomyelitis of the bone lobe following a craniotomy. The therapy requires removal of the affected bone and intravenous administration of antibiotics. After 3–5 months a plastic of the bone defect is performed using an autologous or bone replacement.

## 23.8 Vascular Brain Diseases

Diseases of vessels supplying the central nervous system may be manifested by various types of neurological deficits. The so-called cerebrovascular accident (CVA) is, according to statistics, the third most common cause of death in the Czech Republic. Ischemic CVAs (80%) are more common; hemorrhagic CVAs (20%) are less common. Clinical symptoms of an ischemic CVA are often similar to hemorrhagic CVA, however, the therapy is completely different. It is a sudden neurological deficit with a picture of hemiparesis to hemiplegia, with impairment of the phatic functions, with possible alternating hemiparesis in combination with the affection of cranial nerves, and with a different grade of consciousness alteration. In hemorrhagic accidents the consciousness disorder is far more common compared to ischemic accidents, with gradual worsening.

### 23.8.1 Ischemic Cerebrovascular Accident

An ischemic cerebrovascular accident is caused by insufficient brain tissue perfusion. There may be various causes, the most common of which is the atherosclerotic arterial affection with subsequent embolism or thrombosis of brain arteries.

**Clinical symptoms** – ischemic cerebrovascular accident is classified according to the duration of the neurological deficit. A so-called transitory ischemic attack (TIA) lasts up to 24 hours, and the neurological deficit is mostly recovered **ad integrum** during the first minutes or hours. If the recovery of neurological functions lasts from one day to one week, it is a so-called reversible ischemic neurological deficit (RIND), if some neurological affection persists it is called completed CVA (CS-completed stroke).

**Diagnostics** – in patients with an acute neurological affection it is always necessary to perform imaging examinations – acute native CT examination (and/or MRI examination). The advantage of up-to-date CT examinations is the possibility to add a contrast substance, and thus to display the condition of extracranial and intracranial brain arteries – the CT angiography. The MRI examination provides – through diffusion weighted image – an exact display of the extent of the infarction zone. The CT or perfusion MRI examination identifies the extent of perfusion in the surrounding affected areas of the brain.

**Therapy** – neurosurgical thrombolysis in acute ischemic stroke (intravenous or less commonly intraarterial), acute surgical desobliteration may be performed in exceptional situations. The problem of the therapy of acute ischemic stroke consists in a very short therapeutic window. Major surgical achievements can be achieved upon the so-called **secondary prophylaxis**. Carotic endarterectomy is performed not only in patients with the clinically manifested CVA but also in asymptomatic patients who were diagnosed with arterial constriction mostly in the internal carotid artery.

During the surgery it is necessary to monitor brain perfusion around the closed artery; at some departments surgeries are performed only under regional anesthesia with a co-operating patient. The indication for surgery abides by conclusions of several studies, such as NASCET, ECST, and ACAS. The clinical status of the patient and the finding on the artery are considered; the benefit of the surgery must be higher than the natural course of the disease upon the pharmacological monotherapy. A less common procedure is extra-intracranial anastomosis (EC-IC bypass). This type of surgery was popular until the mid-1980s, and it is currently performed under very strictly indicated conditions. The surgery is indicated in patients with closed internal carotid artery and consists in sewing of the branch of the superficial temporal artery to the peripheral branch of the middle cerebral artery. Moderately wide decompression craniotomies above the swelling brain hemisphere in case of extensive ischemic stroke are a special chapter. The indication must be careful as the surgery improves mortality but does not improve morbidity.

### 23.8.2 Hemorrhagic Vascular Accident

This affection is divided into bleeding directly to the brain tissue (intracerebral hematoma, ICH) and subarachnoid hemorrhage (SAH).

#### ■ INTRACEREBRAL HEMATOMA

Intracerebral hematoma (ICH) develops on the basis of spontaneous bleeding into the brain tissue. It is twice as common as SAH, more often in elderly people; it occurs during physical activity, in contrast to ischemic strokes which often occur during sleep. ICH is divided into the so-called typical hemorrhage in hypertonic patients (basal gangliae and thalamus hemorrhage), atypical hemorrhage in hypertonic patients (hematoma is in the white matter and proceeds below the brain cortex), cerebellar hemorrhage and brain stem hemorrhage. Indication for surgery depends on the neurological and internal condition of the patient and on the location of the hematoma. A small hematoma in the basal ganglia but with a neurological finding of hemiplegia is usually not operated on (the clinical condition does not improve even after the evacuation of the hematoma), a subcortical larger hematoma that compresses the surrounding healthy brain tissue is indicated for surgery. Cerebellar hematomas are urgently removed due to the risk of brain stem impairment with edema, and even a larger destruction of the cerebellum has no major significance for good prognosis of the patient. On the contrary, stem hematomas with a serious deficit are not operated on.

### ■ SUBARACHNOID HEMORRHAGE

Spontaneous bleeding in the subarachnoid space (SAH) is most commonly (in approximately 80% of cases) caused by rupture of a vascular aneurysm. It is manifested by a sudden headache with the impairment of consciousness and the mobility of limbs. Aneurysms are mostly clinically manifested in the age group between 40–60 years of age, often during physical activity. Some patients (about 20%) die soon after the aneurysm ruptures. The risk of repeated bleeding is 20% within 2 weeks and 50% within 6 months. Diagnostic tools include an acute CT examination; in the event of a negative CT finding a small amount of cerebrospinal fluid can be collected (the risk of rupture of an aneurysm in the event of a sudden change of the intracranial pressure!), brain panangiography is the basic examination, digital subtraction angiography (DSA), or easier CTAG or MRAG. When an aneurysm is found it has to be immediately operated on since the risk of rupture in the first hours is the highest. Open surgery is performed with the closure of the aneurysmatic neck by a clamp and elimination of the aneurysm from circulation. The endovascular technique is the method of choice. The so-called coils (metal coils) are used to fill the aneurysm. The advantage of endovascular techniques is that they are minimally invasive; their disadvantage is the possible instability of the closure after a longer time period. A rare source of SAH is **arteriovenous malformation** (AVM). This is a pathologically extended convolute of vessels through which blood flows under high pressure directly from arteries to veins. An AVM hemorrhage affects more commonly brain parenchyma and affects younger people at approximately 20 years of age. AVM is clinically manifested by bleeding or epileptic seizures.

**Diagnostics of hematoma** –CT examination, to display the vascular pathology it is possible to use the non-invasive CT angiography or the MRI angiography. DSA – the digital subtraction angiography is appropriate as a part of therapeutic intervention in edovascular techniques.

**Therapy** – surgical with resection of the AVM or irradiation using a gamma knife or a combination of endovascular and surgical techniques. The risk of repeated bleeding in AVM is approximately 4% per year.

## 23.9 Brain Tumors

Brain tumors represent a serious field of neurosurgery because of their therapeutic challenges and socioeconomic consequences. Their incidence differs based on the geographic location and there are reported to be 5–15 newly diagnosed tumors per 100,000 inhabitants above 19 years of age. In adults supratentorial tumors are more common than infratentorial ones. The brain stem tumors represent less than 2%. From the histopathological point of view the most common are glial tumors (about 50%), meningeomas (12%), schwannomas (12%) and metastases.

From the viewpoint of tumor location and its relationship to the brain parenchyma they are divided into extraaxial (extrinsic) – growing from the tissues outside the pia mater, from the tissues separated from parenchyma of the central nervous system. Intraaxial tumors (intrinsic) grow from the brain parenchyma and they also include intraventricular tumors.

The most common tumor intracranial process in adults are metastases in the brain lobes and meninges. The most common metastatic processes is the hematogenous route, when metastases occur at the same time in the brain and lungs. Lung cancer, breast cancer, Grawitz cancer, GIT cancers and malign melanoma spread out most often. In a large number (up to 15%) the primary process is not preoperatively verified. Solitary surgically approachable metastases are indicated for surgery. With regard to the clinical status only 10–25% of patients undergo surgery. Currently more often operated are several foci, others can be treated stereotactically.

**Symptoms** – sometimes unspecific or insignificant problems, or typical symptoms of intracranial hypertension. The following symptoms are common in supratentorial tumors: headaches, double vision, dizziness, ataxia, behavioral changes, focal epileptic seizures, nausea, vomiting and focal neurological findings. In processes in the sellar area and the III. ventricle there may appear vision impairments and endocrinological disorders. The symptoms of infratentorial tumors include tetanus, forced holding of the head, headaches, vomiting, ataxia, diplopia, nystagmus, bulbar symptoms, affection of head nerves, lateral mixed system and pyramidal lines.

**Diagnostics** – additional examinations such as eye ground (fundus oculi) examination are important, which may find congestion or hemorrhage. The finding in the eye ground may be negative even upon marked intracranial hypertension. The most significant and sensitive imaging method is the contrast MRI. CT is the most widely available examination, but some tumors (low-grade gliomas and brain stem tumors) are not displayed by it. Angiography (DSA) is significant in some highly vascularized processes. The MRI angiography is usually sufficient for the surgical strategy. MRI examination is also necessary for early postoperative check-up of the procedure radicality.

### 23.9.1 Supratentorial Tumors

#### ■ HEMISPHERAL TUMORS

**Benign Glial Tumors**

LG-gliomas (the WHO classification grade I, II) represent 60% of supratentorial tumors of the brain hemispheres. The names are derived from the histological type of cells from which they develop. They include mainly:
- Astrocytary tumors – pilocystic astrocytoma
- Oligodendroglial tumors
- Mixed gliomas
- Benign neuroepithelial tumors (ganglioglioma) and dysembryoplastic euroepithelial tumors

**Pilocystic astrocytoma** is a well delimited, slowly growing tumor that occurs mostly in younger adults and can grow for many years even with symptoms. It usually affects the frontal or temporal lobes. If there is no progression the patient can be monitored with regular MRI check-ups. The neurosurgical therapy consists in radical removal and subsequent monitoring with MRI check-ups without oncological therapy. Re-operation is appropriate in the event of recurrence. Following a non-radical procedure the symptoms of radiotherapy malignization appear.

**Subependymal large-cell astrocytoma** occurs more commonly in patients with tuberous sclerosis. It is a completely benign tumor with slow progression. It occurs in ventricular walls with the propagation intraventricularly. Patients with a finding of an expansive focus with the obstruction of liquor ducts (foramen interventriculare Monroi) are indicated for surgery. Progression of the disease rarely leads to death and radical resection is possible even during re-operation.

**Pleomorphic xanthoastrocytoma, oligodendroglioma, mixed oligoastrocytoma, ganglioglioma and benign neuroepithelial tumors** (dysembryoplastic neuroepithelial tumor – DNET) are benign tumors with very slow progression, well delimited, and often manifested with epileptic seizures.

**Diffusion astrocytoma of grade II** – although it is classified among histologically benign types of neuroepithelial brain tumors its biological behavior is different and it must be differentiated from pilocytic astrocytoma. It can be localized in any region of the CNS and it mostly affects the frontal and temporal lobes. Histopathologically it is the most common fibrillary astrocytoma. There may be nuclear atypias but no mitoses, microvascular proliferations and necroses. Also reported are protoplasmic and gemistocytic variants, of which gemistocytic is more prone to malignization.

**Malign Glial Tumors**

The malign glial tumors are divided into anaplastic gliomas, anaplastic oligodendrogliomas and oligoastrocytomas (mixed gliomas) and glioblastomas. Classification and ranking according to the degree of malignity (grading) is carried out on the basis of the biological nature of the tumor and the grade is specified according to the site with the biggest characteristics of anaplasia. Cell atypia, mitoses, endothelial proliferations and the presence of necrosis are assessed.

The MRI examination displays expansion, sometimes affecting more than one brain lobe. Tumors are characterized by expansive behavior with the shift of midline brain structures, collateral edema, they have inhomogeneous saturation following the administration of the contrast substance, and there are necroses in the center of the tumor in the event of glioblastoma. Histopathologically it is anaplastic astrocytoma of grade III according to the WHO and glioblastoma multiforme (GM) – grade IV. Other types are rare. Based on the localization of the tumor resection or biopsy is performed and it is supplemented by radiotherapy and chemotherapy. The reported average survival rate in astrocytoma of grade III is 1–3 years, in the event of GM about 12 months.

## MENINGEOMAS

Meningeomas represent approximately 20% of all intracranial tumors in adults. The maximum occurrence is in patients of middle age and above with a predominance in women. Multiple meningeomas occur in 8% of cases. They develop from meningothelial cells, cell elements of brain meninges, and they do not grow through the brain tissue but push in the parenchyma as extrinsic tumors. The majority of meningeomas are benign tumors of grade I according to WHO. More aggressive forms also appear – atypical meningeomas of grade II (5–7%) and papillary and anaplastic meningeomas of grade III (1–2.8%).

Anaplastic meningeomas can spread out extracranially. Meningeomas may occur anywhere on the convexity, base, posterior hole and ventricles. The typical locations include olphactory, small wing, parasagitally from falx cerebri and convexity, tuberculi sellae turcicae, tentorium and clivus. The tumor may grow only through contact with the dura mater – globular type, with hyperostosis of the adjacent bone – en plaque, or multicentrically – the so-called menigomatosis – in 90% it is neurofibromatosis type 2.

The treatment of meningeomas is surgical and it is preferred to other treatment modalities. Radicality of the removal of meningioma is classified according to Simpson. In the case of maximal radicality the risk of relapses is up to 10%. The prognosis in the anaplastic variant is completely unfavorable.

## MIDLINE AND INTRAVENTRICULAR TUMORS

Tumors may develop in the ventricle or may sink into the ventricular system as false intraventricular tumors (gliomas, subependymomas). Ependymomas can be found only in lateral ventricles and in the III. ventricle, or they may reach up to the hemisphere without any apparent delimitation.

Benign papilloma of chorioideal plexus of grade I according to WHO and malign cancer of chorioideal plexus of grade III develop from the structures of the chorioideal plexus. Meningeomas occur in ventricles in about 10% of cases and they grow from arachnoid cells of the plexus chorioideus. Intraventricular tumors occur rarely. The first symptoms usually include increased intracranial pressure with obstructive hydrocephalus. The aim of the therapy is removal of the tumor, clearing of liquor paths and temporary or continual ventricular drainage.

### ■ PINEAL REGION TUMORS

The pineal gland is a neuroendocrine organ innervated with sympathetic nerves from the upper cervical ganglion. It produces melatonin and its release from pinealocytes affects the circadian rhythm and mental tuning of the organism; however its exact function remains the subject of research. It is a small formation of 5–10 mm in diameter, sometimes with a cyst, in adult people with calcification. It can be found in the posterior part of the III. ventricle and it is surrounded by a number of structures in this area: quadruplet bodies (tectum), deep venous structures, and ventricular ependyma.

Many tumors of various histological origins develop in this small delimited area. Extrapineal tumors develop from the surrounding neural and mesenchymal structures – astrocytomas, ependymomas, meningeomas, and choroid plexus papillomas. Germinal tumors and pineal parenchymous tumors develop from the pineal gland. Pineal gland tumors occur in 2–8% of cases from the overall number of intracranial tumors. Germinal tumors represent 40–70% of all pineal expansions. Clinical symptoms are mostly caused by hydrocephalus upon the obstruction of the duct and the posterior part of the III. ventricle. Laboratory diagnostics are important to determine tumor markers such as beta-HCG and alpha-fetoprotein in the serum and liquor, both in the primary diagnosis of the tumor and as a symptom of its recurrence.

**Treatment** – histological verification using the stereotactic biopsy, endoscopic approach with ventriculostomy of the III. ventricle, or open surgery, irradiation and chemotherapy as well as irradiation with a gamma knife. Germinal tumors with negative markers have a good prognosis with a survival rate of 80–100%. Tumors with positive markers and pinealoblastomas have a poor prognosis, and the three-year survival is reported to be about 60%. Radical resection is appropriate in benign tumors, such as teratomas, dermoids, choroid plexus papillomas, cystic astrocytomas and meningeomas.

### ■ SELLAR REGION TUMORS

#### Hypophyseal Adenomas

Hypophyseal adenomas represent 10–15% of intracranial tumors in adults and they occur mostly between 30 and 40 years of age, more often in women. They mostly originate in adenohypophysis. The classification of tumors depends on their ability to produce hormones: functional, hormonally active adenomas and afunctional adenomas. According to their size adenomas up to 1 cm are called microadenomas, above 1 cm macroadenomas, and those more than 2.5 cm in diameter gigantic adenomas.

### Afunctional Adenomas
These are bigger and more difficult to diagnose. Symptoms of hypopituitarism develop gradually and the patients often come to the doctor with the symptoms of compression of the visual tract. A late symptom is panhypopituitarism.

Tumors sometimes manifest by a lower prolactin blood level as the so-called pseudoprolactinomas. This is the compression of the pituitary stalk (stalk effect) when the transport of the prolactin-inhibitory factor is reduced. The treatment of afunctional adenomas is surgical and it is focused on the maximum removal of the tumor and release of the visual tract. Radiosurgery may be used in the event of a residuum.

### Functional Adenomas
**Prolactinoma** is the most common type of hormonally active pituitary tumor. In females, it is manifested as the so-called amenorrhea-galactorrhea syndrome, and in males with the reduction of sexual appetence, potency and sometimes with symptoms of expansive behavior. The therapy is almost always pharmacological with the administration of dopamine antagonists (bromocriptine). Surgical treatment is indicated in cases of intolerance of the pharmacological therapy, in the event of low response to the therapy or the progression of visual impairment. Hormonal therapy must continue following the surgery.

**STH producing adenoma** – in young individuals before the closure of epiphyseal plates it causes gigantism, and when the growth is completed the patients with overproduction of STH develop the clinical picture of acromegaly. Besides the increase of acral parts persons with acromegaly are affected by cardiomegalia, hypertension, arthralgias, myopathy and diabetes. A 5-year remission in microadenomas is up to 90% and in macroadenomas it is between 30–60%.

**ACTH producing adenoma** – Cushing disease – increased secretion of cortisol by the suprarenal cortex of a central origin that causes typical disproportional obesity with a moon face, striae, osteoporosis, hypertension, and reduced glucose tolerance. The MRI examination shows microadenoma in 75% of cases. The treatment is surgical with the maximum effort to preserve the healthy pituitary tissue.

It is necessary to determine the origin of Cushing's syndrome – in about 70% of cases it is the typical Cushing disease with a pituitary adenoma. Hypercorticolism also occurs as paraneoplastic in lung cancer, ovarian cancer, breast or pancreatic cancer or in adenoma or adrenal cortex cancer. In the event adrenal cortex is removed in a patient with pituitary adenoma then the so-called Nelson syndrome develops with hyperpigmentation of the skin and the risk of tumor malignization.

## Craniopharyngioma
Craniopharyngioma occurs in 2.5–4% of CNS tumors and in about 20% of suprasellar region tumors in adults. It is a benign epithelial tumor of grade I according to WHO that develops from ectoblastic remains of Rathke's pouch (ductus nasopharyngicus). In adults it can develop from metaplastic cells.

There are two distinct clinical-pathological forms recognized – adamantinomatous and papillary craniopharyngioma. In the adamantinomatous type the MRI examination shows a solid tumor that is saturated inhomogenously after the administration of a contrast substance, and a CT scan shows calcifications. Papillary craniopharyngioma occurs more in adults, and CT and MRI examinations show that it is more homogenous and without calcifications.

The treatment of craniopharyngiomas is one of the most difficult neurosurgical procedures. A radical excision is often difficult and it is associated with high morbidity involving especially endocrinological deficits. Therefore, a subtotal removal with the minimization of postoperative complications is recommended with additional radiotherapy. In our experience macroscopically radically removed tumors with repeatedly negative MRI examinations may also reoccur. Another therapeutic possibility is the intracystic application of radioisotopes – intracavital brachytherapy. Similarly, the intracystic application of bleomycin is used in limited series. Perioperative mortality is relatively high (2–10%), with a higher risk in re-operations. Recidives are reported in up to 20%. A 10-year progression free survival rate is between 50–80% and a 10-year survival rate between 79–93%.

### Visual Tract Tumors

75% of visual tract gliomas affect patients under 10 years of age, exceptionally adults. It is a heterogeneous group of gliomas which may affect the visual tract behind the eyeball (optic nerve glioma), chiasma (chiasmatic glioma) and optic tracts, hypothalamus up to corpora geniculata (optochiasmatic-hypothalamic gliomas – OCHG). Optic nerve gliomas are astrocytomas of a low grade (the WHO grade I), while chiasmatic and hypothalamic gliomas may be more aggressive.

### 23.9.2  Infratentorial Tumors

■ PONTOCEREBELLAR ANGLE TUMORS

**Vestibular schwannoma** (acoustic neuroma) represent approximately 10% of intracranial tumors in adults and it is the most common tumor in the pontocerebellar angle (80%). The tumor grows from the upper vestibular nerve from the Obersteiner-Redlich zone at the site of the junction of the central and peripheral myelin, in the internal auditory passage. It is more common in females with a maximum incidence between the 4$^{th}$ and 5$^{th}$ decade. Clinical symptoms depend on the size of the tumor. Smaller tumors are associated with unilateral hearing loss, tinnitus, disturbed sense of balance without rotational vertigo. The symptoms of large tumors include compression of the cerebellum, lateral mixed system and mainly the brain stem. Four tumor sizes are distinguished – from purely intracanalicular (type 1) to tumors with brain stem compression (type 4) over 3 cm in size. Small tumors without any signs of growth can be followed up with regular MRI check-ups. The only therapeutic approach in large tumors with brain stem compression is their microsurgical excision. In smaller tumors we can decide for irradiation using stereotactic radiosurgery but small schwannomas are the easiest for surgical treatment and their removal leads to permanent recovery. The maximal removal of the tumor with the preservation of the facial nerve function is important.

## CEREBELLAR TUMORS

**Pilocystic astrocytoma** – a benign tumor of grade I according to WHO which occurs mostly in children younger than 10 years of age. In adults it is rare, and occurs usually only in young patients.

The tumor is well delimited, and the typical MRI finding is a cystic tumor with a solid tumor nodule in the wall, it can replace a major part of the cerebellar hemisphere, and sometimes it is polycystic. After the administration of a contrast substance the solid part of the tumor is saturated, the wall of the cyst is saturated only if it contains tumor tissue.

**Malign gliomas** of the cerebellum are rare, anaplastic astrocytomas occur only in 3–5%, and glioblastomas in 1–2%. Oncological therapy follows after a macroscopic radical removal, in the event of a residual tumor the mean survival time is reported to be about 8 months.

**Cerebellar hemangioblastoma** – a benign tumor of grade I according to WHO, of unclear histogenesis. It occurs as a sporadic tumor with rare autosomally dominant affection with high penetration – von Hippel-Lindau disease (capillary hemangioma of the retina, renal and pancreatic cysts, feochromocytoma, carcinoma).

A cerebellar expansion is formed by the cyst with a mural nodule that is markedly saturated after the administration of a contrast substance during the CT or MRI examinations and in the arterial phase during angiography.

The disease is more often diagnosed after the 20th year of age. It has been proved that the risk of incidence occurs in 50% of children of affected patients. Therefore, a detailed screening is needed of affected families. The surgery is associated with minimum risk. Removal of the capillary hemangioma prevents potential bleeding, and radiotherapy or radiosurgery are recommended in recidives in adults, not in children.

**Ependymoma** is a type of tumor that develops from ependymal cells in the wall of the IV. ventricle. Histological classification corresponds to grade II according to WHO. Although it is histopathologially classified under benign tumors, it belongs to the worst curable tumor affections. Radical resection of the tumor is often associated with significant morbidity with a view to the tumor extension. The tumor grows most often from the obex, it fills the dilated IV. ventricle as a cast, spreads out into lateral recesses and often grows into the pontocerebellar angle and overgrows the cranial nerves.

**Anaplastic ependymoma** or malign ependymoma of grade III according to WHO (it has to be differentiated from ependymoblastoma that belongs to embryonal tumors) represents only 7% of ependymomas. Its growth is faster and the histopathological finding shows an increased cellularity and vascular proliferation and mitotic activity.

**Meduloblastoma** – (WHO grade IV) is a highly malign invasive embryonal tumor in children with an incidence of 0.5 per 100,000 children younger than 15 years. It is the most common malign solid tumor in children and represents up to 30% of expansive processes in the posterior hole, and up to 10% of solid tumors of the CNS in children. They can be found in boys between 5 and 8 years of age. In adults it occurs between the 20$^{th}$ and 40$^{th}$ years of age, and later quite exceptionally. In contrast to children it affects more often cerebellar hemispheres. An MRI can display it as isotense or hypotense expansions in a T1-weighted image that is saturated after the administration of a contrast substance.

## BRAIN-STEM TUMORS

For quite a long period of time these tumors were considered as inoperable; MRI examination has made it possible to differentiate stem tumors into subtypes which are appropriate for surgical solution, and those that are inoperable. Out of the total number of tumors of the central nervous system of adults they occur in about 2% of patients. According to the MRI picture they are classified to diffusional, focal, exophytic and cervicomedullary.

**Diffusional tumors** of the brain stem are mostly fibrillary astrocytomas which spread out in the region of the medulla oblongata, pons and cranially to the diencephalon. Histopathologically it is a heterogeneous group of tumors of grade II to IV according to WHO. From the prognostic viewpoint they are the least favorable group with a short period of survival. They are not operable and some departments carry out a biopsy only in order to exactly classify it into the therapeutic protocol.

**Focal tumors** may occur in various parts of the brain stem and their neurological symptoms correspond to their location. Obstructive hydrocephalus are common, impairment of the cranial nerves and lateral mixed system, with or without pyramidal tract affection. Histopathologically they include completely benign up to malign tumors of WHO classification IV. They may be solid or with a cyst. The surgical approach is decided based on the least risk of the neurological affection, in cystic lesions through the wall of the cyst.

**Exophytic tumors** of the brain stem are mostly benign expansions with slow growth, mostly dorsally exophytic with the expansion into the IV. ventricle, or growing laterally from the stem, with the MRI picture in the pontocerebellar angle tumors. They may penetrate only under the ependyma of the IV. ventricle or, as intrinsic tumors with exophytic parts, they can reach with their bigger part to the brain stem.

**Cervicomedullary tumors** have the best prognosis from all brain stem tumors and they are appropriate for neurosurgical treatment. Surgery is indicated before the development of focal neurological symptoms. Peroperative neuromonitoring and stimulation of the brain stem structures are prerequisites for the brain stem surgeries and enable targeted selection of the surgical approach to the tumor and monitoring of the brain stem functions during excision.

## 23.9.3 Intraspinal Tumors and Spinal Cord Tumors

### INTRADURAL TUMORS

#### Intramedullary Tumors

These tumors represent about 20% of the intraspinal processes in adults. Clinical symptoms depend on the size and location of the tumor with benign lesions lasting from several weeks to several years. The location is mostly in the upper thoracic and cervical spinal cord. Mostly observed are gait problems, local pain, kyphoscoliosis, impairment of sensation and urination problems. An X-ray examination of the spine typically detects extension of the spinal canal at the level of several vertebral bodies with erosions or displacement of pedicles. The MRI examination is an excellent method to diagnose intramedullary expansions and it can display a solid part of the tumor and cysts which do not have to be of a tumor character and are located below and above the solid part of the tumor. Based on the extent of the tumor we distinguish three types. The focal tumor affects a small part of the spinal tissue, the elongated tumor affects several levels, and the type that affects the whole spinal cord is the holocord tumor.

Histologically astrocytomas, gangliogliomas and ependymomas occur most often (70%). Ependymomas are always well delimited and their radical removal is easier compared to astrocytomas which may grow infiltratively in the upper or lower tumor pole. The procedure must be performed with pre-operative neuromonitoring. Morbidity is relatively high, especially in glial tumors. Pareses of different grades occur in approximately 1/3 of patients following surgery, and the risk factor is the severity of a neurological affection before the surgery. Most surgeries in the spinal canal are performed from the osteoplastic laminotomy, removed arches are fixed at the end of the surgery and the interspinal ligamentum is reconstructed.

#### Extramedullary Tumors

**Benign tumors** include meningeomas and tumors from nerve sheaths occur – schwannomas and neurofibromas. Symptoms develop slowly – in months and sometimes in years. They are manifested mostly by pain – local or radicular irradiation and weakness of the lower limbs. After removal of the tumor the picture of paresis is recovered. The tumor that grows from the root may spread out through foramina even extracelullary and create a picture of sandglass.

**Malign tumors** are mostly the symptom of dissemination of the intracranial malign process, and they are more common in children. Metastases may occur in medulloblastoma, malign ependymoma, germinal tumors, and primitive neuroectodermal tumors. A delimited focus is indicated for surgery. Diffusional subarachnoid (leptomeningeal) processes are inoperable and their prognosis is poor.

### EXTRADURAL TUMORS

Most often these are metastases. The development of symptoms is often dramatic; paresis to plegia of the lower limbs and impairment of sphincters may develop within several hours to days. In quickly developed weak plegia of the lower limbs the neurological finding persists even after decompression, the spinal lesion is partly caused also by ischemia due to compression of the spinal arteries. Lung, breast, kidney and prostate cancers create metastases most often. Malign tumors from vertebral bodies and soft tissues occur locally, and rarely the primary or metastatic non-Hodgkin lymphoma also appears. The aim of the surgery in extradural tumors is the decompression of the spinal cord and the reduction of the tumor. The up-to-date instrumental technology enables extensive surgical procedures with removal of vertebral bodies at several levels and their replacement with implants and stabilization using splint fixations.

## 23.10 Surgical Treatment of Epilepsy

### TYPES OF SURGICAL PROCEDURES

Epileptosurgical procedures are divided based on the types of epilepsy, demonstrated structural changes of the brain, extent of the procedure and the method used. Surgeries are generally divided into causal and palliative. The causal procedures include resections of the epileptic focus, e.g. anteromedial temporal resection, amygdalohippocampectomy, resection of low-grade gliomas, cavernomas, hamartomas, extratemporal resection due to cortical dysplasia, etc. The purpose of palliative procedures is to interrupt connections which are significant for spreading seizures. The surgical result in the palliative procedures is less satisfactory.

Epileptic surgeries are divided to resection, non-resection, disconnection and stimulation procedures. In resections the principle of surgery is the removal of the epileptogenic focus, the non-resection procedures include disconnection procedures of a callosotomy type, multiple subpial transactions and vagus nerve stimulation. According to the extent of the resection the procedures can be divided into precisely individually targeted (tailored) lesionectomies (e.g. partial frontal resection), and to standard procedures with the removal of a larger part of the brain lobe (mostly epileptosurgrical procedures – anteromedial temporal resections).

### 23.10.1 Anteromedial Temporal Resections

Removal of the anterior part of the temporal lobe is the most common epileptosurgrical procedure with the best post-operative results. The surgery consists in subpial preparation along with a Sylvian fissure, along with the upper edge of the upper temporal gyrus with the opening of the temporal angle of the lateral ventricle.

Following the identification of the mesial structures the anterior part of the temporal lobe should be removed together with the amygdalohippocampal complex. The procedure is technically relatively difficult compared to the two-phase surgery when the anterior part of the temporal lobe is removed first and then the mesial structures are separately removed.

Another possibility is an individually different extent of resection of the temporal lobe based on peroperative electrocorticography (ECoG). In the so called "awake craniotomy" – awaking the patient from the general anesthesia during the procedure – the extent of resection is decided during the surgery following the cortical stimulation. The aim of the procedure is to save as much of the eloquent areas as possible. This procedure is therefore appropriate only for well co-operating patients with affection of the dominant temporal lobe.

### 23.10.2 Extratemporal Resection

In adults the complete resection of the frontal, parietal or occipital lobe is performed only rarely. Most of the procedures are targeted to a partial cortical resection with precise determination of the epileptogenic focus based on the ECoG.

The surgeries are performed at one time in the case of consistent findings in the pre-operative examinations. The peroperative corticography, examination of somatosensory evoked potentials (SEP, i.e. determination of the so called "phase reversion"), and cortical stimulation with functional mapping of eloquent cortical regions are a significant benefit for minimization of the post-operative neurological deficit. Triggering of a seizure upon peroperative cortical stimulation is not desirable and it has no predicative value for the post-operative result. Two-phase surgeries are performed when it is necessary to record the exact stroke findings and the functional cortical mapping must be carried out by means of preoperative stimulation. 50–70% of patients undergoing extratemporal resections are seizure-free, and depending on the type and location of the brain pathology auras may persist in some of the patients. The complications include sensory-motor deficits, mostly reversible, and dropouts in a visual field in occipital resections.

### 23.10.3 Stimulation of the Vagus Nerve

Stimulation of the vagus nerve is today the most common palliative procedure in epileptic surgery. In patients for whom the resection procedure is not appropriate (no epileptic focus defined, the eloquent cortex cannot be resected, failure of previous resections) the implantation is possible of a vagus nerve stimulation. The generator is placed in the supraclavicular region and a subcutaneously inserted electrode is fixed by the spiral ends to the left vagus nerve. The generator provides adjustable electrical stimuli which may affect frequency and strength of the seizures via the brain nuclei, reticular formation and cortex.

# 24 MODERN TECHNIQUES OF CUTTING, DISSECTION, COAGULATION, HEMOSTASIS, SUTURE AND TISSUE ADHESION, VISCEROSYNTHESIS

The basic surgical techniques are cutting and suture of organs and tissues, and hemostasis. Cuts are performed with a scalpel and scissors, sutures are carried out with various techniques and sewing material, hemostasis is achieved by ligation of vessels or by punctures to the sites of bleeding. Besides standard surgical tools, other techniques and technologies are also commonly used to improve the mentioned procedures or reduce blood loss, the extent of damage of the surrounding tissues, the risk of bleeding or failure of sutures or anastomoses or to replace them; other technologies enable changing the performance or concept of the surgery – e.g. stapling of hemorrhoids.

**Electrosurgical (electrocoagulation) units** are used to cut tissues and perform coagulation to achieve hemostasis. The effect is achieved by means of coagulation necrosis caused by releasing Joule heating originating when the electric current passes through the conductor with high resistance, in this case tissue. The units consist of a high-frequency modulated current generator, a working tool and connection (or grounding) cables and have various outputs. Combinations of regimens allow changing the modulations according to the needs of the surgeon, and even a cut with immediate hemostasis is possible (e.g. Force Triad generator, "Valleylab cut" regimen). According to the electric current passing through the tissue they are classified as monopolar and bipolar. To stop the areal bleeding some units have a "spray" regimen, modern units are equipped with automatic suction of surgical smoke.

**Argon-plasma coagulation (APC)** is a monopolar high-frequency technology enabling coagulation and hemostasis through a high temperature plasma beam. It is used in surgery and endoscopy; in endoscopy also for the destruction or recanalization of tumors or other tissue, especially mucous lesions.

**Harmonic (ultrasound) scalpel** (ultracision harmonic scalpel system) uses the energy of the ultrasound frequency. It is used for "hemostatic" cutting, i.e. cutting of soft tissues without hemorrhage. It enables more accurate dissection and coagulation with minimal tissue destruction around the cutting line and with minimal thermal damage of the surrounding tissue, including its desiccation. The basic tools are knives and scissors. The dissected tissue is held by the tool, and the vibrating part of the tool coagulates the tissue and then cuts it.

**LigaSure™** is a permanent vessel sealing system enables fast and hemostatic dissection of tissues, including closure of vessels of 5–7 mm in diameter.

The above-mentioned techniques speed up the procedures, reduce blood loss, limit or avoid ligatures and because of the amount of the suture material left in the tissues they can be used for hemostasis of blood as well as lymphatic vessels which would otherwise be neglected. Consideration should also be given to the concomitant phenomena of which the most important is the aerosol produced during surgery which may contain viable microbial or tumor particles.

**Ultrasound dissector** (CUSA, Sonoca) is a supplementary tool that enables selective tissue removal. Besides tissue cutting it irrigates the cut region and drains out the released tissue. The energy transmitted by the ultrasound vibration probe causes cavitation of the tissue depending on the tissue structure; the dissection is tissue selective. Sutures in vessels, biliary ducts or nerves remain intact during the dissection, and other tissues – liver parenchyma or tumors – are selectively destructed and drained out.

**Tissue adhesives and hemostatics** are used to improve hemostasis or even to stop bleeding, especially areal bleeding, to seal or support sutures and anastomoses in gastrointestinal, thoracic and cardiovascular surgery, neurosurgery, or transplant surgery. They can be used in various levels of hemostasis, or production of coagulum. According to the active substance adhesives are classified as natural or synthetic, and according to the composition as unicomponent or combined. These include:
- Gelatin sponge based (e.g. Spongostan)
- Oxidized cellulose (e.g. Surgicel, Traumacel)
- Bone waxes
- Multicomponent adhesives containing fibrin, thrombin and collagen (e.g. Tachosil, Tachocomb, Tissucol)
- Cyanoacrylate adhesives (e.g. Histoacryl)

Adhesives are administered in the form of a solution that precipitates and after some time is absorbed, or as sponges or knitted fabric that are applied on the treated site or cover the site, e.g. anastomosis or the resection or suture line. With a few exceptions these tools are used as supplementary, i.e. for safety reasons after treatment. One of the exceptions is Tissucol which is used to treat defects of liver parenchyma of various origins separately without suture or other mechanical treatments.

**Staplers** are another routine part of current surgical equipment. Except for some cases – e.g. skin stapler for closure of skin wounds – they enable the performance of anastomosis using clamps (viscerosynthesis) or closure of the resection line, but also interruption of the resected organ or making the anastomosis patent by cutting the opening. According to shape they are classified as linear and circular, and they differ in shape and in the method of suture. Insertion of sutures/anastomosis in the gastrointestinal tract by a linear stapler is performed outside the organ, and by a circular (endoluminal) stapler inside it. After healing when no mechanical support is needed to maintain integrity of the anastomosis/suture some clamps are eliminated **per vias naturales**, while the others remain intact *in situ* without any effect on the anastomosis. To avoid a potential risk of leaving the claps staplers are available with biologically degradable clamps. The staplers are further divided according to surgical fields and organs and expected method of use – for open and mini-invasive surgery.

**Special staplers** are for one purpose only, i.e. hemorrhoidal and prolapse staplers (for surgery according to Long) or rectocele surgery staplers.

Special tools for endoluminal intestinal anastomosis are the compressive endoluminal rings (e.g. BAR – biodegradable anastomotic rings). By means of compression they keep the ends of the anastomosis together during healing and then they are eliminated.

Among the less commonly used tools and devices we should mention anoscope for **DGHAL** "Doppler-guided hemorrhoidal artery ligation" that enables identification of hemorrhoidal arteries by means of ultrasound and ligation of them separately, and the **Buess surgical rectoscope** for endoluminal surgery of the anus.

**Retractors** of various constructions are used to maintain the wound approach and the space in the surgical field, to improve the view and save physical effort.

In abdominal surgery a special role is played by **anti-adhesives** which are expected to reduce or avoid adhesions. Without comparable results irrigations are used routinely, sometimes with the addition of corticoids or hyaluronidase. The demonstrable effect is that of two brands of products: foil which is placed into the abdomen at the end of the surgery and releases hyaluronidase that supports proadhesive activity of mesothel (Seprafilm), and polysaccharide solution which reduces adhesivity and adherence of the organ serous membranes following surgery (Adept).

To treat septic complications we currently use two methods using the suction principle. The first method **VAC** (vacuum assisted closure) consists in the application of a porous material – a sponge with defined porosity – into the wound that is covered by an impermeable foil and connected to a device that maintains stable pressure. The second method is the therapy of anastomotic complications following rectal surgeries when a drain with a sponge is inserted in the defect and connected to the suction system (EndoSponge).

# 25 ORGAN TRANSPLANTATION

> 25.1 Introduction
> 25.2 Issues of Organ Donation – Multi Organ Harvesting
> 25.3 Kidney Transplantation
> 25.4 Liver Transplantation
> 25.5 Heart Transplantation
> 25.6 Lung Transplantation
> 25.7 Pancreas Transplantation
> 25.8 Intestinal Transplantation and Multi Organ Transplantation
> 25.9 Immunosuppression and Complications of Organ Transplantation
> 25.10 Future of Organ Transplantation

## 25.1 Introduction

Transplantology is a very young medical discipline. A successful kidney transplantation experiment was performed in 1902 and Alexis Carrel was awarded the Nobel Prize in 1911 for successful short-term experiments with kidney, heart and intestinal transplantations and for tissue cultures. The immunological mechanism of the reaction of an organism to "alien" tissue was gradually discovered after World War II. It was also revealed that immunological problems are not present between monozygotic twins; this enabled the first successful kidney transplantation from a living donor to his brother, a monozygotic twin with chronic renal failure (Joseph Murray and Hartwell Harrison, Boston, USA) in 1954. This team carried out another 7 kidney transplantations from living donors (some grafts were functioning for more than 30 years!).

### BASIC TYPES OF TRANSPLANTATION

Theoretically, it is possible to transplant organs of different origin. In **xenotransplantation** a graft from other animal species is transplanted. **Allotransplantation** is a graft transplant from the same animal species – and that is what this chapter is dedicated to. In certain situations **autotransplantation** is carried out, i.e. transplantation of one's own organ – for example kidney autotransplantation after treatment of pathology (complicated pyelolithiasis, renal hypertension due

TEXTBOOK OF SURGERY

to peripheral arterial stenoses of renal artery branches in hilus), or autotransplantation of a pulmonary valve and trunk into the aortal position in the Ross procedure in cardiac surgery.

## POSITION OF TRANSPLANTOLOGY IN TODAY'S MEDICINE

In the past fifty years, transplantology has gradually developed and created conditions that have permitted organ transplantations to become a routine therapeutic method. Transplant activities are well analyzed statistically worldwide and the outcomes confirm that it is an effective and economically favorable multidisciplinary field.

In the Czech Republic **transplantology** is undoubtedly part of undergraduate medical education. As of 31 December 2008, there were 5,380 registered living transplanted patients (3,687 after kidney transplant, 750 after liver transplant, 583 after heart transplant, 61 after lung transplant and 199 after pancreas transplant). Therefore transplanted patients constitute a subpopulation that will be commonly met by all medical university graduates that will practice clinical medicine or general practice. Hence **transplant surgery** has become a specific sub-specialization even in the Czech Republic.

## ORGAN COLLECTION, ISCHEMIA AND PRESERVATION

Collection of organs as well as their transplantation is a demanding surgical procedure that must be performed flawlessly within a certain time limit, which is different for individual organs (Tab. 25.1).

The collection of the organ must preserve its function. This means not only to retain important anatomical structures but also to preserve the quality of cells and tissues on the molecular level. Cell metabolic systems are destroyed by **warm ischemia** – the period when the organ is without perfusion of oxygenated blood, and uncooled. In such a situation the mitochondrial enzymes promptly exhaust stocks of high-energy phosphates, suffer from anaerobic metabolism, final meta-

■ **Table 25.1** Tolerated cold ischemia time for transplanted organs*)

| Organ | Tolerated cold ischemia time |
| --- | --- |
| Heart | Up to 4–5 h |
| Lungs | Up to 5–6 h |
| Small intestine | Up to 12 h |
| Pancreas | Up to 16 h |
| Liver | Up to 12–18 h |
| Kidneys | Up to 36–48 h |

*) *generally reported values – some departments have more strict or more liberal limits*

bolic products accumulate resulting in cell death within 30–60 minutes (depending on the type of tissue). Therefore, during the collection of an organ it is imperative to shorten the warm ischemia to a minimum or to avoid it by an early irrigation with a cool (approx. 4 °C) perfusion solution. The period from the organ cooling to the restored circulation in the recipient's body is called **cold ischemia**.

**Organ preservation** is started during organ collection. It is a fundamental process that enables organ transport from the donor's hospital to transplantation departments (even long distances of hundreds and thousands of kilometers) and provides time for the preparation and performance of transplantation of the collected organs.

Organs are routinely preserved by the **method of simple hypothermic preservation.** During the collection they are irrigated with a perfusion solution and until the transplantation they are protected mainly by cold (kept in sterile wrapping in the remaining perfusion solution), kept in polystyrene containers on crushed ice with temperatures just above 0 °C; however, they must not freeze. The tolerated period of cold ischemia can be prolonged and the quality of collected organs can be increased by **preservation with continuous perfusion** in special transport machines.

The composition of current commercially available perfusion solutions is complex (electrolytes, osmotically active substances, colloids, substances protecting against active forms of oxygen, energetic precursors). They represent several decades of basic research , resulting in prolongation of tolerated limits of cold ischemia up to the values mentioned above.

## TRANSPLANT COORDINATION

Respecting the tolerated cold ischemia requires **logistic management** that is **administered by transplant centers (TCs)**. The TCs collaborate on collection and transplantation of cadaveric organs at a national or international level.

Table 25.1 shows why the kidney was the first organ successfully transplanted both in an experiment and in clinical practice and why kidney transplantation from cadaveric donors could have become a program in developed countries. In former Czechoslovakia, the renal transplant program was formed at a national level in the 1970s. At that time a network of regional TCs was established (IKEM – Institute of Clinical and Experimental Medicine / Institut klinické a experimentální medicíny Praha, Plzeň, Hradec Králové, Brno, Olomouc, Bratislava, Banská Bystrica and Košice, then in the 1990s also University Hospital Motol, Praha and Ostrava). Coordination within the republic (mainly organ allocation) is in the hands of the biggest TC, IKEM Praha, which, subsequently, became even an international coordinating center for the member countries of the COMECON (Council for Mutual Economic Assistance) within the scope of the Intertransplant program (only Czechoslovakia, Hungary and former East Germany were really effectively collaborating). All this was possible due to sufficiently long periods of tolerated cold ischemia.

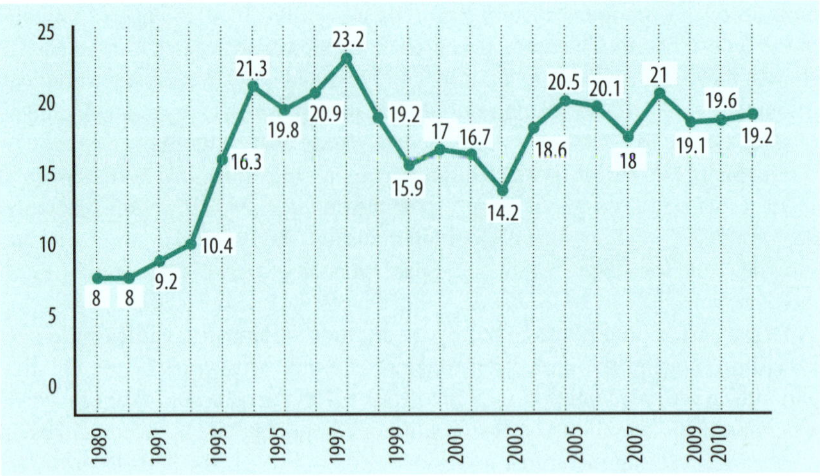

**Fig. 25.1** *Number of cadaveric organ donors in the Czech Republic – related to population of 1 million people (statistics of the Coordinating transplant centre/Koordinační středisko tansplantací)*

Transplantations of other extrarenal organs were gradually introduced utilizing the current network of mutually cooperating regional TCs. However, extrarenal transplantations did not become a program until the 1990s when the (personal and technical) facilities of the TCs and the available communication and transport infrastructure in the country permitted coping regularly with the **distant collection of organs** and their transplantation within the limits of tolerated cold ischemia.

The Czech transplant program currently generates about 20 cadaveric donors per 1 million persons per year, multi organ donors comprising more than a half of them. Fig. 25.1 depicts the collection activity in the Czech Republic in recent years. The graph clearly demonstrates the efficiency of the coordination. In the early 1990s, a permanent emergency duty of a transplant coordinator equipped with a mobile phone was introduced to all centers. With this measure the number of organ donations virtually doubled. Fig. 25.2 shows the outcome of the Czech transplant program in 2009.

The Czech Republic is one of the countries with a modern approach to legislation related to collection and transplantation of organs and tissues – cf. Act on the Donation, Collection and Transplantation of Tissues and Organs, No. 285/2002 Coll. as amended (referred to as the Transplant Act) and the Act on Human Cells and Tissues, No 296/2008 Coll. (as amended).

In compliance with the Transplant Act, an independent **Coordinating Transplant Centre (Koordinační středisko tansplantací – KST)** was established in 2003. It is a transparent and independent institution directed by the Ministry of

ORGAN TRANSPLANTATION

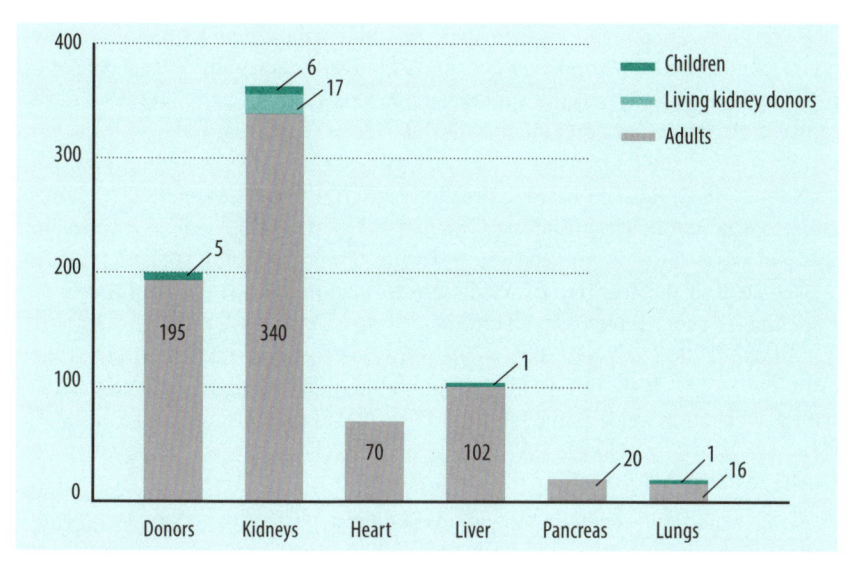

**Fig. 25.2** *Number of transplantations and organ collections in the Czech Republic in 2010 (statistics of Coordinating transplant centre/Koordinační středisko tansplantací)*

Health of the Czech Republic. The mission of KST is to provide and coordinate transplantations in compliance with the knowledge of modern medicine, ethics and law. The purpose of the activity of the KST team is to contribute, to the maximum extent, to the quality of life of a patient to be improved or their life to be preserved. One of the major tasks is the **administration of waiting lists** (WL) **for individual organs** and realization of **organ allocation** according to the rules that were prepared and have been updated **in cooperation with specialists from the Czech Transplant Society (Česká transplantační společnost – ČTS)**. Medical and ethical criteria are respected. **Compatibility of blood groups** (AB0 system) between the donor and recipient **is respected** in the transplantation of all organs. The limit of tolerated cold ischemia **for kidneys** permits this organ to respect even the **compatibility of HLA antigens** between the donor and recipient that are the most significant factor for immunological reaction of the recipient to the tissue of the transplanted organ.

## 25.2 Issues of Organ Donation – Multi Organ Harvesting

**The poor availability of donors represents a limiting factor for the number of organ transplantations.** Donors can be living persons (usually relatives) or deceased people, i.e. cadaveric donors.

Regarding organ donations from deceased adults, the Czech legislation is based on the philosophy of "supposed consent". On the contrary, the organ collection from a deceased child must be approved by his/her parents or legal representative. Those who are not in agreement with the supposed consent have the option to apply for being included into the national register of persons not consenting with a posthumous organ and tissue collection (NROD) that, as stipulated by law, is administered by the Coordinating Center for Departmental Medical Information Systems (Koordinační středisko pro resortní zdravotnické informační systémy) – (Registers of the Institute of Medical Information and Statistics of the Czech Republic – Ústav zdravotnických informací a statistiky ČR – ÚZIS ČR). The registration can be done on-line (https://snzr.ksrzis.cz/snzr/rod/index.html), in person or by means of a legal representative (in children and legally incapable persons) with a declaration made in the presence of an attending physician and a witness.

### ■ LIVING DONORS

A living donor can donate a pair organs (kidneys) or part of an organ, typically part of the liver, lung lobe or part of the small intestine. Most often, living donors donate a kidney or a part of an organ to their direct relative (for example a parent to a child), less often to a personally close person (e.g. donation between husband and wife) but especially outside the Czech Republic, organs are collected for transplant purposes even from unrelated living donors (so-called altruistic donors). This type of donation is unequivocally controlled by legislation and it is mandatory to exclude any pressure on a potential living donor and commercial background.

In the majority of developed countries including the Czech Republic the main source of organs for transplant purposes are cadaveric donors – with functioning circulation or after circulation arrest. Both these alternatives are included and specified in the Czech Republic's Transplant Act. The crucial issue is the definition of death, its diagnostics and confirmation.

### ■ CADAVERIC DONORS

Cadaveric "**heart-beating donors**" (HBD) are deceased persons – originally on mechanical ventilation – who were diagnosed with brain death, however, whose circulation is working (usually with inotropic support) and parenchymatous organs (or at least some of them) are therefore functioning.

Death of such a donor is clinically diagnosed by the attending physician. If an organ collection for transplant purposes is considered, it is stipulated by law that death be confirmed by clinical examination (and recorded in medical files) by two adequately qualified specialists in a mutually independent manner. In deceased adults this examination is repeated after at least 4 hours (in children under 1 year of age after 48 hours). If both committees unequivocally confirm the death of the patient, then the Czech legislation requires proof of brain death by one instrumental diagnostic method that objectively documents the absent perfusion of brain tissue. A brain angiography, brain perfusion scintigraphy and in children under 1 year also transcranial Doppler ultrasound can be used. In deceased persons with an open cranial trauma or after craniotomy brain death can be confirmed by the examination of brainstem auditory evoked potentials. It is mandatory to record the examinations performed, into a form "Protocol of the evidence of death", which forms an appendix to the Transplant Act.

Cadaverous **"non-heart-beating donors"** (NHBD) are deceased people whose death was caused by refractory circulation and respiratory arrest where circulation could not be restored after 30 minutes of adequate cardiopulmonary resuscitation. That is, it is a "death of the heart". These donors can then be used for collection of organs for transplant purposes. The most commonly used organs from these donors are kidneys, but there are centers using liver or lungs collected this way.

Members of the transplant team must not participate in the treatment of potential organ donors or in the diagnostics of brain death.

### PREPARATION FOR MULTI ORGAN HARVESTING

After confirmation of brain death or heart death the potential donor still requires intensive care that, however, should not be called "treatment" (a dead person cannot be treated). Exactly speaking, **measures for preservation of organ viability** are performed. The aim is to get, collect and use as many organs or tissues for transplant purposes as possible – to perform **multi organ harvesting** (MOH).

In the majority of cases, donor identification, the care thereof, diagnostics of brain death and organ collection (at best MOH and tissue collection) are carried out in the donor's hospital. **It is stipulated by law that every hospital has the duty of reporting potential donors of organs or tissues to the regional TC.** The transplant coordinator of the regional TC then provides logistic support to the whole action. He/she informs the Coordinating Transplant Center about the prepared collection and KTS immediately arranges the allocation of extrarenal organs. According to this allocation, collection of the extrarenal organs is performed by the arriving teams that will later transplant these organs (thus, respecting the limit of cold ischemia is the sole responsibility of the collecting and transplanting teams). Kidney allocation is performed last, after an HLA typization of the donor (from lymph nodes and spleen collected during the MOH).

### 25.2.1 Techniques of Multi Organ Harvesting

The core of multi organ harvesting is the collection of all usable organs avoiding their warm ischemia. The anesthesiologist continues to maintain optimum ventilation and stable circulation, i.e. the most physiological perfusion of the collected organs. This is an extensive procedure performed in three phases: preparation, organ perfusion, and explantation.

## 1. Preparation

The standard approach of surgical preparation is the incision from jugulum to symphysis (i.e. median sternotomy together with median laparotomy) which provides access to all organs in the abdominal and thoracic cavities. It is mandatory for the collecting surgeon to inspect the thoracic and abdominal cavities (he/she opens the pericardium and both pleural cavities, inspects the digestive tube in all its length, large vessels and retroperitoneum by palpation), to assess the quality of the collected organs and to describe all pathological changes, since the report on the collection constitutes an appendix to the autopsy report on the mandatory autopsy of the donor. If no contraindication for MOH (for example malignancy) has been revealed, the process continues with the preparation of basic anatomic structures. First the ascending colon and mesenteric trunk are unfastened. This, together with an extended Kocher maneuver (unfastening and removing duodenum and pancreas to the left side), results in wide access to retroperitoneum where the abdominal aorta and inferior vena cava are prepared. Vessels are ligated in tissues and organs that will not be perfused – irrigated (inferior mesenteric artery, splenic artery, superior mesenteric artery, iliac artery). A perfusion cannula is inserted into the abdominal aorta above its bifurcation (for the simultaneous irrigation of the block of kidneys, pancreas and liver) and another wider cannula is inserted into the inferior vena cava for the future drainage of the donor's warm blood out of the body to cool the collected organs faster.

The liver team mobilizes the liver dissecting its suspensory ligaments and prepares the structures in hepatoduodenal ligament – bile duct, hepatic artery and portal vein. Perfusion cannulas are inserted into ascending aorta and trunk of the pulmonary artery. Superior and inferior vena cava and all pulmonary veins are isolated.

## 2. Perfusion

After administration of heparin, the liver team usually cannulates the portal vein, the abdominal aorta is closed with a clamp above the branching of the celiac trunk and perfusion of the block of abdominal organs is started immediately. While the abdominal organs are irrigated, the chest team initiates isolated heart and lung perfusion.

During the perfusion the irrigated abdominal and chest organs are at the same time immediately externally cooled with sterile crushed ice and the donor's warm blood is drained by gravity via the cannula in the inferior vena cava out of the donor's body. This method of MOH is ideal for the preservation of collected organs and the data "warm ischemia 0 minutes" is recorded into the protocol (Fig. 25.3 and Fig. 25.4). The organ perfusion concludes the role of anesthesiologists who accompanied the donor from the identification, through the indication assessment, diagnosis of brain death up to MOH.

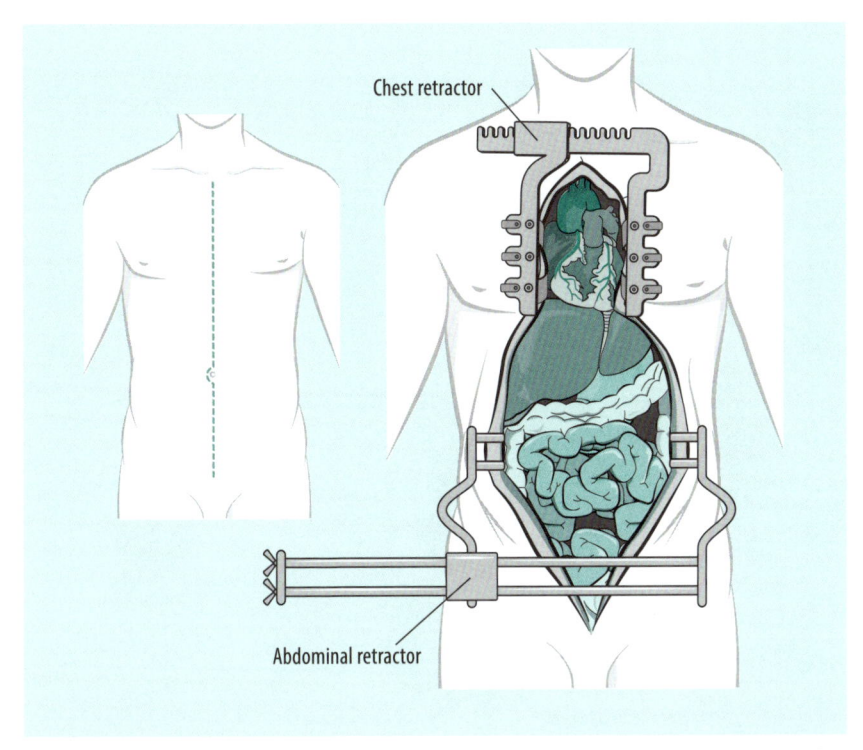

**Fig. 25.3** *Surgical approach for a standard multi organ approach. The incision from jugulum to symphysis (medium thoracophrenolaparotomy with a wide opening of both pleural cavities and retroperitoneum) permits access for inspection and safe collection of all standard collected organs practically avoiding their warm ischemia*

## 3. Explantation

In explantation, the tolerated cold ischemia of collected organs is also respected, thus first of all, the heart surgeon collects the heart and immediately afterwards the chest surgeon collects both lungs. Then the process continues with explantation of the liver, pancreas (in the close future also intestines) and the MOH terminates with kidney collection (in small children both kidneys are collected and then transplanted together – en bloc to one recipient). During the collection of the kidney the donors' mesenteric lymph nodes and spleen are also removed as material for HLA typing of the donor.

At this moment the cold ischemia of all organs begins. Therefore they are examined, possibly also processed on a separate sterile table ("backtable") on crushed ice, labeled and packed in triple sterile wrapping. For the transport they are placed in polystyrene transport containers with ice. Extrarenal organs are

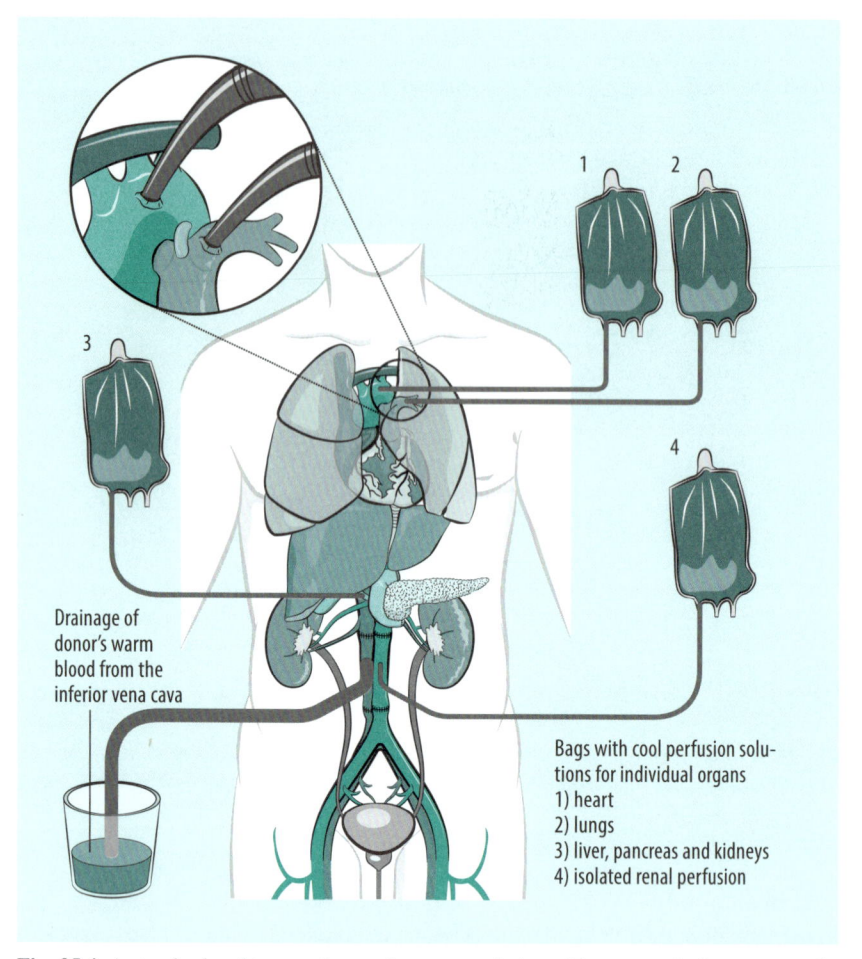

**Fig. 25.4** *A standard multi organ harvesting – cannulation of large vessels for organ perfusion with 4 °C cold preservation solution. Perfusion cannulas are inserted into abdominal aorta, aortic trunk and trunk of pulmonary artery for an immediate perfusion, cooling and preservation of the collecting organs. The wide cannula inserted into inferior vena cava permits a fast drainage of warm blood from the body immediately after the heart arrest. These steps are necessary to avoid warm ischemia of the collected organs.*

transported by the collecting teams to their home departments where the recipient is already waiting in some phase of preparation. Kidneys are kept in the regional TC until the KST gets the result of the donor's HLA typing from the examining laboratory. Afterward the kidneys are allocated by the KST and they are distributed by the regional TC. Usually one kidney is allocated for a recipient from the collecting regional TC.

The above clearly shows how difficult and demanding the process is, including the logistics of identification and indication of organ donors, the diagnosis of brain death and the organization and implementation of MOH. Commonly more than 100 persons of medical and transport professions are engaged during one MOH and subsequent transplantations. That is why statistics providing the number of organ donors and transplantations (for international comparison presented in a number per 1 million persons) do not testify only to the level of healthcare in assessed countries, but they also reflect the level of legislation, transport and communication infrastructure, i.e. the whole level of the assessed country.

## 25.3 Kidney Transplantation

Kidney transplantation is the organ transplantation with the longest tradition. The first kidney transplantation in the Czech Republic was performed in 1961 after thorough preparations (Josef Šváb, Jaroslav Procházka, Pavel Navrátil Sn., Rudolf Klen and Josef Erben, Hradec Králové); the female patient died the 16$^{th}$ day (sepsis and radiation disease). The first successful transplantation followed then in 1966 (Jaroslav Hejnal, IKEM Praha). This procedure as a program was available in the 1970s. Thanks to the availability of renal elimination methods (hemodialysis, peritoneal dialysis) the patient can be prepared for the procedure and in the vast majority of cases the transplantation itself is not life-saving.

Kidney transplantation is **indicated in patients with chronic renal failure** most often caused by chronic glomerulonephritis, diabetic nephropathy, chronic pyelonephritis and malignant nephrosclerosis (in children also congenital renal hypoplasia and congenital uropathy, nephronophtisis, renal polycystosis, hemolytic-uremic syndrome and others).

**Contraindications of kidney transplantation** comprise serious diseases of the cardiovascular system, HIV positivity and AIDS, chronic infection (e.g. tuberculosis), obesity (BMI above 35), active hepatitis, malignancy, marked malnutrition, severe impairment of other organs.

From a technical point of view, **transplantations are heterotopic** (Fig. 25.5). The graft is placed in retroperitoneum, renal vessels are sutured to iliac vessels and the graft ureter is reimplanted to the wall of the recipient's urinary bladder, at present usually by an extravesical technique. Native, non-functional kidneys are usually left *in situ*. Nephrectomy of the recipient's native kidney is indicated only in the situation when the recipient is threatened by the native kidney which can be the source of chronic infection or a cause of hypertension (or in children the reason for uncontrollable proteinuria in congenital nephrotic syndrome).

These are the fundamentals of kidney transplantation in adult patients, i.e. in the situation when the recipient gets a graft from an adult donor with the graft size approximately corresponding to the size of his/her own kidney. Such a graft does not produce mechanical problems caused by its size and after unfastening

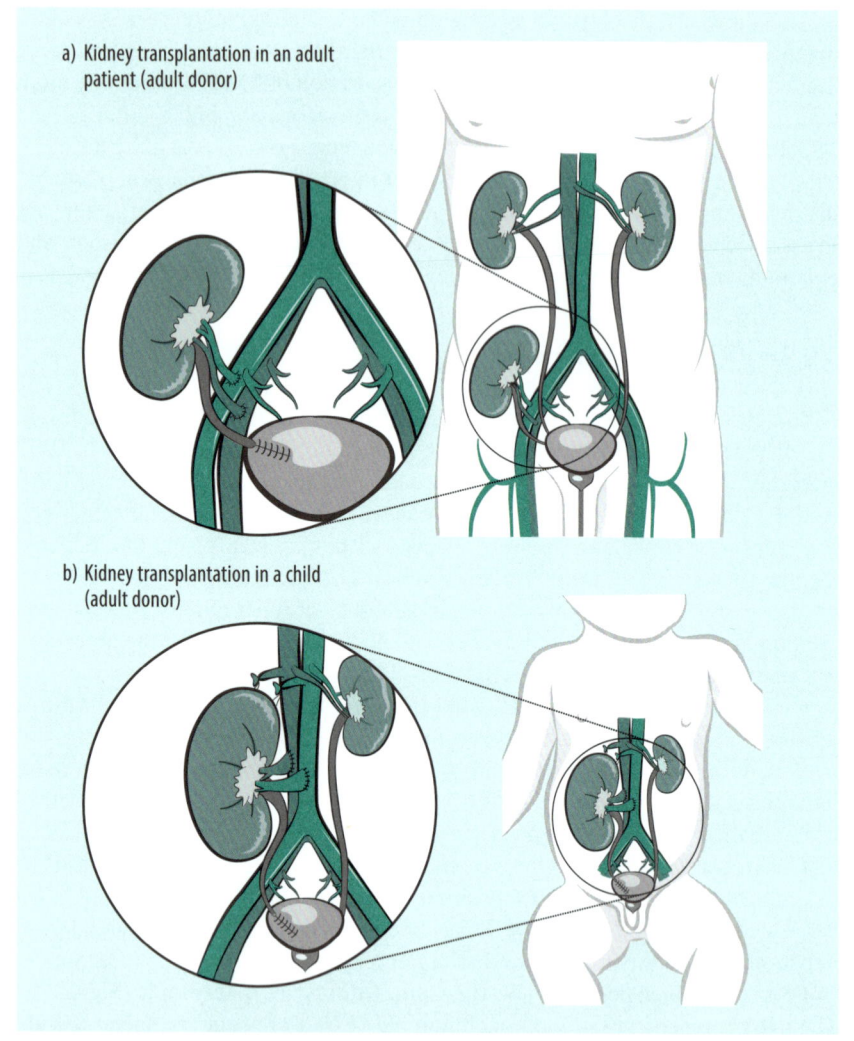

**Fig. 25.5** *Scheme of kidney transplantation: a) Kidney transplantation to an adult recipient – the scheme shows the situation when the recipient gets a kidney of the size corresponding to his/her weight (standard situation in adult recipients); b) Kidney transplantation to a child – scheme of transplantation of a large kidney from an adult donor to a small child recipient (drawn according to the photo of kidney transplantation from an adult cadaveric female donor with the weight of 75 kg to a child of 17 kg)*

the clamps, hemodynamically approximately 10% of recipient's minute cardiac output is required which represents only a minor hemodynamic increment.

However, for a child the ideal kidney donor is not a donor of childhood age. Due to many reasons the optimum donor has a kidney of the size that still fits the retroperitoneum of the pediatric recipient. Such a kidney due to space factors must then be transplanted into the retroperitoneum up to the subhepatic region and vascular anastomoses are sutured directly to the abdominal aorta and inferior vena cava. This graft mechanically elevates the diaphragm and interferes with breathing (small transplanted children with a graft from an adult donor often require mechanical ventilation for several days). From the hemodynamic point of view, such a graft requires a significant part of minute cardiac outcome (even up to 30–45%).

Even in the case of a flawlessly performed MOH, a certain degree of graft damage is always detectable that, in the post-transplant period, manifests itself as a polyuric phase of renal insufficiency. In children this polyuria (often reaching up to 10–15 L of urine per 24 hours) again requires specific postoperative care.

**Kidney transplantation from a living donor** is a planned procedure enabling optimum examination and preparation of both the donor and the recipient, as well as optimum staff and technical management. The procedure can be planned to take place even in the period before the recipient initiates chronic dialysis – **preemptive transplantation**.

The outcomes of kidney transplantations are generally very good; most recipients have a good quality of life.

## 25.4  Liver Transplantation

Liver transplantation has been performed outside the Czech Republic since 1963 (Thomas Starzl, Denver, USA), in the Czech Republic since 1983 (Kořístek and Jan Černý, Brno). Nevertheless, in the Czech Republic liver transplantation as a program was not initiated until the mid-1990s. Currently, livers are transplanted in the Czech Republic in TC IKEM Praha and in the Center of Cardiovascular and Transplant Surgery (Centrum kardiovaskulární a transplantační chirurgie – CKTCH) Brno. In contrast to chronic renal failure, there is no long-term substitution for liver function; therefore liver transplantation is considered a **life-saving procedure**.

Liver transplantation is **indicated in the end stage of liver diseases**:
1. In cholestatic diseases (above all in primary biliary cirrhosis, primary sclerosing cholangitis, secondary biliary cirrhosis, congenital atresia of hepatic ducts, cystic fibrosis, etc.)
2. In parenchymal diseases (especially in chronic hepatitis C and B with the transition to cirrhosis, cryptogenic cirrhosis and chronic alcoholic liver disease)
3. In metabolic disorders (e.g. in Wilson disease, deficiency of $\alpha$1-antitrypsin, hemochromatosis and a number of other rare diseases)
4. In fulminant liver failure
5. In rare diseases such as polycystic disease of the liver and kidneys (where a combined transplantation of kidneys and liver is indicated), extensive liver hemangiomatosis, extensive liver trauma, etc.

TEXTBOOK OF SURGERY

6. A controversial liver transplantation performed for malignancy represents a special topic. Transplantations are performed for example for hepatocellular carcinoma (size up to 3 cm) and only in highly exceptional cases for other malignancies.

**Contraindications of liver transplantation** are as follows:
- **Absolute** – other malignancy including cholangiocarcinoma, HIV positivity and AIDS, active alcoholism or other drug addictions, sepsis and serious infections and significant psychosomatic disorders
- **Relative** – too advanced liver failure, age above 60–65, previous extensive abdominal operation, significant anatomical malformations and thrombosis of the portal vein

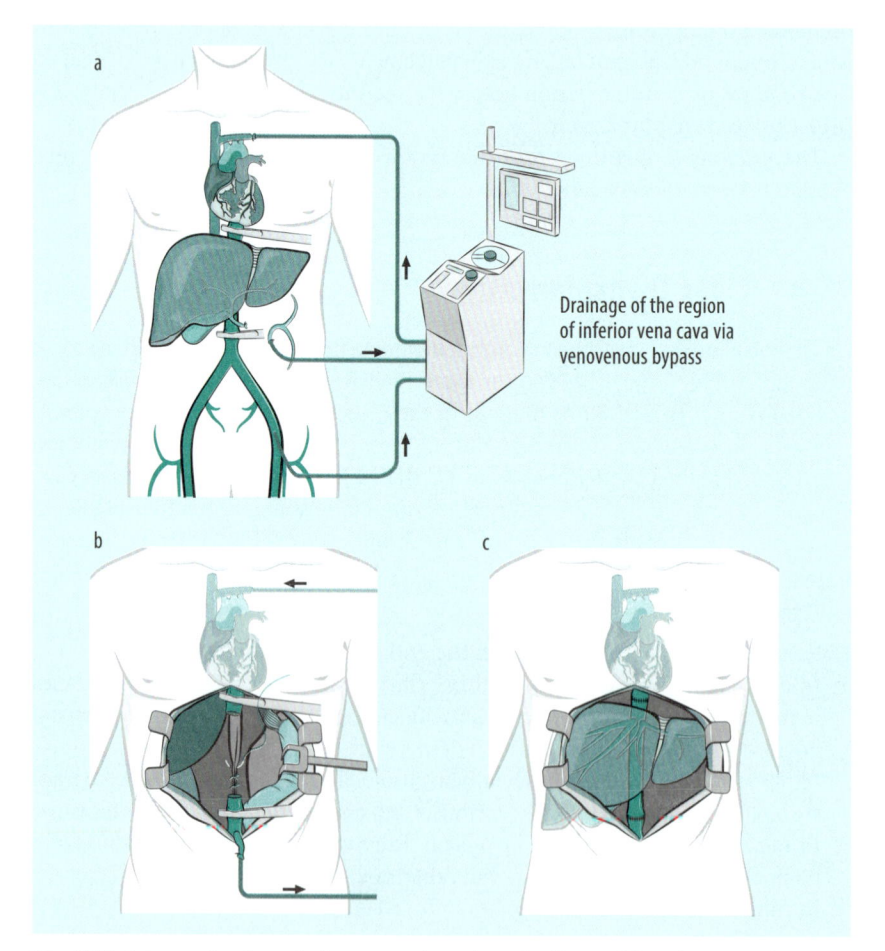

**Fig. 25.6** *Scheme of orthotopic liver transplantation; the diseased liver is removed in all its extent and the donor's liver is sutured in the orthotopic way, it is necessary to restore arterial and venous circulation and also portal bloodstream and biliary ducts – the original technique*

ORGAN TRANSPLANTATION

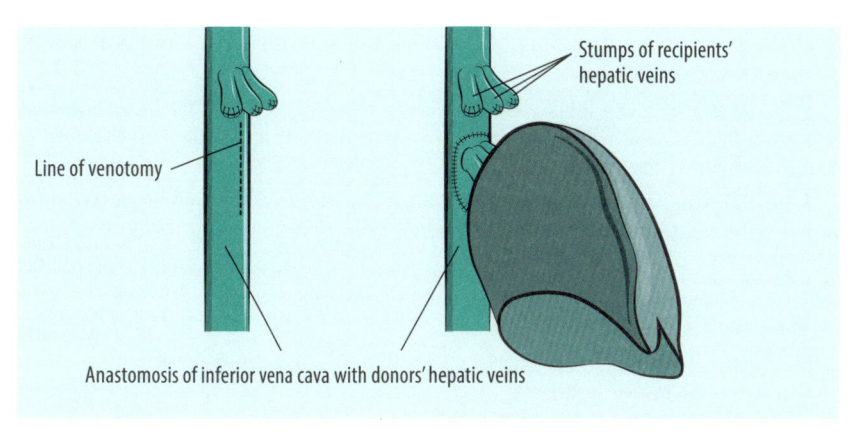

**Fig. 25.7** *Scheme of orthotopic liver transplantation – the currently used technique*

Technically, the transplantation is orthotopic (Figs. 25.6, 25.7) when the pathological liver is completely removed and the donor's liver (or its part) is sutured in its place. Generally, it is the most complicated routinely performed organ transplantation when the surgeon must reconstruct not only arterial supply and venous drainage of the graft, but also the portal bloodstream and biliary ducts. Child recipients usually represent a delicate situation as the number of child donors is very limited (only less than 5% of organ donors in the Czech Republic are children). Therefore, for a child it is usually necessary to allocate part of the liver from an adult donor. Theoretically, the liver from a big donor can be split and used for two smaller recipients or reduced in size. One of the parents can be a suitable living donor of part of their liver. From the point of view of the living donor it is a serious procedure, he/she must be informed about possible complications (including death).

The outcome of liver transplants is also very encouraging and most recipients report a good quality of life.

## 25.5 Heart Transplantation

The first, revolutionary heart transplantation was performed by Christian Barnard in 1967. He used the technique developed by Norman Shumway (Stanford, USA). In the Czech Republic the first heart transplantation was carried out in 1984 (Pavel Firt and Vladimír Kočandrle, IKEM Praha). This therapeutic method was introduced as a program in the early 1990s. Currently heart transplantations are performed in TC IKEM Praha and CKTCH Brno.

The **possibility of short-term and medium-term** (at some departments also of long-term) **mechanical support and heart substitution** are important factors for the program of heart transplantation. This program covers the period when the patient is waiting for a suitable donor (bridge to transplant) and is available also in the Czech Republic.

**The indication** of heart transplantation most often consists of chronic ischemic heart disease with significant impairment of left ventricular function, cardiomyopathy, less often valvular or congenital heart defects.

**Contraindication** is represented mainly by fixed pulmonary hypertension, organ complications of diabetes, irreversible liver failure, malignancy, general cachexia, HIV positivity and AIDS, sepsis or serious infection, malignant hypertension, extreme obesity.

**Relative contraindication** comprises chronic renal failure (combined transplantation of heart and kidney can be considered), age above 60–65.

The transplantation team begins to operate on the recipient after receiving the information that the donor's heart during MOH was found suitable and was collected properly. The operation is performed in an extracorporeal circulation, from the median sternotomy. At present the technique of orthotopic heart transplantation performed by bicaval technique is used. First, the donor's left atrium is sutured to the disk of recipient's pulmonary veins (to the posterior wall of

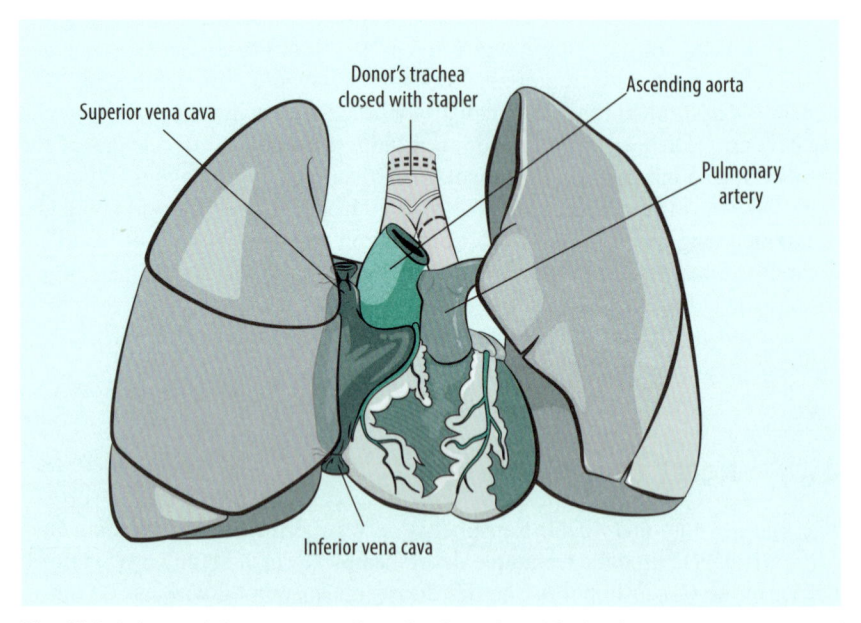

*Fig. 25.8 Scheme of chest organs collected in heart-lung block. After evacuating heart and placing a clamp on aorta, the heart is arrested by a cold cardioplegia (as for a standard procedure on a closed heart with the use of extracorporeal circulation). At the same time the pulmonary trunk is cannulated and the lungs are perfused with an ice-cold preservation solution. After dissecting ascending aorta and venae cavae, the block of chest organs can be separated from esophagus, aortic arch and descending aorta. The heart is separated from the block of both lungs on a crushed ice, outside the operating table (backtable, not depicted)*

# ORGAN TRANSPLANTATION

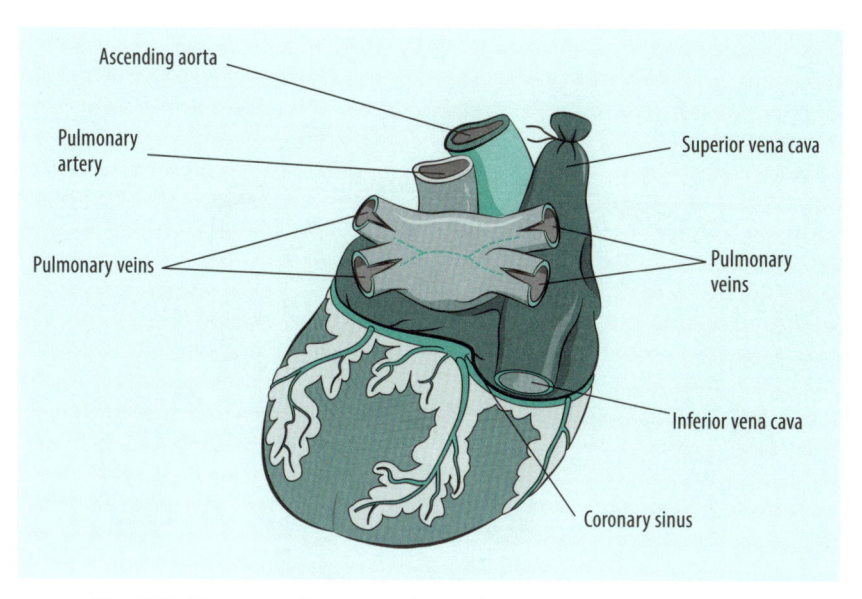

**Fig. 25.9** *Heart transplantation – donor's heart (a view of the dorsal side)*

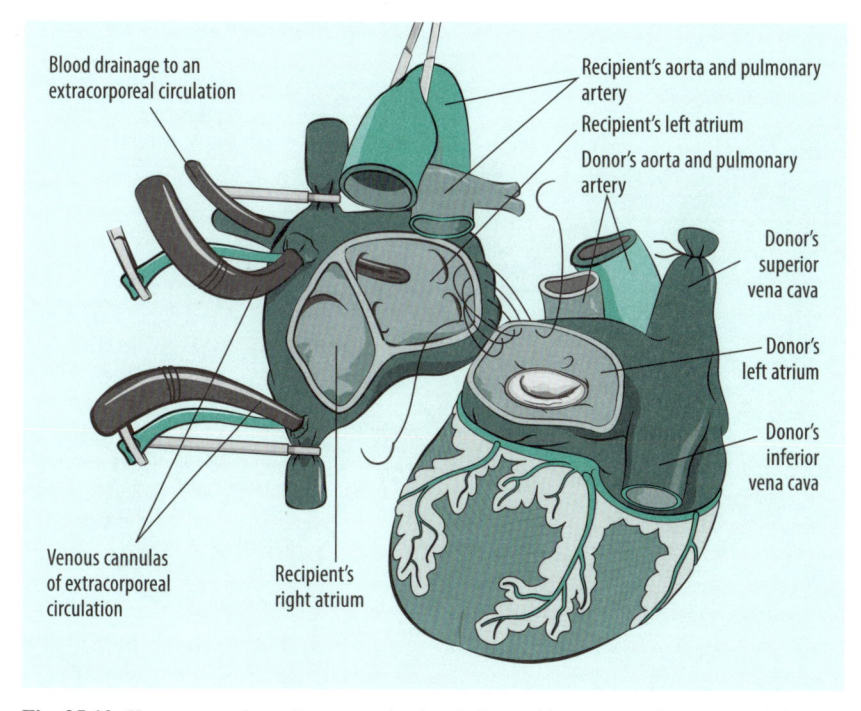

**Fig. 25.10** *Heart transplantation – standard technique of heart transplantation – left atrial anastomosis*

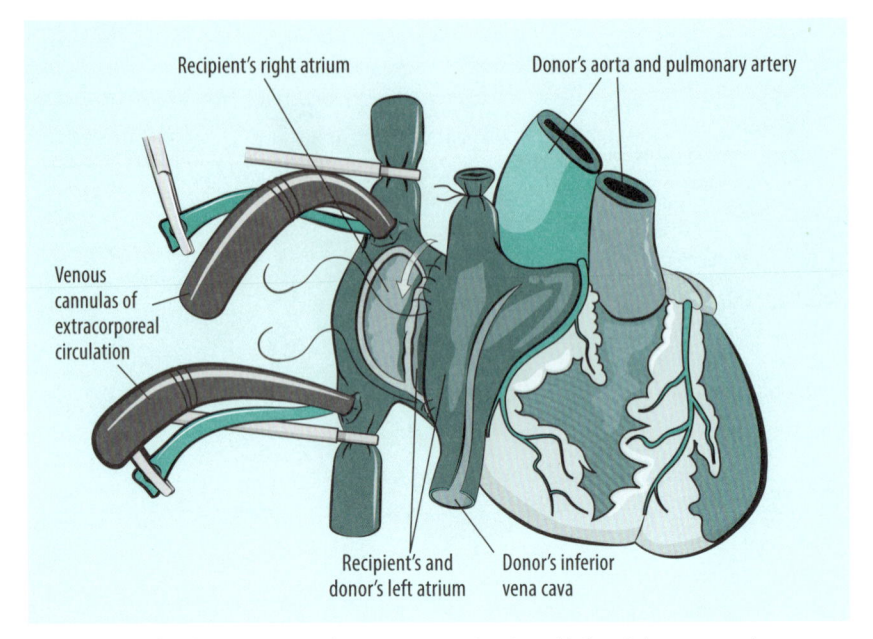

**Fig. 25.11** *Heart transplantation – termination of left atrial anastomosis*

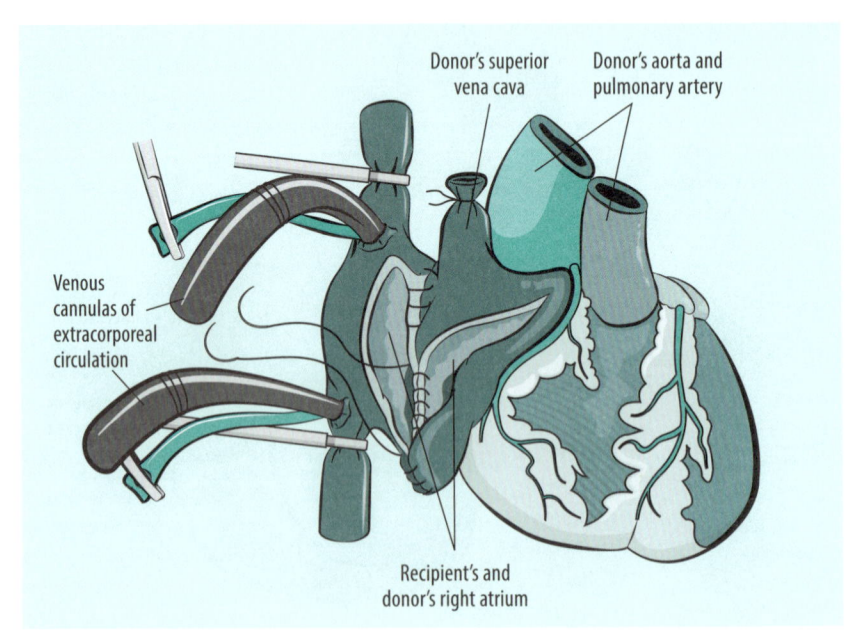

**Fig. 25.12** *Heart transplantation – right atrial anastomosis*

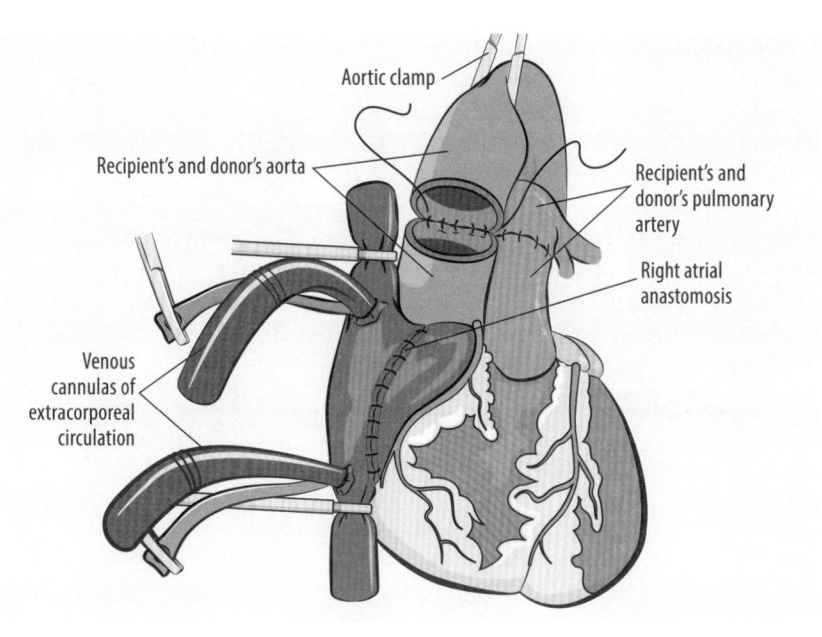

**Fig. 25.13** *Heart transplantation – termination – anastomosis of aorta*

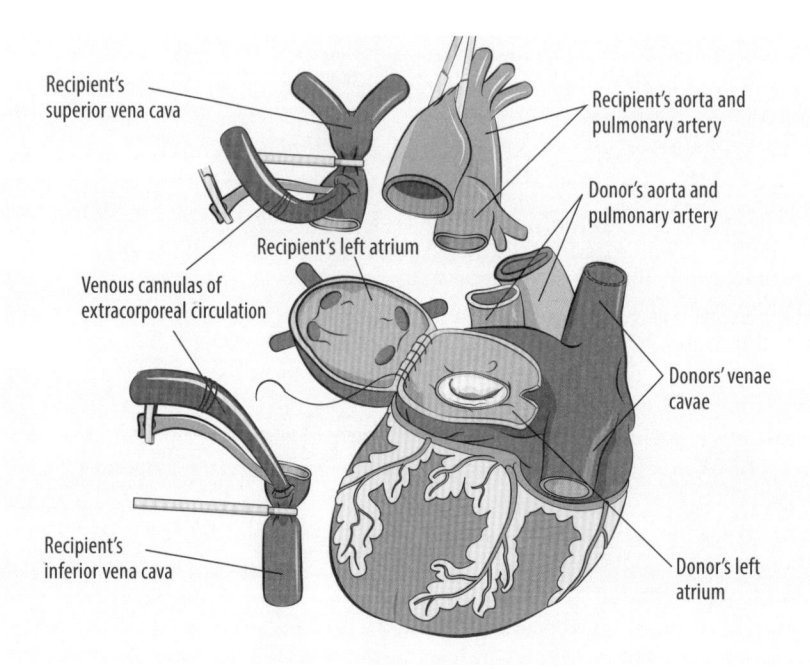

**Fig. 25.14** *Heart transplantation – bicaval technique*

recipient's left atrium which avoids anastomoses of individual pulmonary veins), then the remaining anastomoses of the aorta, pulmonary artery and superior and inferior vena cava are performed. After disconnecting from an extracorporeal circulation the donor's heart must assume the recipient's circulation; this step is followed by the postoperative care usual in cardiac surgery.

In orthotopic heart transplantation, an adequate proportion between the weight of the donor and recipient is necessary. Heterotopic heart transplantation, when the patient's own failing heart is left in place and the graft works as a bilateral heart support, is performed at present quite rarely.

The long-term outcome of heart transplantation is encouraging; most of the surviving patients have a good quality of life.

## 25.6 Lung Transplantation

The first lung transplantation was performed in 1963 (James Hardy, Jackson, USA). However, experience of the involved medical departments showed that practically all the patients died of infection, rejection and most often of dehiscence of bronchial anastomosis. Lungs are (together with the intestine) after the transplantation in a specific situation because they are in permanent contact with infectious material (inhaled air) and at the same time the natural tissue defense is significantly decreased by immunosuppressive therapy. Therefore, similarly to the history of heart transplantation, lung transplantations were practically abandoned until the new immunosuppressive drug cyclosporin A, less aggressive to tissues and healing, was introduced (1976, Jean-Francois Borrel).

In 1980 transplantation of the heart-lung block was performed (Bruce Reitz, Stanford, USA), then in 1983 a single lung transplantation and in 1986 transplantation of both lungs in block (both Joel Cooper, Toronto, Canada). In the Czech Republic the first single lung transplantation was performed in 1997 and bilateral sequential lung transplantation in 1998 (both Pavel Pafko, University Hospital Motol, Praha).

**Indication** of the lung transplantation consists in end-stage diseases of lung parenchyma. That comprises restrictive diseases (idiopathic pulmonary fibrosis, exogenous allergic alveolitis, histiocytosis, sarcoidosis and lymphangioleiomyomatosis), obstructive diseases (primary pulmonary emphysema due to $\alpha 1$-antitrypsin deficiency, chronic obstructive pulmonary disease, bronchiectasias, cystic fibrosis) and also vascular pulmonary diseases (primary pulmonary hypertension, Eisenmenger complex, chronic thromboembolic pulmonary hypertension). The transplant is indicated for an isolated pulmonary disease, after exhaustion of all conservative and surgical therapeutic options, in a patient dependent on oxygen. The best timing of the indication is when patients have a life expectancy of 12–18 months.

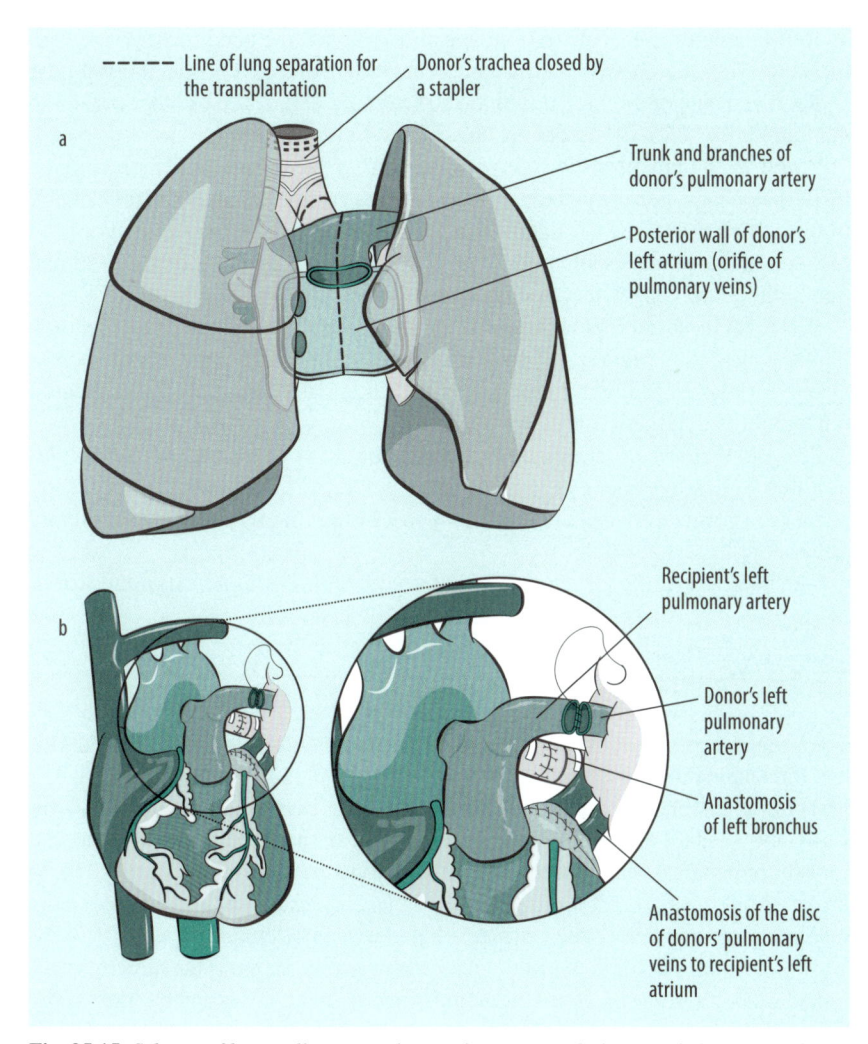

**Fig. 25.15** *Scheme of lung collection and transplantation with the "single lung transplantation" method. Lungs are usually (if collection of one of them is not contraindicated) collected in block of both lungs, trachea after the organ inflation is closed with a stapler and dissected. The posterior part of donor's left atrium is collected together with the disc of pulmonary veins. Then the lungs are separated on crushed ice outside the operating table (backtable)*

**Contraindication** includes malignancy, serious systemic disease, multiple organ failure, HIV positivity and AIDS, sepsis or chronic infection (hepatitis B, C), extreme cachexia or, on the contrary, obesity, long-term corticotherapy with complications, smoking, alcoholism or other drug addiction, progressive neuromuscular disease.

**Relative contraindication** is an age above 60–65, the need for invasive ventilation, serious cardiovascular disease, renal failure and psychosocial instability.

Requirements of the lung donor are stricter than in the case of other organs so that only about 15% of donors are suitable as donors of lungs.

**Single lung transplantation** is performed from the anterolateral thoracotomy. First, the pneumonectomy of the diseased lung is carried out and then the donor's lung is implanted. The bronchus is sutured first, then the anastomosis of the recipient's left atrium is stitched to the disc of pulmonary veins of the graft and finally the pulmonary artery is connected.

**Bilateral lung transplantation** is currently performed as a bilateral sequential transplantation via a transversal sternotomy (clamshell incision), or successively via two anterolateral thoracotomies (bilaterally). Actually, a sequential unilateral transplantation is carried out.

The vast majority of procedures are carried out without extracorporeal circulation that is, however, always ready to use ("stand by"), because it is needed especially in patients transplanted due to restrictive pulmonary disease or primary pulmonary hypertension.

The outcome of the Czech program is comparable with the rest of the world.

## 25.7  Pancreas Transplantation

The program of pancreas transplantation has been closely connected with kidney transplantation (in diabetes, kidneys suffer from diabetic nephropathy). The first combined kidney-pancreas transplantation was performed in 1966 (William Kelly and Richard Lillehei, Minneapolis, USA). In the Czech Republic the first transfer of pancreas was carried out in 1984 (Ivan Vaněk, Vladimír Bartoš, IKEM Praha). The transplantation of the islets of Langerhans that belongs to the transplantation of cells and tissues was developed in a parallel manner.

**Indication** for combined kidney-pancreas transplantation is the already-mentioned diabetes mellitus type 1 with end-stage diabetic nephropathy, preferably still in the pre-dialysis stage, with creatinine levels above 250–300 μmol/l. The essential condition is that the patient profits from the induced normoglycemia.

**Contraindication** consists in any serious cardiovascular disease. Pancreas transplantation is not contraindicated in blind people where, on the contrary, it can make their life easier by elimination of insulin application.

During the transplantation the pancreas graft is placed in the retroperitoneum, in the similar manner as a transplanted kidney. Vascular anastomoses are constructed on iliac vessels and the exocrine secretion of pancreas is drained either into the urinary bladder, or to the loop of the small intestine.

The outcome of pancreas or pancreas-kidney transplantations performed in the Czech Republic is also comparable with international data.

# ORGAN TRANSPLANTATION

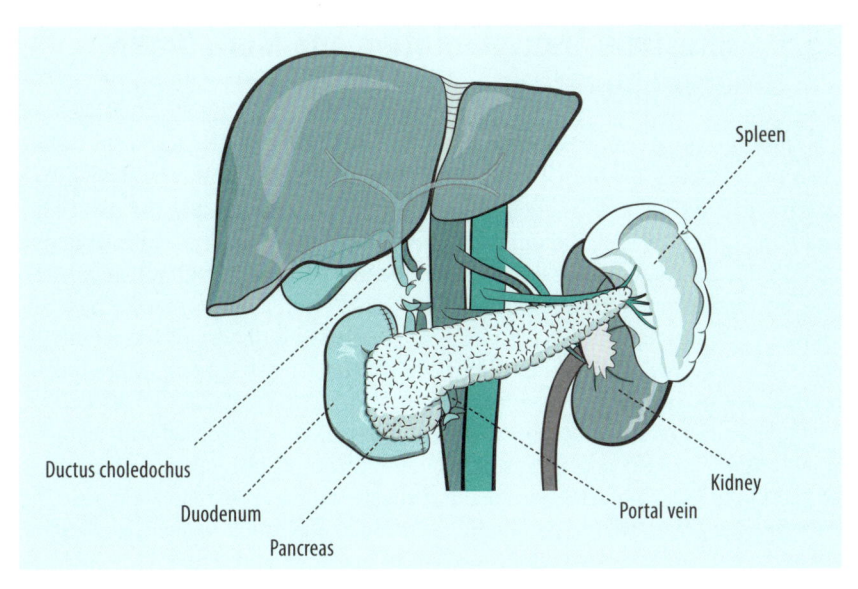

**Fig. 25.16** *Scheme of collection of pancreas; pancreas is collected in multi organ harvesting together with the spleen and duodenum*

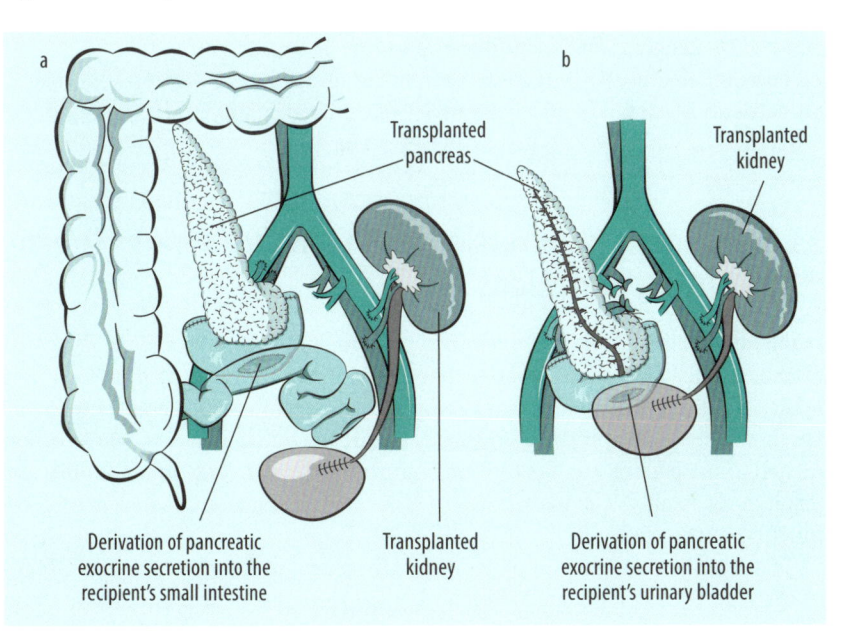

**Fig. 25.17** *Scheme of pancreas transplantation; a) Combined transplantation of pancreas to the right iliac fossa + kidney on the left side; exocrine secretion of the graft is derived physiologically into the loop of small intestine; b) Combined transplantation of pancreas to the right iliac fossa + kidney on the left side; exocrine secretion of the graft is derived into the urinary bladder*

## 25.8 Intestinal Transplantation and Multi Organ Transplantation

The first intestinal transplantation was performed probably by Ralph Deterling (Boston, USA) in 1964. In 1969 another transplantation of the small intestine was published (Richard Lillehei, Minneapolis, USA). Likewise in the case of the heart and lungs, the new immunosuppressive drug cyclosporin A was awaited to be introduced into the clinical practice so that the first successful transplantation was not performed until 1988 (Eberhard Deltz, Kiel, Germany). The next advance in immunosuppression (Tacrolimus) resulted in further improvement of the outcome; nevertheless, the transplantation of small intestines has still remained a clinical experiment.

The intestinal transplantation is **indicated** in patients diagnosed with an intestinal failure and suffering from serious complications during the administration of parenteral nutrition. Also permanent damage of the liver parenchyma resulting from the administration of parenteral nutrition is one of the indications, leading finally to **combined transplantation (small intestine and liver).** This situation is encountered mainly in children. There is a group of patients that, besides the small intestine, suffer from an important impairment of several organs. For them the **multi organ transplantation** is a life-saving procedure – liver, stomach, duodenum, pancreas and small intestines (Fig. 25.18).

The outcome of the best centers is encouraging: 1-year patients' survival is 80–90%, in 5 years it is 60%, and in 10 years 40%. In the Czech Republic, the program is about to be initiated in IKEM Praha.

## 25.9 Immunosuppression and Complications of Organ Transplantations

In the imagination of most laymen (and unfortunately also of some medical staff members) transplantations result in a final solution of the patients' problems. The reality is quite different and that is why the transplant candidate as well as his/her family should be properly informed. Before the transplantation, all the action related to the patient was focused on combating the end-stage organ failure and resulting problems. The main concern after the transplantation is the long-term function of the graft.

The recipient's organism physiologically reacts to the transplant of allogeneic tissue by a complicated immunological response dependent above all on T lymphocytes. The immunological response can be manifested clinically as an **acute rejection** or **chronic rejection**. Immunosuppressive drugs are medication that has enabled the realization of organ transplantation by means of direct or indirect suppression of T lymphocyte response to antigens of allogeneic tissue.

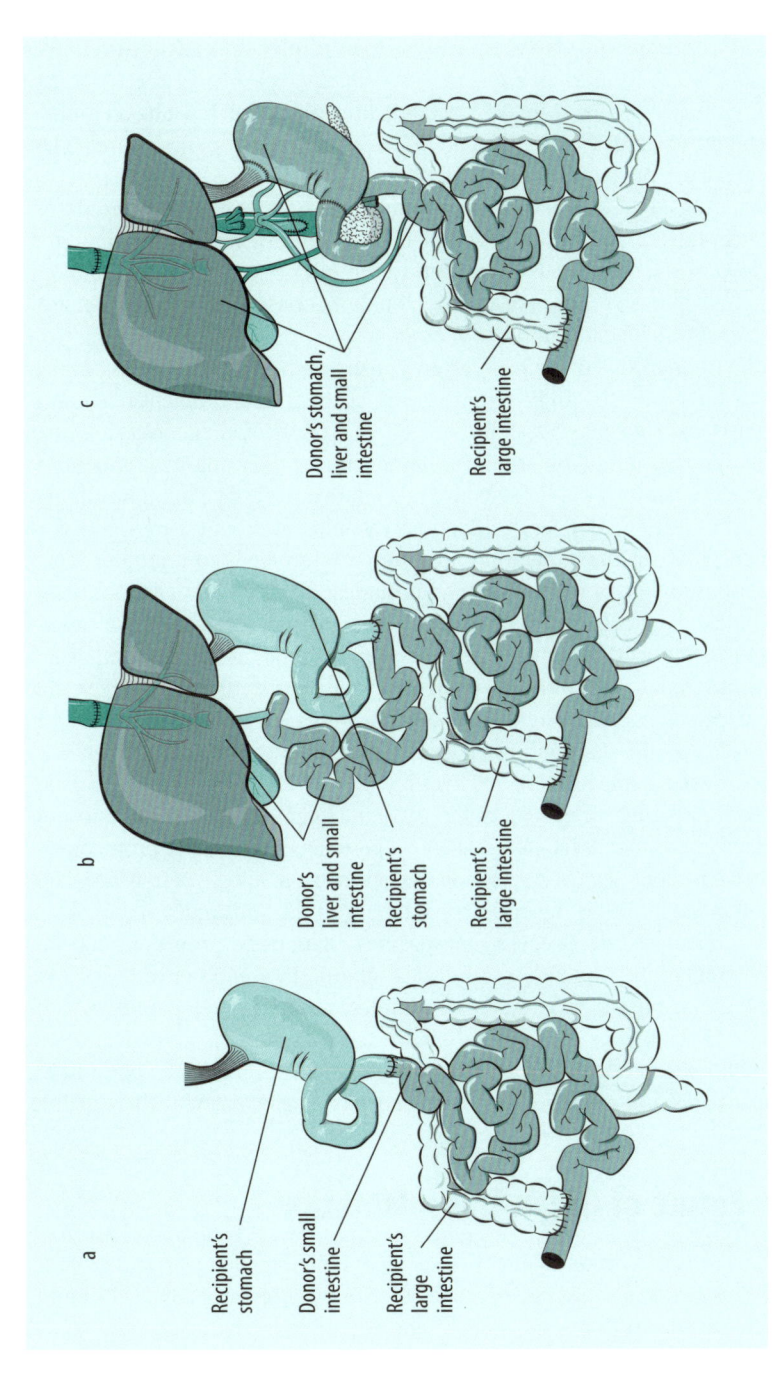

**Fig. 25.18** *Transplantation of small intestine and multi organ transplantation: a) Isolated small bowel transplantation; b) Combined small bowel and liver transplantation; c) Combined transplantation of small intestine, liver and other organs (stomach, possibly others – not depicted in the scheme)*

**The aim of immunosuppressive therapy is to minimize the risk of developing acute rejection.**

All the patients who have undergone organ transplantation must be on lifelong immunosuppressive medication (in patients after a kidney or pancreas transplant this is true during the period of graft function).

Medical drugs used on this account belong to the group of corticosteroids, antimetabolites (e.g. azathioprine, mycophenolate mofetil), calcineurin inhibitors (e.g. cyclosporin A, tacrolimus), macrolide antibiotics (e.g. rapamycin), biological immunosuppressive drugs (e.g. polyclonal or monoclonal antibodies, antibodies against IL2-R) and a number of other drugs with diverse modes of action. Each of the used groups of drugs interferes specifically with the immunological reaction of the organism (in different phases of the immunological reaction to alloantigens) and also has its specific side effects. These medical drugs are practically always used in combination and monitoring of their pharmacokinetics in the particular patient is a part of standard procedures. Excessive immunosuppression means an extreme danger of infectious complications and increased risk of a malignant disease. Inadequate immunosuppression leads to rejection. Thus, both situations endanger not only the graft but also the recipient's life.

The clinical diagnostics of the rejection are usually not simple and it is always essential to distinguish them from infectious complications as the treatment is diametrically different – the rejection is treated with pulses of corticoids and increased immunosuppression whereas infectious complications are treated with antibiotics in accordance with the susceptibility. An excellent method for rejection diagnostics is the graft biopsy. In the kidneys and liver it is performed by means of a puncture, in the heart transplant by transvenous biopsy of the right ventricle (at most hospital departments performed in the post-transplant period as a part of the protocol; and obviously carried out always if rejection is suspected), in lungs via transbronchial biopsy and in the intestines by endoscopic biopsy of the graft mucosa.

Chronic rejection is a process that currently cannot be prevented and that gradually results in complete loss of graft function. In a number of cases a re-transplantation is possible; in the renal transplantation it is even common.

Organ transplantations are obviously burdened with possible complications as any surgical procedure and the transplant surgeon must be an erudite specialist capable both of preventing complications and of detecting and resolving them in time.

## 25.10 Future of Organ Transplantation

Organ transplantation is undoubtedly a medical field that, due to population aging, will be more and more necessary. The primary problem is and will be the **availability of organ donors**.

It is therefore essential to care about the relevant legislation related to organ donations that should permit the development of a positive attitude towards organ and tissue donations throughout the whole society in the future. Another task is to **"overcome" state borders** because correctly managed international collaboration can increase the chance in patients on waiting lists of getting a quality organ as soon as possible – this applies especially to patients with rare blood groups, with a high titer of specific antibodies, patients on both sides of scatter of weight and height, to children and above all to those in urgent need of an organ. At present, talks at the level of the Council of Europe are being held with the aim to support the collecting activity in member countries and to ease international exchanges of organs for transplant uses. The Ministry of Health of the Czech Republic and the Czech Transplant Society (Česká transplantační společnost) are active in this effort.

**The donor pool** can be **expanded** in several ways. Above all, **organs from marginal donors** are still not used according to the existing potential. Also the quality of collected organs (especially those from NHBD) can be further improved by better preservation, i.e. by further improvement of perfusion solutions and above all, introducing the method of **preservation by continuous perfusion** in specialized transport machines into routine work. This machine can improve the quality of collected organs by medical drugs and by optimum perfusion and significantly prolong organ usability.

Also an **improvement of surgery techniques** (broader use of the split of liver and lung grafts – i.e. one organ for two recipients) can increase the number of transplanted organs, especially in children.

Another hope for patients awaiting a heart, lung or liver transplantation will be the advance in techniques and tactics in medium- and long-term substitution of the organ function. From this aspect, mechanical heart support is the most advanced so far.

Basic research has been investigating for more than 30 years the problem of **xenotransplantation** in general, and in recent years also the issue of organ xenodonors for humans. It is difficult to estimate the time when this project will become a reality.

However, it is indisputable that the long-term outcome of transplantations and the quality of life of transplanted patients will further improve with **advances in immunosuppression** – both thanks to research in pharmacokinetics and the efficiency of the combinations of current immunosuppressive drugs, as well as thanks to the development of new drugs.

Thus, beyond all doubt, the sub-specialization of the transplant surgeon has a fascinating future ahead. Nevertheless, it would apply only under the condition that these specialists will get the adequate education and will continue to work under the transplant centers.

# 26 SENTINEL LYMPH NODES

*26.1 Introduction*
*26.2 Possibilities of Detection of Sentinel Lymph Nodes*
*26.3 Importance of the Method in Particular Tumors*
*26.4 In Vitro Examination*

## 26.1 Introduction

Detection of lymph nodes and of lymph node involvement forms a part of surgical treatment of solid tumors. The search for lymph nodes can be difficult because even the affected lymph nodes can be small and easily overlooked in the fat tissue. One of the methods of identification is the so-called sentinel lymph node concept. The sentinel lymph nodes can be detected *in vivo* and *in vitro*. In the first case the aim is to identify the sentinel lymph nodes during the operation, in the second case to detect them in the resected tissue. The principle of this method consists in marking the lymphatic system from the primary tumor to the first lymph node of the lymphatic drainage, called the sentinel lymph node. This lymph node is the first filter that catches metastatic cells released from the tumor, and that is why it is considered the lymph node with the highest risk of metastatic involvement. This lymph node usually cannot be found just on the basis of known anatomy of tumor lymphatic drainage. A dynamic technique of lymphatic mapping permits identification of the lymphatic drainage as well as the first draining lymph node. Detailed analysis of the sentinel lymph node enables more exact detection of lymph node micrometastases. More accurate lymph node staging alters the disease classification to a higher disease stage, and therefore patients profit from adjuvant treatment. Identification of the first draining lymph node decreases the risk of oversight and leaving it *in situ* during a regional lymphadenectomy. In pathology, this enables more detailed histopathological examination that would be difficult in all other lymph nodes removed during a lymphadenectomy. Examination of the sentinel lymph node could become important in the future also in procedures where lymphadenectomy is not standard. An example can be endoscopic resection of mucosa in early stomach cancer. The probability of lymph node involvement is very low in this kind of tumors; however, it cannot be excluded with certainty.

Currently, the method of sentinel lymph node detection is important mainly because it provides the possibility to assess involvement of other regional lymph nodes. The validity of sequential theory of gradual tumor spreading through the lymph nodes is supported by studies of sentinel lymph node biopsies with the dissection of regional lymph nodes. A tumor is supposed to spread via the lymphatic system gradually without "skipping" the first regional lymph node, and so in case of a negative finding in this lymph node the lymphadenectomy can be avoided. Oncological radicality of the procedure remains preserved and the patient can profit from a less extensive procedure with a lower risk of complications. A more exact lymph node staging is also important for postoperative management of the patient, including indication for adjuvant therapy.

## 26.2 Possibilities of Detection of Sentinel Lymph Nodes

Identification of the sentinel lymph nodes can currently be performed with two different techniques. The first one is vital staining when the sentinel lymph node is stained with a lipophilic dye. The most common stain is lymphotropic patent blue which after application in close proximity to the primary tumor is absorbed quickly into the lymphatic system and dyes the lymphatic vessel and the first lymph nodes. If the dye spreads in several directions from the primary tumor, all the first dyed lymph nodes are considered sentinel. The second used technique is the detection of gamma-radiation after the administration of colloid labeled with a radioisotope. Bigger colloid particles spread through the lymphatic system more slowly and in contrast with the diffusing patent blue, in the first lymph node they are phagocyted. This is why radiocolloid must be administered sufficiently in advance, usually in the interval of 2–24 hours before the operation. In a number of tumors both methods are currently considered complementary; the highest efficiency in identifying the sentinel lymph nodes is described in the event of concurrent use of both techniques – the so-called dual mapping procedure. Achievement of high reliability is offset by higher technical and financial demands of the procedure.

## 26.3 Importance of the Method in Particular Tumors

The largest expansion of this method to date has been observed in malignant melanoma and breast cancer.

Upon the operation of breast cancer the examination of the sentinel lymph nodes can restrict dissection of axillary lymph nodes and associated risks, above all lymphedema of the upper extremity. In malignant melanoma the method permits identification of the drained lymphatic region and the first lymph node where the tumor can spread.

Employment of these methods in gastrointestinal tumors is still of an experimental character. The reason is the quite complicated lymphatic system and numerous connections that can lead to false negative findings in the sentinel lymph node and thus to failure of the method. A limiting factor is also the frequent incidence of micrometastases and isolated tumor cells in the lymph nodes, the detection of which is difficult with current histological techniques. Attention is focused on malignant diseases of the esophagus, stomach, large intestine and rectum.

Besides tumors of the gastrointestinal tract, in recent years the detection of sentinel lymph nodes has also been studied in other malignancies. Indication in skin tumors other than malignant melanoma comprises the so-called carcinoma of Merkel cells that often metastasizes with lymphogenic spread. In the orofacial region the method is used mostly in early carcinomas of the oral cavity (T1–T2 N0 M0) planned for transoral resection. In urology this method draws attention in penile carcinoma (metastasis to lymph nodes in both groins) and in testicular carcinomas (lymphatic spreading of the tumor along the vascular supply of the testicle to precaval and paraaortal lymph nodes). In gynecology, the most extensive experience with the use of this method is in vulvar carcinoma (metastizing to lymph nodes in both groins). The number of studies focused on this technique in tumors of the cervix has been on the rise.

## 26.4 In Vitro Examination

Examination *in vitro* means that the stain is administered to the resected tissue immediately after the operation. The capability to distribute the stain is still preserved, the sentinel lymph node dyes in a similar manner as *in vivo*. Easier detection of the involved lymphatic system is of significant help for the pathologist.

# 27 BARIATRIC SURGERY

*27.1 Definition of Obesity*
*27.2 Treatment of Obesity*

## 27.1 Definition of Obesity

Obesity is defined as an excessive deposition of energy storage in the form of fat. Considering the fact that a certain amount of energy deposited in the fat tissue is physiological, WHO defines obesity as such fat accumulation which presents health risks. Individuals suffering from obesity are more frequently afflicted by:
   The development of cardiovascular diseases including hypertension
- Diabetes mellitus type 2
- Dyslipidemia
- Nonalcoholic steatohepatitis
- Sleep apnea syndrome (together with the risks mentioned above it is termed a metabolic syndrome)
- Overload of the musculoskeletal system
- An increased risk of the development of malignant diseases
- In view of the gravity of the above-mentioned conditions it is obvious that obesity shortens the life span

The general cause of obesity is always an unbalance between energy intake and output. There are a large number of factors leading to excessive energy intake or rather to inadequate output, including genetic predisposition, eating and social habits, but also endocrinopathies, etc.

### CLASSIFICATION OF OBESITY

**Classification of obesity** is assessed by BMI (body mass index) which is defined as a weight-to-height ratio where the weight is divided by the square of the person's height.

$$\text{BMI} = \frac{m}{h \times h}$$

where $m$ is body weight in kilograms and $h$ is body height in meters.

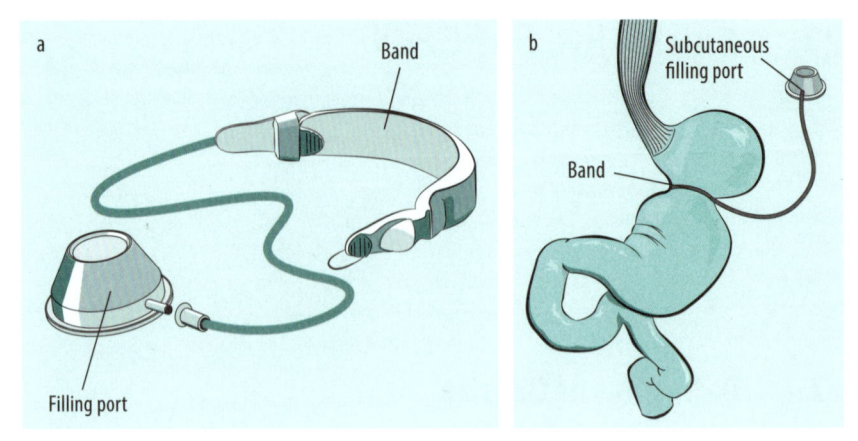

**Fig 27.1** *Gastric banding in the treatment of obesity: a) Silicone band – Swedish adjustable gastric band – SAGB; b) Stomach of asymmetric hourglass shape after the placement of the band*

Physiological values of BMI are 20–25, overweight BMI is 25–30, class I obesity according to WHO is a BMI of 30–35, class II obesity is a BMI of 35–40 and **severe (morbid)** obesity (class III according to WHO) is a BMI above 40. In the Czech Republic about one quarter of the adult population suffers from obesity. Values of BMI above the upper limit of the standard are present in approximately 52% of adults, in the population over 45 years of age the prevalence of overweight and obesity already ranges between 60 and 70%.

## 27.2 Treatment of Obesity

The treatment of obesity is conservative and surgical. The conservative treatment uses dietetic and regimen recommendations, psychotherapy, so-called cognitive behavioral therapy, physiotherapy and pharmacotherapy. With certain exceptions this does not result in the desired effect, i.e. in long-lasting weight loss. Long-term weight reduction of approx. 10–15 kg would be sufficient to reduce health risks. The so-called yo-yo effect is when weight loss is followed by weight increase up to the original value, and repeated failures of treatment result in the patient's resignation. **The only therapeutic method with sufficient and long-lasting effect is the bariatric surgery.**

### BARIATRIC SURGERY

Bariatric surgery is **a surgical treatment of obesity** which at present is probably the only form of treatment that ensures sufficiently large and long-lasting weight loss. The **indication** comprises severe obesity class III according to WHO, so-

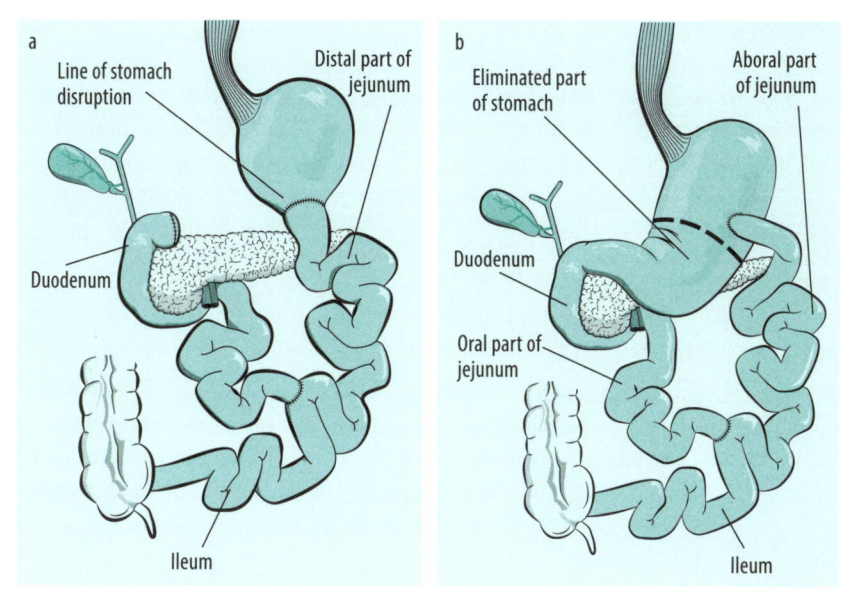

**Fig. 27.2** *Surgical procedures in the treatment of obesity: a) Malabsorptive procedure – biliopancreatic diversion (according to Scopinaro); b) Hybrid "combined" procedure – Roux-en-Y gastric bypass*

called morbid obesity with a BMI of over 40, and obesity with a BMI above 35 with associated diseases. As obesity is a multifactorial disease requiring a multidisciplinary approach, indication for operation should be decided by the obesitologist-internist, psychologist and bariatric surgeon. The experience achieved and the safety required during bariatric operations have changed the timing of surgical treatment. The surgical treatment should not be postponed until a time when it is evident that a nonsurgical approach has not resulted in sufficient effect and when irreversible organ and system disorders have developed.

Bariatric procedures have proved to be important not only for body weight loss but they also have a favorable impact on **metabolic syndrome** and **diabetes mellitus type 2**. Diabetic patients, who cannot further compensate their diabetes with oral antidiabetic drugs, but whose insulin secretion from pancreatic b-cells is still preserved, profit from the treatment most. Currently, the "metabolic surgery" it already classified for example within standard treatments of diabetes mellitus type 2 of the American Association for Diabetes. The explanation of mechanisms by which the operation, besides weight loss, affects metabolism, is not yet quite clear. Changes in gastrointestinal motility, changes of ghrelin level and the effect of cholecystokinin analogs have been reported.

A non-pharmacological and nonsurgical form of the treatment of obesity is **the insertion of an intragastric balloon**. This method is suitable for extremely obese and/or risk patients, or as a preparation for the operation of unacceptable patients. The surgical bariatric procedures can be divided into restrictive, malabsorptive and combined. The effect of restrictive procedures (picture 27.1) is based on the reduction of the stomach capacity. The stomach volume is reduced by placing a soft silicone band around the stomach; hence the stomach is divided in the shape of an hourglass. This results in a mechanical restriction against eating large portions of meal. The procedure – **adjustable gastric band** – leads to slow stomach evacuation and decreases the feeling of hunger. Modern tools enable changing the volume of the band to preserve its efficiency.

### MALABSORPTIVE OPERATIONS

Malabsorptive operations restrict digestion and absorption by means of eliminating the stomach and part of the small intestine from digestion, and separate by anastomoses food passage from duodenal secretion of bile and pancreatic enzymes. Digestion is possible only in the restricted distal part of the small intestine where the food is mixed with bile and pancreatic enzymes. The basic procedures are biliopancreatic diversion (Scopinaro operation) (picture 27.2a) and a hybrid operation – Roux-en-Y gastric bypass (picture 27.2b). Patients are reported to lose 50–60% of their excess weight within 24 months.

Patients with the intragastric balloon do not require mineral or vitamin support. However, after the above mentioned bariatric operations it is necessary to count on such deficiencies and to provide sufficient substitution. Complications of bariatric operations comprise impaired stomach evacuation, stenoses and/or ulcers in anastomoses, stenoses of the small intestine resulting even in ileus. The limited absorption should be kept in mind when oral medication is administered.

# 28 INTENSIVE CARE IN SURGERY

> 28.1 Postoperative Monitoring
> 28.2 Monitoring the Cardiovascular System
> 28.3 Monitoring the Respiratory System
> 28.4 Examination of Blood Gases and Acid-Base Homeostasis
> 28.5 Consciousness

Departments of intensive medicine are intended for patients with threatening or ongoing failure of one or several vital systems. The care of critically ill patients is currently provided not only at inpatient departments of anesthesiology and resuscitation but also in departmental units of intensive medicine.

Intensive care units resulted from the need of specialized care for patients in critical condition in the 1950s. A rapid expansion of intensive care units of various types then followed in the 1960s, and the foundations were also laid for a network of coronary and postoperative monitoring units. Intensive care medicine then specialized in the 1970s in the USA. The Department of Intensive Medicine (Sekce intenzivní medicíny) was established within the Czech Society of Anesthesiology, Resuscitation and Intensive Medicine (Česká společnost anestezie, resuscitace a intenzivní medicíny) in 1966, which is intended for interested persons from various clinical specialties. The specialization "Intensive Medicine" was constituted in the Czech Republic by Act No. 95/2004 Coll., and in 2006 the Czech Society of Intensive Medicine (Česká společnost intenzivní medicíny) was founded. Intensive medicine is currently an independent and rapidly developing discipline with subsequent specialization after completing the specialization in basic clinical branches – anesthesiology, surgery, internal medicine, neurology, and pediatrics.

Departments of intensive medicine can be divided according to the range of care provided:

**1st degree (units of intermediary care)** – enable basic monitoring, urgent cardiopulmonary resuscitation, or possibly short-time mechanical ventilation (usually up to 24 hours).

**2nd degree (specialized/surgical ICU)** – provide surgical intensive care of patients with threatening or ongoing failure of one or several vital organs including mechanical ventilation; the intensivist is permanently present. The standard monitoring of the patient allows for early detection of postoperative complications. The possibility of interdisciplinary cooperation is an inseparable part.

3rd degree (**Department of Anesthesiology and Resuscitation** with Complex Intensive Care) – where specialized diagnostic, monitoring or therapeutic procedures are applied.

Intensive care units can be specialized or multidisciplinary. There are certain economic and organizational arguments in favor of multidisciplinary ICU, especially the possibility of providing intensive care in several specialties if the number of patients in need is not sufficient to fill a specialized ICU. Arguments against are that individual medical specialties are less available and organization of the use of beds, for example with operation schedules, is more complicated.

## 28.1   Postoperative Monitoring

The term monitoring originates from the Latin word monere, i.e. to warn or to remind. Monitoring of physiological functions constitutes an integral part of intensive care. However, the monitoring technique fulfills its function only under the condition that the results are adequately evaluated and responded to.

Monitoring is not a therapeutic procedure; it serves only to focus attention and help in diagnostics. Its importance increases with the use of aggressive and highly invasive procedures to span the period of reversible organ failure. It can contribute to the improvement of prognosis in critically ill patients. The continuous monitoring of vital functions is one of the most frequent indications for admission to ICU.

Monitoring in intensive care is defined as repeated or continuous observation of a patient's physiological functions and of the activity of instruments supporting these functions. Its aim is early detection of abnormalities and facilitation of the deliberation about possible therapeutic intervention. It is an active process (monitoring and evaluation of selected markers), a repeated or continuous action in the course of time, when the human factor is necessary for the evaluation and use of the collected data for diagnostic and therapeutic decisions. Monitoring may also have negative impacts caused by inaccurate measurement, errors in marker monitoring, error of the equipment, or incorrect evaluation of the information (more attention paid to monitors than to the patient).

Non-invasive techniques enable monitoring without disruption of the skin integrity during the monitoring; invasive techniques require contact with patient's body fluids or exhaled gases by disrupting the skin integrity.

The standard monitoring of vital functions comprises monitoring of the basic vital systems – the cardiovascular system, the respiratory system and the state of consciousness. The standard surgical monitoring, depending on the patient's general condition, comprises also the measurement of diuresis, drained fluids and basic laboratory analysis.

# INTENSIVE CARE IN SURGERY

## 28.2 Monitoring the Cardiovascular System

The basic monitoring of the cardiovascular system comprises: ECG monitoring including heart rate and arterial and central venous pressure.

Continuous monitoring of the **ECG curve** is one of the basic monitoring techniques at every department of intensive medicine. It monitors the heart rate. It is intended mainly to detect impairment of heart rate and rhythm. The standard method employs a three- or five-lead ECG. The record corresponding to the lead II or possibly the lead with the best display of the P wave is usually selected on the monitor. Modern systems are equipped with the analysis of ST segments or with the identification of the type and number of arrhythmias. In cardiac patients, a 12-lead ECG should be recorded at least once a day. The normal heart rate is 60–90 pulses per minute.

**Arterial blood pressure** (BP) can be measured by non-invasive or invasive methods. The mean arterial pressure (MAP) provides rough information about the organ perfusion but not about its quality. Normal blood pressure is 140/80 mmHg (18.7/10.7 kPa).

The **non-invasive** method of BP measurement employs the principle of oscillometry registering arterial turbulences under the cuff with the subsequent ultrasound detection of the movement of the arterial wall, recently with the so-called photoplethysmography (the most precise MAP). This method is inconvenient in circulatory instable patients and patients with arrhythmia. When the patient is in a state of shock it does not provide real values.

The **invasive** method of blood pressure measurement requires arterial cannulation. It is used mainly in circulatory unstable patients and in cases when a repeated sampling of arterial blood for analysis of blood gases and acid-base homeostasis is necessary. Its advantages include continuous monitoring of the pulse curve, accuracy and prompt detection of impairment. Radial and femoral arteries are most often cannulated. This approach is not intended for the administration of drugs.

The **central venous pressure** (CVP) is measured usually from the region of the superior vena cava and corresponds to the mean pressure in the right atrium. Subclavian veins and the internal jugular vein are most often cannulated. The normal CVP is 2–8 mmHg (0.27 to 1.07 kPa). This approach is also suitable for the administration of drugs.

## 28.3 Monitoring the Respiratory System

The most commonly used procedures and techniques allowing the monitoring of not only the lung activity with respect to their basic function, i.e. gas exchange

**Table 28.1** Normal values of acid-base homeostasis

| | |
|---|---|
| Normal blood gases in arterial blood | pH 7.35–7.45 |
| | $pCO_2$ 4.6–6 kPa |
| | $pO_2$ 10–13 kPa |
| | $HCO_3^-$ 22–26 mmol/L |
| | BE −2 to +2 mmol/L |
| | Oxygen saturation of Hb in arterial blood 95–98% |
| | Oxygen saturation of Hb in mixed venous blood over 70% |

and their impact on acid-base homeostasis and cardiovascular homeostasis, include: respiratory rate, pulse oximetry, capnometry and capnography, analysis of blood gases and acid-base homeostasis and monitoring during mechanical ventilation.

**Respiratory rate** monitoring represents the basic physical parameter of ventilation. It uses changes of chest bioimpedance during respiratory movements registered with ECG electrodes.

The **pulse oximetry** is a simple non-invasive method that measures oxygen saturation of hemoglobin; as additional data it also registers the heart rate. The principle of this method consists in the fact that the oxidized hemoglobin absorbs less light in the red spectrum than the reduced hemoglobin. It provides basic information about hypoxemia. Advantages of this method include non-invasivity, low cost and absence of any complications. Normal $SpO_2$ is 95–98%. It represents one of the most important means of respiratory system monitoring. The validity of pulse oximetry is limited in conditions associated with impaired peripheral perfusion (low cardiac output, peripheral vasoconstriction, tissue edema, venous congestion), with the presence of abnormal hemoglobins (carboxy- and methemoglobin), anemias, skin pigmentations, jaundice or arrhythmias (absence of regular pulse wave).

**Capnometry** is a non-invasive method measuring the $CO_2$ curve during the respiratory cycle (the value is expressed numerically). **Capnography** then graphically depicts the $CO_2$ curve during the respiratory cycle. The $CO_2$ concentration in the exhaled air at the end of the expiration called ETCO2 (end-tidal $CO_2$) correlates with the alveolar tension of $CO_2$ and thus indirectly allows for the evaluation of alveolar ventilation. The capnography is used mostly during mechanical ventilation. The normal ETCO2 is 35–45 mmHg (4.7–6.0 kPa).

# INTENSIVE CARE IN SURGERY

## 28.4 Examination of Blood Gases and Acid-Base Homeostasis

This examination allows for the assessment of oxygenating lung function, the level of alveolar ventilation and the acid-base homeostasis. The arterial, capillary or venous blood from CVL is usually sampled. The most frequent clinical use comprises detection of hypoxemia or hyperoxemia, hypercapnemia or hypocapnemia and classification of the type of acid-base impairment (tab. 28.1).

## 28.5 Consciousness

The basic rough monitoring of consciousness includes the Glasgow classification of unconsciousness (Glasgow coma scale – GCS) that is recorded and evaluated (see tab. 23.1).

An assessed GCS of 14–15 gives evidence of mildly impaired consciousness, 9–13 of medium to severe and 6–8 of already very severe up to critical unconsciousness.

Special monitoring techniques such as cardiac output monitoring, monitoring in the course of mechanical ventilation, measurement of intracranial pressure, jugular oximetry, and gastric tonometry (regional capnometry) are used only exceptionally in surgical ICU.

Standard monitoring comprises the monitoring of fluid balance including the **measurement of diuresis and the volume of drained fluids.** The losses presented by secretion can be quantitatively assessed by laboratory analysis.

From the organizational point of view, the **basic laboratory tests** can be divided into **basic service** which, in addition to basic tests, performs specialized tests including those with longer analytic procedures, and to **urgent service** when the test results are available continuously 24 hours a day, usually no later than within 2 hours (e.g. blood count, Quick, aPTT, Na, K, Cl, Ca, Mg, osmolality, glucose, urea, creatinine, bilirubin, ALT, AST, ALP, GMT, troponin I, CK-MB, CRP, lactate, acid-base homeostasis and blood gases, urine and sediment, etc.). The knowledge of current laboratory values allows for the substitution of losses of extracellular fluid and the daily electrolyte requirement.

# 29 PERIOPERATIVE NUTRITION

*29.1 Enteral Nutrition*
*29.2 Parenteral Nutrition*

Advances in knowledge about patients' nutrition during the perioperative period have made nutrition an integral part of treatment in surgical patients. Most patients can cope with the operation, although it represents a burden even for a healthy, well-nourished person. If malnutrition or depletion of nutrients is present, this burden increases, the stored nutrients are exhausted and organ functions worsen even more if the disease is serious and complicated. The signs of malnutrition do not have to show overtly — even an obese person can starve!

This is why it is essential to look carefully for signs of malnutrition during admission to the hospital. A number of screening procedures have been developed for this purpose. In practice, the **tables of nutritional screening** have proven to be effective and the resulting score leads to further steps (Tab. 29.1). In profound depletion, the patient must be prepared from the point of view of nutrition; if this cannot be arranged (acute operation), it is necessary to focus on substitution after the operation as soon as possible. A state of insufficient nutrition can even change the surgical or therapeutic strategy and tactics.

Enteral and parenteral nutrition forms the standard part of treatment in patients that, for different reasons, are not capable of being alimented in a natural way. If nutrition can be administered via the gastrointestinal tract, this should always be selected as the basic approach.

## 29.1 Enteral Nutrition

Enteral nutrition represents a natural way of nutrient supply to enterocytes, prevention of atrophy of intestinal mucosa and of damage to the barrier function of the small intestine; it supports intestinal activity, permits higher increment of body weight and decreases the incidence of hepatic steatosis. It improves perfusion of the splanchnic area and reduces the colonization of the gastrointestinal tract with pathogenic strains. Its application is technically easier and cheaper than parenteral nutrition.

The disadvantages of enteral nutrition comprise the risk of aspiration, gastrointestinal intolerance, the impossibility of prompt correction of metabolic disorders, incorrect placement of the enteral tube, food reflux, and mucosal pressure sores.

**Table 29.1** Table of nutritional screening – the data in bold letters are reflected in the total sum

| | | | | | |
|---|---|---|---|---|---|
| Sex | Male × Female | C: Weight loss in the last 3 months | 0–3 kg | 1 | |
| Weight | .......... kg | | 3–6 kg | 2 | |
| Height | .......... cm | | Over 6 kg | 3 | |
| Diagnosis at admission: | | D: Food during the last 3 weeks | Amount unchanged | 0 | |
| | | | Half portions | 1 | |
| | | | Eats sometimes or does not eat at all | 2 | |
| BMI | ............ | E: Manifestations of the disease at present | None | 0 | |
| A: Age | Under 65 years | 0 | | Abdominal pains, anorexia | 1 |
| | Over 65 years | 1 | | Vomiting, diarrhea > 6 a day | 2 |
| B: BMI | 20–35 | 0 | Impossible to specify categories B, C, D | | 3 |
| | 18–20, > 35 | 1 | F: Stress | None | 0 |
| | Under 18 | 2 | | Medium (chronic diseases, diabetes mellitus, minor uncomplicated procedure) | 1 |
| Weight and height cannot be measured | | 2 | | High (acute disease, mechanical ventilation, gastrointestinal bleeding, extensive surgical procedure, postoperative complications, burns, trauma, hospitalization at the department of anesthesiology and resuscitation or ICU) | 2 |
| **Total sum of points:** | | | | | |

*If the sum of points is 0–3 the risk is low, without need of special intervention; 4–7 points mean medium risk, an examination by the nurse nutritionist and a special diet are necessary; 8–12 points represent a high risk with a requirement of special nutritional intervention.*

## CLASSIFICATION OF ENTERAL NUTRITION

a) According to the position of enteral tube – gastric, duodenal and jejunal. Nasal insertion is contraindicated in a fracture of the base of the skull due to the risk that the tube could penetrate intracranially, and due to a higher risk of secondary infection of meninges even if the tube is placed correctly (retention of the secret). Other options of insertion include percutaneous endoscopic gastrostomy (PEG) and jejunostomy by surgical approach if long-term nutrition (months/years) is planned. The nutrition can be delivered into the stomach intermittently or continuously. In duodenal or jejunal entry the administration is always continuous. A break at night can be respected, but is not mandatory.

b) According to its composition – nutritionally defined liquid diets or chemically defined diets that should contain a balanced mixture of basic nutrients

(15–20% protein, 25–35% fat, 45–65% sugars) and in addition to the energy, they must cover the need for vitamins and trace elements.

## 29.2 Parenteral Nutrition

Parenteral nutrition is applied into the venous system. It is non-physiological, the first pass of nutrients bypasses the liver, leads to a prompt atrophy of enteral mucosa and includes more risks and more technical difficulties than enteral nutrition. The necessary cannulation of large vessels can be associated with possible risks; it is also more expensive. It is indicated if enteral nutrition is contraindicated or impossible (gastrointestinal obstruction, bleeding into gastrointestinal tract, etc.).

### 29.2.1 Types of Parenteral Nutrition

**Supportive** parenteral nutrition serves as a supplement of enteral nutrition if enteral nutrition does not cover the requirements of nutrition components. **Total** parenteral nutrition serves as the only means of nutrition if enteral nutrition is contraindicated or impossible. The overall improvement of postoperative outcomes has also been achieved due to a changed strategy of perioperative nutrition. Prolonged preoperative fasting is subjectively perceived as unpleasant by patients and the shortening of this period decreases the postoperative metabolic stress. The dogma of mandatory preoperative fasting has been overshadowed by the **Fast-Track concept** that represents a complex approach to the reduction of perioperative stress.

In the preoperative period, it comprises intensive control of the internal environment, accentuates the surgeon's personal approach, shortens the period of preoperative fasting and allows for individual concessions to the preoperative preparation of the gastrointestinal tract.

In the peroperative period, it accentuates gentle methods of anesthesiology, a gentle, preferably mini-invasive operative approach. It is important to maintain normothermia before, during and after the operation.

In the postoperative period, early mobilization, an active approach to analgesia, a minimum of invasive entries and early oral nutrition should follow.

The early enteral nutrition is introduced individually within 24–48 hours after the operation, even in patients who have undergone a procedure on the gastrointestinal tube; before this was considered as a contraindication of early enteral nutrition.

### 29.2.2 Energy Situation of the Organism in Critical Conditions

**Energy output** increases in critical conditions by 25–100%, the breakdown of muscle mass results in the loss of nitrogen, a hard-to-control hyperglycemia develops as a consequence of extreme gluconeogenesis and decreased utilization of glucose in peripheral tissues in stress.

**Table 29.2** Table of nutritional support – three groups of patients according to their energy requirements

| Daily requirements in adults (per 1 kg of body weight) | Basic | Medium | High |
|---|---|---|---|
| Water (mL) | 30–40 | 40–65 | 65–100 |
| Energy (kJ/kcal) | 120–150 / 28–35 | 150–200 / 35–47 | 200–250 / 47–60 |
| Amino acids (g) | 0.7 | 1.1–1.8 | 2.0–2.5 |
| Glucose (g) | 2–3 | 5 | 6 |
| Fats (g) | 2 | 3 | 3–4 |

Note: *basic*: patients without evidence of catabolism; *medium*: medium catabolism, mild temperatures and stress; *high*: high catabolism, fever, intense stress, sepsis, polytrauma, burns, etc.

## 29.2.3 Energy Requirement in Critically Ill Patients

For each degree of body temperature exceeding 37 °C the energy requirement increases by 10%. The requirement increases also depending on a patient's clinical condition. Generally, energy requirements tend to be underestimated in thin patients and overestimated in obese patients. In most critical conditions the intermediate type of energy substitution suffices. An inadequate or excessive energy intake bears risks, especially in parenteral nutrition (Tab. 29.2).

## 29.2.4 Components of Parenteral Nutrition

### WATER

Water is the basic component of parenteral nutrition; its physiological requirement is 1500 mL/m$^2$ of body surface per day. In critically ill patients the requirement is increased due to fever, sweating, gastrointestinal losses (ileus, diarrhea), tissue trauma, increased volume of transcellular fluid, etc. Diuresis in critically ill patients should be markedly higher than in healthy people (sepsis >3.5 L per 24 hours).

### SUGERS

Glucose – 3–4 g/kg per day – represents the basic source of energy in parenteral nutrition. In critically ill patients insulin must usually be delivered simultaneously (1 unit per 3–4 g of glucose). Sugar solutions are a source of plain water after being metabolized. Their administration is contraindicated in diabetic and hyperosmolar coma.

### FATS

Fats – the basic requirement is 1.5–2 g/kg per day – are used in the form of emulsions; they have high energy content. Therefore, a large amount of energy can be delivered in a small volume of isoosmolar fluid (even into the peripheral vein). They are metabolized relatively quickly. A maximum of 30–40% of the energy requirements can be covered with fats. Contraindications of their administration include a state of shock, significant impairment of coagulation and hemorrhages, severe hyperlipidemia, fat embolism, or a coma of unknown etiology.

### ■ AMINO ACIDS

The amount of 0.7–1.0 g/kg per day is recommended as the basic requirement of amino acids. Nitrogen is irreplaceable in parenteral nutrition. Relative contraindication consists in acute renal or liver failure; however, continuous elimination techniques permit increased administration of amino acids in the nutrition even in these conditions.

### ■ MINERALS, TRACE ELEMENTS AND VITAMINS

Minerals, trace elements and vitamins comprise an important part especially in long-term parenteral nutrition. Standard fabricated mixtures are administered.

## 29.2.5  Operation

**Operations** within the scope of general surgery comprise a wide spectrum of different procedures. In perioperative nutrition it is necessary to keep in mind that even a relatively trivial procedure can affect a person's metabolism and can limit the perioperative nutrition (repeated procedures under total anesthesia).

The location of the surgical procedure strongly affects the options of postoperative nutrition, always reflecting the extent of the procedure, the duration of complaints, associated diseases and the patient's general condition.

## 29.2.6  Conclusion

Critical conditions result in the development of catabolism. A suitable energy-rich substrate should be provided to induce and maintain an anabolic condition. An inadequate supply of energy and nitrogenous substances leads to the development of catabolism, impaired organ functions, disturbed immunity, worsened wound healing, anemia and further complications.

In a hospitalized patient, defects in alimentation must be eliminated (quantity, quality, form, help, monitoring of the intake, etc.), effects of the treatment (chemotherapy, radiation therapy, antibiotics, operation, etc.) should be taken into account, and basic laboratory markers reflecting the nutritional status (usually albumin; the total protein has less validity) should be monitored. A continuity of adequate nutritional support should be provided by all available means of interdisciplinary cooperation, since the early postoperative nutrition does not terminate before a common diet is well tolerated and the signs of malnutrition have disappeared.

# 30 INFECTION IN SURGERY, ANTIBIOTIC THERAPY AND PROPHYLAXIS

> 30.1 Surgical Site Infection
> 30.2 Classification of SSI
> 30.3 Microbiology of SSI
> 30.4 Classification of Operative Wounds According to the Risk of SSI
> 30.5 Risk Factors for Formation and Development of SSI
> 30.6 Microbiological Diagnostics of SSI
> 30.7 Antibiotic Use in the Treatment of SSI
> 30.8 Principles of Antibiotic Prophylaxis During Surgical Procedures

**Infection** is generally caused by dynamic interactions among the host, microorganisms with different grades of pathogenicity and virulence, and environmental factors. If microorganisms overcome the host defense mechanisms, then the infectious process associated with local and/or general signs of variable gravity develops.

**Surgical infections** are complications of surgical (invasive) procedures or infections requiring surgical intervention as a necessary part of the treatment (e.g. abscesses, necrotizing fasciitis, Fournier gangrene, Clostridium gas gangrene, etc.).

The pathogenesis of infection in surgery is often triggered by penetration of bacteria into a primarily sterile localization. The vast majority of postoperative wound infections originate during the operation. The source is usually microflora that permanently or temporarily colonizes in the skin, mucosa of airways, gastrointestinal or genitourinary tract. Etiology of the infection can be polymicrobial, often with anaerobic components, if for example the infection originates in the large intestine. Contaminating bacteria from the external environment can contribute to the development of infections associated with extensive trauma. Critical situations are, for example, contamination with spores of anaerobic bacteria (Clostridium in anaerobic traumas) in the ischemic or devitalized tissue.

## 30.1 Surgical Site Infection

In the current international terminology infections originated in association with a surgical procedure are termed as **SSI** (surgical site infection). They are one of the most frequent nosocomial infections. Their seriousness consists in the significant increase in morbidity, mortality, prolonged hospitalization and consequently in the increased costs of treatment and further healthcare.

Infections are classified as SSI in the event they develop within 30 days after the operation; in procedures associated with the implantation of foreign material (e.g. artificial joints, vascular prostheses) the limit is extended to one year.

## 30.2 Classification of SSI

Depending on the extent, SSIs can be divided into **superficial** affecting skin and subcutaneous tissue and **deep** when the infectious process spreads on fasciae and muscles. The most serious form is **organ** SSI, affecting one or more organs and/or body fluids (peritonitis, mediastinitis, etc.).

## 30.3 Microbiology of SSI

The most frequent agent causing SSI is *Staphylococcus aureus*; enterococci and enterobacteriae, especially *E. coli* and *Klebsiella spp.* are often involved. Coagulase negative staphylococci and mycotic agents (*Candida spp.* and filamentous fungi) are gaining importance, above all in severely immunocompromised patients. The range of potential agents is quite wide; in nosocomial infections it reflects the local epidemiological situation. The microbial etiology is directly associated with the type and localization of the surgical procedure. The extent of the risk of contamination of the operating field which determines the probability of subsequent development of infection is classified into four basic groups.

## 30.4 Classification of Operative Wounds According to the Risk of SSI

**Clean operations** are not associated with the opening of airways, gastrointestinal or gynecological tracts. The most frequent infectious agents are staphylococci, especially *Staphylococcus aureus*. The source of infection can be the patient's body surface or contamination from the external environment. The risk of infectious complications is very low, below 1% on the average. Some of these infectious complications can be very serious (e.g. mediastinitis after a cardiac surgery procedure).

**Clean - (potentially) contaminated** operations are associated with the opening of respiratory, gastrointestinal or genitourinary tracts under controlled conditions and without unusual contamination (gastric resection for ulcer, cholecystectomy, etc.). The incidence of infectious complications usually should not exceed 5%.

**Contaminated** wounds comprise recent random injuries associated with significant external contamination, or operations when the spillage of gastric or intestinal content or urine into the operating field cannot be avoided. The probability of the development of infection ranges between 10 and 17%.

**Infected dirty wounds/operations** are massively contaminated already before the operation (peritonitis, pleural empyema, abscesses, anaerobic infections of abdominal wall, etc.). The development of infection can be expected in up to 30%.

## 30.5 Risk Factors for the Development of SSI

The development of wound infections is determined by the above-mentioned patient's susceptibility to infection that is influenced by age, nutritional status, presence of primary disease (diabetes mellitus, malignancies, etc.), simultaneous therapy with corticosteroids, immunosuppressive or cytostatic drugs; also habits (smoking, drug addiction) and psychological factors play a certain role.

The pathogenesis significantly reflects the bacterial burden, the virulence of microflora that contaminates the operating field, and the wound microenvironment – especially ischemia, acidosis and the presence of foreign (e.g. sutures) material can play a negative role. The risk of infectious complications can be decreased by adequately indicated and properly applied antibiotic prophylaxis preferably limited only to the period of the procedure itself (see below).

**SSI diagnostics** are generally based on the local signs (presence of inflammatory signs, wound dehiscence, purulent secretion, presence of abscess in deeper layers or in an organ), or possibly on the general clinical manifestation and laboratory findings including microbiology.

## 30.6 Microbiological Diagnostics of SSI

### SKIN AND SOFT TISSUES

With bacterial infections of skin and skin adnexa, swabs from skin lesions are examined; tissue samples (incision, biopsy) diagnosed by aerobic and anaerobic cultivation may also be analyzed. In fulminant life threatening infections of soft tissues (streptococcal fasciitis, clostridium gas gangrene, etc.) the biological material obtained during the surgical treatment (pus, tissue samples) must be urgently examined. The result, although just preliminary (microscopy), must be immediately reported to the attending physician. Apart from the complex microbiological culture from the site of infection, in the systemic manifestation it is essential to take a blood sample for hemoculture.

### WOUNDS AND DEFECTS

The sample is taken directly from the sites of ongoing active inflammation; parts of the tissue and pus from the base of the wound may also be taken. Hemoculture is indicated above all in infections of organs and body cavities. Surgical defects (crural ulcers, decubiti) are usually colonized on their surface with microorganisms. The common swab from the surface does not provide a representative picture of probable infectious etiology, and therefore can be misleading also from the viewpoint of the selection of antibiotics. If an ongoing infection is suspected that would invade the surrounding structures and possibly manifest with general symptoms, a radical swab from the edge of the lesion should be performed at the boundary between the affected and the healthy tissue.

### PRIMARY STERILE BODY FLUIDS

These represent diagnostically valuable samples of biological material – pleural, pericardial, peritoneal and articular fluids, ascites, etc. If the presence of microorganisms is finally demonstrated, the finding is usually highly significant, giving evidence for etiology of the infectious process. The sample collection should always be performed by an aseptic puncture. The finding can be rather misleading if the biological material is obtained from drainage, since a positive finding is often only a contamination from the surface of the synthetic material. Besides the classical bacteriological methods (microscopy, culture, antigen positivity), also molecular methods (PCR) can be helpful in these situations.

### CONTENT OF PATHOLOGICAL CAVITIES

This topic refers mainly to pus from abscesses and empyema or to the content of fistulas and pseudocysts with suspected presence of infection. In such situations not only the swab from the focus should be collected but the laboratory should always be provided with a sufficient volume of liquid material (preferably several milliliters). The material must be protected from air oxygen, since these samples usually contain mixed bacterial flora with the presence of anaerobic bacteria.

### FOREIGN MATERIAL

The insertion or implantation of foreign material is a significant risk factor for the development of infection. Some microorganisms (staphylococci, pseudomonas, candidas, etc.) tend to form a biofilm on the surface of foreign bodies. This problem mainly applies to **vascular catheters**, **prosthetic material** in surgery (joint replacement, vascular prostheses, artificial valves, filters), or possibly to **stimulation electrodes** (cardiostimulation and neurostimulation systems) or **drainage** (for example infection of drains and shunts inserted into the CNS). Apart from the routine methods, sonication of synthetic materials (vascular catheters, joint replacements) prior to their removal is recommended to increase the culture sensitivity, if the presence of biofilm is suspected as the source of infection.

## 30.7 Antibiotic Use in the Treatment of SSI

Surgical infections always require early and exact diagnosis with adequate subsequent treatment. The administration of antibiotics often represents an indispensable part; however, their effect in many situatio+ns only complements the surgical therapy and should not be overestimated. The strategy of antibiotic use can basically be divided into three principal approaches: empiric, initial and targeted therapy.

### EMPIRIC THERAPY

Empiric therapy is the strategy based on general criteria for antibiotic choice when no results of microbiological examination are available before starting the treatment that would clarify the infectious etiology. From the standpoint of the principles of antibiotic policy, the empiric approach is the least suitable. It is associated with the risk of polypragmasia, but also with treatment failure. Broad-spectrum antibiotics are preferred, leading to the risk of the selection of resistant strains.

### INITIAL ANTIBIOTIC THERAPY

In the event of serious infections that require starting the treatment urgently, so-called **initial antibiotic therapy** is used. Its initiation is preceded by the collection of clinically relevant samples of biological material for microbiological examination if they are available. The initial therapy usually uses antibiotics of a broader spectrum that should with higher probability affect the supposed etiological agent. Their selection is based on qualified consideration, taking into account all available clinical and epidemiological data.

### TARGETED ANTIBIOTIC THERAPY

It is crucial to switch as soon as possible to **targeted therapy** that has a narrower spectrum, is selectively targeted on the proved infectious agent and is based on the results of an antibiogram. This means the **principle of de-escalation** which requires an organized interdisciplinary approach; it is a professionally demanding but efficient therapy, clinically and epidemiologically safe and cost effective.

## Indication Algorithm of Antibiotic Therapy

Despite the causal character of antibiotic treatment the reasons for its initiation are often very superficial; antibiotics paradoxically belong among the most frequently misused medical drugs. They are often administered just for subfebrile temperatures or other non-specific symptoms; otherwise they are given "just in case". The proper indication and therapeutic algorithm should be based on responses to and consideration of the following questions:

### 1. Is it Really an Infection and are Antibiotics Indicated?

There are relatively many conditions with a clinical picture that can give the impression of infection. Hence, a thorough differentially diagnostic approach is always appropriate. The most common symptom of infectious diseases is fever that can, however, result from different non-infectious causes that must be excluded (drug interactions, collagenosis, brain hemorrhage, pancreatitis, vasculitis, neoplasm/metastasis, etc.).

### 2. Where is the Infection Localized?

For the optimum strategy of antibiotic treatment, defining the place of infection is essential. The selected mode of therapy must enable antibiotics to get to the place of infection in a concentration sufficient enough to affect bacterial microflora, using knowledge of the pharmacological (pharmacokinetics/pharmacodynamics) properties of particular medical drugs. If the place of ongoing infection remains unknown and the antibiotics are given only on the basis of general symptoms or laboratory inflammatory markers, the risk of treatment failure increases. It is always necessary to assess whether the infection is focal or systemic. In diseases with a clinical picture of sepsis of different gravity it is important to start the antibiotic therapy in time and with sufficient intensity.

### 3. Is the Infection of Community-acquired or Nosocomial Origin?
Epidemiological criterion related to the development of an infectious disease is valuable for the assessment of infectious etiology. The range of agents causing community-acquired and nosocomial infections is rather characteristic and should be taken into account when antibiotic therapy is indicated. Significant resistance or multiresistance can be expected especially in nosocomial microorganisms.

### 4. Is the Systemic Application of Antibiotics Indispensable for Curing?
If the disease is caused by a localized process that can be eliminated by surgical methods, the treatment with systemic antibiotics can be avoided; possible options include local antibiotics or antiseptics. The proper interpretation of microbiological examination differentiating between colonization and infection is of crucial importance. In a number of cases, the microbiological finding *per se* is not the reason for the initiation of the systemic antibiotic therapy.

### 5. When can the Clinical Effect of Treatment be Expected?
At least 24 hours and sometimes up to 72 hours must elapse before the clinical effect can be evaluated. Also the nature of infection and the character of the effect of the selected antibiotics (primary bactericidal or bacteriostatic) play a role. If the treatment evidently fails, the determined diagnosis including infectious etiology should be revised, examinations should be repeated or extended, and on the basis of the new information the change of the previously selected antibiotics or other, e.g. a surgical solution, should be considered.

### 6. The Optimum Dose and Dosing Interval
The current trend prefers use of higher or even maximal doses of antibiotics reflecting the seriousness of the infection, without extending unnecessarily the total period of application. The aim is to achieve a prompt eradication of the causative agent and to limit antibiotic side effects and their epidemiological risks (resistance selection). The dosing interval results from pharmacodynamics of the particular antibiotics. The optimum effect of the drug depends either on the concentration (aminoglycosides, fluorochinolones, etc.) or on time (beta-lactams, etc.).

### 7. What Length of Treatment is Necessary to Safely Clear up Infection?
The length of antibiotic treatment depends on clinical diagnosis, disease gravity, characteristics of the causative agent, presence of risk factors (immunosup-

**Table 30.1** Basic parenteral antibiotics – brand names, basic therapeutic doses

| Antibiotics | Brand names | Usual dose (p.e.)* |
|---|---|---|
| Ampicillin | Ampicillin, Ampo-Ampi Penstabil | 1–4 g every 4–6 hours |
| Ampicillin/Sulbactam | Unasyn | 1.5–3 g every 6 hours |
| Amoxicillin/Clavulanate | Augmentin, Amoksiclav, Curam, Forcid | 1–2 g every 6–8 hours |
| Penicillin G | Penicillin G | 1–5 MIU** every 4–6 hours |
| Cefazolin | Kefzol, Cefazolin, Vulmizolin | 1–2 g every 6–8 hours |
| Cefuroxime | Zinnacef, Zinnat, Axetin, Lifurox, Xorimax | 0.75–1.5 g every 8 hours |
| Cefotaxime | Claforan, Sefotax, Taxcef | 1–2 g every 8 hours |
| Ceftazidime | Fortum, Kefadim, Ceftazidim | 1–2 g every 8 hours |
| Clindamycin | Dalacin C, Klimicin | 300–900 mg every 6 hours |
| Lincomycin | Neloren, Lanocin | 1–2 g every 6–8 hours |
| Metronidazole | Entizol, Klion, Efloran, Metronidazole | 500 mg every 8 hours |
| Gentamicin | Gentamicin | 240 mg once daily |
| Amikacin | Amikin | 1–1.5 g once daily |
| Ciprofloxacin | Ciprobay, Ciprinol, Ciphin, Ciplox, Cifloxinal | 400 mg every 12 hours |
| Ofloxacin | Tarivid, Ofloxin, Taroflox, Zanocin | 200–400 mg every 12 hours |
| Vankomycin | Vancocin, Edicin | 1 g every 12 hours |

\* p.e. – parenteral administration,  \*\* MIU – international units

pression, presence of foreign material), secondary diseases and the state of the patient's natural immunity. Antibiotic therapy on average lasts seven or ten days at the maximum, however, some infections must be treated for weeks or even months (for example osteomyelitis, actinomycosis).

### 8. Toxicity and Side Effects of Selected Antibiotics
Medical drugs with minimal toxicity and low incidence of side effects should always be preferred. The cumulative toxicity can occur especially if two or more different antibiotics are combined (nephrotoxicity in the event of the combination of aminoglycosides with vancomycin).

## 30.8 Principles of Antibiotic Prophylaxis during Surgical Procedures

**The main aim** of prophylaxis in surgery is to decrease the risk of SSI that might result from bacterial contamination of the operating field. The **principle** consists in the achievement of efficient, i.e. optimum bactericidal concentration of antibiotics in the operating field during the whole surgical procedure. The spectrum of antibiotic effect should correspond to the bacterial flora that could most probably be present in the particular place.

Application of broad-spectrum antibiotics is improper since it does not increase the efficiency of prophylaxis but significantly impairs the patient's natural bacterial flora with all the possible negative consequences (dysmicrobia, superinfection, etc.).

### THE PRINCIPLES OF APPROPRIATE PROPHYLAXIS INCLUDE

- The optimum spectrum of the drug in relation to the place and type of procedure
- Preferably bactericidal effect
- Adequate pharmacokinetics, i.e. achievement of adequate concentration in the target tissue
- Appropriate timing in most drugs requires 20 to 30 minutes after IV application prior to the incision
- A sufficient dose corresponding to at least the usual therapeutic dose and taking into account the patient's weight
- Repeated peroperative administration in longer lasting procedures (more than 3 hours) and in the event of large blood loss
- Short-time application, i.e. a maximum of 24 hours. Postoperative administration loses its justification and evidently does not decrease the incidence of postoperative infections

### PROFYLAXIS IS INDICATED IN THE EVENT OF:

- A high risk of contamination of the operating field (colorectal surgery)
- Significant disposition to develop infection (immunosuppression, implanted foreign material)
- Threat of serious infectious complications with devastating consequences (even in situations when the risk of SSI is low, like mediastinitis in cardiac surgery)

The most frequently used antimicrobial drugs, suitable for prophylaxis and reflecting the type of procedure and its localization are: aminopenicillins, inhibitor-protected aminopenicillins (ampicillin/sulbactam, amoxicillin/clavulanate), $1^{st}$ and $2^{nd}$ generation cephalosporins, imidazoles (metronidazole), clindamycin (in the case of allergy to penicillins and cephalosporins).

Other groups of antibiotics are selected individually as an alternative in situations when the above mentioned drugs cannot be used, most often due to allergy or because of a reasonable risk of infection with highly resistant bacteria (MRSA – methicillin resistant *Staphylococcus aureus*).

# 31 HEMATOLOGICAL ISSUES IN SURGERY

> 31.1 Antithrombotic Prophylaxis in Surgery
> 31.2 Operation on Patients Receiving Chronic Anticoagulant and Antiaggregant Therapy
> 31.3 Surgical Treatment in Patients with Neutropenia and Thrombocytopenia
> 31.4 Significant Acquired Bleeding Disorders in Surgical Patients
> 31.5 Splenectomy and its Management

## 31.1 Antithrombotic Prophylaxis in Surgery

Thromboprophylaxis applied in surgical procedures has significantly decreased the incidence of postoperative venous thromboembolism (VTE) and pulmonary embolism. Its management is based on the international "Guidelines on Antithrombotic Prophylaxis and Antithrombotic and Thrombolytic Therapy in Conditions Associated with Thrombophilia and Thrombosis" published regularly by the ACCP (American College of Chest Physicians). The 8th ACCP conference was held in 2008. This recommendation is based on the risk assessment of postoperative thrombosis according to the type and duration of the operation, patient's age (Tab. 31.1), and the presence of additional risk factors (Tab. 31.2). Apart from the antithrombotic effect of therapy, the risk of bleeding and economic cost of the treatment is assessed here (Tab. 31.3).

■ Table 31.1 Stratification of VTE risk based on the type and duration of the operation and the patient's age

| Type of operation |  |
| --- | --- |
| • Minor surgical procedure, duration less than 30 min. |  |
| • Major surgical procedure |  |
| Patient's age |  |
| • Under 40 years |  |
| • 40–60 years |  |
| • Above 60 years |  |

**Table 31.2** Important additional risk factors in surgical patients

| Risk factors |
| --- |
| Obesity, smoking, VTE in patient's history, varices |
| Significant internal diseases |
| Heart and respiratory failure |
| Congenital thrombophilia |
| Tumors and their treatment |
| Pregnancy and puerperium |
| Contraception and hormonal substitution |
| Immobility |

### EXTENDED THROMBOPROPHYLAXIS

In patients who have undergone an extensive surgical procedure, in high risk patients with a history of deep venous thrombosis or in those operated on for a malignant tumor, extended administration of LMWH is recommended up to 28 days after discharge from hospital.

## 31.2 Operation on Patients Receiving Chronic Anticoagulant and Antiaggregant Therapy

### 31.2.1 Preoperative Management in Patients on Warfarin Therapy

Patients on warfarin therapy must be prepared for the surgical procedure. Chronic anticoagulant therapy always has its own reasons. Its discontinuation with the aim to achieve normal INR values represents a significant risk of thromboembolic complications. A temporary reduction of the warfarin dose for several days with a target INR value just below 2.0 allows for a minor surgical procedure only. In major surgical procedures, the preoperative management consists in warfarin discontinuation concurrently with initiation of LMWH prophylaxis.

In indicated cases in patients with a high risk of VTE, LMWH is administered in therapeutic doses as a bridge anticoagulant therapy. The duration of postoperative LMWH administration and the time to switch back to warfarin depends on the extent of the surgical procedure, the patient's condition and other factors that reflect the risk of VTE.

**Table 31.3** Prophylaxis in surgery based on the risk assessment of VTE depending on the type of procedure, patient's age and additional risk factors, adapted according to a possible risk of bleeding, and the method of prophylaxis on the basis of the 8th ACCP

| Risk of VTE | Type of procedure | Recommended prophylaxis |
|---|---|---|
| Low risk of VTE (≤ 10% risk without prophylaxis) | • Minor surgical procedure<br>• Procedure in local anesthesia in fully mobile patients | Without specific prophylaxis, only early and consistent mobilization |
| Medium risk (10–40% risk without prophylaxis) | • Minor procedure in a patient with additional risk factors, under 40 years<br>• Surgery at the age of 40–60 years without additional risk factors | LMWH in prophylactic dose once a day s.c. or<br>Compressive stockings / IPC or<br>LDUH 3× daily s.c.<br>Fondaparinux once a day s.c. |
| Medium risk (10–40% risk without prophylaxis) and *high risk of bleeding* | • The same type of operation with a medium risk of venous thrombosis | Compressive stockings / IPC |
| High risk (40–80% risk without prophylaxis) | • Operation on a patient over 60 years of age<br>• Operation at the age of 40–60 years with multiple additional risk factors<br>• Major procedure (hip or knee replacement, polytrauma, spinal cord trauma) | LMWH once a day s.c. or<br>LDUH 3× daily s.c.<br>or<br>Fondaparinux once a day<br>+ combination with gradient compression / IPC |
| High risk (40–80% risk without prophylaxis) and *high risk of bleeding* | • The same type of operation with a high risk of venous thrombosis | Individual approach and compressive stockings / IPC |

*LMWH – low-molecular-weight heparin, LDUH – low-dose unfractioned heparin (5000 U), IPC – intermittent pneumatic compression*

## 31.2.2 Reversal of Anticoagulant Effect of Warfarin Before an Urgent Operation

An urgent operation on a patient on warfarin therapy requires special action since the anticoagulant effect of warfarin must be reversed within several hours to reach the target INR under 1.5.

This can be achieved by the administration of vitamin K (Kanavit) in a slow IV infusion (½–1 vial). The decrease of INR can be reached faster if a fresh plasma (1–2 units) IV is delivered at the same time. In emergency situations substitution therapy with prothrombin complex can be administered. Prothromplex Total is a product containing vitamin K-dependent coagulation factors II (prothrombin), VII, IX, and X. The dosage depends on the value of INR. Repeated coagulation tests are essential. The surgical procedure can be started once the INR value declines to 1.3–1.5. Subsequent administration of LMWH prophylaxis or bridge therapy (the dosage and timing) is individual and depends on the actual condition of hemostasis and the degree of VTE risk.

### 31.2.3  Antiaggregant Therapy in Surgical Patients

In patients on long-term Aspirin or clopidogrel therapy (patients suffering from a chronic form of ischemic heart disease, ischemic disease of the lower extremities, conditions after cerebral stroke) the treatment should be discontinued 7–10 days before the planned procedure. The therapy can be resumed 24 hours after the procedure if the state of hemostasis is satisfactory. A special approach is necessary in patients with a high risk of heart events (patients with coronary stents) where Aspirin therapy should not be interrupted. The risk assessment and perioperative management is provided by a cardiologist. Bleeding in patients on antiaggregant therapy can be resolved by a platelet transfusion.

## 31.3  Surgical Treatment in Patients with Neutropenia and Thrombocytopenia

**Neutropenia** is a decrease of the absolute neutrophil count (ANC) $<1.5 \times 10^9$/L. It is associated with a risk of severe infections that increases with the grade of neutropenia. In patients with ANC $<0.5 \times 10^9$/L the risk is extremely high.

The risk of infection in neutropenic patients depends on:
- The grade of neutropenia
- Its duration
- The primary cause that resulted in neutropenia
- The patient's general condition

The etiology of severe neutropenia comprises bacterial sepsis, viral infections and aplasia after medication. Neutropenia also accompanies systemic diseases and hypersplenism; it is frequent in oncological patients after chemotherapy, whereas in hematological malignancies it is associated with the disease itself as well.

In patients with neutropenia a surgical procedure represents a significant problem. In elective operations, neutropenia is a contraindication to surgery. In acute

# HEMATOLOGICAL ISSUES IN SURGERY

conditions, operation on a neutropenic patient is acceptable only under vital indications.

The perioperative management consists in administration of broad-spectrum antibiotics with sufficient effect anaerobic organisms. The most frequent combinations: beta-lactam antibiotics (penicillins, cephalosporins, and carbapenems) with aminoglycosides administered by IV. The antibiotic prophylaxis should be consulted with the hospital's antibiotic center.

Granulocyte-colony stimulating factor (G-CSF) is used in indicated cases.

**Thrombocytopenia** accompanies many diseases and it can result from a large number of diverse causes.

The risk of spontaneous bleeding is associated with a profound decrease of thrombocytes to lows of $10–20 \times 10^9/L$. Higher platelet counts must be reached for a surgical procedure, depending on the operation type, the nature of thrombocytopenia and the general state of hemostasis (plasmatic coagulation and platelet function).

A minimal required platelet count varies depending on the extent of the operation:
- Minor surgical procedures, skin biopsies, endoscopies without tissue sampling:
  – Thrombocytes above $20 \times 10^9/L$
- Major abdominal and chest operations, lung and liver biopsies, endoscopic procedures with tissue sampling, central cannulation, etc.:
  – Thrombocytes above $60 \times 10^9/L$
- Orthopedic, urological and neurosurgical operations:
  – Thrombocytes above $100 \times 10^9/L$

The most efficient method is a transfusion of thrombocytes collected by apheresis, 1 TU leading to an increase of platelet count by up to $30 \times 10^9/L$. In patients permanently treated with platelet transfusions, a transfusion of 1 TU usually does not suffice. In extensive procedures associated with a high risk of bleeding (orthopedics, urology, spine surgery), platelets must be transfused even during the operation and the platelet transfusion should also be available for the postoperative period.

A special approach in preoperative management is required in patients with immune thrombocytopenia that usually do not respond to substitution therapy. In patients with refractory ITP, collaboration between the hematologist and surgeon prior to a splenectomy is essential.

## 31.4 Significant Acquired Bleeding Disorders in Surgical Patients

### 31.4.1 Hepatic Insufficiency

Surgery on patients suffering from hepatic cirrhosis is more often associated with the risk of bleeding than with thrombotic complications.

This is caused by a hypocoagulation state resulting from:
- Thrombocytopenia (increased platelet sequestration in the spleen) or thrombopathy
- Hypoproduction coagulopathy (decreased synthesis of coagulation factors, dysfibrinogenemia)
- Consumption of coagulation factors in chronic DIC syndrome
- Increased fibrinolytic activity

The indication for surgery must be carefully considered, a detailed hemocoagulation analysis is essential. The preparation of a patient for the operation consists in the substitution of all deficient components. Apart from the administration of vitamin K, frozen plasma and concentrate of prothrombin complex, a platelet transfusion and correction of the level of antithrombin is usually needed.

### 31.4.2 Disseminated Intravascular Coagulopathy (DIC)

DIC is a feared bleeding complication of surgical procedures and injuries, above all of those that lead to extensive tissue devastation, last for a long period of time or are accompanied by marked blood loss. This coagulation disorder is always acquired; it results from a pathological activation of systemic coagulation with a gradual exhaustion of the coagulation potential of blood. Typically, DIC has three phases:
- Activation
- Consumption
- Hyperfibrinolysis, defibrination phase

Clinical manifestations of DIC vary. In the phase of hypercoagulation, the formation of microthrombi, microcirculatory impairment and organ dysfunction develop. This clinically correlates with different manifestations of organ failure as a part of MOF. DIC usually does not manifest until the phase of bleeding diathesis, with an evident decrease of plasmatic coagulation factors, fibrinogen, antithrombin and the platelet count, and with the presence of fibrinogen degradation products in laboratory tests. The treatment consists mainly in prompt elimination of the primary cause of DIC. Correcting coagulopathy that has already developed is difficult. In patients treated in ICU, the monitoring of laboratory values, prompt response to changes and a multidisciplinary approach are essential. In the initial phase of coagulopathy, the administration of heparin (usually prophylactic doses of LMWH) and above all a consistent antithrombin substitution are effective. In the phase of hypocoagulation, replacement of individual components of the coagulation system (transfusion of frozen plasma, fibrinogen, and platelets), the administration of prothrombin complex concentrate, recombinant activated factor VII or antifibrinolytics are necessary.

## 31.5 Splenectomy and its Management

A splenectomy represents a risk for the patient due to two reasons: the first being thrombosis, the second infection.

### 31.5.1 Thrombocytosis and the Risk of Portal Vein Thrombosis

Postsplenectomy thrombocytosis represents an example of reactive thrombocytosis where the thrombocytes can reach genuinely high values (platelets > 1000 × $10^9$/L). It can develop during the first postoperative week and can persist over a long period of time. In otherwise healthy patients the thrombotic complications usually do not emerge; the usage of Anopyrin is, however, recommended. In hematological patients with myeloproliferative disease or hemolytic anemia, the prophylactic usage of LMWH for a splenectomy is necessary. The decrease of the platelet count is gradual and it is not a mistake to extend the LMWH administration even after discharge from the hospital if the platelet count does not decrease below 800 × $10^9$/L. Anopyrin administration can be continued until hematologic tests show normal results.

### 31.5.2 Risk of Infection

The spleen architecture, circulation and presence of immunocompetent cells determine the cardinal role of the spleen in the immunity of the organism. A risk of serious infections increases after a splenectomy, their fulminant course is called **OPSI syndrome** (overwhelming post-splenectomy infection). The most feared pathogens are *Streptococcus pneumoniae* (in adults), *Haemophilus influenzae* (in children) and *Neisseria meningitidis*. The incidence of the OPSI syndrome is approximately 4%, however, its mortality is high. The risk of OPSI is higher during childhood and in hemato-oncological patients where the disease itself and its treatment cause further immunosuppression. Due to the risk of OPSI, **immunoprophylaxis** with recommended vaccines is carried out: 23-valent pneumococcal, conjugated haemophilus and meningococcal vaccines.

Before performing an elective splenectomy, there is enough time to administer all three vaccines, preferably 3–4 weeks prior to the surgery. After an unplanned, for example a traumatic splenectomy, or forced splenectomy during another operation, patients should be vaccinated as soon as possible after the operation. All three vaccines can be administered together at the same time or with a minimum interval in between. Recommended prophylactic antibiotics comprise V-Penicillin, amoxicillin/clavulanate, cefuroxime and second-generation cephalosporins. Long-term antibiotic prophylaxis is questionable.

# 32 ANESTHESIOLOGY AND RESUSCITATION IN SURGERY

*32.1 Terminology Used*
*32.2 Anesthesiological Techniques*
*32.3 The Most Widely Used Pharmaceuticals*
*32.4 Providing for Anesthesiological Care*
*32.5 Collective Cooperation with the Anesthesiologist*

**The perioperative care** of surgical patients has a multidisciplinary character, with the participation of physicians and other health care professionals of many disciplines.

Successful operation indispensably requires that the operated patient be anesthetized; without it the surgical treatment, just as with certain complicated diagnostic procedures, would be unthinkable. In a small portion of minor surgical procedures, local anesthesia can be provided by the operating surgeon him/herself, infiltrating the operating field with local anesthetics. Nevertheless, in the vast majority of operations anesthesia is provided by an anesthesiologist. Hence the collaboration between anesthesiologist and surgeon is crucial for the patient's successful treatment with minimum associated risks.

**An anesthesiologist** is a specialist in anesthesia and intensive care medicine. Preoperatively, he/she evaluates the patient's condition; assesses the risks and collaborates in preparing the patient for a surgical procedure. He/she provides anesthesiological care during the operation. In the course of the operation, he/she delivers anesthesia – he/she provides for a painless course of the operation, minimizes the impact of operative trauma on the patient's condition and maintains the stability of basic vital functions. He/she takes cares of airway patency, respiratory and circulatory stability and controls the internal environment and maintenance of body temperature. He/she monitors the patient's condition visually and with technical instruments, evaluates the obtained data and maintains mandatory medical records. He/she also participates in the postoperative care, focusing mainly on the painless course, respiratory and circulatory stability and homeostasis.

Hence **anesthesiological care** comprises not only the period of the surgical procedure itself, but also the preoperative and postoperative periods.

ANESTHESIOLOGY AND RESUSCITATION IN SURGERY

## 32.1 Terminology Used

**Anesthesia** – the loss of perception and sensation

**Analgesia** – the loss of perception of pain
Anesthesia and analgesia can be **general** or **local**:
- **General anesthesia** – a complete loss of perception and sensation affecting the whole organism; it is associated with decreased consciousness. General anesthesia also includes muscle relaxation and immobility of the operated patient.
- **Local anesthesia** – the loss of perception and sensation is limited only to the anesthetized area, consciousness is not primarily affected
- **General analgesia** – perception of pain is suppressed by systemic medication with analgesics
- **Local analgesia** – suppressed perception of pain only in the specified area. Techniques of local anesthesia are employed using a lower concentration of local anesthetics.

**Analgosedation** – pharmacological procedure leading to the patient's sedation, amnesia and decreased perception of pain. During the analgosedation the consciousness is minimally suppressed; protective reflexes and the patient's capability of cooperation are preserved.

**Anesthesiological supervision** – monitored anesthesiological care. It is usually required for procedures where other forms of anesthesia are not necessary or applicable (e.g. in diagnostic procedures), or in situations where the operating surgeon him/herself carries out local infiltrative anesthesia. The anesthesiologist takes care of the general condition of the operated patient and observes him/her in the same way as in the event of other anesthesiological techniques, and maintains the same documentation.

## 32.2 Anesthesiological Techniques

### 32.2.1 Methods of General Anesthesia Used

**Monoanesthesia** – anesthesia induced with a single active pharmaceutical (anesthetic). According to the route of administration of the anesthetic into the body, we distinguish several types of anesthesia:
- Inhalational (via the lungs)
- Intravenous (via intravenous administration)
- Intramuscular (rarely, only in exceptional situations)
- Rectal (quite rarely, usable only in children)

**Complementary anesthesia** – individual components of anesthesia (loss of consciousness, painlessness, muscle relaxation) are affected selectively by different drugs. Anesthetic complementation may be concurrent – administration of inhalational anesthetic is complemented with intravenous analgesics and myorelaxant drugs, or sequential – intravenous induction is usually followed by inhalational anesthesia. Complementary anesthesia also exists in a purely intravenous form: hypnotic and analgesic administration via an infusion complemented with drugs that potentiate muscle relaxation. In contrast to monoanesthesia, complementary anesthesia is globally more effective while having fewer risks of local anesthesia side effects.

**Combined anesthesia** – techniques of global anesthesia are combined with techniques of local, usually epidural anesthesia.

### 32.2.2 Methods of Local Anesthesia Used

Nowadays the most frequently used methods comprise epidural and subarachnoid anesthesia and nerve blocks.

#### EPIDURAL ANESTHESIA

In epidural anesthesia, the local anesthetic is administered into the vertebral canal, outside the spinal dura mater. Then it defuses along the spinal roots and partially through the spinal dura mater into the cerebrospinal fluid – having the proper effect on the spinal roots and spinal structures. The route of administration of the local anesthetic can be situated at various levels of the spine after penetrating the yellow ligament.

According to the spinal level of puncture, epidural anesthesia can be divided into **thoracic** and **lumbar**; cervical anesthesia is used quite rarely. The epidural space can also be penetrated through the hiatus canalis sacralis puncturing the membrana sacrococcygea – so-called **caudal anesthesia**.

The level of puncture, i.e. the entry into the epidural space, is the most important factor defining the anesthetized field. Concentration of administered local anesthetic determines the intensity of the anesthesia –anesthesia or analgesia can be induced depending on the concentration. The volume of local anesthetic used determines the segmental extent or width of the operating field. The initial effect of the administered anesthetic is rather slow, lasting 15–35 minutes.

Local anesthetics can be administered as a **single dose** or as a **continuous infusion** via an epidural catheter. This enables the extension of epidural anesthesia to epidural analgesia just by a simple change in the concentration of the active drug.

#### SUBARACHNOID ANESTHESIA (SO-CALLED SPINAL ANESTHESIA)

In subarachnoid anesthesia, after performing a lumbar puncture, the anesthetic is delivered directly into cerebrospinal fluid and from there it diffuses into the spinal structures where it acts. The puncture is carried out in the region of the lumbar spine. A very small amount of local anesthetic (several milliliters) is used. The character of anesthesia depends on the character of the administered solution (a hypobaric solution rises through capillary action upwards, and on the contrary, hyperbaric solution falls downwards) and the position the patient takes shortly after the application of the local anesthetic. Within a short period of time the active substance fixates to the spinal structures and takes effect promptly – within minutes. For practical reasons (the risk of cerebrospinal fluid leakage and the risk of infection) only a one-time application of the local anesthetic is used. The advantage of the subarachnoid (spinal) anesthesia is its high intensity including excellent muscle relaxation. Regarding the place of anesthetic administration and the risk of respiratory suppression, this type of anesthesia can be used only in operations distally from the navel and on the lower extremities.

In epidural and subarachnoid anesthesia other active substances, usually morphine and opioids, can be added to the solution of the local anesthetic. The analgesic effect is increased and deepened and the risk of side effects of local anesthetics is reduced.

### NERVE BLOCKS

The application of a sufficient amount of local anesthetics into fascial spaces in immediate proximity to the main nerve trunks results in anesthesia in an innervated area of corresponding nerves, enabling an operation. Due to its character, this anesthesia is intended mainly for procedures on extremities. In a nerve block the procedure itself as well as the assessment of a sufficient amount of the local anesthetics is difficult, which results in the risk of toxicity. It is crucial that the active substance be administered properly in close proximity to the main nerve or nerves. Identification of a suitable place for administration just based on surrounding anatomical structures is not reliable. The administration based on previous induction of paresthesias is more reliable; however, this is associated with a risk of nerve damage with potential long-term consequences. Currently, the most appropriate method of identification of the correct place of administration is the determination of the position of the needle and surrounding structures by an ultrasound.

An intravenous local anesthesia (the so-called Bier block) used to be employed for procedures on extremities; however, due to the high risk of side effects has been practically abandoned.

## 32.3 The Most Widely Used Pharmaceuticals

- For intravenous **induction** of general anesthesia: thiopental, methohexital, propofol, etomidate, midazolam, ketamine
- For **maintenance** of general anesthesia: (in a mixture with nitrous oxide or separately) isoflurane, sevoflurane, desflurane
- For intensification of **analgesia**: phentanyl, sufentanil, alfentanil, remifentanil

TEXTBOOK OF SURGERY

- For **muscle relaxation**
  - At the beginning of anesthesia and during tracheal intubation: suxamethonium
  - In the course of anesthesia: vecuronium, pancuronium, pipecuronium, rocuronium (can also be used in the induction of anesthesia), atracurium, cis-atracurium, mivacurium
- The most frequent **antidotes** used during global anesthesia: atropine, neostigmine, naloxone, flumazenil
- **Local anesthetics**: trimecaine, bupivacaine, levobupivacaine, articaine, tetracaine, prilocaine, lidocaine

Note: Propofol or midazolam can be administered continuously together with alfentanil, remifentanil or ketamine to maintain global, solely intravenous anesthesia. For induction and maintenance of intramuscular anesthesia (for example under extraordinary conditions) ketamine can be administered.

## 32.4 Providing for Anesthesiological Care

### 32.4.1 Preoperative Period

■ CONSULTATION PRIOR TO THE PLANNED PROCEDURE

The anesthesiologist meets the patient in advance prior to a planned procedure, preferably at the outpatient Department of Anesthesiology. The examination has the character of a consultation. During the examination the anesthesiologist:
- Gets acquainted with the preoperative internal examinations and other additional tests and evaluates them
- Gets acquainted with the surgical findings, indication for the procedure, the operation plan, the patient's placement in the operation program and with the quantity of reserved transfusions (if needed)
- Performs a basic examination of the patient at least by aspection and gets information that may be significant for the management and safety of anesthesia
- Assesses the risks according to the American Society of Anesthesiologists (ASA) score, classifying the patient into one of the groups (see below)
- Determines the anesthesiological preparation: fasting, respiratory gymnastics, administration of parenteral medication instead of oral drugs, etc.
- Specifies pre-premedication and premedication
- Determines the plan of anesthesia
- Provides the patient in a reassuring and comprehensible manner with an explanation of the planned medical procedure, stimulates the patient's motivation for cooperation and obtains his/her informed consent.

■ CONSULTATION PRIOR TO AN URGENT PROCEDURE

In the event of urgent procedures, unconscious patients, patients in serious conditions, and the risk of delay, the consultation can exceptionally take place even at admission or in the operating room. It is reduced just to the basic examination that allows an estimation of the gravity of the patient's condition. The anesthesiologist promptly gets acquainted with the planned procedure, determines the premedication and the manner of performance of the anesthesiological procedure. A conscious and stressed patient is approached with the utmost consideration and the anesthesiologist always tries to provide a comforting atmosphere without pain.

## ASA CLASSIFICATION

Preoperative and subsequent anesthesiological examinations result in the patient's categorization into one of five ASA classification groups that express the risk level:
- ASA 1: a patient without complicating chronic diseases under 50 years of age
- ASA 2: a patient with a stabilized and fully compensated chronic disease which does not limit the patient's activity, or a patient over 50 years of age
- ASA 3: a patient with a systemic disease that limits the patient's activity
- ASA 4: a patient with a severe, insufficiently compensated or decompensated systemic disease that is life-threatening
- ASA 5: a moribund patient for whom the operation represents the last chance for saving his/her life

(Bulletin of the Ministry of Health of the Czech Republic part 8, 7/1997)

In the event of an urgent procedure (where there is no time available for all the required examinations or proper preoperative preparation) a letter E (emergency) is added to this classification. It expresses that the patient's condition is worse than the corresponding grade of ASA.

## SELECTION OF ANESTHESIA

**Selection of anesthesia and its provision** during the operation is affected by a number of circumstances:
- The character and extent of the surgical procedure
- Whether the procedure is urgent or elective
- The patient's general condition
- Whether the patient is treated on an outpatient basis (i.e. whether he/she is discharged for home care on the day of operation), or on an inpatient basis
- The patient's preferences (in the event the procedure can be performed under both general and local anesthesia, the patient may choose)

## ANESTHETIC PLAN

The main task of the anesthesiologist in the preoperative period is to utilize all available time to improve the patient's general condition and thus to provide for the maximum safety of the upcoming surgical procedure. The anesthesiologist thereby contributes to a good outcome of the surgical therapy. He/she cooper-

ates with a number of other medical consultants and incorporates results of their examinations and their recommendations into preoperative preparation and modifies the **anesthetic plan**. The anesthetic plan includes the following elements:
- Whether the anesthesia is general or local
- In the event of general anesthesia the decision whether to apply inhalational, intravenous, complementary or combined anesthesia
- What medical drugs, tools and instruments are to be prepared
- What infusion solutions (crystalloids or colloids) and what transfusions are to be prepared or reserved
- The position in which the operation will be performed, potential requirements of the operating surgeon in the course of the procedure
- What equipment to prepare to cope with possible complications.

The anesthesiologist **records** the main data on the findings, the assessed risk and a conclusion into the medical documentation.

### PREPARING THE PATIENT FOR SURGERY

Before the planned operation, the patient is required to **fast for at least 6 hours**. Fluid intake (water, tea, mineral water, fruit juice) in adequate quantity is permitted until 2 hours before the induction of anesthesia. During this period fluids can also be used to wash down oral premedication.

The patient's preparation for the planned procedure culminates with the administration of **pre-premedication** and **premedication**. The medication induces tranquilization up to mild sedation, and a relaxed feeling. It enables good sleep and rest prior to the procedure. Nevertheless, pharmaceuticals cannot replace a hospitable environment, empathic behavior and the professional approach of the medical staff. They block some of undesirable circulatory and other reflexes of vagal innervation and decrease excessive salivation. Selection of pharmaceuticals, the route of administration and dose assessment are the anesthesiologist's tasks.

The operating surgeon's responsibilities include indication for the procedure and its timing. In emergency events the required length of fasting cannot be met and the anesthesiologist must make every effort to minimize the **risk of vomiting, regurgitation and aspiration of the gastric content** at the beginning of anesthesia and during its course. Analogously, in emergency situations premedication can be modified or even omitted.

### 32.4.2 Peroperative Provisions and Administration of Anesthesia

Before the administration of anesthesia the patient must be always correctly identified, his/her planned surgical procedure must be confirmed (in pair organs also the operated side must be confirmed) and all necessary instruments, tools and medication must be properly examined to assure that they are ready for the operation. Also all necessary equipment and medication for extended life support must be available.

## ANESTHESIOLOGY AND RESUSCITATION IN SURGERY

Providing for painlessness and loss of consciousness are not the only aspects sufficient for the performance of the operation. Abdominal surgery also requires the relaxation of abdominal wall muscles. Opening of the abdominal or chest cavity is an indication for mechanical ventilation. After opening the chest cavity, the anesthesiologist employs a special technique that enables lung ventilation only on the side contrary to the side of the operation. The operation on an open heart is performed with the use of extracorporeal circulation. The anesthesiologist also has at his/her disposal other adjuvant methods that facilitate surgical performance or decrease its risks (e.g. induced hypotension, etc.).

The peroperative **anesthesiological care** is the principal task of the anesthesiologist. The **main components** are:
- Anesthesia (provision of the loss of consciousness if the procedure is performed under general anesthesia)
- Analgesia (provision of painlessness)
- Muscle relaxation
- Stabilization of the patient's condition (adequate ventilation – mechanical ventilation if needed, maintenance of bloodstream pressure, maintenance of body temperature, vegetative stabilization)

**The patient's monitoring** during all procedures is focused mainly on his/her vital functions. The basic monitored functions include:
- Heart rate, its regularity and quality, blood pressure
- Perfusion and color of the skin and mucosa, acral capillary perfusion, capillary refill
- Airway patency or quality of its provision, respiratory rate and volume
- Sufficient suppression of reflex activity and adequate depth of unconsciousness (in general anesthesia)

The monitoring includes a summation ECG lead (usually lead II), pulse oximetry ($SpO_2$) and in laparoscopic procedures employing capnoperitoneum and in neurosurgical intracranial procedures also $CO_2$ concentration at the end of expiration (capnometry or capnography). The range of monitored parameters depends on the extent of the operation, its risks and the patient's condition.

The anesthesiologist carefully monitors the course of operation phases and without delay informs the operating surgeon about serious changes in the patient's condition. He/she controls circulatory stability which is conditioned by sufficiently deep anesthesia, good analgesia and adequate bloodstream pressure. Episodes of hypotension and tachycardia are very dangerous, as they are often followed by significant cardiovascular complications in the postoperative period. The anesthesiologist **maintains body temperature** by technical means.

Basic information about the patient's condition prior to anesthesia, in its course, and at discharge from anesthesiological care are recorded in writing. The record forms part of the patient's medical documentation.

The anesthesiologist takes care of the operated patient **from the moment of his/her arrival** at the operating room where he/she receives the patient, until the patient **wakes up from anesthesia**, his/her condition stabilizes and his/her protective reflexes recover, or he/she can possibly be transferred to another member of the medical staff.

After serious procedures and after operations on high risk the patients are transferred to surgical ICU for monitoring and treatment.

In the event of peroperative life-threatening complications, after resuscitation, if long unconsciousness is expected requiring mechanical ventilation, and in conditions requiring extracorporeal eliminating methods, the patients are usually transferred to the inpatient Department of Anesthesiology and Resuscitation.

### 32.4.3   Postoperative Period

From the safety viewpoint, the postoperative period is a risky phase when the **state of consciousness, circulation and breathing must be closely observed and monitored, and in indicated situations homeostasis should be examined**. This is the phase of terminating and subsiding anesthesia and transition from anesthesia and operation trauma into a stabilized condition with recovered consciousness and alertness.

**A quality postoperative analgesia** is essential. It continuously extends the subsiding effect of postoperative analgesics and local anesthetics.

The exact duration cannot be specified. It usually ranges from 2 hours after termination of an uncomplicated procedure performed in an uneventful general anesthesia, to the interval of 4–6 hours which is typical for outpatient procedures, up to several postoperative days during which even a patient with a severe medical condition after a complicated operation should be stabilized.

**The main risks** in the immediate postoperative period include:
- Hypoventilation due to subsiding anesthesia if the muscle relaxation is not terminated or is not subsiding adequately
- Hidden shock with borderline blood pressure and circulatory centralization due to insufficient replacement of general losses
- Surgical complications, mainly bleeding requiring surgery

After a short uncomplicated procedure, the patient should be capable of responding and reliably fulfilling a simple task – to loll his/her tongue, press a hand, raise the head 5 cm above the pad and maintain it without effort in this position while coughing. Intensity of the patient's monitoring should reflect his/her risk and even in the category of common risks observation for a certain period of time is necessary. A recovery room where operated patients are gathered is appropriate.

**An outpatient** is discharged once he/she achieves self-sufficiency in dressing, if he/she does not suffer from pain, does not vomit, has spontaneously voided and when there are no evident signs of surgical complications. He/she is brought home by an accompanying person after being instructed on how to behave at least during the first 24 hours; during such period he/she is not allowed to stay at home without being supervised by an adult and properly instructed person.

### POSTOPERATIVE ANALGESIA

Providing for maximum pain relief is not only a necessary precondition for the patient's comfort, but it is directly associated with the incidence and degree of circulatory and respiratory complications, with wound healing and with the patient's capacity for early mobilization and rehabilitation. The course of the disease of a patient who does not suffer from pain is usually milder. Pain is a significant pathogenetic factor and its suppression requires utmost efforts. Self-perception of pain should be assessed by the patient (e.g. with a visual analog scale – VAS) and the obtained data should be entered into the patient's medical records.

The most common type of postoperative analgesia comprises **systemic medication** with parenteral opiates or opioids supplemented with non-opioid analgesics. Since the pain perception and the effect of analgesics markedly vary between individual persons, the dose must always be titred to achieve the desired effect. The route of administration is usually intramuscular injection; however, in ICU the continuous intravenous administration of analgesics by a linear perfusor can be used.

**Continuous epidural analgesia** is a very efficient technique of postoperative analgesia. It usually follows a previous combined anesthesia and uses an epidural catheter already inserted on this occasion. The epidural catheter can also be inserted postoperatively.

**Patient controlled analgesia** (PCA) allows the patient to regulate the supply of analgesics at his/her discretion reflecting his/her own pain perception. PCA can be used together with intravenous or epidural administration of other pharmaceuticals. The method is technically demanding, nevertheless, it is efficient and safe – the attending physician defines the maximum administered dose and after an additional dose for a defined period of time the machine does not react to the patient's further attempts to increase the dose. The risk of overdose is thus eliminated; however, within the defined limits the patient has the option to adjust the dosing to his/her needs.

## 32.5 Collective Cooperation with the Anesthesiologist

The collective cooperation can have basically two forms.

The anesthesiologist is frequently asked by the surgeon to assess the risk of the considered operative solution in a polymorbid patient. More often he/she is asked to attend a patient who has already been operated on and whose course of recovery is getting complicated. The reason for collective examination is usually a newly emerged disorder of consciousness, respiratory and circulatory insufficiency, or the development of a sepsis syndrome or renal insufficiency. The anesthesiologist is expected to examine the patient properly and to get acquainted with available results of laboratory and imaging examinations. He/she suggests other examinations if needed, assesses the seriousness of the patient's condition and on the basis of differential diagnostic analysis determines a preliminary diagnosis. He/she proposes measures to avert imminent danger, recommends other therapeutic procedures and decides whether the patient can continue the treatment at the given department or should be transferred to the Department of Anesthesiology and Intensive Medicine. In the event that the transfer is necessary, he/she arranges for it. He/she enters all findings and recommendations into the patient's medical records.

On the contrary a surgical patient can be, on a planned or unplanned basis, admitted or transferred to the Department of Anesthesiology and Intensive Medicine. The reason for admission is a present or imminent failure of basic vital functions – consciousness, breathing or circulation that are to be supported or compensated. At the same time the patient must be observed and monitored by technical means. At this point the surgeon becomes the cooperating physician. In collaboration with the attending doctor he/she assesses the patient's condition and recommends examinations or therapeutic measures including operations if needed. The Department of Anesthesiology and Intensive Medicine provides the patient with complete care – mechanical ventilation, pharmacological or even mechanical circulatory support, extracorporeal eliminating methods compensating insufficient renal function, parenteral or enteral nutrition, and anti-infective medication. The patient's consciousness and pain perception is pharmacologically suppressed and contact with him/her is very limited. In such situations, the clinical picture and course of surgical complications significantly varies, often with atypical development. The surgeon's orientation in the situation and his/her recommendations about further steps are difficult. From the viewpoint of communication and content, interdisciplinary collaboration is thus becoming an exceptionally demanding dimension.

# 33  MULTIMODAL ONCOLOGICAL TREATMENT

*33.1 Surgical Treatment*
*33.2 Chemotherapy*
*33.3 Radiotherapy*
*33.4 Hormonal Therapy*
*33.5 Biological Targeted Therapy*

Cancer undoubtedly belongs to the most serious pathological conditions. The number of patients with malignancies has been permanently increasing both worldwide and in the Czech Republic, where every third person suffers from and every fourth one dies of a malignancy. Cancer affects individuals of any age and is the second most frequent cause of death in adulthood after cardiovascular diseases. The diagnostic-therapeutic process is demanding, which reflects the serious nature of cancer.

At the starting point of the diagnostic process of the cancer, there is always a detailed **history** of the patient with emphasis on family history of malignancies and with an active inquiry about **warning signs** that can accompany a malignant tumor. These comprise general signs and symptoms such as tiredness, weakness, loss of appetite, weight loss, sweating or changed behavior. Local signs are related to particular tissue or organ involvement, for example swallowing and digestive problems, difficulty in defecation, respiratory complaints, hoarseness, long-lasting cough, difficult urination, bleeding presenting as blood in sputum, nose bleeds, blood in vomit, stools, urine, gynecological bleeding beyond the regular cycle, also any visible or palpable resistance, alteration of a birthmark and last, but not least, pain. **Physical examination** is an essential part of the diagnostics. Thereafter, basic laboratory tests and imaging methods are performed as well as endoscopic examinations if needed. These methods can reveal a suspected tumor focus. Sampling of the suspected tissue for histopathological examination is the next essential step. The pathologist has a decisive role in distinguishing if the finding is a real malignant tumor; he/she examines the sample macroscopically and microscopically and makes the **histological diagnosis**. By these means the diagnosis of a malignant tumor is confirmed.

The essential part of the diagnostics of a malignant tumor comprises methods of molecular biology that further specify the tumor tissue and assess the risk and therefore prognosis of the disease. They can also detect whether a specific type of systemic therapy (for example hormonal therapy, particular types of biological therapy) can be used. These so called **prognostic and predictive factors** are important for making a therapeutic plan in a patient with a malignant disease.

To make the therapeutic plan, **staging** must be assessed. The above-mentioned methods of physical examination, laboratory tests including levels of tumor markers, and imaging and endoscopic examinations are employed for staging assessment. The stage is determined by the extent of the primary tumor (T tumor), presence or absence of tumor cells in lymph nodes of the drained lymphatic region (N noduli) and the presence or absence of distant metastases (M metastasis). The first and second clinical stages represent a localized disease; the third stage relates to patients with a large primary tumor or with the involvement of lymph nodes in the drained lymphatic region, and the fourth stage corresponds to a generalized disease with the presence of metastases.

The decision about the sequence of therapeutic modalities planned for the entire treatment – assessment of therapeutic plan – always relies on a team of physicians. The **medical team** consists of a clinical oncologist, a surgeon, a specialist in imaging methods, an endoscopist, a pathologist, a radiation oncologist and possibly other specialists depending on the nature of the disease. The clinical oncologist should be the main coordinator of the treatment. When choosing a therapeutic strategy, the patient's biological condition should be evaluated with secondary diseases as well as the patient's attitude towards the treatment to be taken into account.

Basic **therapeutic modalities** used in the treatment of malignancies are:
- Surgical treatment (operation)
- Chemotherapy
- Radiotherapy
- Hormonal therapy
- Biological targeted therapy

A supportive therapy enabling better tolerance of antineoplastic treatment, psychosocial care, and physiotherapy represent an indispensable part of the treatment of malignant diseases.

## 33.1 Surgical Treatment

Early clinical stages of malignant tumors are resolved mainly by surgery – performing a radical surgical procedure, the tumor is resected with an adequate rim of healthy tissue, and lymph nodes of the drained lymphatic region are removed.

If the tumor is completely removed, the **procedure** is **curative**. Surgical treatment is also indicated in advanced diseases when the tumor cannot be removed completely but the major tumor volume can be reduced, a metastasis can be removed, etc. In this case the **procedure** is **palliative**. The purpose of palliative intervention is mainly to improve the patient's quality of life and to extend the asymptomatic period of the disease. Surgical treatment also contributes to diagnostics – bioptic excision, diagnostic laparotomy or laparoscopy.

## 33.2 Chemotherapy

In advanced carcinomas with tumor cells infiltrating lymph nodes of the drained region, or if the primary tumor is too large, surgical treatment itself is usually insufficient and the patient requires further treatment: systemic or locoregional radiotherapy or a combination of both methods. This is known as **adjuvant chemotherapy** – treatment of microscopic residual disease that cannot be identified with imaging or endoscopic methods but its presence can be expected due to the stage of the disease. At the time of application of adjuvant therapy, the patient has no signs or symptoms of malignant disease and the treatment aims to extend the asymptomatic period, to prolong the overall survival or even to cure the patient.

In a locally advanced tumor, even with possible lymph node involvement in the drained region, if its operability is limited, the method of **neoadjuvant chemotherapy** is used. The aim of this treatment is to reduce the tumor while improving its operability; in advanced stages of the disease it is to destroy possible microscopic foci that can be expected in other tissues or organs – metastases. Occasionally, this therapy leads to complete tumor destruction, and after a subsequent operation the pathologist no longer identifies tumor cells in the resected tissue sample. Again, the treatment results in the extension of the asymptomatic period and the patient's overall survival or even healing. In some diagnoses neoadjuvant chemotherapy can be administered together with radiotherapy.

If distant metastases are present in tissues or organs other than in those of the primary tumor, **palliative chemotherapy** is indicated. Its main purpose is to achieve partial or total tumor response to the administered drug, to extend the asymptomatic period and to prolong life with the disease. The principal requirement is a preserved and improved quality of life.

Chemotherapy as a therapeutic systemic method consists in administration of cytostatics, chemical compounds that, by means of different mechanisms, are able to destroy the effects of tumor cells but also of those cells of healthy tissues that multiply and divide quickly. As its activity is not exclusively limited by tumor tissue, it results in a number of side effects. The cytostatics are used in monotherapy or in combinations, most often they are applied intravenously but some can be administered orally, or applied into the peritoneal or pleural cavity, intramuscularly, subcutaneously, or even intra-arterially.

Chemotherapy is applied in cycles; the intervals between them serve for the recovery of healthy tissue. Supportive therapy represents a part of chemotherapeutic treatment that moderates the side effects of cytostatics and improves the patient's quality of life during the treatment.

## 33.3 Radiotherapy

Radiotherapy is one of the basic methods of antineoplastic therapy, applying electromagnetic or corpuscular radiation. The radiation source is outside the patient's body at a defined distance – **teletherapy**, or the radiation source is in close contact with the tumor tissue – **brachytherapy**. Both of these methods can be combined and they mutually potentiate the effect of the treatment. The basic aim of the therapy is to apply a curative dose of radiation into the tumor focus or into the area from where the tumor focus and drained lymphatic region were surgically removed, sparing the surrounding healthy tissues to the maximum extent. Tumor tissues are classified according to their response to radiotherapy as **radiosensitive** and **radioresistant**. This corresponds in direct proportion to the reproductive activity of tumor cells and in indirect proportion to the degree of tumor tissue differentiation.

Radiotherapy is used as a single therapy method with the purpose of complete destruction of neoplastic focus – **curative radiotherapy**, or with the aim to reduce the tumor mass, to eliminate metastasis, to stop bleeding, to eliminate pain – **palliative radiotherapy**.

Radiotherapy performed after the surgical removal of a tumor and regional lymph nodes is called **adjuvant radiotherapy**. It aims to destroy the possible and/or expected microscopic disease in the area where the tumor tissue has been extirpated. The radiation is delivered in separate fractions, with a defined dose per fraction and in defined time intervals. In **standard fractionation,** one fraction of 1.8–2 Gy is administered 5 days a week. **Hyperfractionation** is the application of 2–3 doses per day with an interval of 6–8 hours in between, using a dose of 1.0–1.2 Gy. It is suitable in fast growing undifferentiated radiosensitive tumors. In **hypofractionation**, less than 5 doses per week are delivered, with a dose over 2 Gy per fraction, and it is used in slow growing, well differentiated, radioresistant tumors.

The radiation sources used at present in teletherapy include isotope cobalt units and linear accelerators. Brachytherapy employs the technique of afterloading, placing hollow applicators in close proximity of the neoplastic focus, and after radiographic verification of their position and calculation of the dose, the

# MULTIMODAL ONCOLOGICAL TREATMENT

radiation source is inserted into them. The application is performed via applicators – needles (interstitial brachytherapy, for example in the breast); into cavities (intracavitary brachytherapy, e.g. uterus); intraluminal brachytherapy (for example trachea, esophagus); surface brachytherapy applying the source on the skin (dressing, in skin cancer).

Radiotherapy can be delivered together with chemotherapy – **concomitant adjuvant chemotherapy** where the methods potentiate each other (as in rectal cancer) or as a part of **neoadjuvant therapy** in advanced tumors, separately or concomitantly with chemotherapy in an effort to reduce the tumor mass and to improve its operability. The result can be curative – complete pathological response in the treatment of breast or rectal cancer.

Radiotherapy causes side effects that are associated with the irradiated place – skin and mucosa changes; it has an impact, above all, on the lymphocyte count. These side effects must be managed adequately.

## 33.4 Hormonal Therapy

Hormonal therapy is indicated only in tumors composed of cells bearing specific cell receptors – hormonal dependent tumors, as in breast cancer or cancer of the prostate gland. The basic principle of therapy is to prevent receptors from being affected by hormones that, after binding to a receptor of the tumor cell, can cause its division, and thus the cell multiplication and tumor growth. The effect of hormones as a growth factor can be eliminated by removing the organ responsible for hormone production, **ablative therapy**, by means of surgical or radiation therapy or by drug treatment blocking the organ function. **Competitive therapy** inhibits the hormone responsible for tumor growth using other hormones with an antagonist effect. **Inhibitory therapy** inhibits production of the hormone that potentiates the growth (e.g. aromatase inhibitors inhibit conversion of testosterone to estrone and estradiol and thus cause estrogen depletion in women after menopause with breast cancer).

Hormonal therapy is used in hormone dependent tumors in adjuvant therapy, neoadjuvant therapy as well as in palliative treatment of metastatic disease. In solid tumors hormonal therapy is not usually combined with chemotherapy in adjuvant or palliative treatment but it can be administered together with radiotherapy as a part of palliative treatment.

## 33.5 Biological Targeted Therapy

This is a newly developing method that uses particular targets on tumor cells or tumor tissues, resulting in growth and division suspension of tumor cells as well as neovascularization suspension; it degrades tumor vascularization, leading to tumor necrosis due to lack of nutrition and oxygen.

Specific targets on tumor cells can be detected by methods of molecular biology and tumors potentially sensitive to particular targeted therapy can be identified. Biological therapy is indicated mostly in the fourth clinical stage of the disease, in monotherapy or together with chemotherapy, i.e. as a palliative treatment. The treatment extends the asymptomatic period in a significant manner and improves overall survival. In only one situation the biological targeted therapy is indicated in adjuvant treatment: therapy with monoclonal antibody trastuzumab is indicated in women with breast cancer with high expression of HER2 receptors on tumor cells.

Targeted therapy is more selective than cytostatic treatment and is not associated with a wide range of side effects, except allergic reaction to an active substance.

❖ ❖ ❖

It should be emphasized that oncological therapy is a multidisciplinary treatment. It should always be performed by teams of specialists and should be concentrated in specialized centers that are competent to provide a complex therapeutic service from quality diagnostics up to intensive care. The treatment should be performed according to Czech therapeutic standards that originate from international recommendations based on large randomized studies.

In each particular patient, an individual approach to the therapeutic plan should be discussed by the medical oncological team, reflecting the patient's biological condition and comorbidities.

The therapeutic plan must be explained in detail to the patient so that in the course of treatment he/she can act as the doctors' partner. Subsequent lifelong specialized follow-up – dispensarization – is an indispensable part of the care of a patient who has suffered a malignant disease. It aims to detect the progression of a treated malignancy early, to monitor post-treatment sequelae and to reveal possible secondary malignancies.

# 34 TUMOR GENETICS

*34.1 Hereditary Non-Polyposis Colorectal Cancer (HNPCC, Lynch Syndrome)*
*34.2 Familial Adematous Polyposis (FAP)*
*34.3 Hereditary Breast and Ovarian Cancer Syndrome*
*34.4 Multiple Endocrine Neoplasia Type 1 (MEN 1 Syndrome)*
*34.5 Multiple Endocrine Neoplasia Type 2 (MEN 2 Syndrome)*
*34.6 Medullary Thyroid Carcinoma and MEN 2 Syndromes*

The surgeon plays a crucial role in the therapy of neoplasms, especially of solid tumors. Most malignant diseases are **sporadic, nonhereditary** (90%). A primary initiating genetic event (mutation or knockout, usually of a tumor suppressor gene) can arise in any somatic/stem cell. This event is passed on to descendant cells giving rise to a tumor clone (monoclonal theory). The mutation provides clone cells only with a selective growth advantage. Achievement of fully developed malignant phenotype (independence of external growth signals, insensitivity to external anti-growth signals, escape from apoptosis, ability of infinite replication, support of neoangiogenesis, invasivity and metastatic potential) requires on average the accumulation of at least 6–7 additional mutations of critical genes in the cell (proto-oncogenes, tumor suppressor genes including genes responsible for mutation repair and other genes whose products regulate cell cycle) and other so-called epigenetic events (e.g. methylation of promoter gene regions decreasing or eliminating their expression). No other mutation that escapes antineoplastic mechanisms (mutation repair, apoptosis, and immunological mechanisms) is able to change a normal cell into a tumor cell. It is obvious that the accumulation of the described unrepaired changes in a tumor clone requires a certain lapse of time. Therefore, the incidence of sporadic nonhereditary malignancies depends on age, and they usually appear in the post-reproductive period when effectiveness of antineoplastic mechanisms decline.

**At least 10% of tumors have hereditary etiology** caused by mutations of highly penetrant "tumor" genes. In contrast to sporadic tumors, a person is born with one mutated allele of a certain critical gene. He/she inherits the predisposing mutation from germ cells (germline mutation). In a carrier, mutation of critical allele is present in all somatic cells, leading to a substantially increased risk of developing certain malignancies (depending on the type of tumor gene whose mutated allele was inherited). Mutation or elimination of the second allele in the target tissue (and rarely even without it – haploinsufficiency) usually suffice to initiate a multi-step tumorigenic process. The predisposing allele, or tumor predisposition, is transmitted via the carrier's germ cells to the next generations, usually in autosomal dominant or less frequently recessive or X-linked traits. This process results in the accumulation of malignant tumors of certain types in several generations, giving rise to so-called **cancer families**. It is indispensable that the surgeon is able to distinguish between sporadic and hereditary malignancies.

Cancer families of a certain type should be suspected if typical features in a family tree are present. Genealogical criteria for certain hereditary malignancies are specifically defined (e.g. in colorectal cancer – Amsterdam criteria I, II, Bethesda criteria, in breast and ovarian cancer – criteria in families without Jewish ancestors, in families with Jewish ancestors, etc.). Meeting these criteria (assessed by a clinical geneticist) selects patients/families indicated (after obtaining informed consent) for **genetic testing** (detection of germline mutations of corresponding genes). The aim of this testing is to identify carriers of germline mutation who are at risk but still unaffected, and to provide them with internationally developed preventive monitoring programs focused on prevention of the development of malignancy, or on its early diagnostics while the tumor is more treatable.

Generally speaking, **repeated occurrence of malignancies in several generations** of the same genealogical line (paternal, maternal), occurrence of malignancies **at a young age** (under 45 years), **bilateral** or **multiple** tumors and accumulation of populationally **rare tumors** should raise suspicion of some types of hereditary tumors.

The importance of a carefully taken **family history** and its evaluation must again be emphasized. Upon respecting this undoubtedly lege artis medical rule, an attending physician/surgeon is the pivotal person to refer the patient/family to genetic examination.

However, families also exist with accumulated malignancies that do not meet the criteria of monogenetic type of inheritance of the cancer predisposition, and even mutation analysis does not bring a positive result. The explanation probably consists in the existence of as yet unknown predisposing genes with low penetrance or polymorphisms. The fact that families share the same lifestyle that can predispose to cancer should be also kept in mind. Family members from families with increased incidence of tumors should be followed up with in the same way as in the case of corresponding hereditary forms.

Briefly specified below are the main syndromes with hereditary tumor predisposition that are important from the surgical viewpoint.

# TUMOR GENETICS

## 34.1 Hereditary Non-Polyposis Colorectal Cancer (HNPCC, Lynch Syndrome)

HNPCC is germline mutations of repair genes MLH1, MSH2, MSH6, PMS2, with autosomal dominant inheritance of tumor predisposition. HNPCC is associated with a 28–75% probability of a lifelong risk of colorectal cancer (CRC) in men and a 24–52% risk in women. Women with HNPCC have a 27–71% probability of developing cancer of the endometrium and approximately a 3–13% risk of ovarian cancer. HNPCC is also associated with an increased risk of carcinoma of the stomach, urinary tract, hepatobiliary system and small intestine and of cerebral tumors. In HNPCC, tumors arise at a young age and can be multiple.

Other forms of HNPCC: **Muir-Torre syndrome** (internal malignancies + sebaceous skin cancer), **Turcot syndrome** (CRC + brain tumors).

**Indication for genetic examination/testing** includes genealogical Amsterdam criteria I and II, genealogical characteristics of families, and if the criteria are met, patients and their family members are indicated for genetic testing. The revised criteria (Bethesda) for testing microsatellite instability and immunohistochemical analysis of protein expression of MLH1, MSH2, MSH6 and possibly PMS2 in tumors are also available. They are based on genealogical characteristics and clinical and histological findings of **colorectal** cancer.

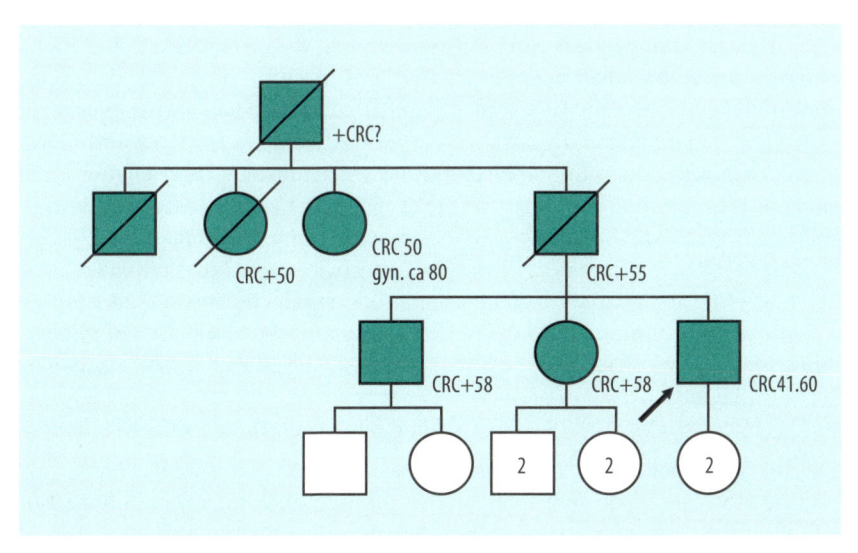

**Fig. 34.1** *Genealogical tree of a tumor family with hereditary non-polyposis colorectal cancer (HNPCC, Lynch syndrome). The arrow indicates the affected patient recommended for genetic consultation. Germline mutations were detected in all tested affected family members; five out of eight unaffected members of the last generation were diagnosed as germline mutation carriers, the preventive monitoring protocol was initiated.*

**The follow-up recommendation for unaffected germline mutation carriers** is repeated physical examination, colposcopy (from the age of 20), fecal occult blood testing, gynecological examination, abdominal ultrasound including transvaginal examination, examination of marker CA 125, aspiration endometrial biopsy, gastroscopy, breast self-examination, breast ultrasound, and urological examination including PSA.

**The options of prophylactic surgical procedures** include hysterectomy (female carriers of MSH6 gene after menopause); prophylactic hysterectomy with bilateral adnexotomy (female carriers of mutations in MLH1, MSH2, PMS2 genes, preferably between the ages of 35–40; prophylactic colectomy is not commonly indicated due to markedly worsened quality of life).

## 34.2 Familial Adenomatous Polyposis (FAP)

FAP is germline mutation in the APC gene (chromosome 5q21–q22), with autosomal dominant inheritance of tumor predisposition.

**Syndrome characteristics:** Classic form of FAP, occurrence of more than 100 adenomatous polyps in the large intestine, or less polyps but at a younger age. In the classic form, polyps begin to develop at approximately 5 years of age, and at the age of 35 polyps are present in 95% of patients. There is a high risk of colorectal cancer (100% risk before reaching the age of 50), often multifocal, even at a very young age. It can be also associated with congenital hypertrophy of retinal pigment epithelium, osteomas, redundant teeth, odontomas, desmoids, epidermoid cysts, duodenal adenomas, papillary thyroid cancer, hepatoblastoma, pancreatic carcinoma, and gastric carcinoma. Affected families should be referred for genetic counseling. If FAP is suspected, all first degree relatives should undergo the colonoscopy as part of the clinical diagnostics (parents, siblings; children from 10 to 15 years of age only sigmoidoscopy). Predictive genetic testing can be offered at any age. Prenatal diagnostics is possible. Preimplantation diagnostics is possible only in serious cases and in selected institutions.

**Follow-up recommendation:** The follow-up should be based on team collaboration between the oncologist, gastroenterologist, surgeon and other specialists.

### A) CLASSIC FAP AND ATTENUATED FORM (UNAFFECTED MUTATION CARRIERS)

The algorithm includes repeated sigmoidoscopy, colposcopy, polypectomy, gastroduodenoscopy, enteroscopy, abdominal ultrasound, in the event of hypertrophy of retinal pigment epithelium also ophthalmological examination, urological examination including PSA, stomatological examination, etc.

**Prophylactic surgery:** Proctocolectomy with ileal reservoir (ileal-pouch anal anastomosis – IPAA), proctocolectomy with ileostomy – however, the patient's follow-up must continue due to the risk of extra-intestinal malignancies, colectomy with postoperative ileorectal anastomosis (findings in a stoma, pouch, adjacent ileum, suture, rectum).

### B) MAP – MYH ASSOCIATED POLYPOSIS

It is a recessive hereditary polyposis caused by germline mutation in the MYH gene (chromosome 1p32.1).

**Clinical picture** comprises multiple intestinal polyposis with an increased risk of colorectal cancer.

**Familial occurrence** – sporadic polyposis, in some families with occurrence in siblings. Follow-up is similar to FAP.

## 34.3 Hereditary Breast and Ovarian Cancer Syndrome

Germline mutations in BRCA1 and BRCA2 genes.

**Syndrome characteristics:** Mutations cause an increased risk especially of breast and ovarian cancer. The lifelong risk in female carriers of mutations on both genes ranges from 40 to 85%. The risk of secondary breast tumor reaches up to 60%. The lifelong risk of ovarian cancer in carriers of BRCA1 gene mutation is up to 60%, in carriers of gene BRCA2 mutation it is about 10–20%. Carriers of BRCA1 mutation also demonstrate an increased risk of uterine and cervical cancer and other malignancies: colorectal carcinoma, carcinoma of the prostate, tumors in the stomach and pancreas. BRCA2 mutation carriers demonstrate an increased risk of colorectal carcinoma, prostate, pancreas, gallbladder, biliary ducts, or stomach melanomas. The risk of breast cancer in male carriers of BRCA2 gene mutation is increased up to 100 times. Gene CHEK2 (two mutations tested) can increase the risk of breast cancer approximately 2–4 times.

**Indication for BRCA gene testing:**
- **Familial forms** – at least 3 direct relatives (including the proband) diagnosed with breast and/or ovarian cancer (bilateral cancer counts for two tumors), or 2 first degree (or paternal second degree) relatives (including the proband) with breast and/or ovarian cancer if at least one was diagnosed under the age of 50.
- **Sporadic forms** are patients with bilateral breast or ovarian cancer with the first diagnosis under the age of 50, or patients with breast and ovarian cancer at any age, or sporadic occurrence of unilateral breast or ovarian cancer under the age of 35, or a man with breast cancer. Testing is indicated by a geneticist. Predictive testing is not performed before reaching the age of legal majority. Prenatal diagnostics is not indicated. Preimplantation diagnostics is not currently performed as a routine examination.

**Follow-up recommendation and other potential prophylactic measures** include regular breast self-examination, general physical examination by an oncologist, ultrasound and MRI of breasts, mammography, examination of markers, gynecological examination, fecal occult blood testing and others.

**Options of prophylactic surgical procedures:** bilateral prophylactic adnexotomy, preferably at the age of 35–40 in mutation carriers, or immediately if the mutation is detected at an older age; according to the finding and the patient's age, the gynecologist also always considers a hysterectomy; prophylactic bilateral mastectomy whenever requested by the patient, after consulting with an oncologist and after complex preventive examinations.

**Men:** dispensarization – repeated self-examination of testicles and breasts, oncological examinations, ultrasound, mammography, examination of markers, urological examinations, colonoscopy, gastroscopy, fecal occult blood testing and others.

**For women at risk of developing breast cancer according to Claus tables** with various risk levels, the corresponding dispensarization is recommended (www.linkos.cz).

## 34.4 Multiple Endocrine Neoplasia Type 1 (MEN 1 Syndrome)

Responsible gene: menin; MEN 1 – chromosome 11q13, autosomal dominant inheritance and predisposition.

**Syndrome characteristics:** different combinations of more than 20 types of endocrine and non-endocrine tumors. The pathognomonic feature of MEN 1 is hyperparathyreosis (adenoma of parathyroid glands in 90–95% of patients). 50–65% of patients suffer from tumors of endocrine pancreas and 40–50% of patients from pituitary tumors; cortical tumors of the suprarenal gland and skin tumors are also frequent. The tumors are usually benign; nevertheless, they cause clinically manifesting hyperfunction of affected glands.

**Diagnostic criteria:** the presence of at least two types of the above-mentioned endocrine tumors. The familial form of MEN 1 is defined as the presence of at least one patient with MEN 1 and at the minimum one first degree relative with at least one of the above-mentioned endocrine tumors.

**Clinical picture** – the most frequent manifestation comprises primary hyperparathyreosis that in contrast to sporadic form begins at an earlier age, affects both sexes, adenomas are multiple and affect several parathyroid glands. Tumors affect mainly the pancreas, but also the duodenal wall, and in contrast to sporadic forms, are multiple. Tumors associated with MEN 1 appear approximately

10 years earlier than sporadic tumors. Metastases occur frequently in regional lymph nodes and the liver, and possibly also in bones.

**Indication for MEN1 gene testing** – patients with MEN 1 syndrome, patients with familial isolated hyperparathyreosis, Zollinger-Ellison syndrome and primary hyperaldosteronism. If the patient was diagnosed with a causative germline mutation in the MEN1 gene, a targeted molecular genetic examination of his/her at-risk relatives should be performed.

**Therapy and prevention** – treatment consists in surgical removal of tumors and in pharmacotherapy of hormonal overproduction.

### RECOMMENDED PROTOCOL OF PREVENTIVE FOLLOW-UP

The protocol relates to preventive follow-up, both of persons with MEN 1 syndrome and of persons at risk of the disease. Family members carrying the MEN1 gene mutation, or, in the case of a non-informative result of genetic analysis, all consanguineous relatives must be followed up with the aim to detect the tumor early, in accordance with the recommended protocol.

## 34.5 Multiple Endocrine Neoplasia Type 2 (MEN 2 Syndrome)

Responsible gene: RET; proto-oncogene chromosome 10q11.2, type of inheritance: autosomal dominant.

**Syndrome characteristics** – multiple endocrine neoplasias (MEN) are diseases with familial occurrence when the patient develops simultaneously or successively neoplastic involvement of several endocrine glands; **the presence of medullary thyroid carcinoma is typical** and may combine with pheochromocytoma and/or primary hyperparathyreosis (MEN 2A syndrome), or in MEN 2B with pheochromocytoma and a number of other lesions (neurinomas, ganglioneuromatosis in the gastrointestinal tract, ocular anomalies) and marphanoid habitus with typical symptomatology.

## 34.6 Medullary Thyroid Carcinoma (MTC) and MEN 2 Syndromes

Medullary thyroid carcinoma is a tumor originating from the parafollicular cells (C-cells producing calcitonin) of the thyroid gland and represents 4–10% of all thyroid tumors. MTC usually occurs in the sporadic form (75%), less frequently in the familial form (25%). The familial form is inherited in an autosomal dominant trait and has three variants: familial MTC (FMTC), multiple endocrine neoplasia type 2A (MEN 2A) and multiple endocrine neoplasia type 2B (MEN 2B).

**Clinical picture** – medullary thyroid carcinoma is usually localized in the middle and upper thyroid lobes where the concentration of C-cells is physiologically the highest. Early metastases are frequently found in regional lymph nodes. Distant metastases develop mainly in the liver, lungs and bones. Also typical is the age-depending occurrence of the disease: MEN 2A affects middle-aged patients, while MEN 2B is diagnosed earlier, usually in childhood.

### 34.6.1 Gene Nature and Correlation Genotype-Phenotype

The MTC and MEN 2 syndromes are caused by activating point mutations in RET proto-oncogene. Individual mutations in the gene differ in their manifestations, i.e. in their impact on phenotype and in their aggressivity.

**Indication for RET gene testing** – all patients with pathologically confirmed MTC (including sporadic MTC) should be genetically tested for the presence of RET germline mutation. Relatives at risk of the disease should also be examined. Genetic consultation and signed informed consent must precede such examination. Prenatal diagnostics is possible. Preimplantation diagnostics is possible in serious cases and in selected institutions.

**Therapy and prevention** – the primary therapy of MTC is total thyroidectomy (TTE). In 50–80% of patients with hereditary MTC, metastases to regional lymph nodes are already present at the time of diagnosis. Hence further prognosis of the disease depends on early diagnostics, successfulness, extent and radicality of the primary operation, the size of the tumor, and the patient's age. Last but not least, lifelong follow-up with regular clinical and laboratory check-ups play a key role in the prognosis, since they may reveal potential relapses (up to 10%) early.

**Follow-up recommendation** –patients should receive further follow up, even after a performed TTE, since they can possibly develop residual or relapsing MTC or pheochromocytoma; in the event of postoperative hypoparathyrosis in post-operative patients this should also be followed up and treated.

Descriptions of certain additional hereditary tumor syndromes, e.g. Li-Fraumeni syndrome, Gorlin syndrome, Peutz-Jeghers syndrome, Recklinghausen neurofibromatosis, hereditary pancreatitis, Cowden syndrome, Von Hippel-Lindau syndrome – are mentioned in the journal of Clinical Oncology (Klinická onkologie) 22, 2009, Supplement.

# 35 PATHOLOGY

> 35.1 The Discipline of Pathology in Surgery
> 35.2 Autopsy
> 35.3 Bioptic Pathology
> 35.4 Generalization of Optimum Practice in Clinical Pathology

## 35.1 The Discipline of Pathology in Surgery

The collaboration between the surgeon and the pathologist has been evolving for centuries and it remains close and indispensable. The discipline of pathology arose mainly from the curiosity of the ancestors of present surgeons who tried to verify their treatment, performing autopsies of their deceased patients. The amount of documented information has been increasing since the first university centers in Europe were established and since anatomy and pathology emerged and started to develop as significant medical disciplines, especially since the end of the 18$^{th}$ century.

In current medicine, the professional relationship between the pathologist and the surgeon has two levels: biopsy and autopsy.

## 35.2 Autopsy

Autopsy helps to confirm the etiology of a disease and its complications as well as the outcome of a surgeon's work. It represents the basis of feedback in clinical practice. Post mortem examination is helpful nowadays, even in the time of rapid progress and usage of imaging methods. Currently, imaging methods with computer tomography or magnetic resonance substantially replace the proper macroscopic tissue evaluation. However, autopsy has proven to be important in evaluating clinical practice. It is widely known that despite apparently flawless imaging methods and their interpretation, autopsy not only provides more detailed information, but often reveals surprising findings. The autopsy is indicated by a clinical surgeon, with the aim to **verify a therapeutic outcome, clarify unexpected complications**, or as an examination with **potential forensic impact**. The latter relates not only to the justification of a doctor's therapeutic procedures for him/herself and for the hospital, but also as a means of defense against often unsubstantiated objections and complaints from the bereaved. Autopsies help to identify various insufficiencies or even errors in clinical practice. Post mortem findings, above all the unusual ones or those showing new information about the patient's disease, should be discussed in **clinical-pathological seminars**. A surgeon's **participation in an autopsy** (but also that of other specialists) is beneficial. Confirming the cause of death by an autopsy is often required by the deceased patient's relatives for various reasons. The autopsy and the results as well as the evaluation of pathological findings in organs have an **educative value** in undergraduate medical education as well as in postgraduate education in various medical specialties.

## 35.3   Bioptic Pathology

Bioptic activities currently represent the **major part of a pathologist's work**, analyzing cells and tissues collected from patients during their life. In the European concept, "biopsy" comprises examinations regardless of the type and form of tissue/cell collection. The term "biopsy" expresses both the proper tissue collection and its subsequent examination, possibly specifying the form of collection, for example: a fine needle biopsy, endoscopic forceps biopsy, etc. In the USA and in other countries, the term biopsy means minor sampling collected with a needle, forceps or excision. Major excisions and resections are called "surgical collections" (or simply "surgicals"). That is why bioptic pathology, in the Czech Republic understood as a histopathological examination of cells and tissues, is called "surgical pathology" in some countries.

Tissue examination in surgery can be divided into the following groups according to timing, type of tissue collection and the technique used by a pathologist: **preoperative examination, perioperative bioptic examination, bioptic examination after a surgical procedure,** examination of surgically resected tissues **after neoadjuvant oncological therapy** and specialized pathological examination **after organ transplantation**. In the traditional form of pathology and according to general medical understanding, the pathologist's basic tool is a microscope and examinations are based on histological tissue processing (the term "**histopathological examination**" is also used). However, pathological examination in this time of medical advances is not limited to **microscopic examination** of cells and tissues; **molecular diagnostics at the gene level** (DNA diagnostics e.g. of chromosomal translocations in sarcomas), at the level of gene expression detecting the **mRNA expression** (qualitative and now also quantitative) and at the **protein** level are gaining growing importance and practical usage in the field of pathology. In detecting particular molecules, its practical usage is only in the beginning. The development of a considerably more complex approach can be expected in the near future, simultaneously measuring the expression of tens up to thousands of cell products and evaluating the activity or suppression of cellular metabolic paths. Newly, a pharmacologically oriented

## PATHOLOGY

aspect in the so-called **therapeutic-indicative** area (see below) is gaining importance in pathology. As a result of the above-mentioned findings, the examination that a pathologist can offer to a clinical partner and, above all, to a patient (although indirectly) provides a more complex view of the pathological process, and the diagnosis is made assembling **results of different examinations** often including several methods (histopathology, flow cytometry, blotting techniques of protein detection, DNA and RNA diagnostics).

### 35.3.1  Preoperative Examination

Often **cytological** preoperative analysis precedes histological examination. Cytological analysis obtains specimens by **needle puncture** (trepanobiopsy in bone marrow), endoscopic examination with **forceps collection** of tissue samples, or the diagnosis is made on the basis of the **excision** of a suspected area.

The above-mentioned examinations usually provide information of diagnostic value that can serve as the basis to plan a resection and consider its extent. In some oncological indications, histopathological diagnostics from a small collection (puncture, excision, curettage) are followed by adjuvant oncological therapy and the resection is planned for a later period, depending on the tumor response.

Practical examples include:
a) **Fine needle aspiration biopsy** with **cytological smears** from thyroid gland and cytological examination of a specimen from a suspected focus collected under ultrasound supervision
b) **Puncture biopsy** of cylindrical tissue specimens collected from a suspected tumor focus, e.g. from the prostate, mammary glands, liver or brain, and mold specimens examined histologically
c) **Curttage/excisioen** of the tissue from a bone or soft tissue tumor, gynecological curettage performed to assess pathological changes of endometrium. Diagnostic excision is performed even in inoperable tumors to assess the nature of the pathological process, which is necessary for the sake of deciding on further oncological treatment.

**From the technical point of view**, these examinations use methods of **cytological smears**, **cytocentrifugation** and subsequent staining, or methods of the classic **histological technique**. The latter term means fixation of tissue (usually 10% formol, i.e. 4% solution of formaldehyde), subsequent infiltration with paraffin, embedding into a paraffin block and slicing and placing the cross sections on histological glasses, followed by staining. The so called **histological staining** currently employs classic histological staining methods. Combined staining with hematoxylin and eosin, silver impregnation methods to detect reticulin fibers or some pathological agents *(Helicobacter pylori)*, and various staining to detect the production of mucins (essential in epithelial tumors) are the most frequent methods. The list is mentioned by way of example, since there is a wide range of usage of histological staining. The presence of various cell-specific proteins is analyzed by **immunohistochemical methods** directly in the tissue and this examination is used in diagnostic practice routinely to a larger extent. Less frequently, **blotting techniques** are employed, after the homogenization of the tissue and after extraction of proteins from these homogenized cells (Western blotting). In some indications, even methods of **flow cytometry** and **analysis of nucleic acids** can be used.

### 35.3.2 Perioperative Bioptic Examination

Perioperative bioptic examination is carried out with the purpose of confirming the primary preoperative diagnosis, and is often performed as a part of the surgical resection. The aim of this examination is:

a) **Diagnostic purposes**
b) **To confirm suspected** diagnosis so that the surgeon can continue the surgical procedure radically
c) **To define** the **margins of resection** – i.e. to evaluate healthy tissue versus tumor margin, or its potential microscopic propagation **per continuitatem** or via vessels into the resection line or beyond
d) **To evaluate findings in sentinel** lymph nodes; this applies in selected indications, focusing on the presence or absence of tumor propagation into the lymph nodes. The extent of the surgical procedure is based on this finding. Perioperative examination is performed not only as a part of resection, but always when the surgeon needs to analyze the nature of tissue during an operation, i.e. for example in endoscopic examinations like thoracoscopy with tissue sampling from mediastinal organs.
e) In these cases, the main aim is to **confirm the quality of sampling** for further analysis, e.g. if the collection is intralesional, or if it contains only fibrous or necrotic tissue. If the perioperative sample does not contain diagnostic tissue, the collection can still be continued with the instruments in place, therefore pathologically changed and diagnostically evaluable tissue can be collected in a single session.

The surgeon provides the laboratory with fresh tissue for the perioperative examination; the extent of examination relies on the pathologist who is responsible for making the diagnosis. In the majority of cases, perioperative examination is evaluable and is in agreement with the final diagnosis assessed after classic histological analysis. However, in certain situations, not even a rough diagnosis can be made on the basis of the perioperative examination, such as sometimes in carcinoma and atypical hyperplasia of mammary glands, or chronic pancreatitis and adenocarcinoma of the pancreas. In these cases the operation must be finished and the so-called definitive processing of samples must wait until fixation, embedding in paraffin and processing enables further specialized, but time-consuming analyses leading to diagnosis.

The technique used in perioperative examination is one that "fixates" the collected sample of fresh tissue by fast freezing. At present this is usually achieved in liquid nitrogen, cooling the tissue to –195.8 °C. Freezing prevents the tissue from autolytic processes and at the same time it hardens the tissue, enabling the specimen to be sliced to histological cross-sections of 4–5 µm of width using microtome kept in a cooled room, usually –18 to –21 °C (so called cryostat). This technique of histological preparation including staining lasts approximately 10–15 minutes. It enables analyzing the tissue while the patient is being operated on, during the course of operation, and even repeatedly.

For a perioperative biopsy and evaluation, the pathologist requires extensive experience across the whole area of pathology, fast decision making and good command of the pros and cons of the frozen section biopsy technique. Preparations are never as perfectly evaluable as in classic histological processing after fixation and paraffin embedding. They usually have less clear contours; cross-sections are often thicker and less evaluable than cross-sections of the same tissue from paraffin blocks. Not only the pathologist, but also the surgeon should be aware of this fact. Since fast perioperative decisions have significant consequences for the patient, mistakes must be eliminated as much as possible. Timing and space organization of a perioperative biopsy should be organized in such a way that not only the pathologist who makes the diagnosis is available (carrying out the **perioperative bioptic service**), but that this pathologist can promptly ask another experienced pathologist for consiliary advice, above all a specialist in examining particular organs or types of pathological processes. This organization of work reduces errors in interpretation. A special room in the vestibule of operating rooms or a separate room at the department of pathology is usually reserved for perioperative biopsies, and in this room all cooperative activities are available thanks to professionals employed there.

Besides the direct impact of perioperative biopsy on the further steps of the surgeon during an operation, the fresh tissue collection and its delivery to the hands of the pathologist have other advantages. The tissue can be divided by the pathologist for **further specialized examinations**. A part of the fresh tissue, e.g. from an excised lymph node, can be sent for homogenization and **flow cytometry** examination (to identify antigen epitopes) or for homogenization and extraction of nucleic acids for subsequent **pathological/genetic** examinations. In practice, a part of the tissue can be used for cytogenetic examinations (karyotypization) and for further genetic examinations. An obvious advantage is the fact that the **pathologist can provide these specialized examinations with confirmed tissue** from a mirror image that he/she froze and evaluated with the use of a microscope. This procedure enables the biologist-geneticist to work with a diagnostically valuable, histologically confirmed tissue sample, which he/she usually examines in the form of homogenized cells and he/she does not have another possibility to assess the nature and quality of the processed specimen.

### 35.3.3 Bioptic Examination after Surgical Procedures

If the resected tissue or major excision has not been sent in a native state for pathological examination, the surgeon fixates the tissue to prevent its autolysis and to preserve the tissue for further histopathological processing. In the same way, the pathologist treats parts of a major excision that he/she has received from a surgeon in a native state, after making diagnosis from this tissue, with the frozen section technique. He/she fixates the tissue in a fixative solution. This step is **often associated with mistakes**; therefore some necessary rules are worth mentioning. Fixation in a fixative (most often in formol) depends on the ability of the fixative to penetrate the tissue. Penetration of one millimeter through the tissue takes approximately one hour; therefore the tissue should be fixated in a sufficiently large volume of the fixative for a sufficiently long period. For example, tissue cross-sections of 3–4 mm thick are considered convenient; the surface can be substantially larger, even several centimeters. Thinner cross-sections are penetrated by the fixative faster (if needed), however, they become distorted in the fixative and further steps of the definitive processing, i.e. dehydratation and paraffin embedding, result in excessive or even undesirable reduction. Besides these rules, the volume of the fixative should be at least 20 times greater than the volume of the fixated material, otherwise penetration of the fixative is slowed down and the center of the tissue is autolyzed and therefore destroyed for evaluation.

There are many examples of improper tissue processing in practice. For instance, spleen processing after splenectomy can be mentioned. Usually the whole spleen, regardless of its size, is placed in a container of almost the same volume as the resected organ, and several tens of milliliters of formol are poured over it. In the lapse of time before reaching the hands of the pathologist, i.e. for several hours up to 24–48 hours (e.g. in an urgent operation at a weekend time), the resected tissue except a thin subcapsular zone is completely autolyzed and practically unusable.

An alternative manipulation with resected tissue in an operating room can be the procedure when, after arrangement with the pathologist, a major resected tissue is wrapped in mull moistened with saline solution and sent to the laboratory for further processing. The pathologist evaluates and labels the resected tissue, makes photo documentation and cuts the specimen adequately – slicing and fixating the tissue. The surgical team in the operating room can act likewise. It depends on the agreement between the surgeon and the pathological laboratory and on the pathologist's availability during the operation and afterwards. It is suitable to cut some major resected tissues longitudinally, above all hollow organs (stomach, intestine), to rinse them and to spread them on an appropriate surface (e.g. cork) with the mucosa side upwards and to fasten their position with pins. This procedure is laborious; however, with its use, both the proper pathological finding as well as the margins of excision can be evaluated correctly. Fixation of mesenterium should be performed in a similar manner, as well as fixation of omentum where lymph nodes must be examined. Orientation in the tissue can be made easier and more precise by stitches at the margin or another part of the resected tissue according to an agreed scheme. The histological request form should preferably contain a schematic picture of the tissue position. It is well known that after removing a part of an organ from the body, the orientation is very difficult even for the surgeon who removed it and much more for someone who has not seen the removed tissue *in situ*. The assessment is even more difficult due to fixation, resulting in changed tissue shape and color. It is **rather undesirable** to place an easily deformable resected tissue into an inadequately large container (bottle) with fixate. The tissue hardens due to the formol fixative and often cannot even be removed from the container, so that the container must be broken first, the result being that it becomes difficult or even impossible to evaluate the tissue for a proper evaluation and description. Therefore the pathologist is not able to respond to crucial questions of the surgeon related to the assessment of surgical margins, oral-aboral, or questions about the presence of lymph nodes in apical or lateral parts of resected tissue. Hence mutual information and knowing the limits of the surgeon's and pathologist's work are essential.

The pathologist and his/her team (in fact specialized technicians) proceed with the help of the classic histological technique (see above). The pathologist as a segment of the work chain analyzes the tissue by microscopy. The basis of this technology was already well known in the middle of the 19$^{th}$ century and is still practical and widely usable. The paraffin embedded tissue in blocks can be preserved for many tens of years, the blocks can easily be stored and, if needed, they can be retrospectively found and examined.

If the pathologist works with **frozen tissue**, it can also be stored on a long-term basis. Nevertheless, this activity is demanding in terms of space possibilities as well as the accessibility of freezing – usually carried out in special containers with liquid nitrogen or in deep freezing boxes (–80 °C). Moreover, the frozen tissue at these low temperatures gets dry within months of storage (it lyophilizes) and its usability for histological processing decreases. Nucleic acids suitable for molecular biological examinations are, however, preserved for a prolonged time even in such tissue. The applicability and practical impact of isolation and examination of nucleic acids has been increasing during the last decades, see below.

The attending surgeon should count on a much **longer period of time** required for **tissue processing with histological technology** of paraffin embedding in blocks and subsequent tissue staining in contrast to the freezing technique. Properly fixed tissue of a smaller size (e.g. originated from puncture or forceps collection) delivered during morning hours can be processed by dehydration and embedding with paraffin the very same day. Under these circumstances, the next day the tissue is embedded in paraffin and further processed so that pathologist gets these small specimens of tissue the day after collection and can provide the surgeon (or other specialist) with the definite or at least provisional diagnosis. However, the majority of specimens need longer fixation, usually overnight, and further processing is carried out after the so-called **cutting of samples** and their **labeling** by the pathologist. **Photo documentation** is beneficial in some specimens. In most samples it should be kept in mind that the pathologist gets histological preparations the following day, i.e. not earlier than 48–54 hours postoperatively. If, for example, the situation requires immunohistochemical examination in addition to the standard histological staining, the sample processing takes longer, at least further 24 hours, in practice probably 48 hours. Hence a complex examination of more complicated cases lasts 4–5 working days, sometimes even more. Procedures such as the demineralization of solid tissues (e.g. bone) enabling them to be further examined histologically, are time consuming as well, e.g. the first preparation of basic staining can be made after a week-long demineralization of the tissue.

Since pathology is based on an empiric approach and the interpretation of results lies in the hands of the pathologist, the examination can take several days, particularly in problematic cases even over a week. This system is influenced by other facts that should be taken into account. The number of examinations at a particular moment is very important. The clinical partner of a pathologist can usually adequately regulate the number of planned procedures and he/she knows how many patients can be attended in a certain period of time. The pathologist is not in the same position and his work speed together with the diagnostic outcomes depends, besides other factors, on the productivity of clinical departments. As he/she provides a service not only for the department of surgery, but for the whole hospital (in larger hospitals, material for perioperative examination can be sent from several departments at the same time), and the number of sent specimens on a particular day or days can exceed the technological capacity of the department or a pathologist's time capacity. This situation can lead to a prolonged time needed for tissue processing and assessment of the diagnosis. The proper way to cope with this situation is mutual communication and the sharing of information between the surgeon and the pathologist to prevent the patient being harmed as a result of a delay.

In resections performed on oncological patients, the assessment of the extent of a disease is extremely important not only regarding tumor propagation **per continuitatem**, but also with respect to dissemination via blood and lymphatic vessels and to lymph nodes. The descriptions by the pathologist should be exact not only in relation to diagnostics of the pathological process (in the sense of tumor versus non-malignant disease, the exact tumor classification according to internationally accepted criteria, tumor grade assessment), but also regarding its propagation. This information is provided not only in the form of a descriptive report, but also classifying according to internationally accepted tumor classification criteria in oncology TNM where, after examination by the pathologist, the tumor extent is assessed and then expressed as pTpNpM. From the perspective of a bioptic pathologist, the local extent of the disease and lymph node involvement are crucial.

There are **two basic schemes** of collaboration with a surgeon in **lymph node examination**. The first one consists in a procedure performed by the surgeon (and specialists of other fields of surgery): **the individual lymph nodes** are prepared and **extirpated** and are provided to the pathologist in separately labeled containers. Then the lymph node examination is topically localized according to the surgeon's description and the extent of metastases into lymph nodes, if present, can be specified exactly. This technique is often chosen by surgeons in operations of malignancies in the area of the head and neck or by gynecologists in tumors of the internal genitals. The second alternative is the **resection of lymph nodes "en bloc"**. Here the pathologist must assess the resected tissue him/herself to locate the lymph nodes and to evaluate them. If the lymph nodes are enlarged their identification does not cause problems and they can easily be excided from the tissue and examined, such as in axillary lymph nodes in mammary gland cancer. In such a situation it is recommended to mark the resected tissue with a stitch as it permits determining which part of the fat tissue is proximal and which is distal even after removing the lymph nodes. Also various levels can be marked. Lymphatic drainage in intestinal tumors represents another example of removing the mesenterium together with the part of the intestine affected by the tumor. Good pathological examination of lymphatic drainage requires that the resected tissue be stretched on a flat surface, or at least placed in a sufficiently large flat container to prevent rolling, if proper processing cannot be achieved. In this situation it is also convenient to mark apical, oral-aboral parts and extremities of the resected tissue with stitches, under an agreement between the surgeon and pathologist. When examining resected intestinal mesenterium, the pathologist faces a problem with the **identification of lymph nodes**. Lymph nodes are small in size and they are often subject to fat atrophy, so that they can easily be overlooked even when they are carefully looked for, both with palpation and by cutting mesenterium. Only enlarged lymph nodes, often already markedly affected by tumor metastases, are easily identifiable. The so-called **tissue clearance** is a technique that, after formol fixation, can improve identification of lymph nodes localized in fat tissue. In practice, after fixation in formol the tissue is placed in a solution of 96% ethanol with formaldehyde and acetic acid. As a result of this procedure, lymph nodes change color to pure white, while the color of fat tissue remains stable. Then a careful slicing of the specimen can reveal lymph nodes even if the size is only several millimeters and these can be excided and examined. This method confirms or excludes the metastatic involvement of lymph nodes and the extent, above all in lateral margins and in apex of the resected tissue, and therefore plays a decisive role in a patient's subsequent oncological treatment.

### 35.3.4 Examination of Resected Tissue after Neoadjuvant Therapy

In many indications of onco-surgical practice, the procedure is sequential. First, the diagnosis is made with the help of histopathological analysis, e.g. from puncture or excision; then a conservative oncological treatment with systemic chemotherapy or local radiotherapy focused on the tumor follows, and finally, surgical resection is carried out. This procedure is also common in the treatment of breast cancer, cancer of the prostate, the rectum, in the therapy of some bone malignancies (e.g. osteosarcoma) and in other oncological indications. The evidence of vital tumor tissue unaffected by therapy, and on the other hand assessment of the degree of tumor regression has an impact on prognosis. The tumor can necrotize, fibrotize, and if it is present in residua, then it often has a modified morphological appearance. The pathologist receives the tissue already modified by the treatment, and should be aware of a changed appearance of the tissue. Sometimes it is quite difficult to identify residua of modified but vital tumor tissue. Also subsequent specialized examinations of this bioptic material are difficult to evaluate. If the tumor has not responded to previous therapy with expected regression, an alternative procedure, both conservative and onco-surgical, should be considered. **The degree of regression** after neoadjuvant therapy is expressed by various classifications and has a prognostic impact.

### 35.3.5 Specialized Pathological Examinations after Organ Transplantations

In surgical practice, in addition to the basic diagnostics, consecutive examinations include sequentially collected samples after organ transplantations (heart, lungs, and kidneys). Histopathological examination is important in the assessment of the degree of acute or chronic **rejection immune reaction**, or it can identify inflammatory changes in developing infectious disease (e.g. after lung transplantation). Microbiological and successive molecular biological examination focused on the detection of a pathogen play a key role in confirming infection.

### 35.3.6 Detection of Diagnostically and Prognostically Significant Molecules in Pathology and Therapeutic-Indicative Pathology

In the last decades, the molecular basis of various diseases has been identified. This knowledge enables detecting specific molecules with pathogenetic and often also diagnostic or prognostic importance. Protein expression is often analyzed and this makes the diagnostics more precise. In tumors, this examination is also important for prognostic assessment and subsequent indication for oncological treatment. Proteins are routinely identified with immunohistochemical analysis, detecting proteins directly in tissues or cells of histological preparations. Results of these examinations are recorded in histology reports. The surgeon with the help of a pathologist or molecular biologist should study how to gain insight into these descriptions.

For a long time, the number of mitoses in a tumor has been considered important for surgical practice. It is applied for instance to distinguish between leiomyoma and leiomyosarcoma, or to assess potential risks of progression in gastrointestinal

PATHOLOGY

stromal tumors, or it forms part of tumor grading, e.g. in breast cancer or in some brain tumors. Since only nuclei with already spiralized chromosomes (mitotic figures) can be identified in basic histological staining when mitotic activity is assessed, immunohistochemical methods analyzing the expression of molecules of the cell cycle or apoptotic cascade are also used. The surgeon usually obtains an estimation of the number of cells (in %) in an active cell cycle after testing the worldwide accepted standard molecule Ki-67. ("Ki" comes from the city of Kiel in Germany where this molecule was identified in a university laboratory in a certain order and a diagnostically usable antibody against it was obtained).

Advanced methods of the **biological (targeted) therapy** aim to suppress gene functions and to assess expression intensity of these genes. Benefits of biologics are evaluated depending on detecting these molecules. Breast cancer can serve as an example, as the pathologist assesses the degree of expression of **ERBB-2 (Her-2/neu)** – a receptor protein on tumor cell membranes. If positive, therapy with humanized monoclonal antibodies against the mentioned protein is started and the treatment is effective. If negative it has no effect. Typically, the tissue of a colorectal carcinoma is examined in a similar way. The examination includes the detection of the membrane receptor **EGFR** in tumor cells. If it is expressed, the subsequent molecular assessment of mutation status of the **ras gene** is relevant.

In regulatory cascades the constitutively activated membrane receptor EGFR stimulates the submembrane protein $p21^{ras}$ and this activated protein transmits signals of growth activation into the cell nucleus. If the **ras gene** is not mutated, administration of monoclonal antibodies against EGFR has a therapeutic effect, since it is logical that in the preserved regulatory cascade the EGFR block also suppresses the function of $p21^{ras}$. If the **ras gene** is mutated, it behaves in an independent manner as constitutively active and stimulates an autonomous tumor cell to proliferate. Then the therapy with monoclonal antibodies targeted at blocking the activation of EGFR would be unjustifiable.

The Identification and detection of key molecules in cells has been advancing gradually. Biological therapy is effective and represents **one of the alternatives of** a patient's **individualized therapy**. On the other hand, it substantially increases the cost of healthcare; hence it must be justifiable and specifically indicated. This has led to the development of a new diagnostic **therapeutic-indicative** branch oriented toward pharmacology.

## 35.4 Generalization of Optimum Practice in Clinical Pathology

The pathologist is one of the closest collaborators of many clinical physicians specialized in operations or in collection of bioptic samples in general. He/she works for many specialized medical disciplines from general surgery to neurosurgery, orthopedics and many others. Since he/she usually is not in touch with the patient, he/she must rely on the data provided by the attending physician. Therefore the collaboration between the pathologist and the clinician should be very close. The pathologist must be provided with relevant information to have an idea about the nature of the disease before starting microscopic examination. The pathologist's clinical partners often make the mistake of not providing any information on the histology request form. The pathologist then attempts to deduce the nature of the disease from the microscopic presentation, which is often possible, but fails in a number of cases.

The following case report represents one of hundreds of examples from everyday practice: a 46-year old female patient with the information of "tumor of the thigh" reported in the histological request form has a tumor that could be histologically interpreted as low grade squamous cell carcinoma. As this kind of tumor is not a primary tumor of soft tissues, epitheloid sarcoma can be considered in differential diagnosis, i.e. completely different nosologic entity. The request form mentions sex and age, but the localization is not specified, i.e. the compartment of tumor resection (thigh not specified in more detail). After several phone calls, the pathologist uncovers that the patient terminated therapy for extensive squamous cell carcinoma of the uterine cervix a year ago, previously undergoing biopsy in another hospital. The excision of the thigh tumor was performed from the ventral proximal part. Hence the biopsy can be justifiably concluded as a progression of the original tumor – a squamous cell carcinoma to the region of proximal groin/thigh. Proper information about the patient's anamnesis would have saved time for diagnostics and avoided the hesitation of the pathologist over an unusual finding.

**Clinical-pathological correlation** in the form of a collective consultation (or possibly seminars related to individual cases) is effective in complicated cases, as it often helps to make the diagnosis or to specify the diagnosis in more detail. The participation of the surgeon and the specialist in imaging methods is very beneficial. These seminars have a diagnostic and educative character and are motivated by an effort to help patients to the maximum extent.

The surgeon should know the needs of the pathologist, above all in the preparation of tissue for pathological examination (see above). If the entry of the tissue to the laboratory is adequate, high quality and exact results can be expected. On the other hand, pathologists should be able to answer questions posed by surgeons, not only related to the exact nosologic diagnosis, but also about the extent of the disease in the patient.

The range of diagnostic, prognostic and monitoring tests in the area of pathology together with therapeutic-indicative examinations have been developing quickly and the topic should be studied and new information introduced into clinical-pathological practice.

# 36  IMAGING METHODS IN SURGERY

> 36.1 Radiodiagnostics
> 36.2 Interventional Radiology

## 36.1  Radiodiagnostics

### 36.1.1  Neck

■ THYROID GLAND

Ultrasound enables examining superficially localized neck structures such as the thyroid gland, salivary glands or lymph nodes. In the thyroid gland, the size of both lobes and isthmus, echogenity and cystic and solid foci are evaluated. Distinguishing between benign and malignant nature of a solid focus cannot be based only on hypo- or hyperechogenicity; scintigraphy or fine needle biopsy is necessary.

CT is indicated in restrosternal goiter to assess its caudal demarcation and compression of trachea or aortic arch vessels. In superior vena cava syndrome, it is helpful in assessing the compression of the subclavian vein or internal jugular vein.

CT or MRI with application of a contrast agent is indicated to detect ectopically localized parathyroid gland (often in upper mediastinum) in patients with hyperparathyreosis.

■ SALIVARY GLANDS

Ultrasound is the method of first choice and the size and echogenity of parenchyma permit to distinguish acute inflammation (enlarged, hypoechogenic gland) from chronic inflammation (smaller, hypoechogenic gland). Sialography evaluates the salivary gland duct, its intraparenchymal branches and the presence of calcifications. CT or preferably MRI help to identify salivary gland tumors, their relation to surrounding structures (nerves and vessels) and their infiltration.

■ LYMPH NODES

Imaging methods (ultrasound, CT, MRI) do not distinguish lymph nodes altered by inflammation from lymph nodes infiltrated with a tumor. The preserved oval shape of a lymph node, or color Doppler imaging of its vascularization, or formation of lymph node packets are not sufficiently specific, hence a lymph node biopsy is necessary in indicated cases. The search for a primary tumor in the neck or ENT region can be further modified, reflecting individual regions drained by neck lymph nodes. Benign inflammatory lymphadenopathy is usually associated with hyperplasia of lymphatic tissue in **Waldeyer's ring**.

Tissue specific contrast agents that would be specific for lymphatic tissue are promising for the future.

### 36.1.2 Chest Imaging

Summation **radiography in posteroanterior and lateral projections in a standing position** represents the basic examination of the chest; oblique projection is used to evaluate the chest skeleton. Horizontal beam projection of the patient lying on his/her side (Rigler projection) is usually indicated to prove free fluid. This projection can sometimes also detect pneumothorax. Chest radiography can reveal pathological changes of the chest organs. The size of the heart and vessels and changes in their arrangement indicate the character of the disease. Radiography of lung parenchyma can demonstrate inflammation, tumor, abscess, congestion, emphysema, trauma, pneumothorax, and foreign bodies. In the diaphragm, the position and condition are evaluated. In patients confined to bed or in patients incapable of the standing position, radiography is performed on bed; however, the pictures are of less diagnostic value. Another diagnostic method is chest **skiascopy** targeted on the examined lesion, assessing its shape, size, homogeneity, possible pulsations and its localization. The **ultrasound** can assess, besides heart and vessels, also chest wall structures, pleura and peripheral atelectatic lung lesions. **CT** is quite indispensable in complex diagnostics of the chest. Acute indications for CT comprise, above all, chest traumas. In comparison to MRI, the CT is faster and permits native examination without contrast agents as well as interventions such as puncture, drainage, abscess evacuation or local injections close to the spinal canal. The type of fluid can be assessed on the basis of its density. **MRI** examination is used, above all, in the diagnostics of major chest structures, especially in the area of pulmonary hila and mediastinum and also in some indications in the region of the chest wall. **Digital subtraction angiography** is used mainly in the treatment of acute hemorrhage into the chest wall in hemodynamically stable patients: in bleeding from intercostal arteries, hemoptysis or arteriovenous malformations of pulmonary arteries.

■ CHEST WALL

**Summation radiography** of the chest in anteroposterior and lateral projections is the basic examination to evaluate the chest wall skeleton and soft tissues or foreign bodies in chest trauma. Pathological conditions of the chest wall are examined by an **ultrasound**. This is a fast method, less arduous for patients, not requiring any special preparation of the patient prior to examination. It permits assessing pathological processes of the chest wall – hematomas, abscesses, malignant and benign tumors, structure and demarcation of lesions, and it enables assess to their propagation into surrounding structures and vascularization of the process; a targeted biopsy can be performed if needed. In fractures of ribs and the sternum, the trauma can be presumed on the basis of indirect signs such as hematoma, pleural effusion and lung contusion in the proximity of the fracture. **CT** is also used to examine the chest wall, providing a detailed picture of anatomical-pathological relations of bone structures and pathological findings with gas content – e.g. subcutaneous emphysema in traumas and postoperative conditions. CT is essential in the diagnostics of tumors and congenital deformities of the chest wall, including pectus excavatum, in biopsies of focal lesions and in drainage of pathological collections.

## PLEURA

Pathological processes of the pleural cavity are better evaluated with the help of an ultrasound than on the basis of summation chest radiography. The volume and character of pleural effusions can be roughly estimated. The effusion can be demonstrated in the sitting or lying positions, if its volume exceeds 5 mL; the ultrasound has 100% sensitivity and 99% specificity, radiography 71% sensitivity and 98% specificity. Ultrasound cannot evaluate processes in the interlobium and in lung parenchyma; nevertheless, it can distinguish between solid and fluid processes on the pleura. It can also assess some peripheral pulmonary consolidations such as atelectasis, abscess, tumor or infarction. The CT scan is irreplaceable for diagnostic assessment of pathological processes on the pleura – effusions, solid lesions, limited pneumothorax cavities including interlobia. CT helps to specify the character and nature of fluid collection, septation of collections, size and localization of the pneumothorax cavity and as the case may be also vascularization of solid expansive formation and calcifications. CT enables targeted biopsies of focal lesions and drainage of pathological collections and cavities. Ultrasound examination can assess the mobility of the diaphragm in real time, which can also be evaluated with skiascopy. The diaphragm is well evaluable on CT, especially in traumas. Magnetic resonance can also be employed in the assessment of the pleura and diaphragm.

## LUNGS

Summation chest radiography is the basic imaging method. CT has a fundamental value for surgery. Indications for CT are wide and comprise practically all diagnoses. The most frequent indication is the exclusion or confirmation of focal lesions (tumors, metastases) and their classification. Important indications are lung trauma, lung contusion, laceration and trauma of the trachea and bronchi.

### Chest Traumas
Basic imaging examination in chest trauma comprises a standard radiography of the chest and subdiaphragmatic region. It permits the diagnosis of rib frac-

tures (simple, serial, window), pneumothorax or hemothorax and assessing the mediastinal width. If the patient is hemodynamically stable and does not have any associated injuries, an ultrasound of the chest wall and organs, above all subdiaphragmatic, can be used as a subsequent imaging method, while chest and abdominal CT with or without contrast is employed in serious injuries. CT enables identifying lesions of soft tissues, the skeleton, lungs, bronchi, diaphragm and mediastinum including the aorta and large vessels.

Lung contusion is visible on radiography as irregular mild cloudy shadows, evident within several hours up to days; they can be absent immediately after the trauma, but develop within hours. The affected lung can be enlarged and the diaphragm lowered and flattened. Pulmonary laceration is well visible on CT as a pneumocele with hemothorax which can be extensive, with the volume of up to 1,000 mL. Trauma of the trachea and bronchi can be revealed by the presence of a sickle-shaped lucent streak outlining the pericardium, corresponding to the pneumomediastinum.

Aortic injury is diagnosed with **CT angiography**. It is visible as a traumatic aortic transection, most often in the aortic isthmus, with formation of a pseudoaneurysm. It is usually associated with hematoma in the mediastinum or in the left pleural cavity. The injury requires urgent endovascular treatment with implantation of a stent graft.

### Other Frequent Surgical Diseases

Other frequent surgical diseases comprise pulmonary inflammations and abscesses, gangrene, chronic pneumonia, middle lobe syndrome, bronchiectasia, tuberculosis and cystic fibrosis.

The abscess has a typical cavity resulting from tissue disintegration, with a gas-fluid level and with a thick irregular demarcating membrane communicating with the bronchus. Chronic pneumonia is difficult to radiologically distinguish from a tumor. A typical CT scan shows bronchiectasia with widened peripheral bronchi adjacent to the accompanying pulmonary artery.

## ■ LUNG TUMORS

- Benign – bronchial adenomas
- Semimalignant – carcinoids – on CT typically detected intraluminally in the bronchus
- Malignant lung tumors – carcinomas. Radiographic diagnosis in early stages is difficult; a simple summation picture does not always reveal tumors of central localization. Then a CT scan must be performed in both the native form and with a contrast agent

### Pulmonary and Bronchial Anomalies and Cysts

Agenesis, aplasia and hypoplasia can be detected on summation radiography with shadowing on the affected side; the diagnosis can be more specified with the help of CT. Bronchogenic cysts and cystic adenomatoid malformations are visible on radiography as a sharply demarcated homogeneous shadowing. CT specifies the diagnosis of cystic formation in more detail and also helps in differential diagnostics of lobar and bullous emphysema – pneumothorax and pulmonary cyst should be taken into account. Pulmonary sequestration – interlobar – is shown on radiography as a number of changes from a simple shadowing up to cystic lesions with levels. Extralobar sequestration is separated from the lung parenchyma and usually has its own visceral artery dividing from the aorta.

### ■ MEDIASTINUM

In the posteroanterior chest picture, the mediastinum forms a middle-line shadow with an individual variability. The shadow is constituted mainly by heart and large vessels with lucent streak, trachea and large bronchi. A detailed assessment of anatomical-pathological processes in mediastinum is enabled by CT or magnetic resonance. CT is always performed with application of an i.v. contrast agent.

The diagnosis of mediastinal tumors is based on radiography and especially on CT scans. Tumors of the thymus are typically situated in the anterior mediastinum. Mediastinal cysts – bronchogenic, esophageal, gastroenteral and pericardial – have a typical localization and the diagnosis is made with the help of CT and MRI. Teratomas contain cellular structures of all three embryonic layers and their image on CT and MRI is typical. Diagnostics of other neoplastic mediastinal diseases, mesenchymal tumors, carcinomas and lymphomas require examination by CT or MRI.

## 36.1.3   Mammary Glands

Mammography and ultrasound represent two basic imaging methods of breast examination. Each of these methods has its indication, pros and cons. They complement each other yet they are not mutually interchangeable or replaceable.

### ■ MAMMOGRAPHY

Mammography is the basic examination method in women over 40 years of age. The mammograph is a special radiographic device enabling to visualize and distinguish particular structures of breast tissue.

The mammographic image of breast tissue structure changes with the years. In the Czech Republic, a classification of breast tissue composition into five groups according to the ratio between fat tissue, gland and connective tissue is used. Mammographic diagnostics is based on three types of changes – **focal changes, microcalcifications and asymmetrical structural changes** of breast tissue composition.

Benign foci – cysts, fibroadenomas and papillomas – usually have typical appearance with a sharp and regular contour. Their contour can sometimes join with adjacent structures.

Detection of microcalcifications is the major benefit of mammography. They can be the first sign of mammary ductal carcinoma in the *in situ* stage, i.e. without infiltration of adjacent tissues and without propagation via the lymphatic system. These microcalcifications can be revealed exclusively by mammography. Only some calcifications and microcalcifications visualized by mammography are of a malignant nature. Microcalcifications are often associated just with changes of mammary tissue corresponding to the wide group of "mastopathic changes".

Asymmetry and structural changes of breast tissue revealed on the mammogram belong to other signs of breast tissue diseases. These changes are sometimes discrete and their assessment requires much experience in mammographic diagnostics (e.g. lobular carcinoma).

### ■ ULTRASOUND

Ultrasound belongs to basic examination methods in women under 40 years of age and represents a complementary examination method to mammography. In women over 40 years of age, the ultrasound alone does not replace mammography. Ultrasound can distinguish solid and cystic foci and show intracystic solid structures.

A simple cyst has a sharp and regular contour, anechogenic content, fine wall and dorsal acoustic enhancement. Solid foci have homogeneous or non-homogeneous internal structure which is usually hypo- or isoechogenic with the surrounding tissue. The contour in benign foci is sharp and regular, in malignant foci irregular and blurred. In contrast to mammography, ultrasound does not permit the diagnosis of microcalcifications or the incipient stage of carcinoma.

### ■ INTERVENTIONAL METHODS

Basic interventional diagnostic methods comprise cyst puncture, biopsy of solid foci and vacuum-assisted biopsy of microcalcifications. These interventions are carried out under direct supervision through an ultrasound or mammograph which enables to target even minor foci. The second group of interventions is constituted by ultrasound localization methods. The localization of minor non-palpable foci is possible by several means – a mark on the skin above the focus, staining with dye, placing a little piece of wire or a clip – and is performed preoperatively.

## 36.1.4  Soft Tissues

Ultrasound is the method of choice for soft tissue assessment. It permits distinguishing between cystic and solid hypoechogenic or hyperechogenic lesions. Doppler ultrasound enables the assessment of the vascularization of the focus localized in soft tissue, its supplying arteries, draining veins and bloodstream velocity.

X-ray helps to visualize calcifications in the focus. Expansion can have different transparency in comparison with surrounding soft tissues (lipoma is more transparent).

MRI provides the most complex information about soft tissue involvement. It can show the focus in all three mutually perpendicular projections, distinguishing, if the lesion is intramuscular and specifying its relation to intramuscular septa, intermuscular fasciae and subcutaneous tissue. Biopsy is necessary when specific or even differential diagnostics of the focus cannot be provided by MRI.

## 36.1.5   Abdominal Wall

Ultrasound is the method of choice in imaging of abdominal wall lesions. Due to the thickness of the abdominal wall, a probe of higher frequency with higher spatial resolution is suitable. Ultrasound shows individual layers of the abdominal wall – subcutaneous tissue, muscular layers, differentiated defects of the abdominal wall e.g. herniation. The content of the hernia sac can be examined as well as peristalsis of a herniated intestinal loop and thickness and the vascularization of its wall.

Magnetic resonance can examine the thickness of the muscular layer, atrophy of abdominal muscles and can reliably assess their defects.

High signal of fat in T1 sequence demonstrates fat tissue, e.g. content of mesenterium in the hernia sac, in a relatively specific way. Dynamic MRI sequences in cinematographic loop can show discoordination of muscular contractions and can contribute to the diagnostics of intermuscular hernias. Radiographically non-contrast foreign objects in the abdominal wall are best visible on MRI. **Prior to MRI examination, it is vital to exclude the presence of a ferromagnetic foreign body.** (If the composition of a foreign body is not clear, an ultrasound examination should be performed first!)

## 36.1.6   Esophagus and Gastroduodenum

Radiographic imaging of the esophagus, stomach and duodenum is usually performed with a contrast medium. This enables assessing the localization and character of the lesion, its length and anatomical relations to adjacent structures. Barium contrast is used if leakage outside the lumen of gastrointestinal tube is not expected; otherwise a water-soluble contrast is used in situations comprising the perforation of the gastrointestinal tube or the control of suture tightness and anastomosis patency after surgical procedures. The examination of the esophagus, stomach and duodenum with a barium contrast agent is suitable if an impaired passage of benign or malignant etiology is suspected, in patients with suspicion of peptic ulcer disease of the duodenum, gastric herniation and malrotation. If a foreign body in the esophagus is suspected, a native chest radiography is always performed first, searching for the foreign body or free gas in the mediastinum or subcutaneously. Only after performing the above-mentioned, the water-soluble contrast agent is administered with a small, contrast-soaked piece of cotton that can get stuck on the non-contrast foreign body and help to localize it. In tumors of the esophagus, stomach, and duodenum, the chest and abdominal CT examination is essential, providing more detailed information on the propagation of the tumor into adjacent structures or on its generalization.

### 36.1.7 Small and Large Intestine

■ SMALL INTESTINE

The examination of the small intestine – enteroclysis – is carried out with the use of the so-called double contrast. A duodenal tube is inserted, a barium contrast agent is applied and then methyl cellulose as a negative contrast agent is administered.

A radiographic enteroclysis is the most reliable examination to confirm stenoses and fistulas.

CT or MR enterography is performed after the administration of a 2% solution of hyperosmolar agent (mannitol) that leads to an increased amount of fluid in the lumen of the small intestine causing its distension. Chronic inflammatory changes can be detected if the wall of the small intestine is widened more than 4 mm. An active inflammation is visible as a postcontrast signal enhancement of the intestinal wall; the intensity of enhancement is directly proportional to the seriousness of the inflammation. CT or MR enterography can also reveal abscesses between intestinal loops. Both examinations are also used in the diagnostics of small intestine tumors.

■ APPENDICITIS

Imaging methods (ultrasound, CT) can contribute to complex diagnostics of appendicitis. Ultrasound is used, performing graded compression on the right meso- and hypogastrium, at the end of a routine abdominal examination. An appendix affected with inflammation is a non-compressible blind tubular structure without peristalsis. The wall has a thicker muscular (hypoechogenic) layer of a width over 3 mm and a wide external diameter. Hyperemia of the appendix and adjacent structures can be seen on a Doppler ultrasound. However, even with a graded compression, some cases of appendices affected by inflammation pass unnoticed, as they are overlapped with gas present inside extended intestinal loops. CT finding in appendicitis: evident circular thickening of the appendix wall, mild edema in its surroundings, inflammatory infiltration or abscess.

■ LARGE INTESTINE

Irrigography is performed as a radiographic examination with a double contrast, applying barium contrast medium **per rectum** with subsequent air insufflation. The whole large intestine must be displayed including the reflux of the contrast agent into the terminal ileum.

Tumors of the large intestine lead to the development of stenosis; barium stagnates before stenosis and the narrowing is displayed with a delay. A picture of the typical "claw sign" is usually visible at both sides of the affected part of the bowel.

CT and MRI examinations play a role in the staging of colorectal carcinoma.

Constipation and impaired defecation can be examined by other contrast radiographic methods. In constipation, velocity of the large intestinal passage can be evaluated by **transit time**; the examination consists in the administration of contrast marks by mouth and in observing their passage through intestinal segments. **Defecography** enables examining the function and anatomy of the anorectum and pelvic floor including the course of defecation. This radiographic examination is performed with a contrast enema.

## 36.1.8 Liver

A native abdominal radiography can display only major hepatomegaly or the diaphragm surface domed by an expansive process or calcifications. The presence of gas in the biliary tract or in abscesses can be detected.

Ultrasound is one of the basic examination methods in diagnostics of both focal and diffuse lesions. Doppler ultrasound can distinguish vessels from other tubular structures. A resistance index in the portal vein can be assessed, or collaterals in the case of liver cirrhosis. Usage of intravenous contrast medium in ultrasounds helps in the differential diagnosis of vascularized focal lesions.

CT shows the liver and its adjacent area in more detail than ultrasound; usage of an i.v. contrast agent increases its sensitivity in the case of focal liver impairment. Magnetic resonance in dynamic T1 sequence after the application of gadolinium is more suitable for differential diagnostics than CT due to its high sensitivity and specificity, above all to minor focal lesions. It also permits distinguishing vascularized structures from avascular ones.

**Angiography** is carried out to detect vascular anomalies, bleeding or to reveal vascularized foci. The procedure enables subsequent application of therapeutic embolization or chemoembolization in tumorous vascularized foci, above all in HCC, colorectal metastases, metastases of carcinoma of the mammary gland, pancreas, and melanoma.

Ultrasound or CT is employed for targeted navigated biopsy of foci, for drainage of pathological collection and to insert a radiofrequency probe (RFA).

**Percutaneous portography** is used for targeted embolization of portal vein branches and before resection in the liver.

## 36.1.9 Gallbladder

Only radiocontrast concrements can be visualized on a native radiography of the subhepatic region; however, only 10–15% of all concrements are radiocontrast. Hence an ultrasound is the method of choice for stomach and biliary tract imaging. It can show concrements, thick bile, inflammation and tumors of the gallbladder and its surroundings as well as the gallbladder wall. Before the examination, patients are required to fast.

CT is suitable in some pathological processes of the intrahepatic biliary tract (Caroli syndrome), if a tumor of the gallbladder or biliary tract is suspected, and the method also permits assessing the extent of inflammation in the subhepatic region.

**Endoscopic retrograde cholangiopancreatography** (ERCP) is performed if a total or partial obstruction of the extra- or intrahepatic biliary tract is suspected, which can result from concrements, tumors, or in chronic inflammatory and fibrotizing changes of the Vater's papilla or biliary ducts. It can also clarify postoperative conditions. The procedure can be diagnostic or therapeutic, with the possibility to remove concrements or to insert an internal plastic drain.

**Percutaneous transhepatic cholangiography** and drainage (PTC and PTD) can be performed in patients with an obstructive jaundice where ERCP could not be carried out. The intrahepatic biliary tree is punctured under skiascopic supervision through skin and liver parenchyma and visualized with a contrast agent. After detecting and localizing the obstruction, an external or external-internal drain can be inserted into the duodenum. A **self-expanding metal stent** can be placed into the site of a malignant stricture as a definitive solution. If the bile flow to the duodenum is blocked by a concrement, it can be removed with a Dormia basket inserted percutaneously into the duodenum.

**Percutaneous cholecystotomy** is performed in patients with hydrops or empyema of the gallbladder. A thin drain is inserted under CT or MRI supervision into the lumen of the gallbladder to drain bile into a collection bag. This procedure is less arduous for patients than the operation, especially in elderly patients.

Peroperative and postoperative cholangiography via a T-drain is performed to control the biliary tract after its surgical revision. If remanent concrements persist, they can be extracted with a Dormia basket through the canal after the T-drain. MRI of biliary tract (MRCP) is indicated if an attempted ERCP is not successful.

### 36.1.10 Pancreas

Imaging methods in the diagnostics of pancreatic diseases comprise a native abdominal radiography, ultrasound, computerized tomography and MRCP (magnetic resonance cholangiopancreatography) as an alternative to diagnostic ERCP. Indications of individual imaging methods differ depending on the expected diagnosis.

■ ACUTE PANCREATITIS

Simple abdominal radiography in the standing position reveals the presence of so-called sentinel loops that indicate peritoneal irritation in acute pancreatitis.

# IMAGING METHODS IN SURGERY

In an acute stage, ultrasound has a limited validity. The area of the pancreas is often covered with artifacts of intestinal content and edema of its surroundings. However, the ultrasound reliably displays biliary ducts, their dilatation or presence of concrements in the case of pancreatitis of biliary origin.

CT examination with an i.v. contrast agent reliably distinguishes between the edematous and necrotizing forms of pancreatitis. The whole pancreas is enlarged, its structure is blurred, its contours are blunt and necrotic parts of parenchyma do not increase their density after the application of a contrast agent. In further course, fluid, inflammatory or necrotic collection can be visualized and eventually drained under CT supervision.

### ■ CHRONIC PANCREATITIS

Ultrasound and CT enable follow up on patients with a chronic form of pancreatitis and monitoring its manifestations like pancreatic atrophy, parenchymal calcifications, dilatation of the pancreatic duct or acute exacerbation of pancreatitis.

### ■ PANCREATIC TUMORS

The ultrasound or CT displays tumors as expansions of non-homogenous structure and blunt demarcation. The pancreatic duct is often dilated due to its compression. Intravenous application of a contrast agent during a CT examination helps to differentiate the tumor from the surrounding parenchyma.

Pancreatic tumors are often associated with chronic pancreatitis; the difference of structure between chronic inflammatory changes and tumor are usually discrete.

## 36.1.11 Spleen

Radiography has practically been abandoned as an imaging method of the spleen. Calcifications in the spleen develop after traumas, infarctions, in the walls of cysts, rarely also after a cured tubercular process. Calcifications are situated in the vessel walls in the splenic hilum. The preferred imaging method is the ultrasound that enables assessing the spleen size, shape, character of the parenchyma, number and size of foci and possible changes in the surroundings. Doppler ultrasound displays perfusion of the splenic parenchyma, pseudoaneurysms or posttraumatic arteriovenous fistulas in the splenic parenchyma. The CT is similarly helpful as the ultrasound; however, it is more precise and enables examining the spleen even in patients where the spleen cannot be properly visualized by the ultrasound for various reasons. Magnetic resonance has similar benefits. Both CT and MRI can be used to assess arterial perfusion of the spleen, above all with the aim to exclude aneurysms and pseudoaneurysms in acute pancreatitis. Examination of the spleen with imaging methods is usually indicated in blunt abdominal trauma and in hematological diseases.

Splenic lesion is a frequent consequence of blunt abdominal trauma. Both examinations can usually provide exact diagnostics of the character and extent of capsular and parenchymal injury. Angiography is performed only if an aneurysm or pseudoaneurysm of the splenic artery is suspected, with the aim to embolize the aneurysm or to implant a stent graft.

### 36.1.12 Ileus

■ NATIVE RADIOGRAPHY

Native radiography represents the basic examination. In the picture in a standing position, the ileus is characterized by distended intestinal loops with gas-fluid levels. The distribution of distended loops enables to distinguish between mechanical ileus resulting from an obstruction (bowels are distended above the obstruction) from paralytic, functional ileus where both small and large intestinal loops are distended. If a patient's condition does not permit carrying out radiography in a standing position with a horizontal beam, the position on the patient's left side is preferred.

■ APPLICATION OF WATER-SOLUBLE IODINATED CONTRAST BY MOUTH

This method is used to localize the site of an obstruction and to distinguish obstructive and paralytic ileus.

■ ULTRASOUND

In ileus conditions, the ultrasound is markedly limited by increased intestinal gas content; therefore it usually does not provide any helpful information about the site of obstruction. Nevertheless, it can be helpful in distinguishing between mechanical ileus, where the peristalsis of bowels is visible above the obstruction. In paralytic ileus, the bowel peristalsis is markedly slower.

### 36.1.13 Abdominal Trauma

■ ULTRASOUND

In blunt abdominal trauma, the ultrasound is the basic examination. It enables assessing the presence of free fluid in the peritoneal cavity. In a patient in the lying position, the free fluid is usually situated in the lowest site of the peritoneal cavity, i.e. in the Douglas space. Less often the fluid is in the surroundings of an injured intra-abdominal organ.

■ CT

CT is indicated, if the ultrasound finding is unclear or if a patient's clinical condition is worsening. In CT, the patient's usual preparation with iodinated contrast fluid **by mouth** prior to examination is not necessary.

CT is helpful in showing fissures and contusions of parenchymatous organs. They are displayed as postcontrast hypodensities, in comparison with organ parenchyma that has normal density. The native density of the contusion focus depends on the extent of bleeding; acute hemorrhage causes hyperdensity (60 HU) of the contusion focus.

Liver trauma can be associated with the laceration of the biliary tract and with the development of bile collection in the site of a laceration or in the subhepatic region.

Pancreatic trauma is rare.

## 36.2 Interventional Radiology

Significant advances in imaging methods based on X-rays, ultrasound and magnetic resonance led to the development of interventional radiology. This specialization, which currently belongs to postgraduate medical education, enables treatment of some diseases and conditions with minimum disruption of the external integrity of the human body. Mini-invasiveness of the procedure is associated with lower morbidity. The method was founded by Charles Dotter in 1964 when he carried out the first percutaneous recanalization of an artery; the term interventional radiology originated in 1977.

Interventional radiology comprises procedures on the vascular system as well as non-vascular interventions; both are possible on transplanted organs as well. Continuous improvement of machine equipment, used materials, techniques as well as the introduction of new therapeutic procedures has altered indications in favor of interventional procedures.

### 36.2.1 Arterial Interventions

■ PERCUTANEOUS TRANSLUMINAR ANGIOPLASTY (PTA)

PTA is a treatment of stenoses. In adults, stenoses and occlusions are most often caused by atherosclerosis. PTA is carried out through a sleeve or using a guide catheter inserted close to the stenosis. If PTA fails, metal stents are implanted to maintain good vessel patency. In some localizations, the stent implantation is a primary procedure, as in PTA of internal carotids, ostial stenoses of renal arteries or impairment of pelvic arteries.

Intraluminal PTA is recommended for occlusions of up to 10 cm, since the primary effect and long-term outcome in long atherosclerotic lesions are poor. The technique of subintimal recanalization (extraluminal method) can be used in longer occlusions on limbs (10 cm and above, but also for instance 40 cm), when a new canal is created in subintimal space. Subintimal intervention can also be performed in patients who have undergone repeated bypasses or in older arterial occlusions after 5 years or more.

Coated stents, so called **stent grafts**, are used in some types of arterial impairment. Their insertion is indicated in aneurysms of the descending part of the thoracic aorta, in thoracoabdominal aneurysms, in aneurysms of arteries in other localizations, in dissected aneurysm type B, in traumatic transection of the thoracic aorta or in pseudoaneurysms. Fenestrated grafts are used if visceral arteries must be implanted. These are also newly developed for the implantation of aortic arch branches where, up to now, only hybrid procedures with vascular surgery have been performed. Stent grafts are also inserted in iatrogenic lesions, e.g. in arteriovenous shunts resulting from subclavian vein puncture. Nevertheless, stent grafts are not used in similar impairment in groins where a surgical treatment is preferred due to increased physical exertion.

A low-molecular-weight heparin and permanent antiaggregant therapy is administered after an arterial PTA.

### ■ THROMBOLYSIS

Local thrombolytic treatment represents a significant part of the therapy of acute arterial occlusion caused by embolism or thrombosis. It is usually performed together with percutaneous aspiration thromboebolectomy and PTA; in some cases also with surgical treatment. Local thrombolysis is also carried out in patients with thrombosis of a peripheral arterial bypass. A catheter is inserted into the site of the occlusion; the dose of thrombolytic is low. In the Czech Republic, the only thrombolytic pharmaceutical for local application is a recombinant form of tissue plasminogen activator, rt-PA (Actilyse, Boehringer-Ingelheim Pharma KG). The dose ranges between 0.5 and 1 mg rt-PA per hour. Simultaneously, a small amount of heparin is administered intravenously (500 units per hour). Similar dosing is used in local thrombolysis in the venous system.

The incidence of bleeding complications associated with thrombolysis has been decreasing since the introduction of low doses of thrombolytics together with lower doses of heparin. In application of rt-PA, a subsequent targeted surgical procedure can be performed practically immediately after finishing the thrombolysis.

### ■ EMBOLIZATION

Generally speaking, embolization should be performed in the maximum proximity to the target region. Microcatheters and coaxial systems are employed. A proximal embolization of the filling artery with coils must be avoided as this would prevent access in the future. A number of embolization materials are used: gelfoam, polyvinyl alcohol particles, microcoils, ethanol and tissue glues. For example, in trauma of the liver, spleen or pelvis with hemodynamic instability, a gelfoam is applied in the form of a mixture or as so-called torpedoes, i.e. temporary embolization materials. This enables control of bleeding with the possibility

IMAGING METHODS IN SURGERY

to reconstruct the bloodstream several days or weeks later. Pulmonary arteriovenous malformations are embolized with special occluders which are also used in other shunt defects, heart septal defects and patent arterial ducts.

A combination of regional intra-arterial chemotherapy with tumor ischemization via embolization, the so-called chemoembolization, is used in some types of tumors (e.g. HCC).

## 36.2.2 Venous Interventions

### ■ DEEP VENOUS THROMBOSIS OF LOWER EXTREMITIES

The intervention is based on duplex ultrasound under the supervision of conventional venography. Endovascular therapy is routinely used in deep venous thrombosis of lower extremities (≤ 10 days from the onset of symptoms) and phlegmasia coerulea dolens. It comprises various forms of local **application of thrombolytics** and in recent years also **mechanical thrombectomy**. A more aggressive approach is suitable in younger and highly active patients. A temporary **vena cava filter** should always be considered to prevent pulmonary embolism. The endovascular therapy is highly successful. Stent implantation is necessary in compressive syndrome (May-Thurner syndrome) or in aplasia of the inferior vena cava (to improve the flow), or possibly also in residual stenosis non-responding to PTA.

Endovascular therapy of deep venous thrombosis has replaced surgical thrombectomy that was associated with relatively high peroperative mortality. Surgical thrombectomy is performed only if endovascular treatment fails or in situations when the venous bloodstream is severely impaired but thrombolytic therapy is contraindicated and mechanical thrombectomy is not accessible.

After the intervention, the patient is converted from heparin to warfarin anticoagulation and wears compressive stockings. Long-term ultrasound controls are necessary.

In the less common thromboses of the upper extremities, the interventional treatment is performed likewise.

Not only acute deep venous thrombosis, but also symptomatic patients with chronic venous occlusion of central bloodstream and with post-thrombotic syndrome can be treated. Because of the painfulness, the procedures are performed under general anesthesia; a higher number of stents (three or more) is required.

### ■ CENTRAL VENOUS CATHETERS

Central venous catheters can be inserted via the periphery, mainly through forearm and arm veins, or via central entry through jugular or subclavian veins or possibly through common femoral veins.

## ■ PORTAL HYPERTENSION – TRANSJUGULAR INTRAHEPATIC PORTOSYSTEMIC SHUNT

Transjugular intrahepatic portosystemic shung (TIPS) represents an artificial communication that conveys blood from the portal systemic bloodstream; it is the most effective method to decrease portal hypertension. Under ideal conditions, the shunt should decrease portal pressure preventing bleeding and ascites, but at the same time hepatic portal perfusion should be maintained and the risk of encephalopathy should not increase.

The possibility of percutaneous creation of an artificial portosystemic shunt has extended indications of this therapy also to patients that could not undergo a surgical treatment due to an unacceptably high risk resulting from their poor general condition. Currently, TIPS represents the first choice in patients with a patent portal vein and with acute thrombosis of the portal vein.

TIPS is indicated in bleeding into the gastrointestinal tract caused by portal hypertension, in refractory ascites, acute or subacute thrombosis of hepatic veins and in hepatorenal syndrome, above all with a perspective of liver transplantation. In emergency procedures performed because of endoscopically unstoppable bleeding, the procedure is performed together with embolization of portosystemic collaterals. Currently, instead of the formerly used flexible stents, the intrahepatic canal is reinforced with a stent graft leading to a lower risk of developing stenosis.

### 36.2.3 Intervention on Transplanted Organs

Intervention on transplanted organs refers, above all, to interventions after kidney and liver transplantations. In transplanted organs, intervention on the vascular system as well as neovascular procedures can be performed.

In the liver, the PTA is carried out at the site of the anastomoses; arterial and venous stenoses emerging over a longer period of time after transplantation are treated with stent insertion. Indications for neovascular interventions comprise biliary obstruction based on stenosis in anastomosis or in intrahepatic biliary ducts and biliary fistula. The interventions consist in balloon catheter dilatation, external/internal drainage or insertion of a metal stent. Surgical drainage is the basic therapy of extrahepatic biliomas.

**IMAGING METHODS IN SURGERY – GALLERY**

**TEXTBOOK OF SURGERY**

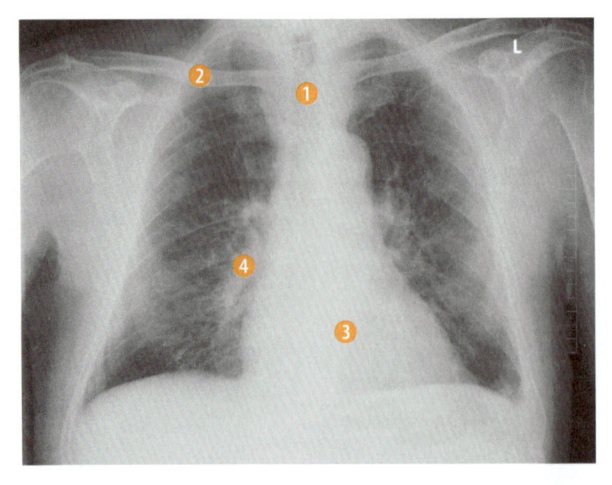

Fig. 1a   Retrosternal goiter, chest radiography
1) Cup shaped widening of upper mediastinum
2) Clavicle
3) Heart
4) Right pulmonary artery

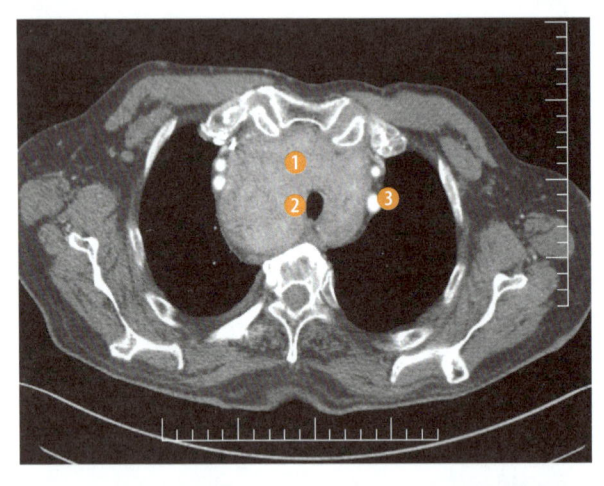

Fig. 1b   Retrosternal goiter, chest CT with application of contrast agent, transverse plane
1) Retrosternal goiter
2) Compressing and dislocating trachea
3) Pushing aside arteries of aortic arch

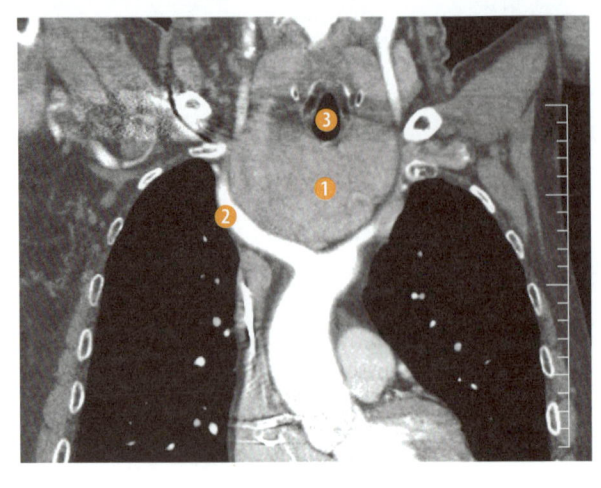

Fig. 1c   Retrosternal goiter, chest CT with application of contrast agent, coronal plane
1) Retrosternal goiter
2) Pressure on large vessels of aortic arch
3) Goiter encircling trachea

IMAGING METHODS IN SURGERY – GALLERY

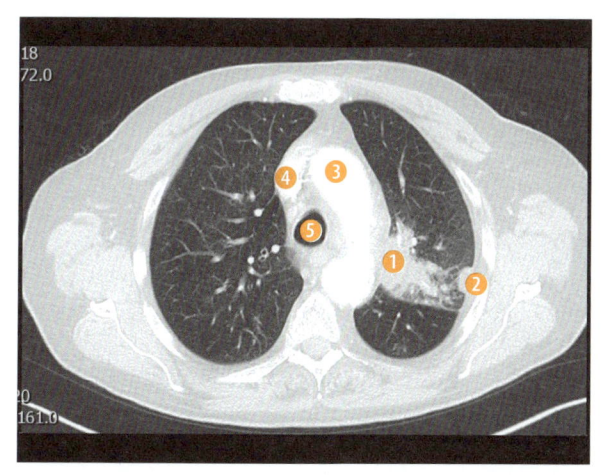

**Fig. 2a** Bronchogenic carcinoma, lung CT, lung window
1) Tumor (bronchogenic carcinoma) in left parahilar area
2) Lung metastasis on the left side in subpleural area adjacent to chest wall
3) Aortic arch
4) Superior vena cava
5) Trachea

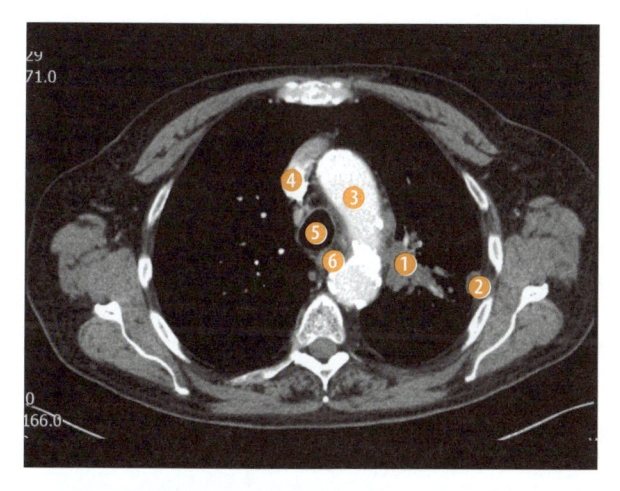

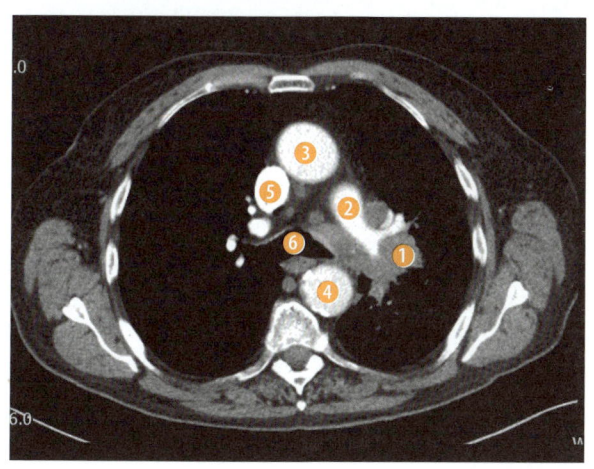

**Fig. 2b** Bronchogenic carcinoma, lung CT, mediastinal window after application of contrast agent
1) Tumor (bronchogenic carcinoma) in left parahilar area
2) Lung metastasis on the left side in subpleural area adjacent to chest wall
3) Aortic arch
4) Superior vena cava
5) Trachea
6) Esophagus

**Fig. 2c** Bronchogenic carcinoma, lung CT, mediastinal window after application of contrast agent
1) Tumor (bronchogenic carcinoma) in left parahilar area
2) Encircling left pulmonary artery
3) Ascending aorta
4) Descending aorta
5) Superior vena cava
6) Tracheal bifurcation

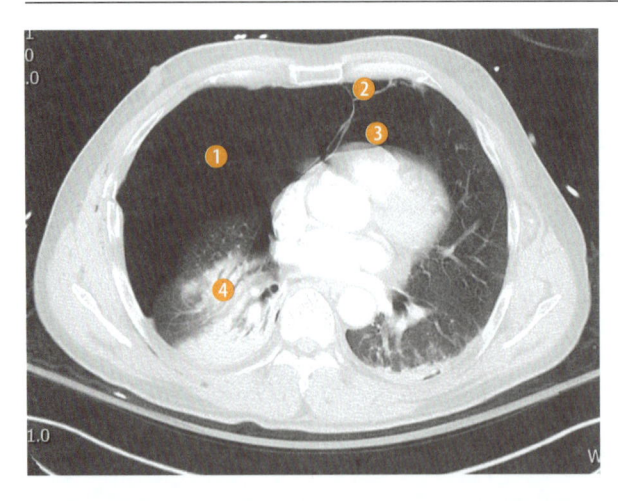

**Fig. 3a** Pneumothorax on the right side, chest CT, lung window
1) Marked pneumothorax on the right side
2) Pneumomediastinum
3) Pneumopericardium
4) Collapsed lung, atelectasis

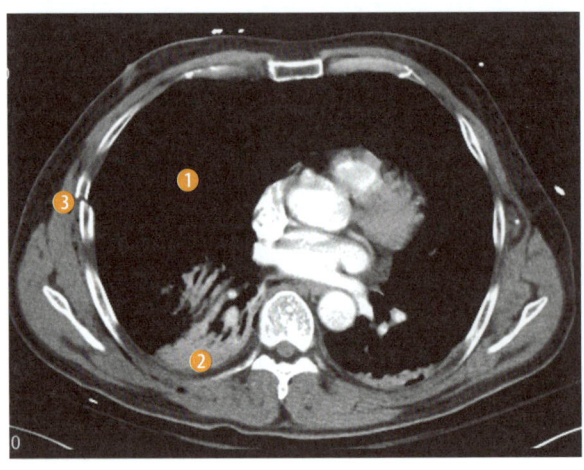

**Fig. 3b** Pneumothorax on the right side, chest CT, mediastinal window, with application of contrast agent
1) Pneumothorax on the right side
2) Atelectasis of inferior lobe of the right lung
3) Rib fracture on the right side

## IMAGING METHODS IN SURGERY – GALLERY

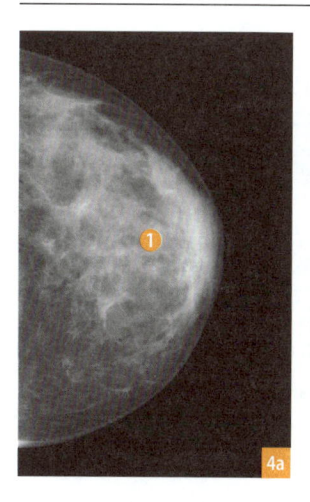

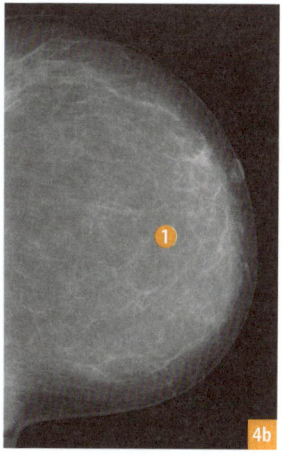

**Fig. 4a** Tabar's typology of breast tissue composition – Tabar I, mammography
1) Image of breast in a young woman

**Fig. 4b** Tabar's typology of breast tissue composition – Tabar II, mammography
1) Image of fat involution

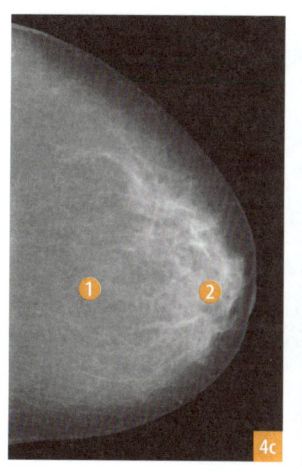

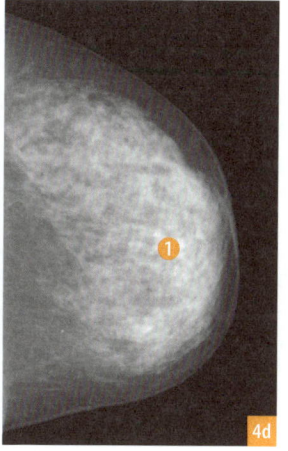

**Fig. 4c** Tabar's typology of breast tissue composition – Tabar III, mammography
1) Image of fat involution
2) Residues of fibroglandular tissue only in retroareolar localization

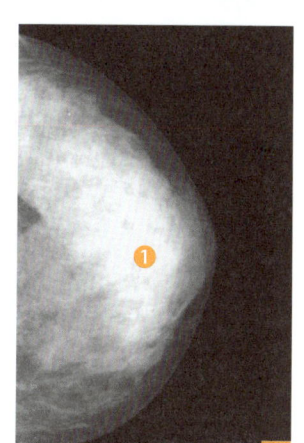

**Fig. 4d** Tabar's typology of breast tissue composition – Tabar IV, mammography
1) Predominance of connective tissue with diffuse non-homogenous shadowing

**Fig. 4e** Tabar's typology of breast tissue composition – Tabar V, mammography
1) Dense breast with predominance of fibroglandular tissue and intense, almost homogeneous diffuse shadowing

Chapter 36

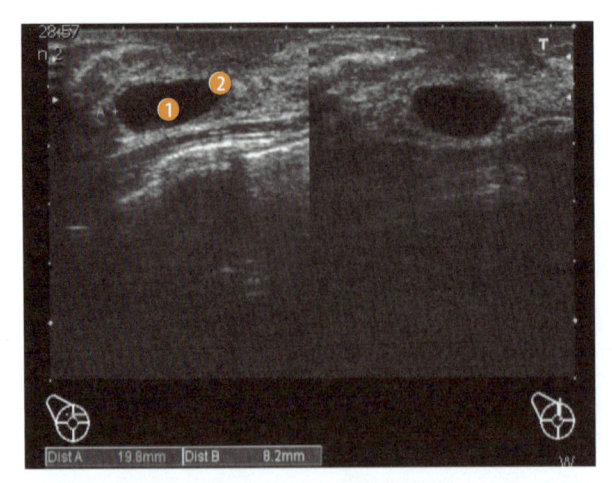

Fig. 5 Breast cyst, ultrasound
1) Anechogenic content
2) Smooth cyst wall

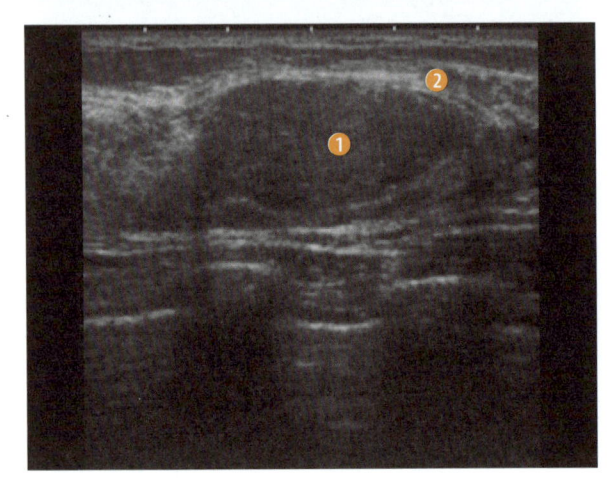

Fig. 6 Breast fibroadenoma, ultrasound
1) Hypoechogenic oval focus with homogenous structure
2) With sharp contour

IMAGING METHODS IN SURGERY – GALLERY

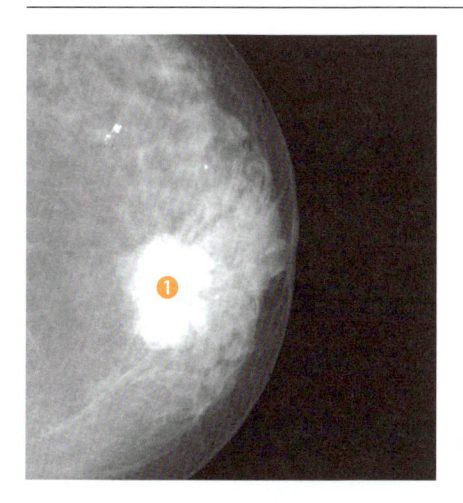

Fig. 7a  Breast carcinoma, mammography
1) Large breast carcinoma in retroareolar localization

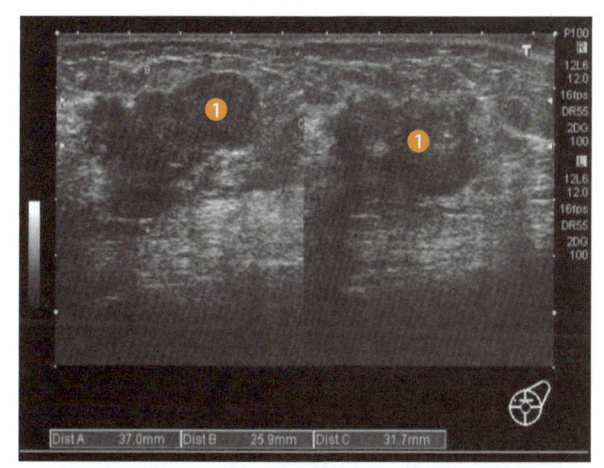

Fig. 7b  Breast carcinoma, ultrasound
1) Hypoechogenic focus with irregular and lobulated contour

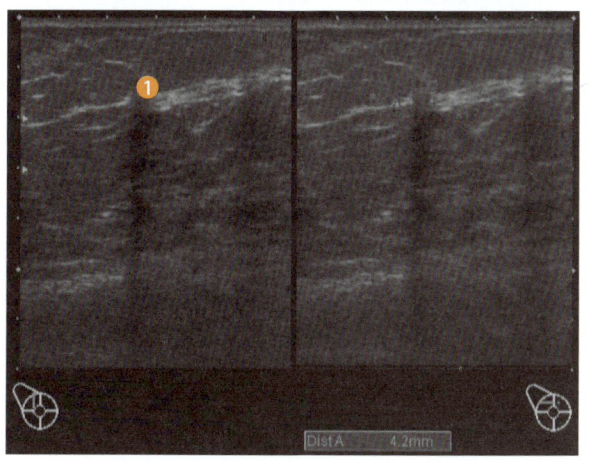

Fig. 7c  Minimum breast carcinoma, ultrasound
1) Tumor hardly differentiable, except by acoustic shadow

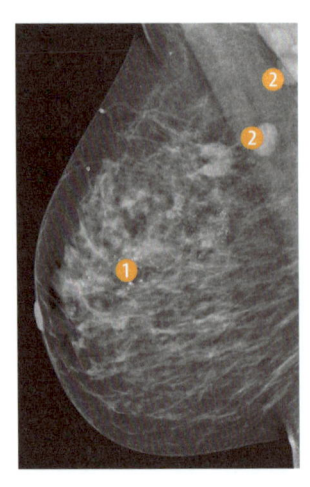

**Fig. 8a Microcalcifications in ductal carcinoma, mammography**
1) Dense focus with microcalcifications
2) Involvement of axillary lymph nodes

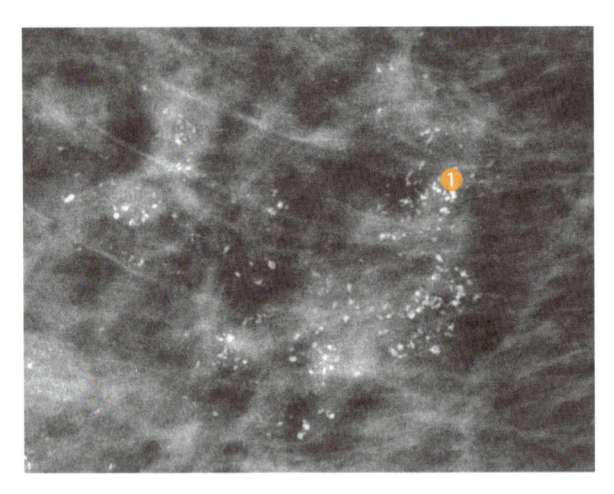

**Fig. 8b Detail of malignant intraductal microcalcifications**
1) Irregular shape, variable density, in some places hints of branched calcifications

**IMAGING METHODS IN SURGERY – GALLERY**

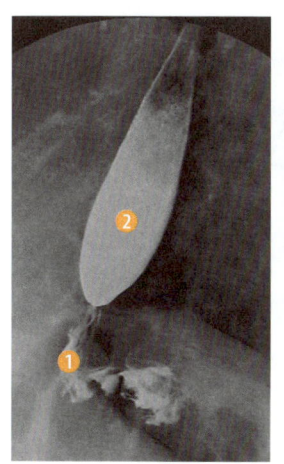

Fig. 9  Tumor of aboral esophagus and cardia, radiography – barium swallow
1) Narrowed aboral esophagus and cardia with irregular contour of the wall
2) Dilatation of oral part of esophagus above stenosis

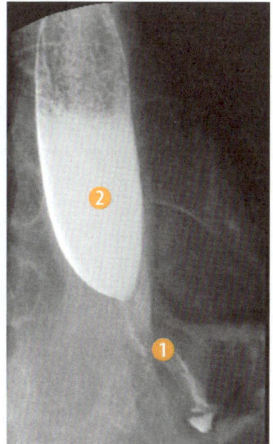

Fig. 10  Condition after operation of esophagus with a tight stenosis in anastomosis, radiography – barium swallow
1) Hairline stenosis of aboral esophagus
2) Prestenotic dilatation

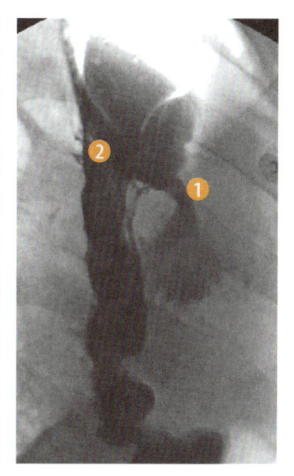

Fig. 11  Esophageal fistula, radiography – barium swallow
1) Extra lumination of contrast agent – fistula
2) Esophagogastroanastomosis

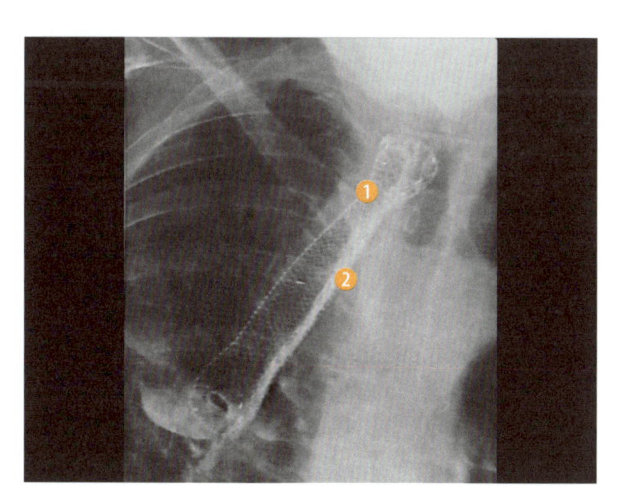

Fig. 12  Stent in esophagus, radiography – barium swallow
1) Stent in the place of original esophageal stenosis
2) Contrast agent in stent lumen – skiascopic control of stent patency

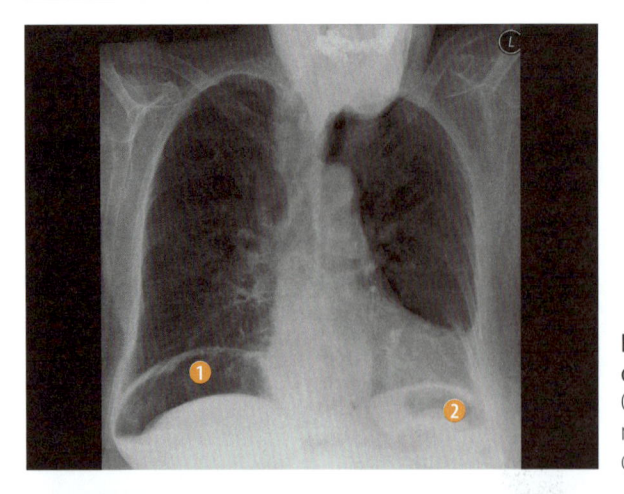

**Fig. 13 Pneumoperitoneum, chest radiography**
Crescent lucency – free gas below right (1) and left (2) half of diaphragm

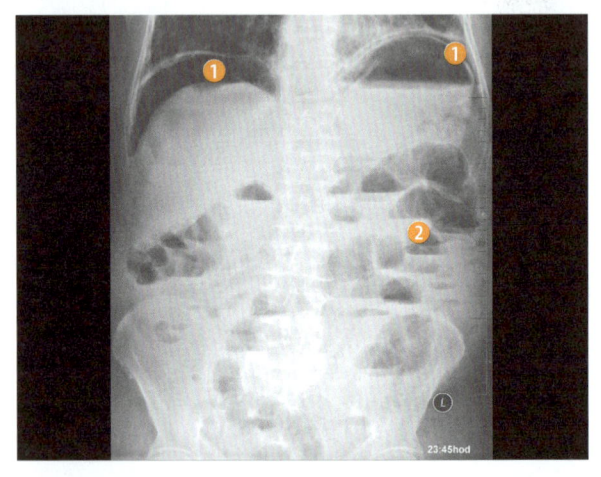

**Fig. 14 Pneumoperitoneum and ileus, native abdominal radiography**
1) Pneumoperitoneum with lucency in both subphrenic regions
2) Subileus condition with dilatation of small intestine loops and with levels

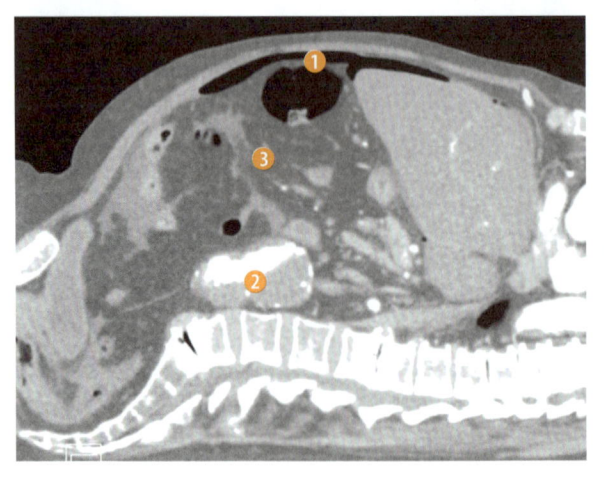

**Fig. 15 Pneumoperitoneum, abdominal CT, multiplanar reconstruction in sagittal plane**
1) Rim of air below abdominal wall – pneumoperitoneum
2) Dissecting aneurysm of abdominal aorta
3) Visceral lipomatosis

IMAGING METHODS IN SURGERY – GALLERY

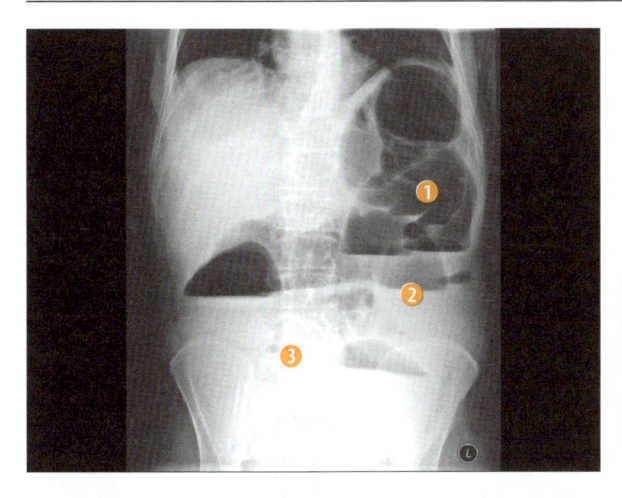

Fig. 16 Mechanical ileus of small intestine, native abdominal radiography in standing position
1) Dilatation of small intestine loops
2) Gas-fluid levels
3) Diffuse shadowing of peritoneal cavity below obstruction

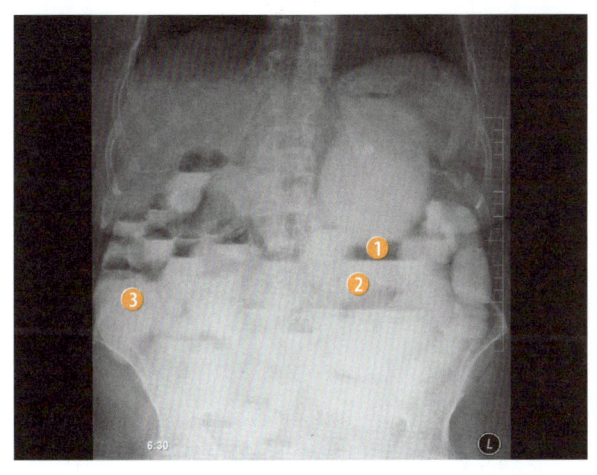

Fig. 17 Functional ileus of small intestine, abdominal radiography after application of water-soluble contrast agent
1) Dilatation of small intestine loops
2) With levels of contrast agent
3) Levels of contrast agent also in large intestine

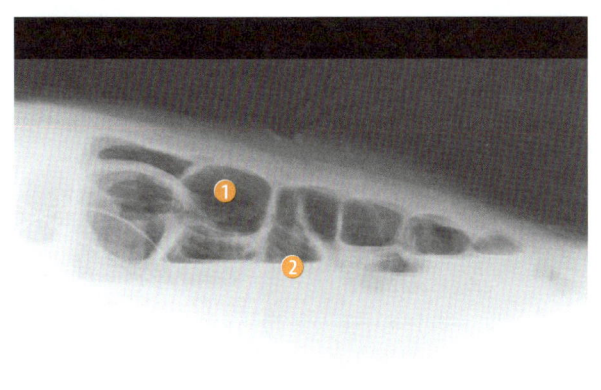

Fig. 18 Ileus of small intestine in a lying patient – radiography in a lying position on patient's side with a horizontal beam
1) Dilatation of small intestine loops
2) Gas-fluid levels

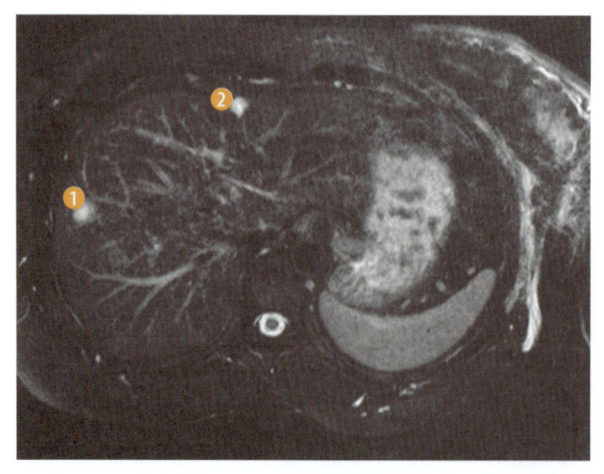

Fig. 19a Liver cysts, MRI of liver, T2 turbo spin echo sequence with fat suppression
1) Hypersignal focus in right liver lobe – cyst
2) Hypersignal focus in left lobe – cyst

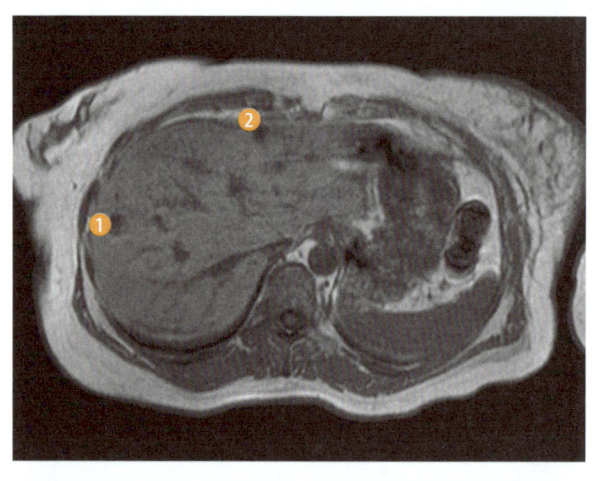

Fig. 19b Liver cysts, MRI of liver, native T1 VIBE sequence
1) Hyposignal focus in right liver lobe – cyst
2) Hyposignal focus in left lobe – cyst

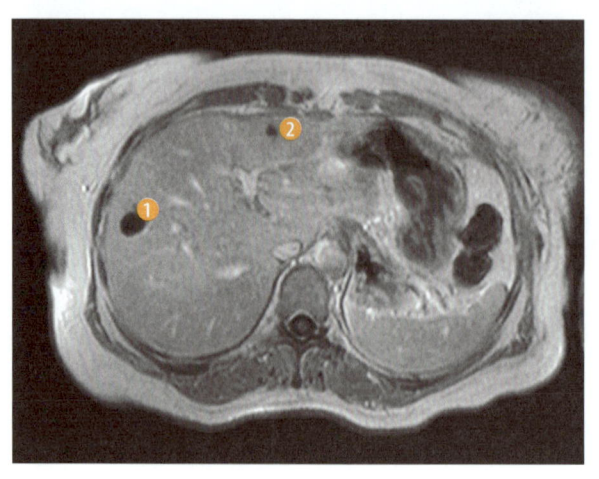

Fig. 19c Liver cysts, MRI of liver, T1 VIBE sequence after application of gadolinium
1) Focus in the right lobe, no enhancement after application of gadolinium – cyst
2) Focus in the left lobe, no enhancement after application of gadolinium – cyst

IMAGING METHODS IN SURGERY – GALLERY

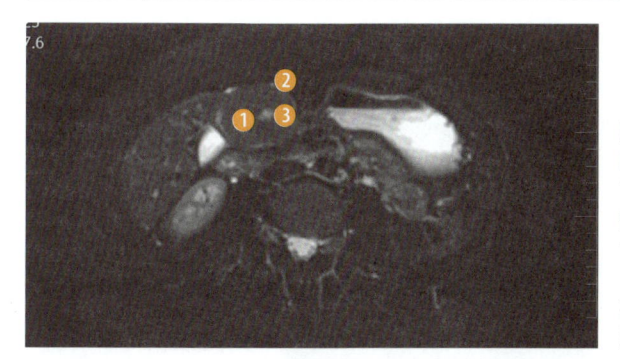

**Fig. 20a** Focal nodular hyperplasia, liver MRI, T2 turbo spin echo sequence with fat suppression
1) Mildly hyposignal focus in the left liver lobe
2) Hypersignal peripheral capsule
3) Hypersignal central scar

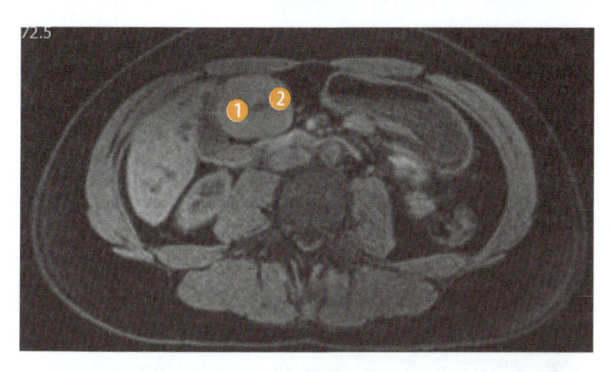

**Fig. 20b** Focal nodular hyperplasia, liver MRI, native T1 VIBE sequence
1) Mildly hyposignal focus in left liver lobe
2) Markedly hyposignal central scar

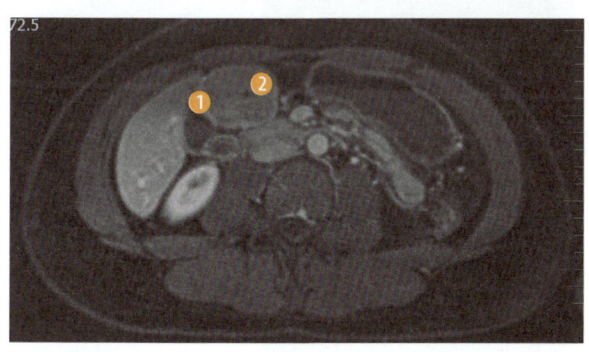

**Fig. 20c** Focal nodular hyperplasia, liver MRI, T1 VIBE sequence after application of gadolinium, arterial phase
1) Higher signal of capsule
2) Central scar remains hyposignal

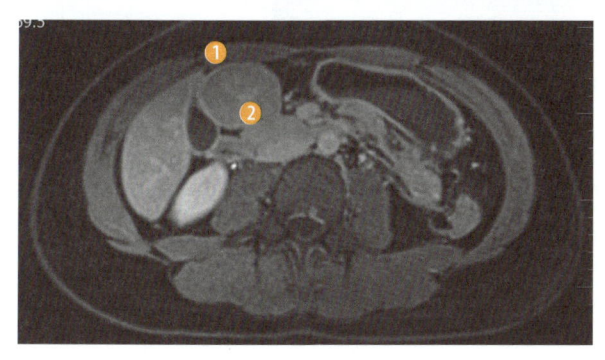

**Fig. 20d** Focal nodular hyperplasia, liver MRI, T1 VIBE sequence after application of gadolinium, late phase
1) Enhanced capsule of the focus
2) Markedly enhanced central fibrous scar

Chapter 36

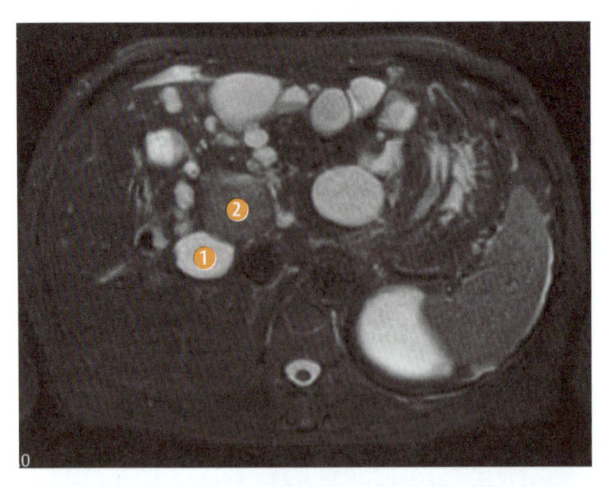

Fig. 21a Cystic and hemorrhagic liver metastases in GIST, liver MRI, T2 turbo spin echo with fat suppression in transverse plane
1) Markedly hypersignal focus – cystic metastasis
2) Mildly hypersignal focus – hemorrhagic metastasis

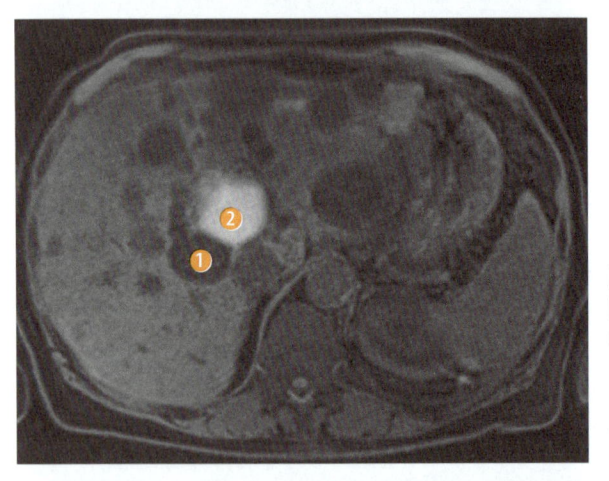

Fig. 21b Cystic and hemorrhagic liver metastases in GIST, liver MRI, native T1 VIBE
1) Markedly hyposignal focus – cystic metastasis
2) Hypersignal focus – hemorrhagic metastasis

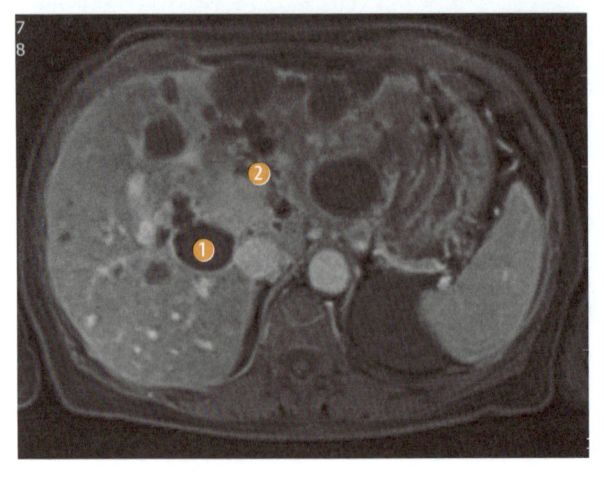

Fig. 21c Cystic and hemorrhagic liver metastases in GIST, liver MRI, T1 VIBE with application of contrast agent
1) Cystic metastasis not enhanced; enhancement of peripheral rim
2) Mildly hypersignal focus – hemorrhagic metastasis

IMAGING METHODS IN SURGERY – GALLERY

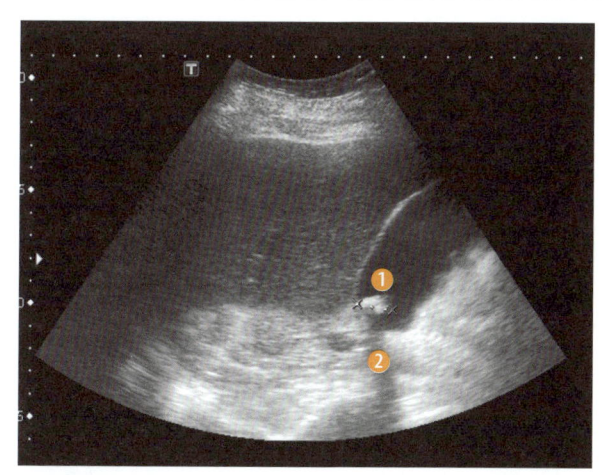

**Fig. 22 Solitary cholecystolithiasis, Ultrasound of gallbladder**
1) Solitary stone in gallbladder lumen
2) Distal acoustic shadow

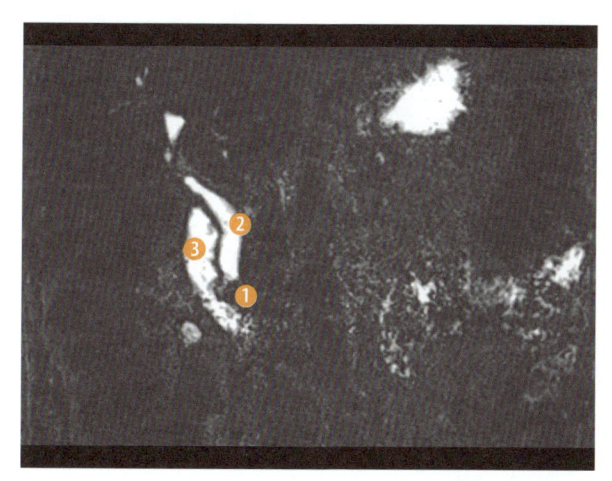

**Fig. 23 Dilatation of biliary tract, MRCP (magnetic resonance cholangiopancreatography)**
1) Suprapapillar stenosis of choledochus
2) Dilatation of biliary tract
3) Duodenum

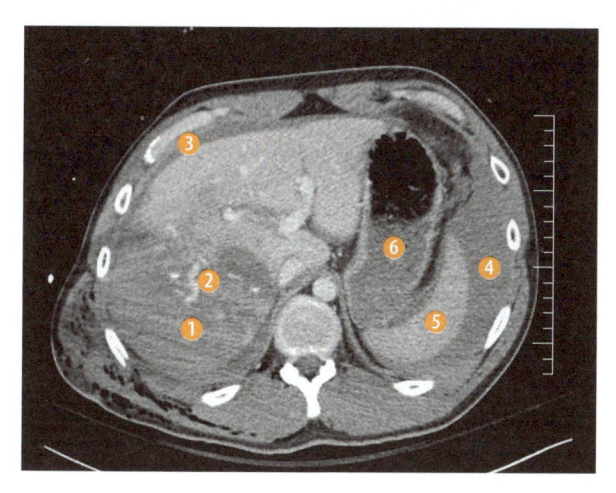

**Fig. 24a Liver trauma, CT after intravenous application of contrast agent in transverse plane**
1) Hypodense contusion focus – contusion
2) Contrast-enhanced site of hepatic vessel injury – leakage of contrast agent
3) Fluid around liver
4) Fluid around spleen
5) Spleen
6) Stomach

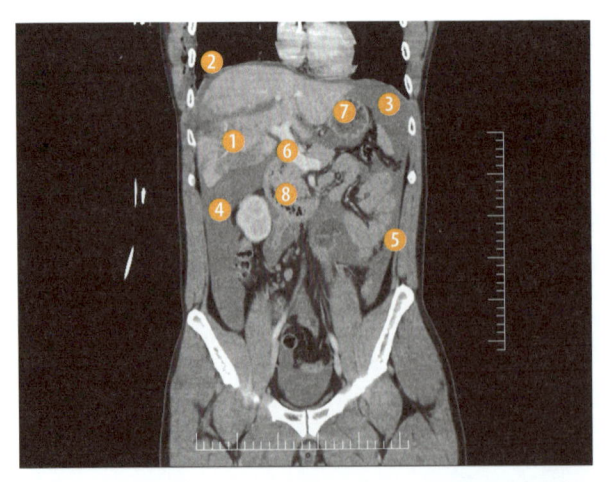

**Fig. 24b** Liver trauma,
CT after intravenous application of contrast agent, in coronary plane
1) Irregular hypodense focus in the right liver lobe – contusion
2) Fluid around liver
3) Fluid around spleen
4) Fluid in right paracolic space
5) Fluid in left paracolic space
6) Portal vein
7) Stomach
8) Duodenum

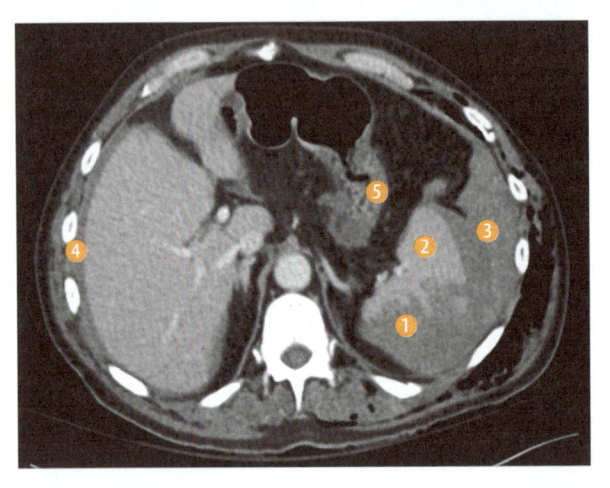

**Fig. 25a** Spleen trauma,
CT after intravenous application of contrast agent, in transverse plane
1) Hypodense, contrast non-enhanced focus in the spleen – contusion
2) Spleen
3) Rim of fluid around the spleen
4) Rim of fluid around the liver
5) Stomach

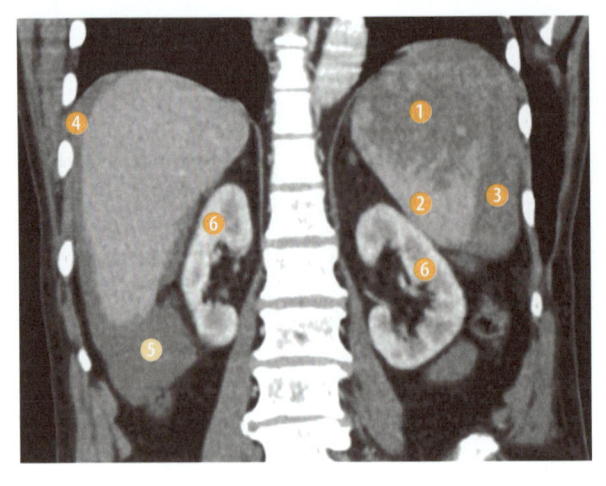

**Fig. 25b** Spleen trauma,
CT after intravenous application of contrast agent, MPR in coronal plane
1) Hypodense contrast non-enhanced focus in the spleen – contusion
2) Spleen
3) Rim of fluid around the spleen
4) Rim of fluid around the liver
5) Fluid in subhepatic region
6) Kidneys

## IMAGING METHODS IN SURGERY – GALLERY

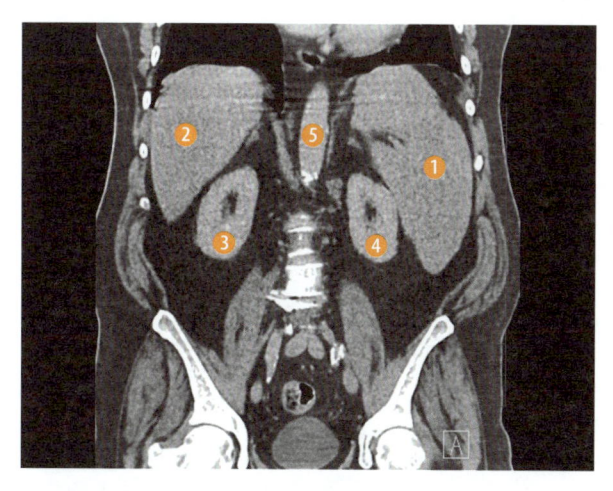

**Fig. 26 Splenomegaly, native CT, MPR in coronal plane**
1) Enlarged spleen – inferior pole extending caudally deep below the hilus of the left kidney
2) Liver
3) Right kidney
4) Left kidney
5) Abdominal aorta

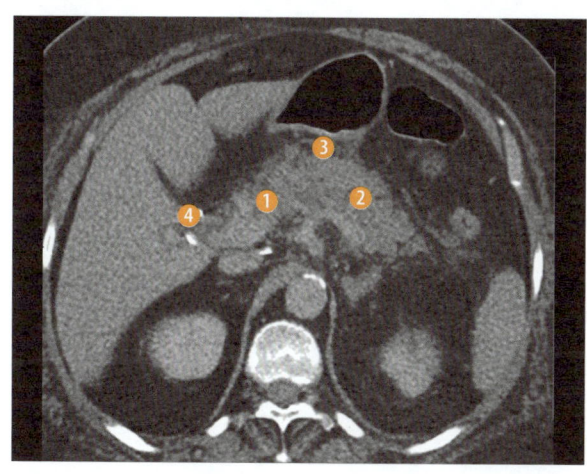

**Fig. 27a Acute pancreatitis, native CT, transverse plane**
1) Enlarged pancreas
2) Hypodense patches in pancreas
3) Edematous pancreatic fat
4) Metal staples after cholecystectomy

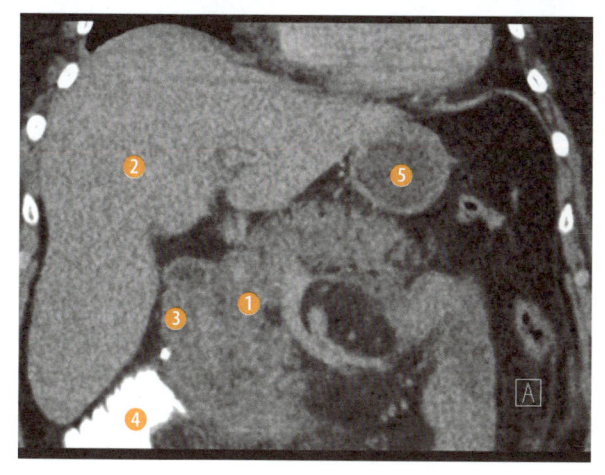

**Fig. 27b Acute pancreatitis, native CT, coronal plane**
1) Enlarged pancreas especially in the region of the head
2) Liver
3) Duodenum
4) Hepatic flexure of large intestine
5) Stomach

Chapter 36

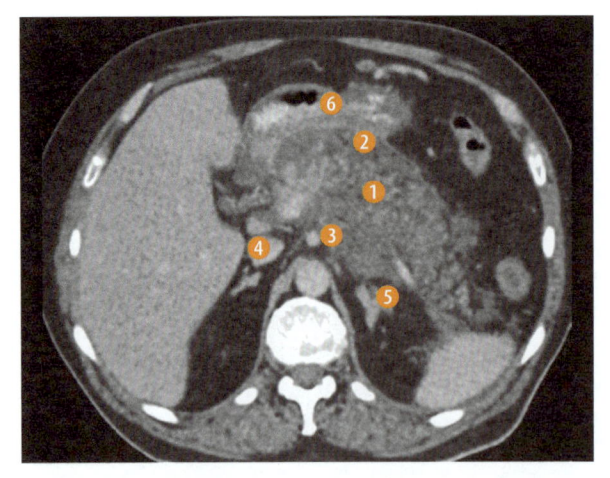

**Fig. 28** Acute pancreatitis, CT with application of contrast agent, transverse plane
1) Enlarged pancreas with hypodense patches
2) Edematous peripancreatic fat
3) Superior mesenteric artery
4) Inferior vena cava
5) Suprarenal gland
6) Stomach

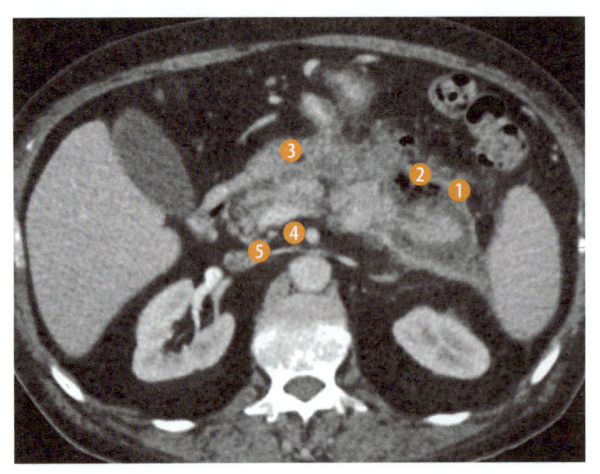

**Fig. 29a** Acute necrotizing pancreatitis, CT with application of contrast agent, transverse plane
1) Hypodense non-enhanced area in the tale of the pancreas – tissue necrosis
2) Air bubbles
3) Viable pancreatic tissue with contrast enhancement
4) Superior mesenteric artery
5) Left renal vein

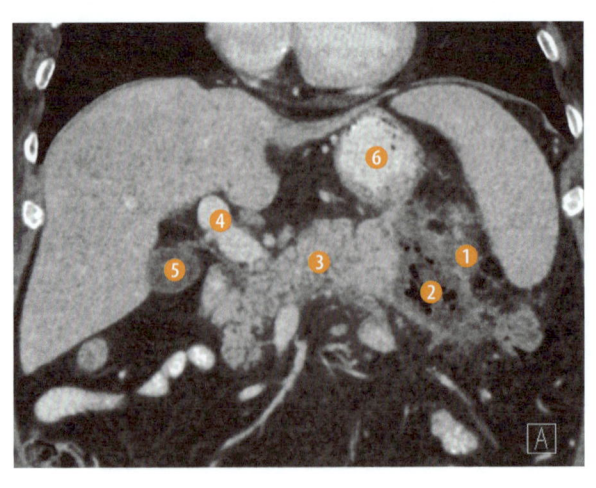

**Fig. 29b** Necrotizing pancreatitis, CT with application of contrast agent, coronal plane
1) Hypodense non-enhanced area in the tale of the pancreas– tissue necrosis
2) Air bubbles
3) Viable pancreatic tissue with contrast-enhancement
4) Portal vein
5) Gallbladder
6) Stomach

IMAGING METHODS IN SURGERY – GALLERY

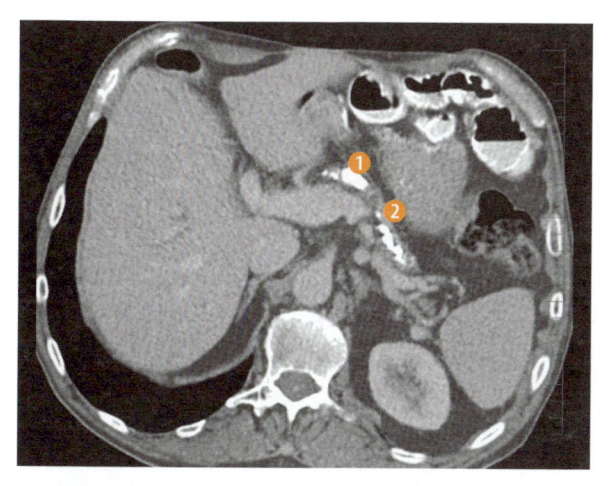

Fig. 30 Chronic pancreatitis with calcifications, CT, transverse plane
1) Multiple calcifications
2) Atrophy of body and tail of pancreas

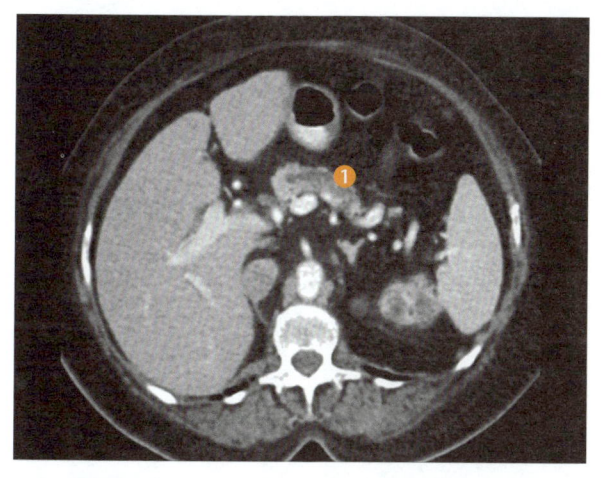

Fig. 31 Chronic pancreatitis, CT, transverse plane
1) Dilation of pancreatic duct

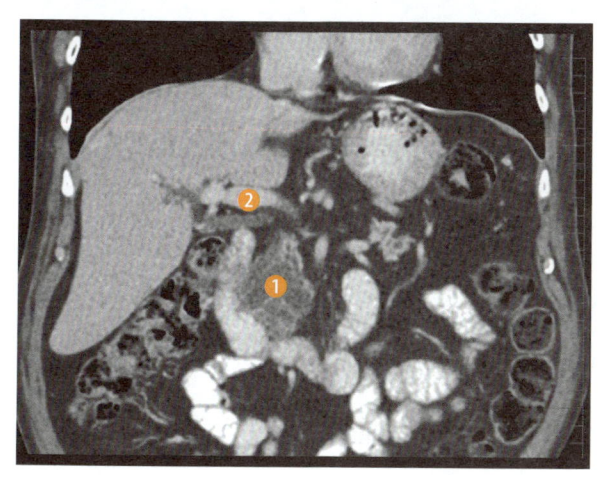

Fig. 32 Chronic pancreatitis with pseudocyst, CT with application of contrast agent, coronal plane
1) Septated pseudocyst in the area of the head of the pancreas
2) Portal vein

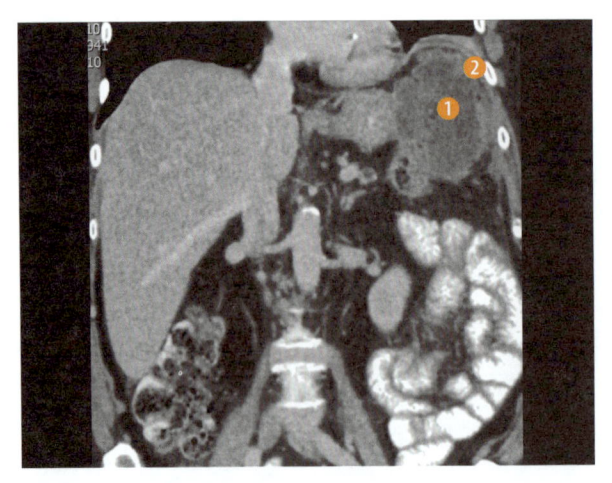

**Fig. 33a** Subphrenic abscess, CT with application of contrast agent, coronal plane
1) Cystic hypodense structure on the left side below diaphragm
2) Thicker irregular capsule on periphery with postcontrast enhancement

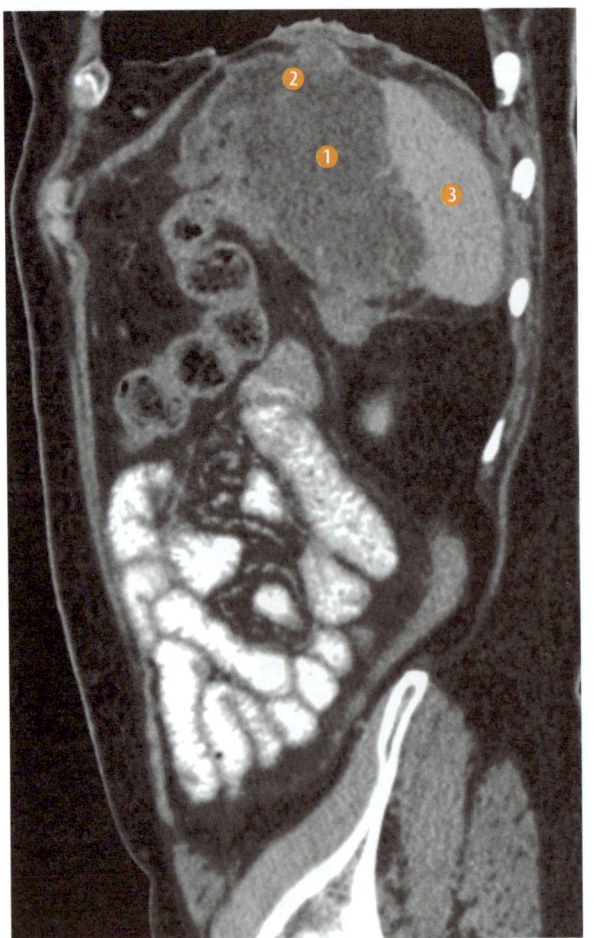

**Fig. 33b** Subphrenic abscess, CT with application of contrast agent, sagittal plane
1) Cystic hypodense structure on the left side below diaphragm
2) Thicker irregular capsule on periphery
3) Spleen

IMAGING METHODS IN SURGERY – GALLERY

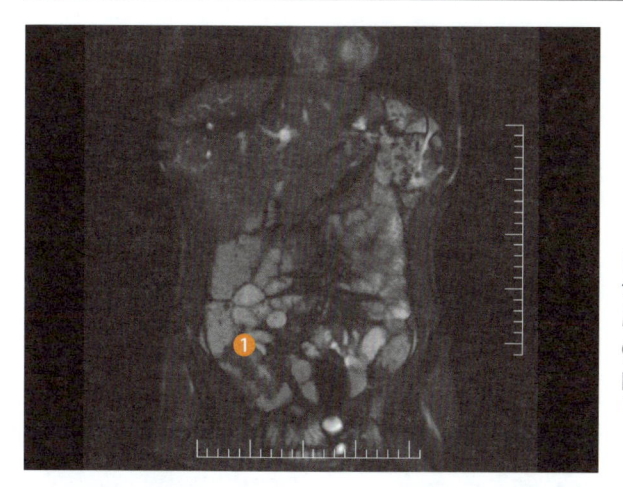

Fig. 34a Crohn's disease, affected terminal ileum,
MR enterography – balanced gradient-echo sequence, coronal plane
1) Markedly thicker walls of terminal ileum – chronic inflammatory changes

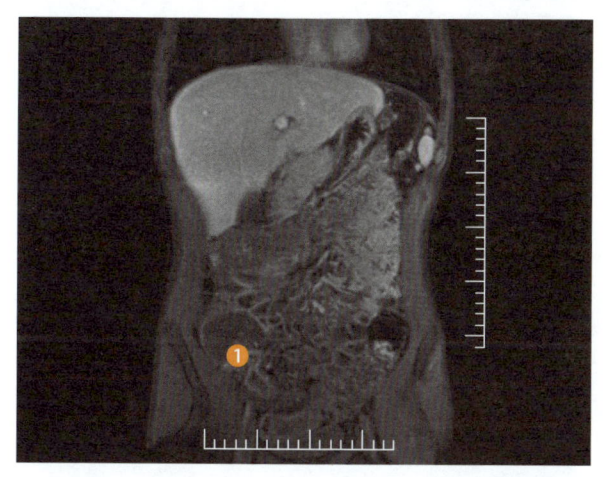

Fig. 34b Crohn's disease, affected terminal ileum,
MR enterography T1 VIBE sequence after application of gadolinium, coronal plane
1) Enhanced signal of the wall of terminal ileum – acute inflammatory changes

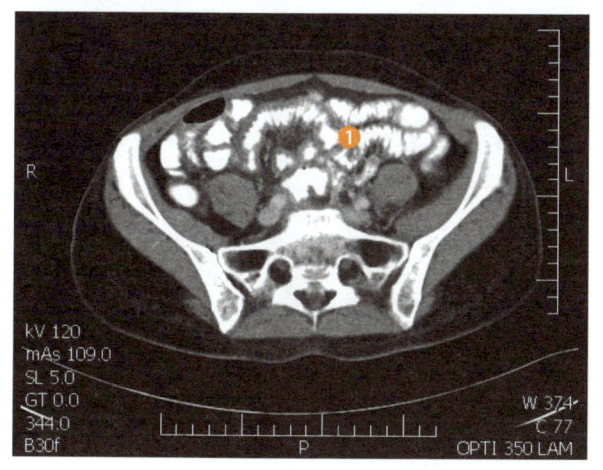

Fig. 35a Enteritis of small intestine, CT, transverse plane
1) Thicker wall of small intestine loops

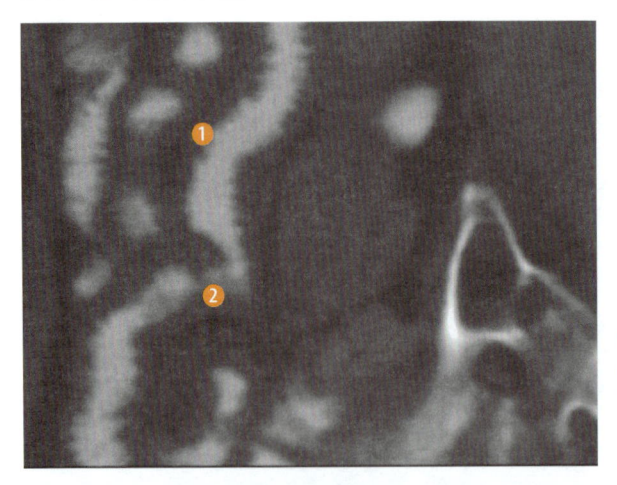

**Fig. 35b Enteritis of small intestine, CT, sagittal plane**
1) Thicker wall of small intestine loops
2) Stenosis

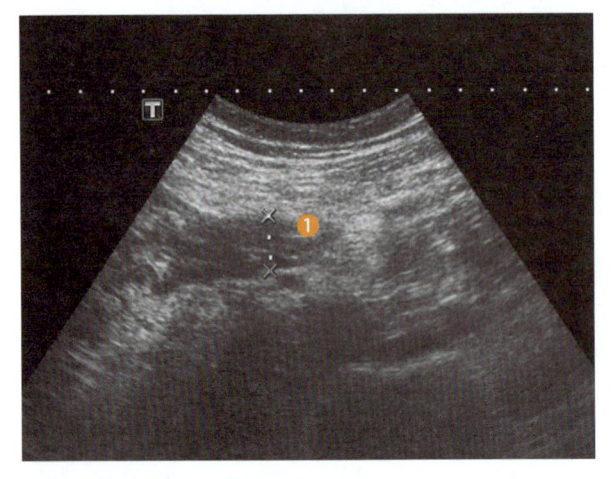

**Fig. 36a Appendicitis, ultrasound**
1) Thickening of the wall of appendix

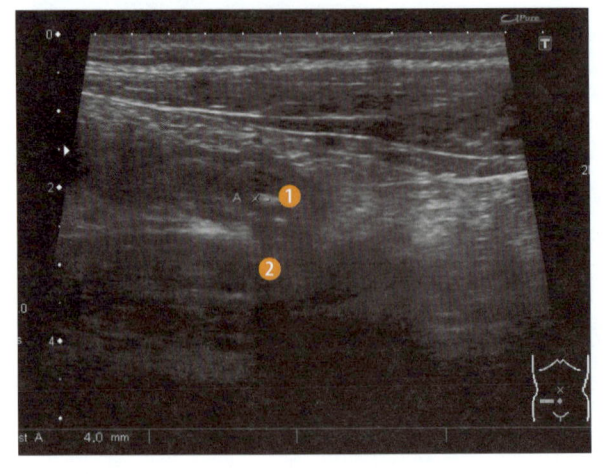

**Fig. 36b Appendicolith, ultrasound**
1) Echogenic structure in appendix
2) Distal acoustic shadow

IMAGING METHODS IN SURGERY – GALLERY

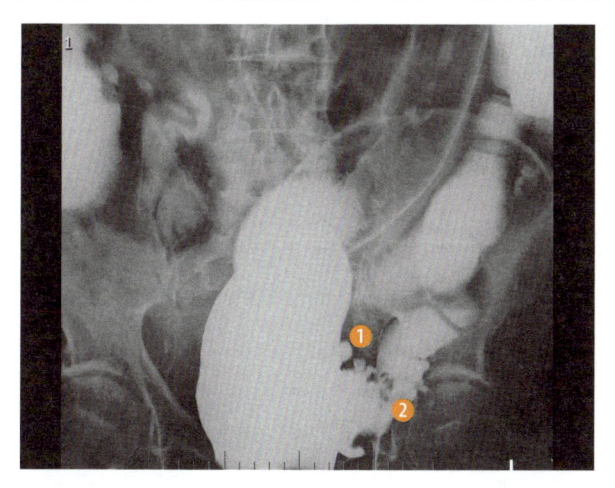

Fig. 37 Diverticulosis and diverticulitis, irrigography
1) Diverticula in sigmoid colon
2) Stenosis in sigmoid colon

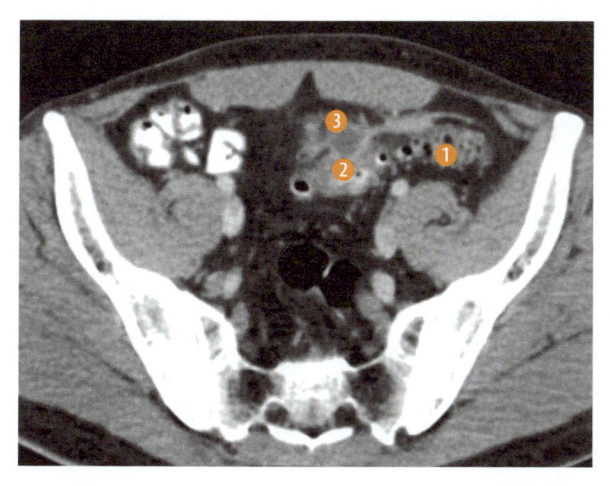

Fig. 38 Diverticulitis of sigmoid colon, CT with application of contrast agent, transverse plane
1) Pouches on the wall of sigmoid colon filled with air – diverticula
2) Thickened wall of sigmoid colon with stenosis of its lumen
3) Perisigmoid abscess

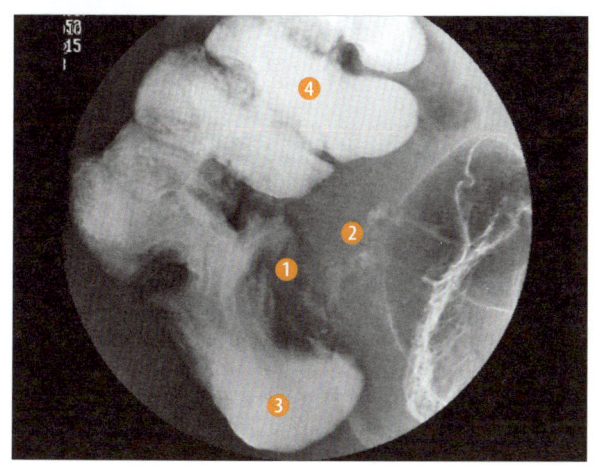

Fig. 39 Tumor of cecum, irrigography
1) Filling defect in lumen – tumor
2) Stenosis of terminal ileum
3) Base of cecum
4) Ascending colon

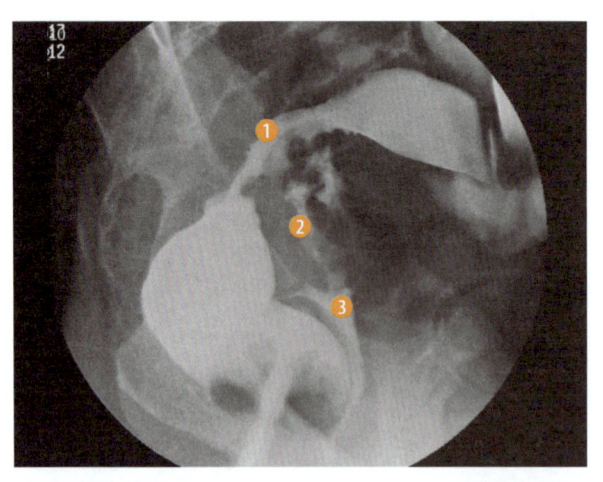

**Fig. 40 Tumor of sigmoid colon with fistula to vagina, irrigography**
1) Tumor stenosis of sigmoid colon
2) Fistula
3) Vagina filled with contrast agent

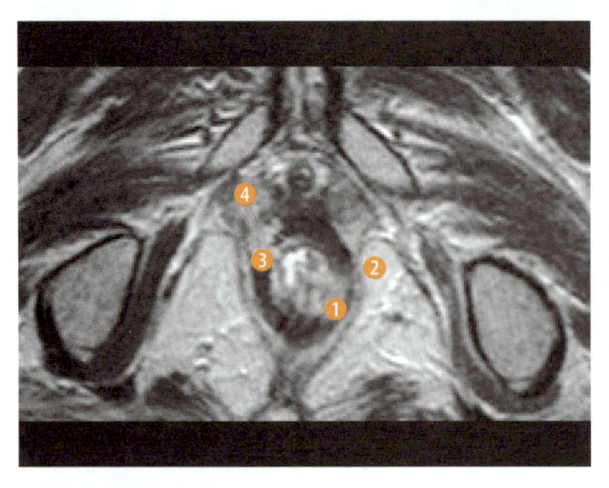

**Fig. 41a Rectal carcinoma, MR T2 sequence in transverse plane**
1) Infiltration of rectal wall
2) With infiltration of external capsule on the left
3) Transsphincteric fistula on the right side
4) Minor perirectal abscess

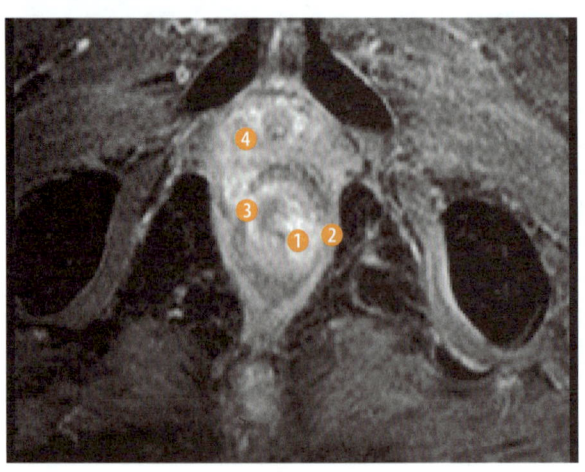

**Fig. 41b Rectal carcinoma, MR T1 sequence in transverse plane with fat signal suppression**
1) Infiltration of rectal wall
2) With infiltration of external capsule on the left
3) Transsphincteric fistula on the right side
4) Minor perirectal abscess

IMAGING METHODS IN SURGERY – GALLERY

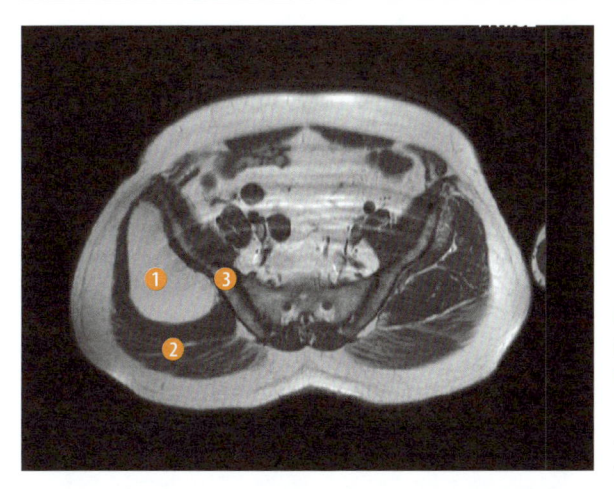

Fig. 42a Lipoma of right gluteal muscle, MR T1 spin echo in transverse plane
1) Hypersignal focus - lipoma
2) Right gluteus maximus muscle
3) Ala of ilium

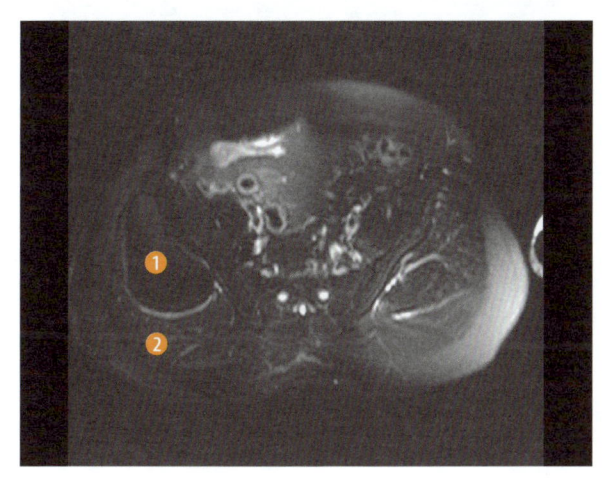

Fig. 42b Lipoma of right gluteal muscle, MR T2 turbo spin echo with fat suppression in transverse plane
1) Focus of low signal after fat signal suppression
2) Gluteus maximus muscle

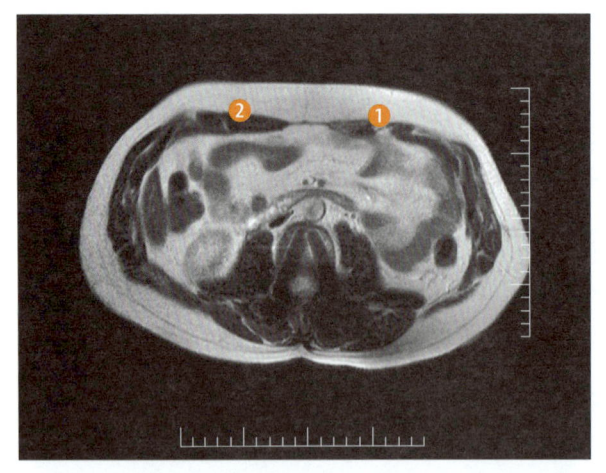

Fig. 43a Atrophy of rectus abdominis muscle on the left side with increased fat tissue, MRI in transverse plane in T1 turbo gradient sequence
1) Narrower left rectus abdominis muscle with hypersignal portions
2) Adequate width and signal of right rectus abdominis muscle

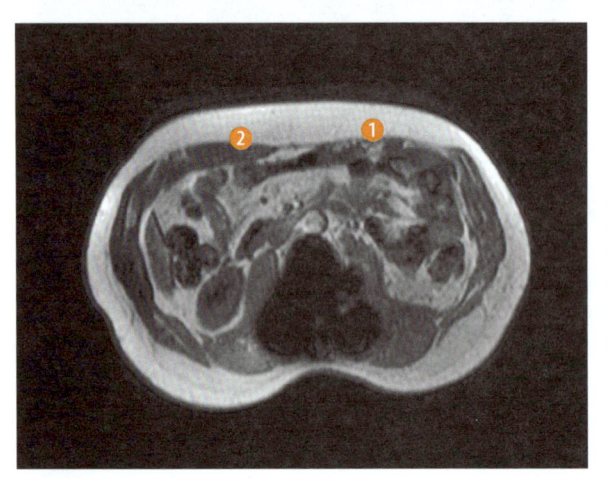

Fig. 43b Atrophy of rectus abdominis muscle on the left side with increased fat tissue, MRI of abdominal wall in transverse plane in T2 turbo spin echo sequence
1) Narrower left rectus abdominis muscle with hypersignal portions
2) Adequate width and signal of right rectus abdominis muscle

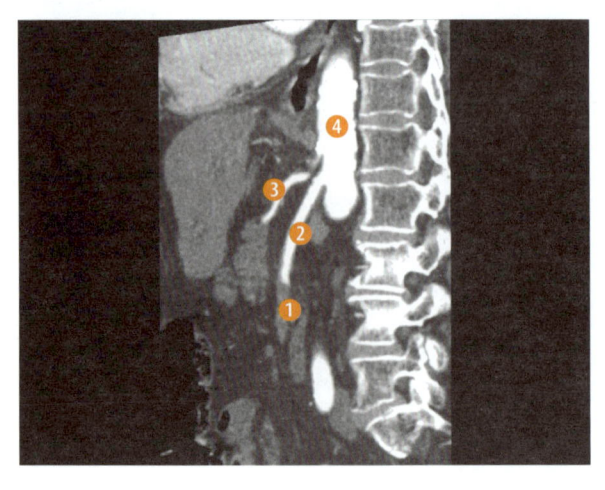

Fig. 44 Acute occlusion of superior mesenteric artery, CT angiography, sagittal plane
1) Defect in contrast filling of distal part of superior mesenteric artery
2) Division of superior mesenteric artery
3) Celiac trunk
4) Abdominal aorta

IMAGING METHODS IN SURGERY – GALLERY

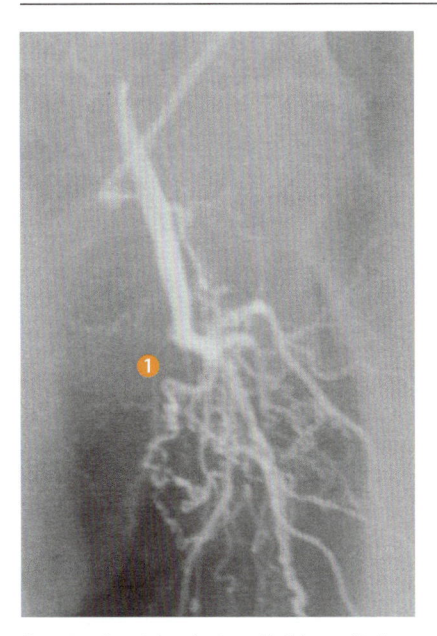

Fig. 45a Arterial occlusion of left lower limb, angiography (critical ischemia)
1) Occlusion of superficial femoral artery

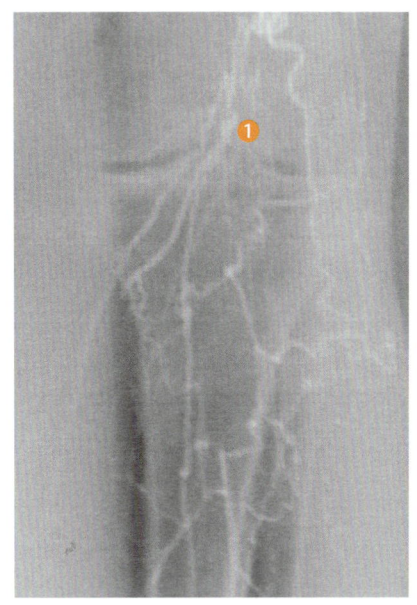

Fig. 45b Arterial occlusion of left lower limb, angiography (critical ischemia)
1) Occlusion of popliteal artery

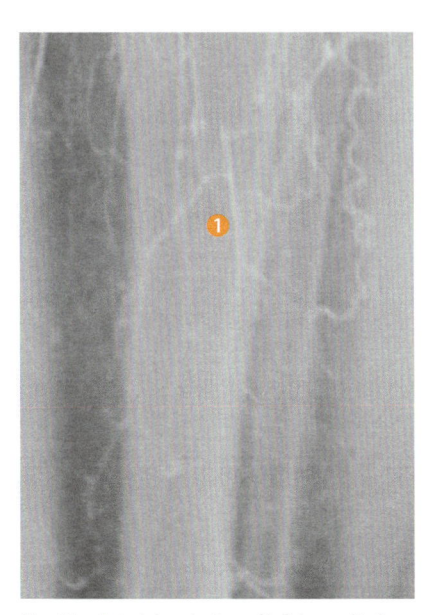

Fig. 45c Arterial occlusion of left lower limb, angiography (critical ischemia)
1) Occlusion of crural arteries

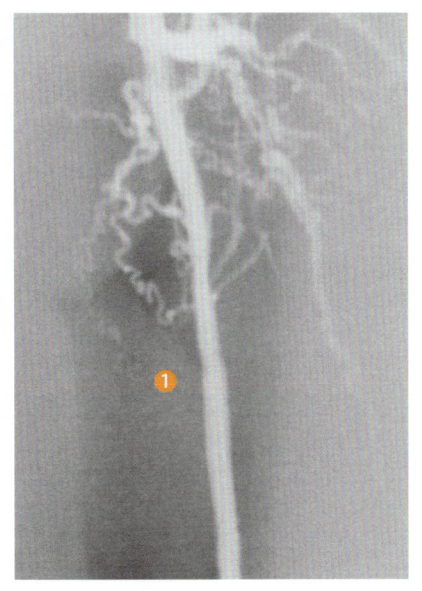

Fig. 45d Restored arterial patency in left lower limb, percutaneous recanalization (critical ischemia)
1) Patent superficial femoral artery after subintimal recanalization

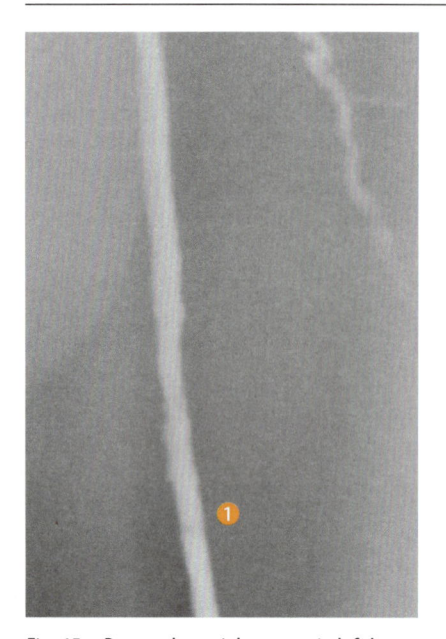

**Fig. 45e** Restored arterial patency in left lower limb, percutaneous recanalization (critical ischemia)
1) Patent distal part of superficial femoral artery

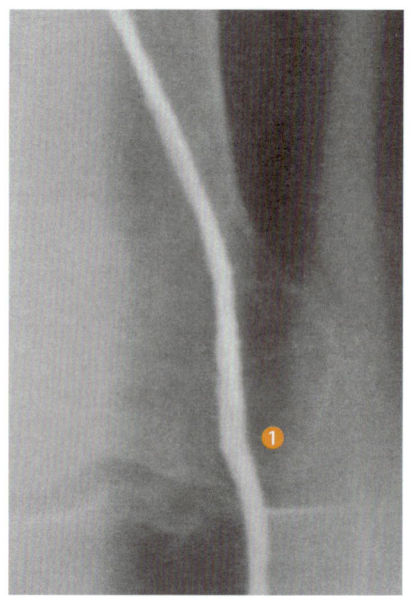

**Fig. 45f** Restored arterial patency in left lower limb, percutaneous recanalization (critical ischemia)
1) Patent popliteal artery after intervention

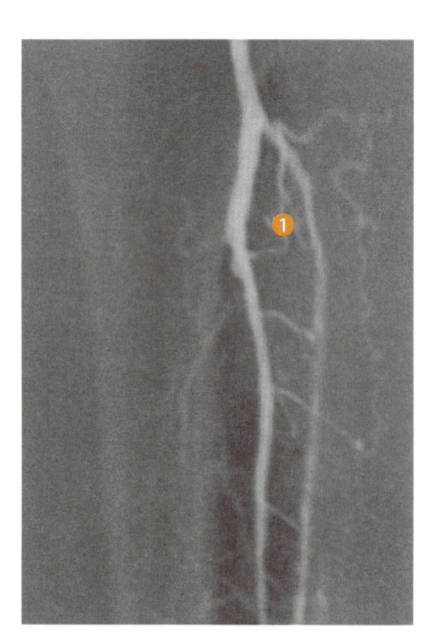

**Fig. 45g** Restored arterial patency in left lower limb, percutaneous recanalization (critical ischemia)
1) Patent two crural arteries after treatment

**IMAGING METHODS IN SURGERY – GALLERY**

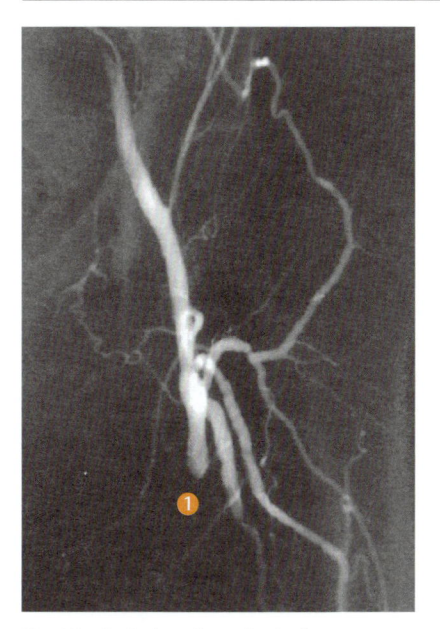

Fig. 46a  Occlusion of prosthesis of femoropopliteal bypass, thrombolysis
1) Stump of femoropopliteal bypass

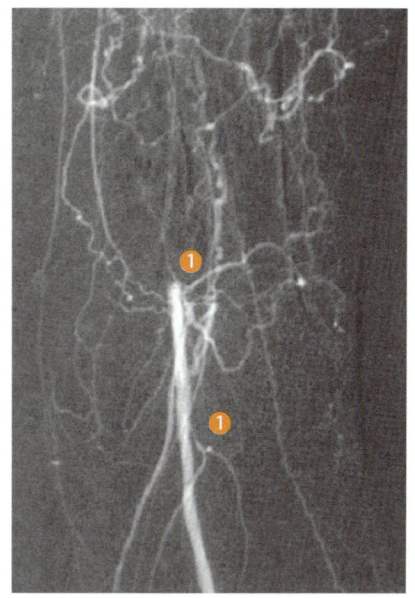

Fig. 46b  Occlusion of prosthesis of femoropopliteal bypass, thrombolysis
1) Popliteal artery patent via collaterals

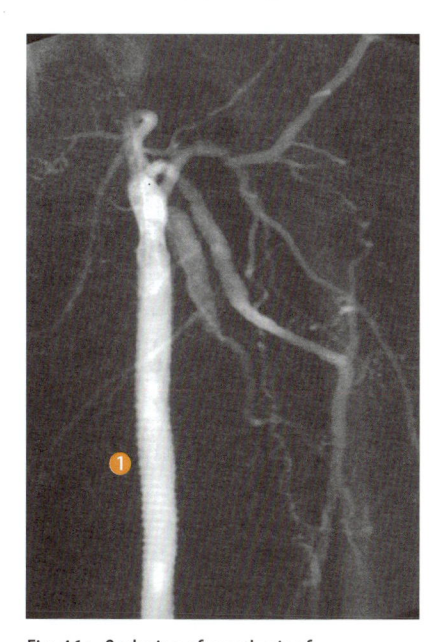

Fig. 46c  Occlusion of prosthesis of femoropopliteal bypass, thrombolysis
1) Bypass patent after local thrombolysis with 20 mg rt-PA

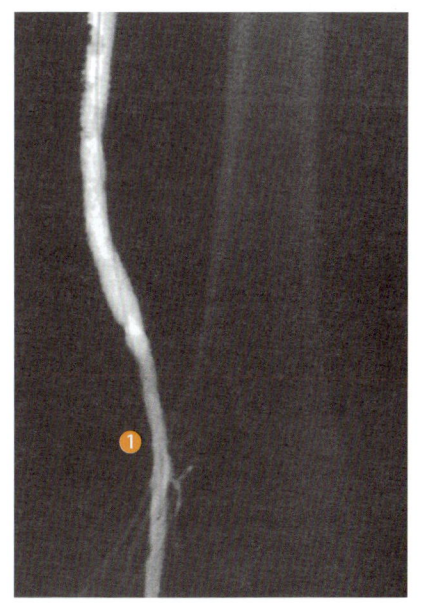

Fig. 46d  Occlusion of prosthesis of femoropopliteal bypass, thrombolysis
1) Popliteal artery fills via patent bypass

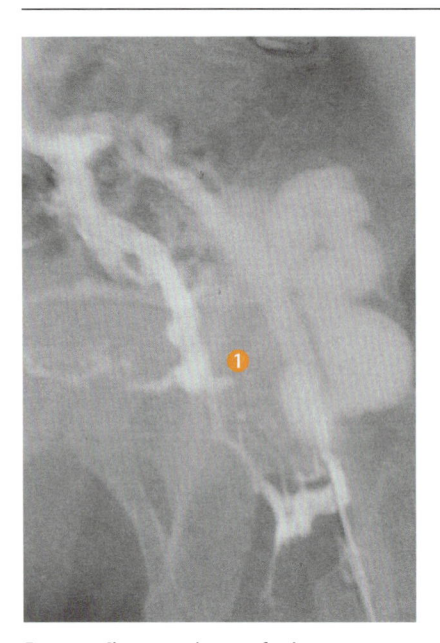

Fig. 47a  Chronic occlusion of pelvic veins on the left side, percutaneous recanalization
1) Insufficient collateral circulation on the left side

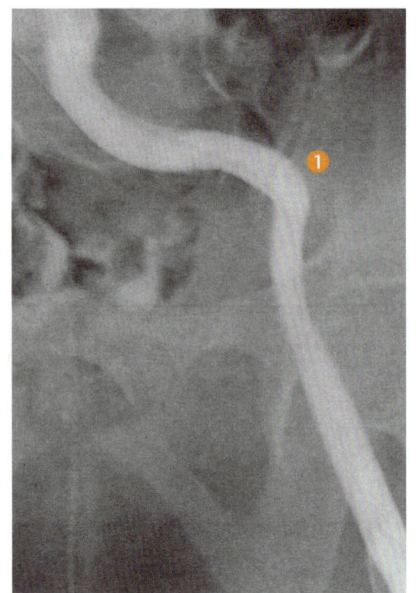

Fig. 47b  Chronic occlusion of pelvic veins on the left side, percutaneous recanalization
1) Good patency of pelvic veins after insertion of stent

IMAGING METHODS IN SURGERY – GALLERY

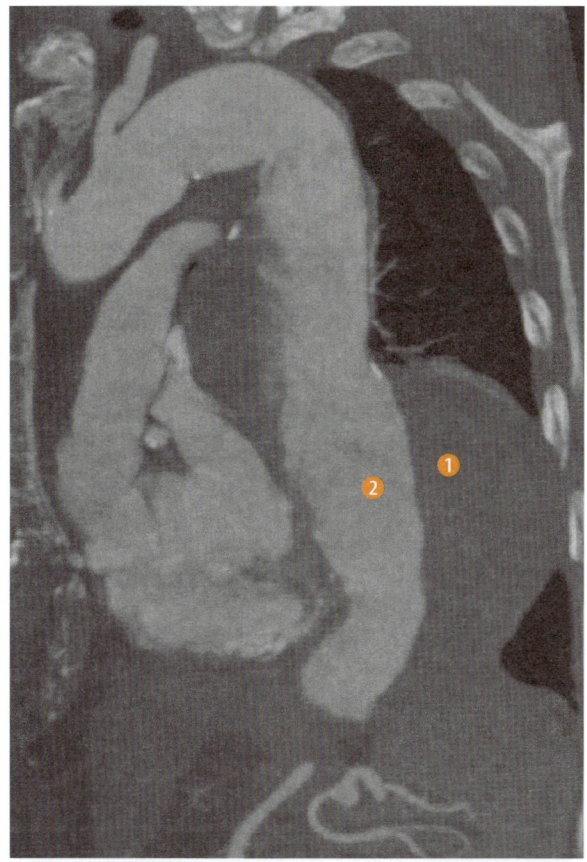

Fig. 48a  Aneurysm of chest aorta, CT angiography
1) Large sclerotic aneurysm
2) Lumen of descending aorta

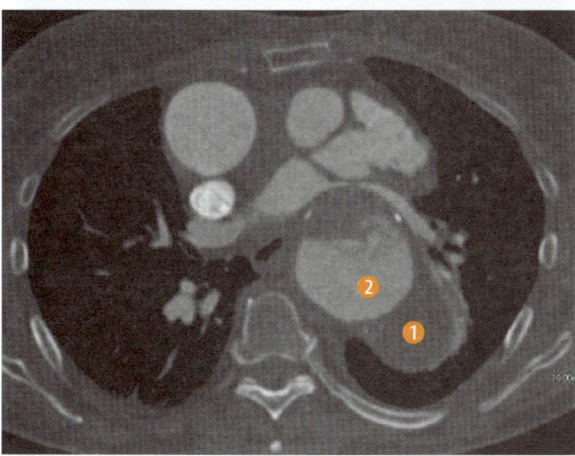

Fig. 48b  Aneurysm of chest aorta, CT angiography
1) Aneurysm in axial plane
2) Descending aorta

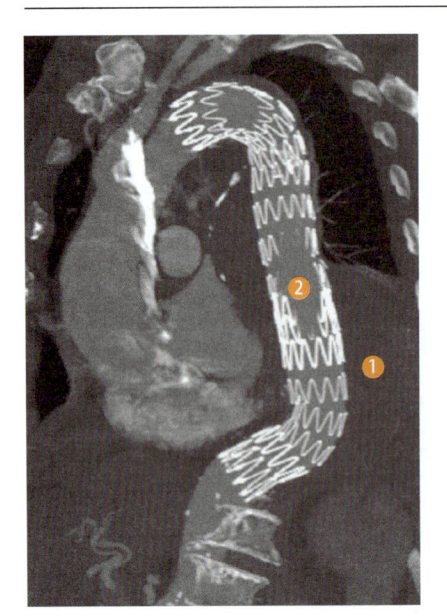

**Fig. 48c** Aneurysm of chest aorta, CT angiography
1) Covered aneurysm
2) Stent graft

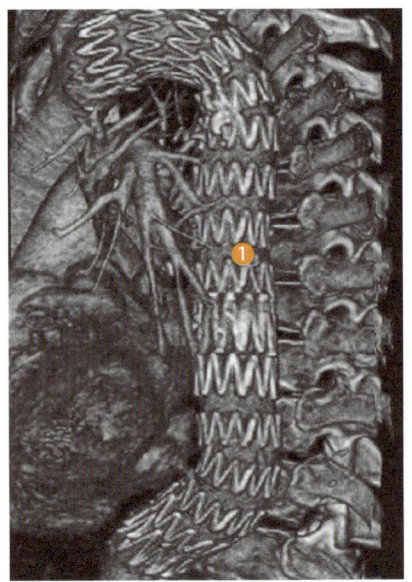

**Fig. 48d** Aneurysm of chest aorta, CT angiography 3D imaging
1) Confirmation of stent graft patency during other imaging examination

**Brava®**

**Coloplast**

## Brava® - nová řada produktů Coloplast
## Extra péče o kůži v okolí stomie

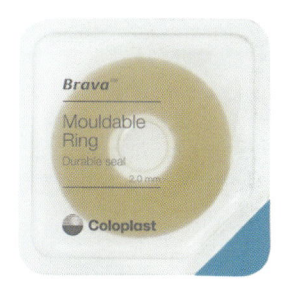

### Těsnící tvarovatelný kroužek Brava® (30 ks v balení)
- vytvaruje se pomocí prstů kolem stomie
- vytvoří extra utěsnění mezi stomií a pomůckou

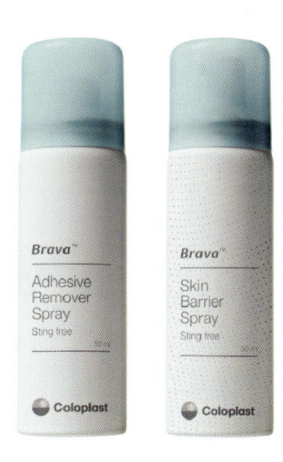

### Odstraňovač adheziv Brava® (sprej, 50 ml)
- nastříká se kolem podložky na kůži, pomůcka se bezbolestně odlepí
- je vyroben na bázi silikonu, nedráždí kůži

### Ochranný film Brava® (sprej, 50 ml)
- vytvoří na kůži ochrannou vrstvu, chrání před agresivními sekrety
- je vyroben na bázi silikonu, nedráždí kůži

Volejte bezplatnou linku 800 100 416 a vyžádejte si další informace ohledně nových výrobků Brava od společnosti Coloplast.

**800 100 416**
bezplatná informační linka

**Coloplast**

Coloplast A/S
odštěpný závod
Radlická 740/113d
158 00 Praha 5
tel.: 244 470 212
fax: 244 472 106
czsensura@coloplast.com
www.coloplast.cz

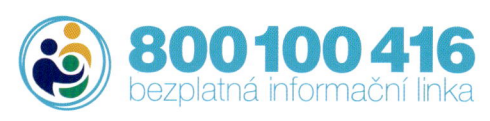

Společnost Coloplast vyvíjí výrobky a služby, které usnadňují život lidem s velmi osobními a soukromými zdravotními obtížemi.
Protože neustále pracujeme a komunikujeme s lidmi, kteří naše výrobky používají, vyvíjíme řešení citlivá k jejich mimořádným potřebám. Toto my nazýváme intimní zdravotní péčí.

Coloplast je registrovaná ochranná známka společnosti Coloplast A/S. © 2013-11
Všechna práva vyhrazena pro Coloplast A/S, 3050 Humlebaek, Dánsko.

**COLOR IMAGE GALLERY**

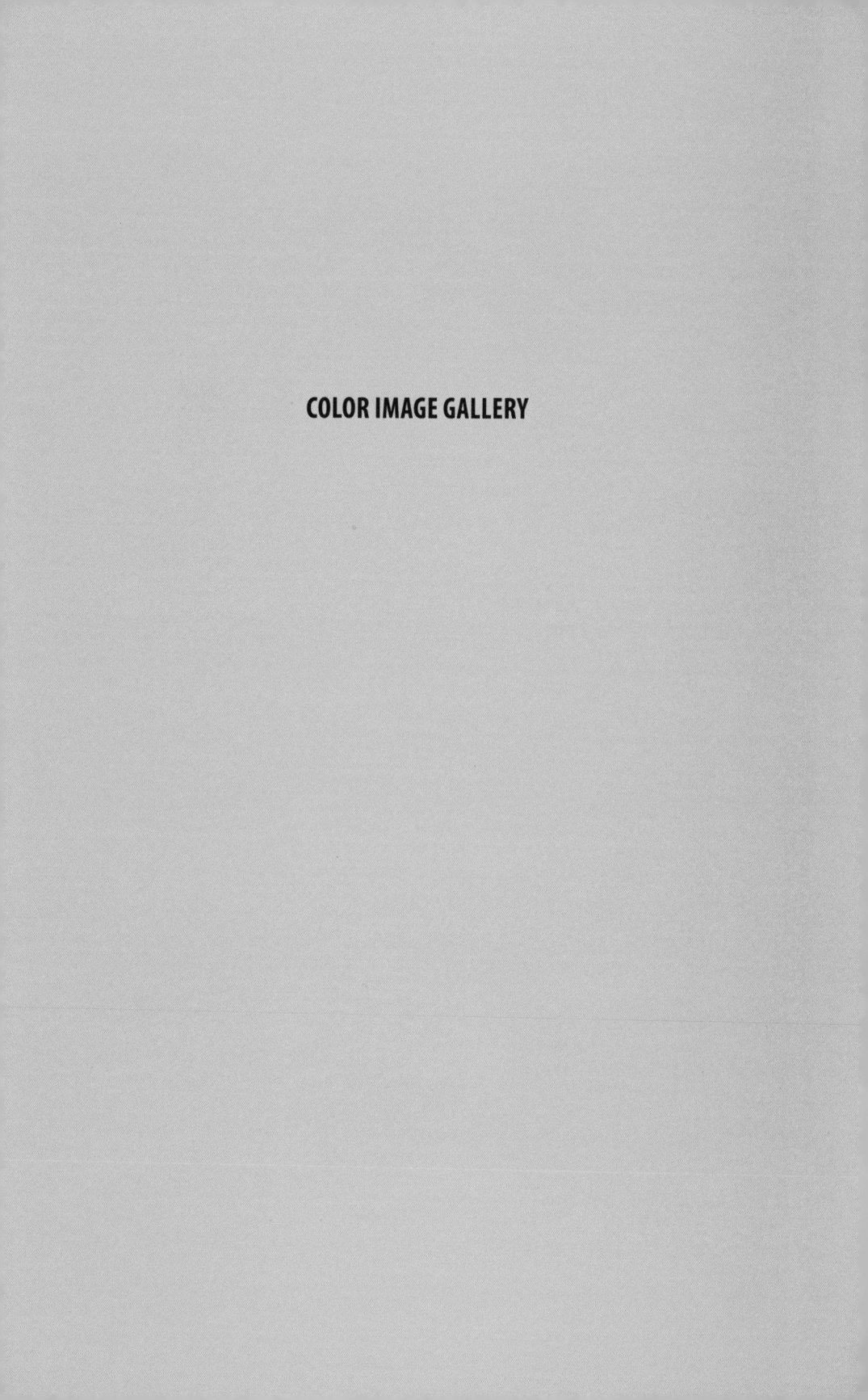

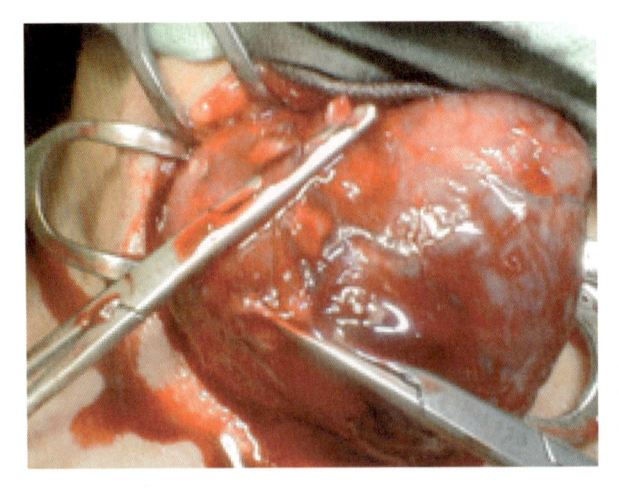

**Fig. 49 Retrosternal goiter**
Peroperative picture:
Part of a large goiter is removed outside the operative wound

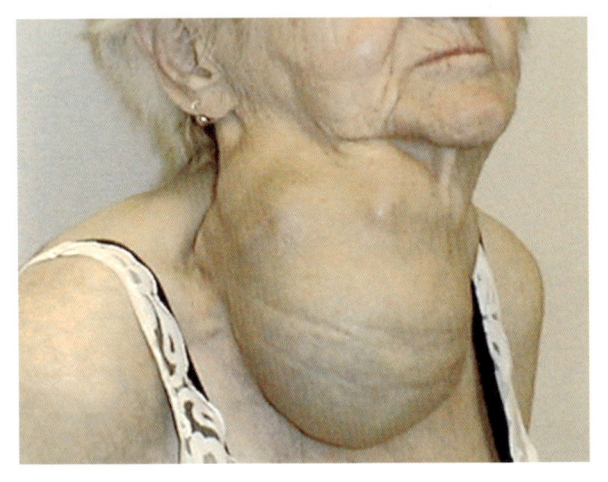

**Fig. 50 Endemic polynodular goiter**

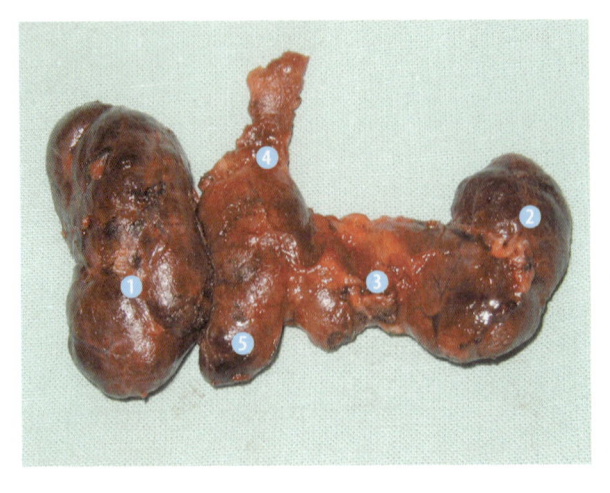

**Fig. 51 Polynodular goiter**
Postoperative picture, TTE:
1) Right lobe
2) Left lobe
3) Isthmus
4) Pyramidal lobe
5) Paraisthmic nodule

**NECK SURGERY**

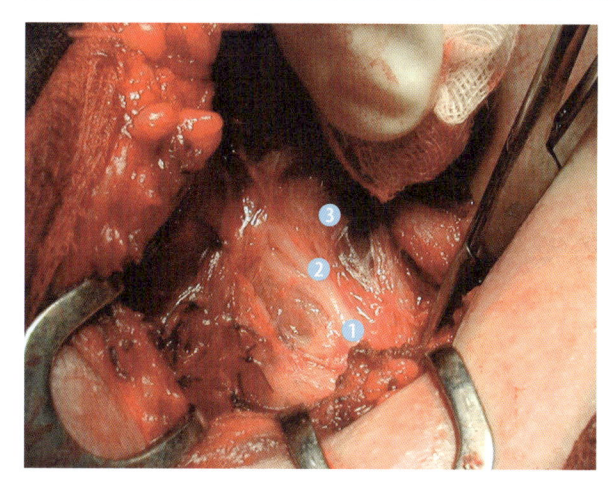

**Fig. 52 State after right-side lobectomy of thyroid gland**
Peroperative picture:
1) Recurrent laryngeal nerve
2) Extralaryngeal branching of recurrent laryngeal nerve
3) Anterior surface of trachea

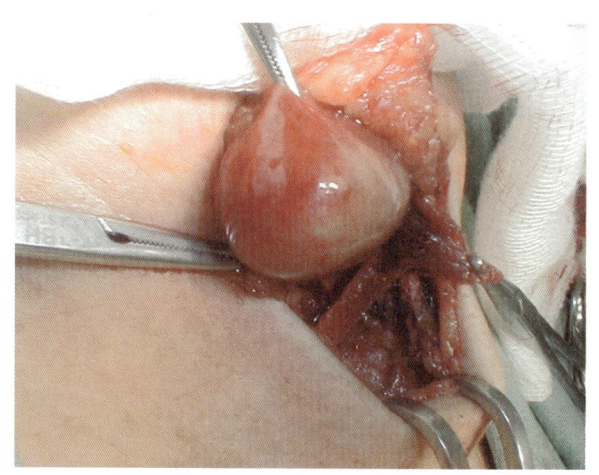

**Fig. 53 Adenoma of suprathyroid gland**
Peroperative picture

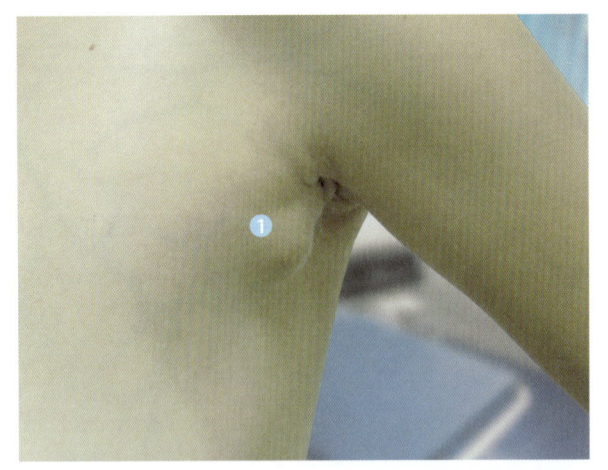

Fig. 54 Accessory mammary gland (1) at the edge of left axilla

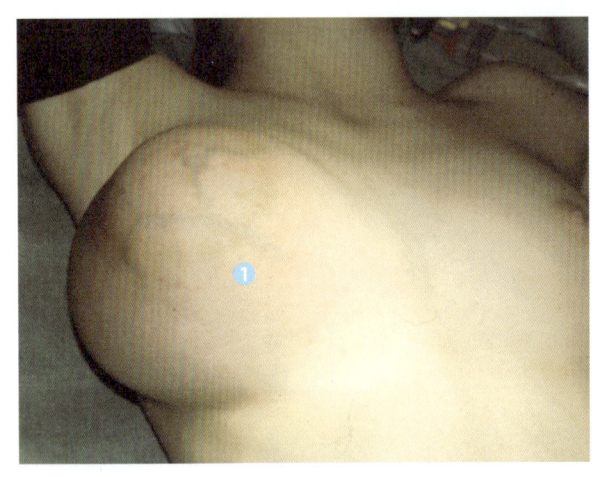

Fig. 55 Benign fibroadenoma of right breast (1)

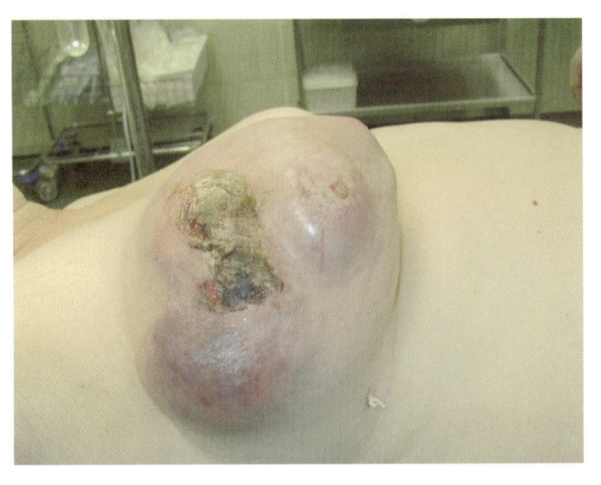

Fig. 56 Advanced exulcerated breast tumor

MAMMARY GLAND SURGERY

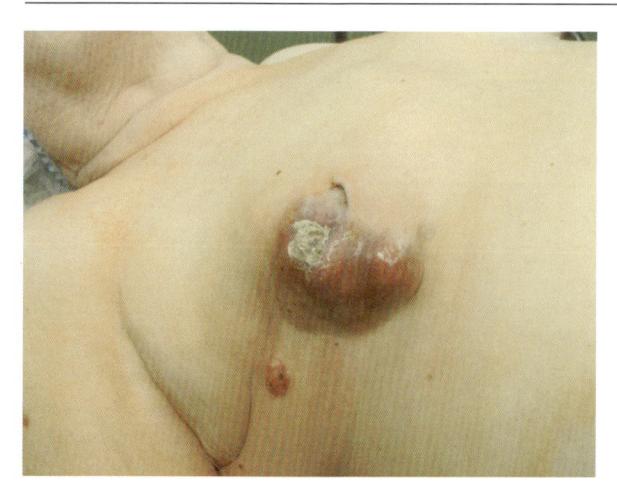

Fig. 57 Advanced exulcerated breast tumor

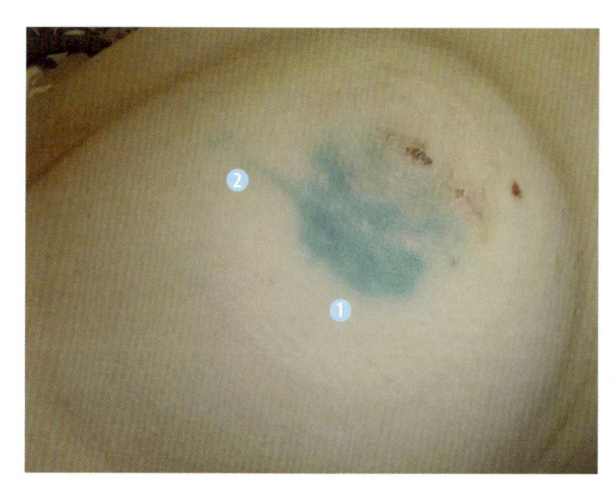

Fig. 58 Marking of the focus in breast with dye (1) and identification of lymphatic drainage in axilla (2)

MAMMARY GLAND SURGERY

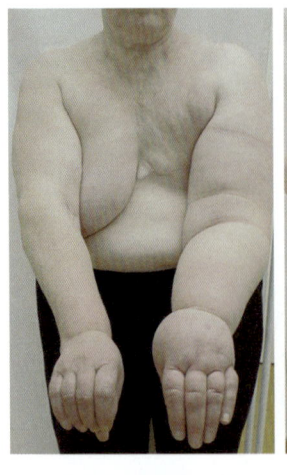

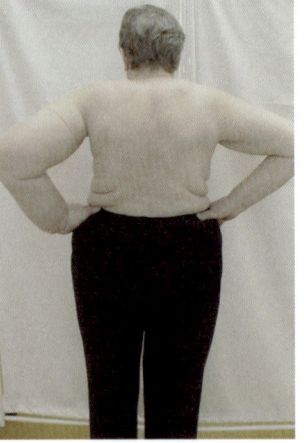

**Fig. 59 Secondary lymphedema (elephantiasis) of left upper extremity**
State after left-sided mastectomy with exenteration of axilla and radiotherapy

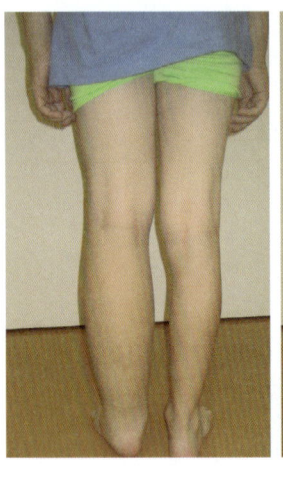

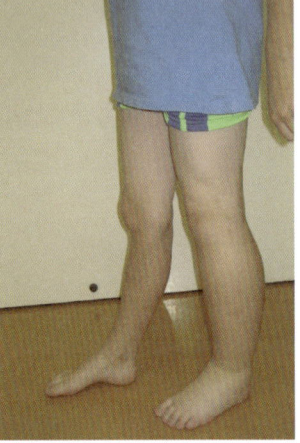

**Fig. 60 Secondary lymphedema of left lower extremity**
State after left-sided orchidectomy with subsequent radiotherapy for rhabdomyosarcoma of left testicle (at the age of 4). Condition of left lower extremity at the age of 14.

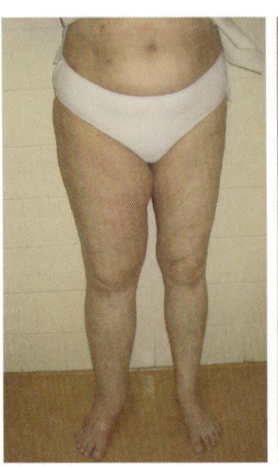

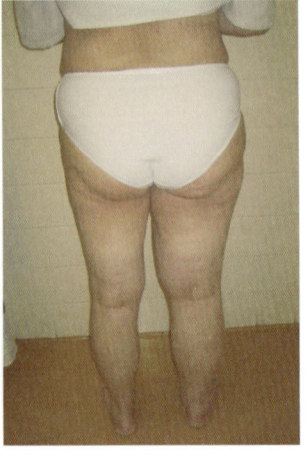

**Fig. 61 Secondary lymphedema of right lower extremity**
State after right-sided nephrectomy and adnexectomy, partial cystectomy and pelvic lymphadenectomy with subsequent radiotherapy for tumor of right kidney

SOFT TISSUE TUMORS IN ADULTS

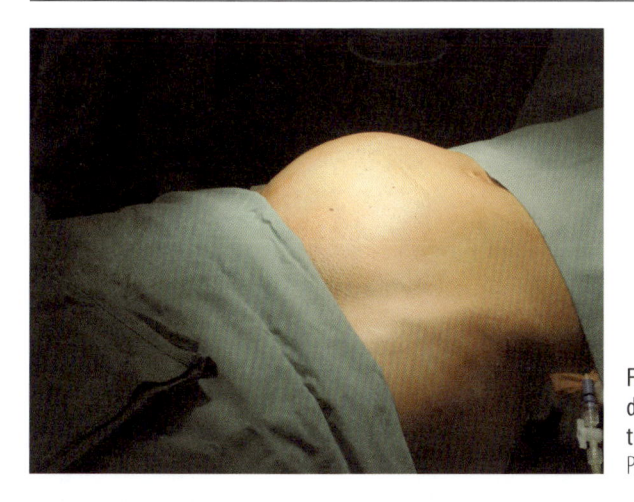

**Fig. 62  Abdominal disfigurement due to extensive retroperitoneal tumor**
Preoperative finding

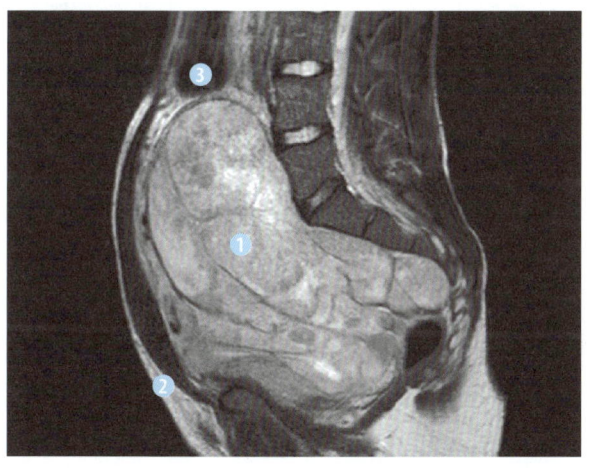

**Fig. 63  Large retroperitoneal tumor**
The same patient as in previous picture. MRI scan, reconstruction in sagittal plane:
1) Tumor masses
2) Bulged anterior abdominal wall
3) Visceral dislocation into epigastrium

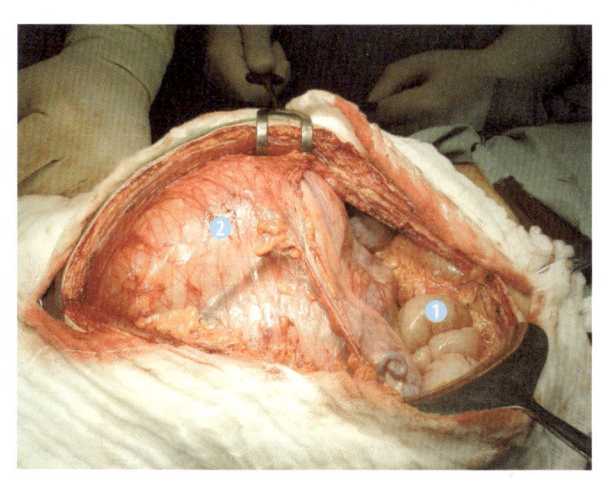

**Fig. 64  Large retroperitoneal tumor**
The same patient as in previous picture. Peroperative picture:
1) Dislocated loops of small intestine
2) Tumor

SOFT TISSUE TUMORS IN ADULTS

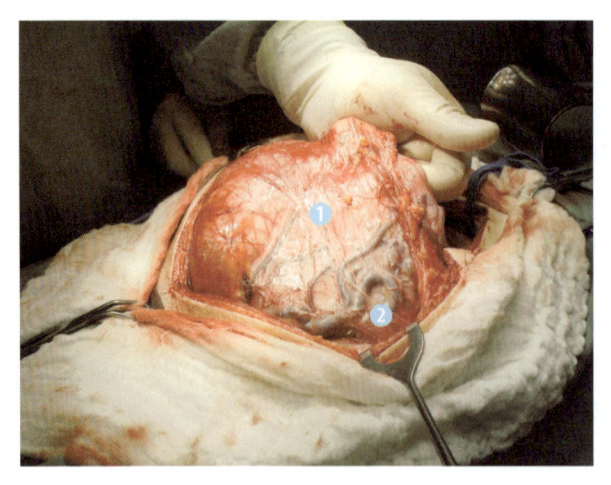

**Fig. 65  Large retroperitoneal tumor**
Peroperative picture:
1) Tumor mass
2) Pathological vascularization

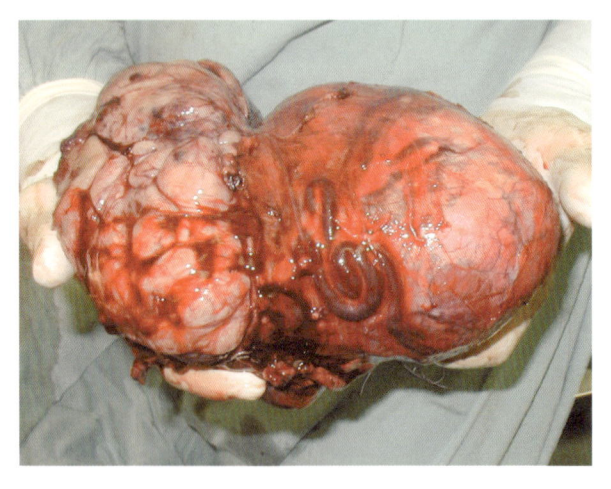

**Fig. 66  Retroperitoneal tumor**
Postoperative picture – resected tissue.
Schwannoma was diagnosed.

## MALIGNANT MELANOMA

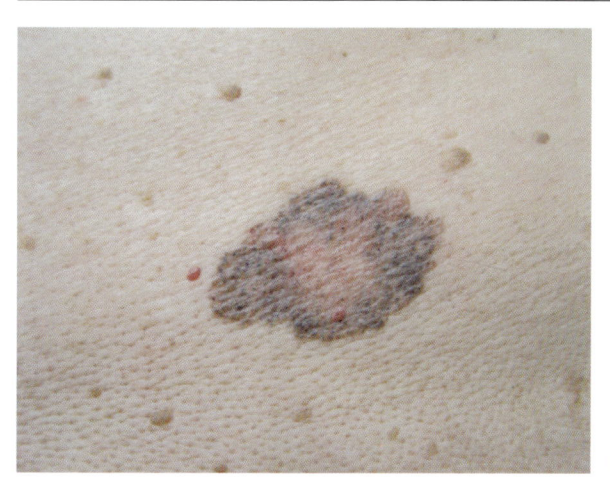

Fig. 67  Skin melanoma

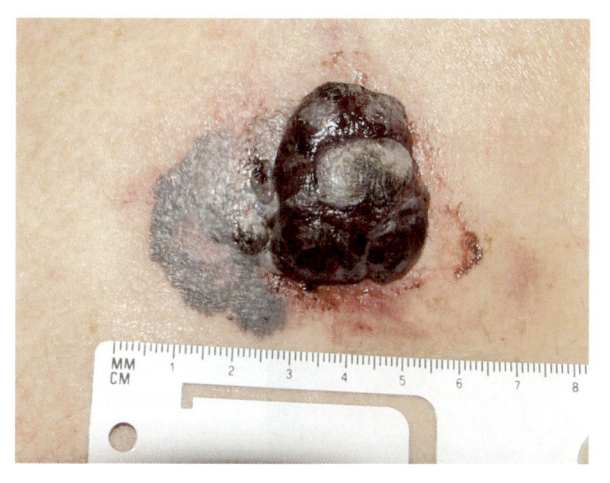

Fig. 68  Nodular melanoma

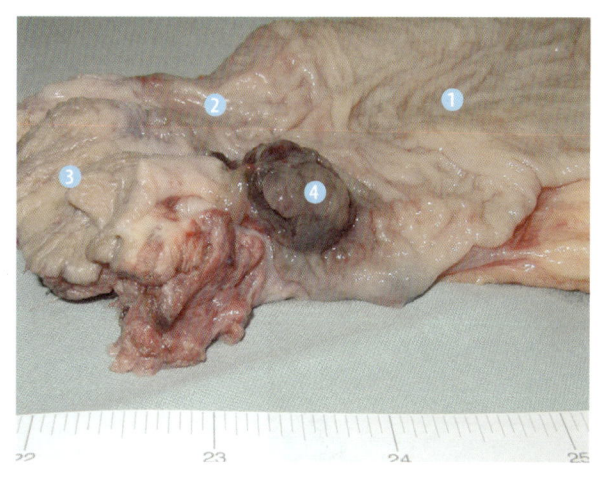

Fig. 69  Anorectal melanoma
Postoperative picture, resected tissue:
1) Mucosa of rectal ampulla
2) Dentate line in anal canal
3) Skin anal margin
4) Melanoma in anorectal junction

ESOPHAGUS AND DIAPHRAGM SURGERY

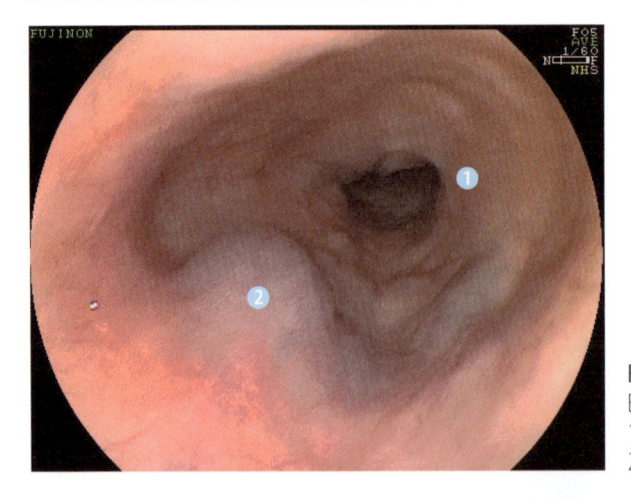

**Fig. 70   Esophageal varix**
Endoscopic finding:
1) Lumen of gastric cardia
2) Esophageal varix

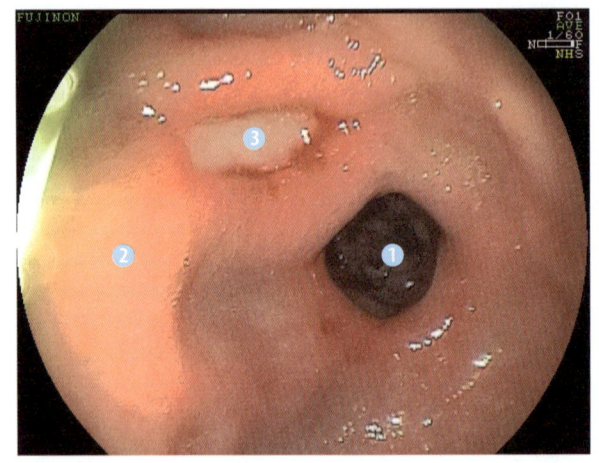

**Fig. 71   Prepyloric ulcer**
Endoscopic finding:
1) Lumen of pylorus
2) Gastric mucosa
3) Gastric ulcer

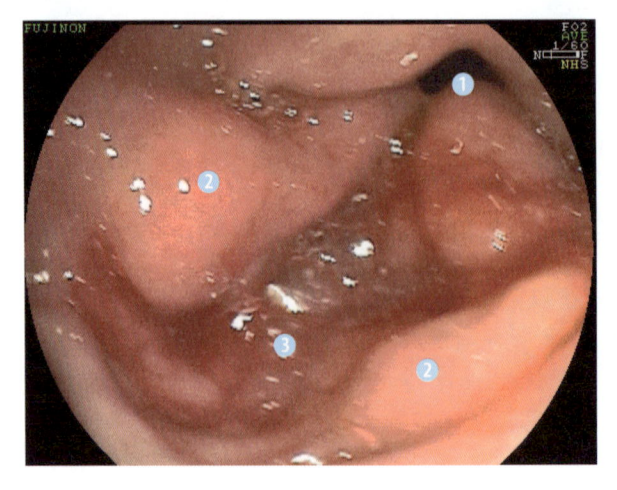

**Fig. 72   Bleeding gastric ulcer**
Endoscopic finding:
1) Lumen of pylorus
2) Mucosal plicae
3) Bleeding ulcer

## GASTRIC AND DUODENAL SURGERY

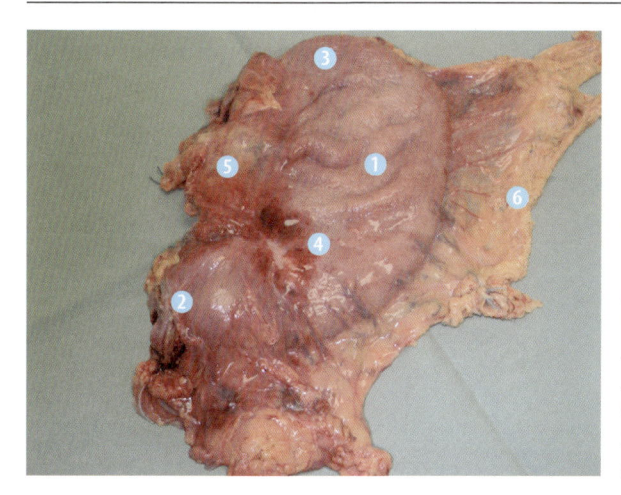

**Fig. 73  Gastric tumor**
Postoperative picture, resected tissue after gastrectomy:
1) Body of stomach
2) Pylorus
3) Cardia
4) Tumor
5) Lesser curvature and mesenterium
6) Residue of gastrocolic ligament

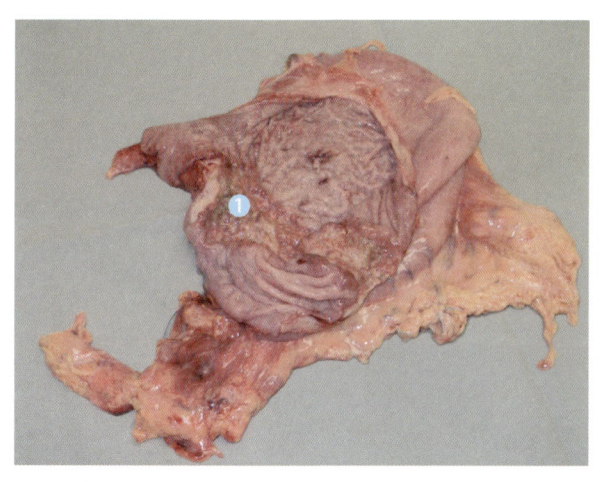

**Fig. 74  Gastric tumor**
Postoperative picture, resected tissue cut open:
1) Large gastric tumor

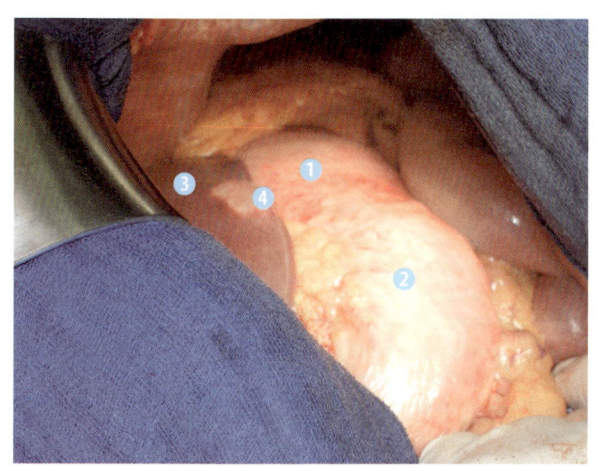

**Fig. 75  Advanced gastric tumor**
Peroperative picture:
1) Stomach
2) Tumor infiltration
3) Liver
4) Metastasis in the edge of left lobe

GASTRIC AND DUODENAL SURGERY

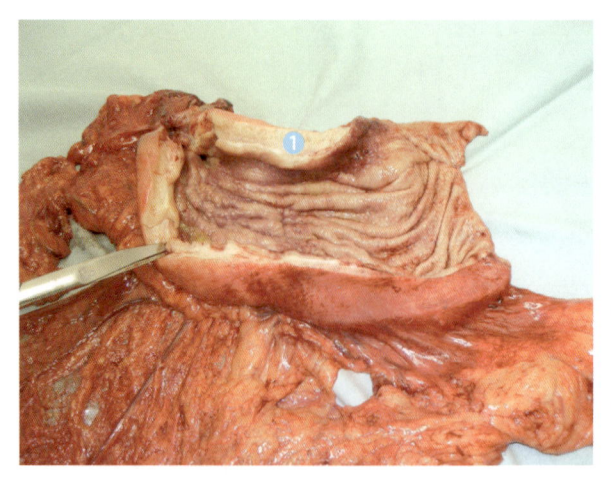

**Fig. 76  Diffuse gastric carcinoma**
Postoperative picture – resected tissue:
Thickening of gastric wall by a tumor growing below mucosa can be observed on the cross-section (1)

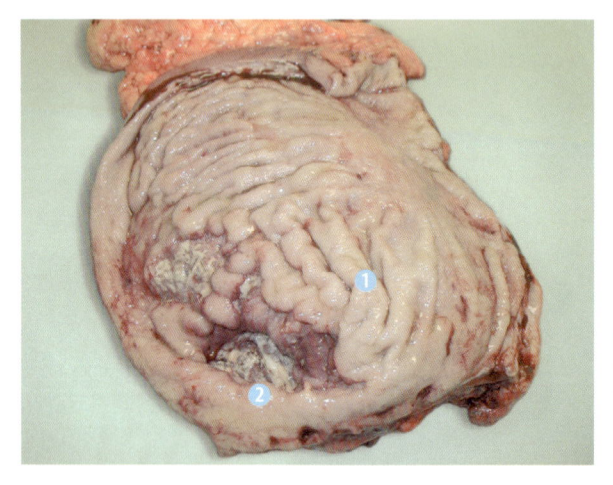

**Fig. 77  Gastric carcinoma**
Postoperative picture – resected tissue:
1) Gastric plicae
2) Tumor imitating ulcer

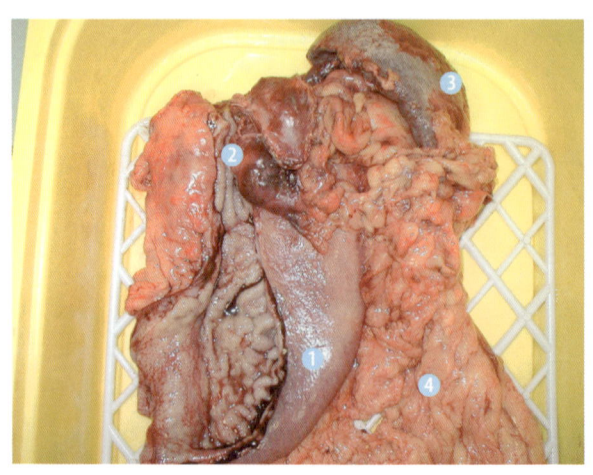

**Fig. 78  Carcinoma of cardia**
Postoperative picture – resected tissue of stomach with spleen and omentum:
1) Stomach
2) Cardia with tumor
3) Spleen
4) Greater omentum

GASTRIC AND DUODENAL SURGERY

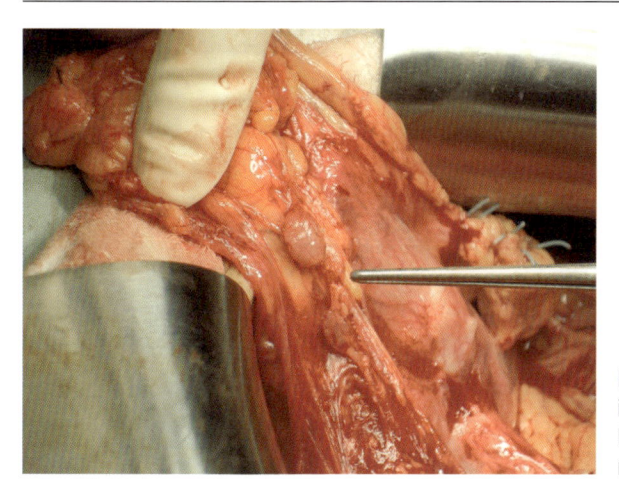

**Fig. 79 Lymph node involvement in gastric carcinoma**
Peroperative picture: Enlarged lymph node at the tip of pincers

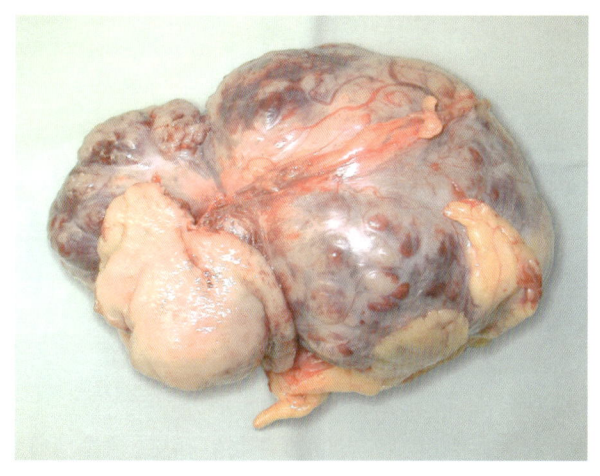

**Fig. 80 Gastric GIST**
Postoperative picture – resected tissue

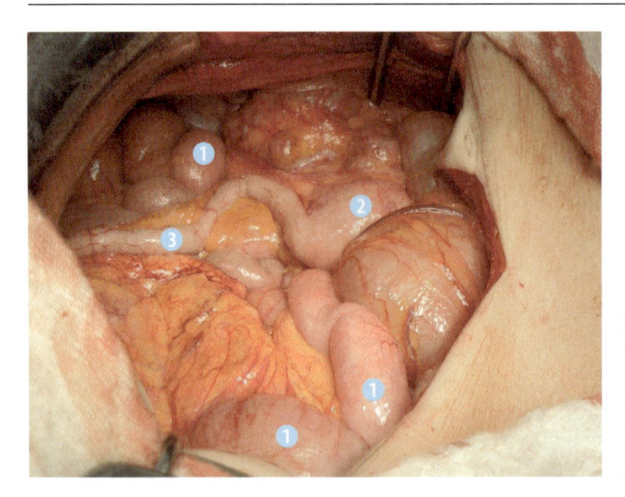

## SURGERY OF THE SMALL AND LARGE INTESTINES, RECTUM AND ANUS

**Fig. 81 Appendix**
Peroperative picture during laparotomy:
1) Small intestine
2) Cecum
3) Appendix

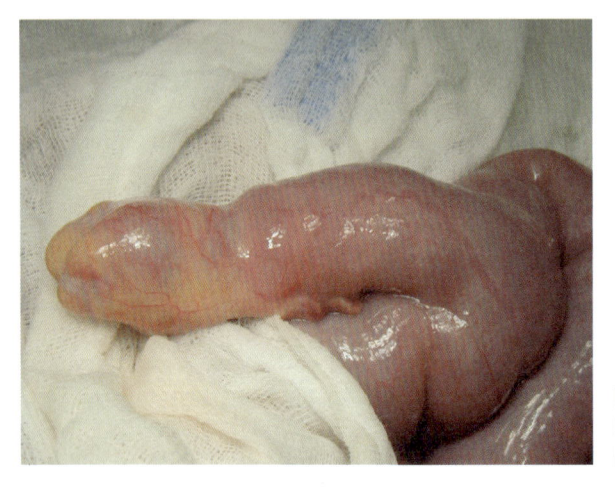

**Fig. 82 Meckel's diverticulum**
Peroperative picture during laparotomy

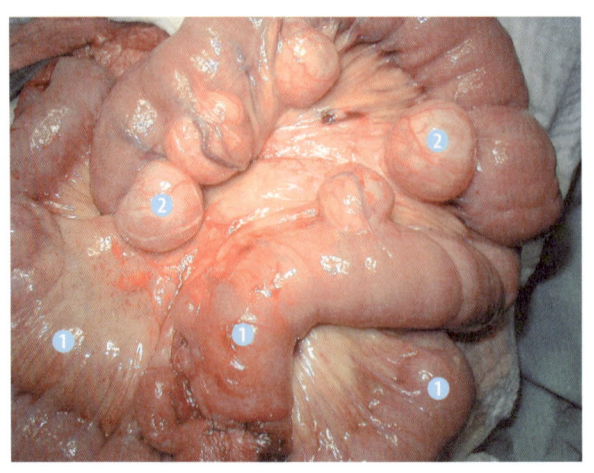

**Fig. 83 Diverticulosis of small intestine**
Peroperative picture:
1) Loops of small intestine
2) Diverticula

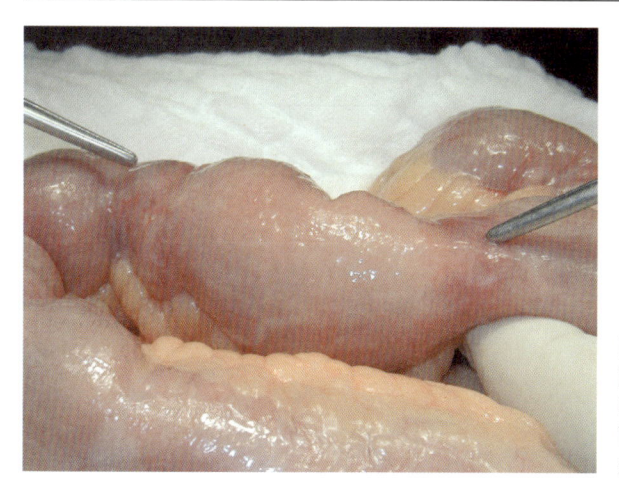

## SURGERY OF THE SMALL AND LARGE INTESTINES, RECTUM AND ANUS

**Fig. 84  Crohn's disease, affected ileum**
Peroperative picture:
Tips of both pincers indicate sites of stenoses – "skip" lesions

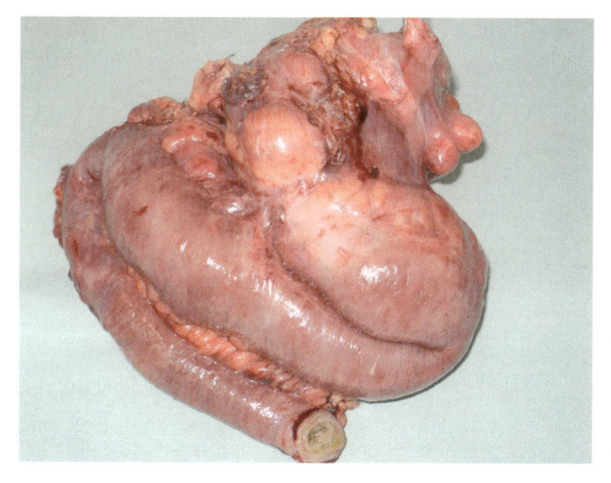

**Fig. 85a  Crohn's disease, affected ileum**
Postoperative picture.
Resected tissue of affected segment with inflammatory infiltration

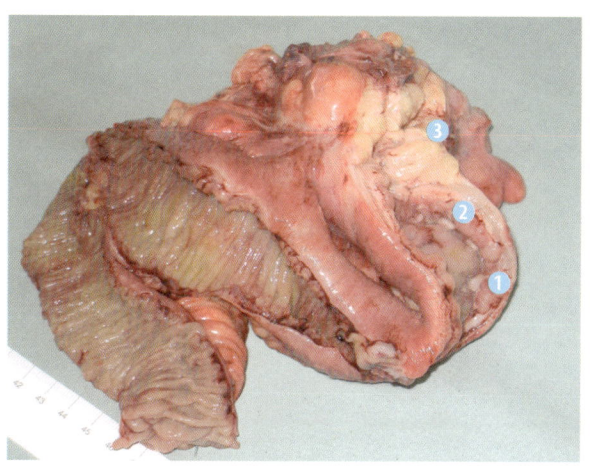

**Fig. 85b  Intestine cut open**
1) Thickened wall
2) Affected mucosa
3) Stenotic segment

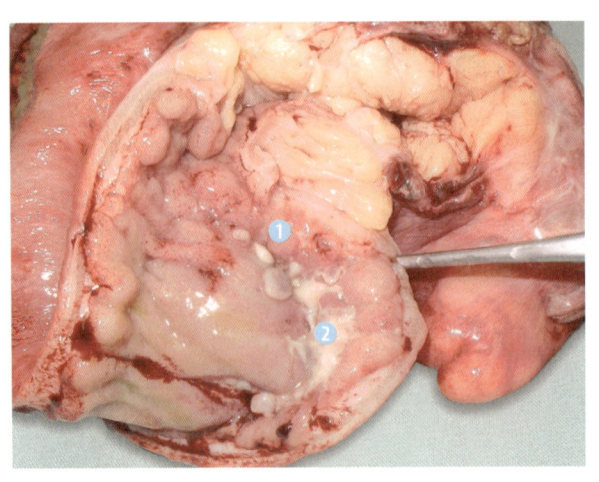

Fig. 85c  Resected tissue in detail
1) Mucosa altered by inflammation with superficial ulcerations
2) Purulent pseudomembranes

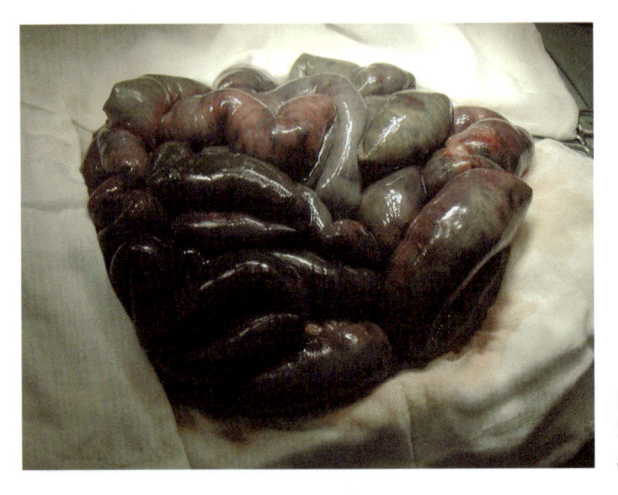

Fig. 86a  Necrosis of small intestine. Ischemia after superior mesenteric artery embolism

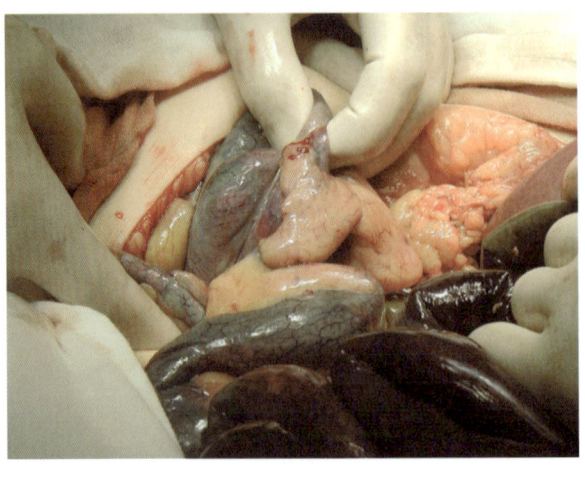

Fig. 86b  Necrosis of small intestine
Detail: intestinal segments with unequally advances necrosis

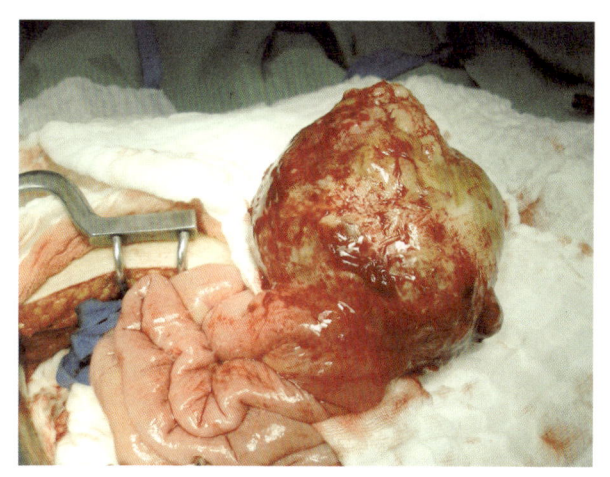

## SURGERY OF THE SMALL AND LARGE INTESTINES, RECTUM AND ANUS

**Fig. 87  Jejunal GIST**
Peroperative picture

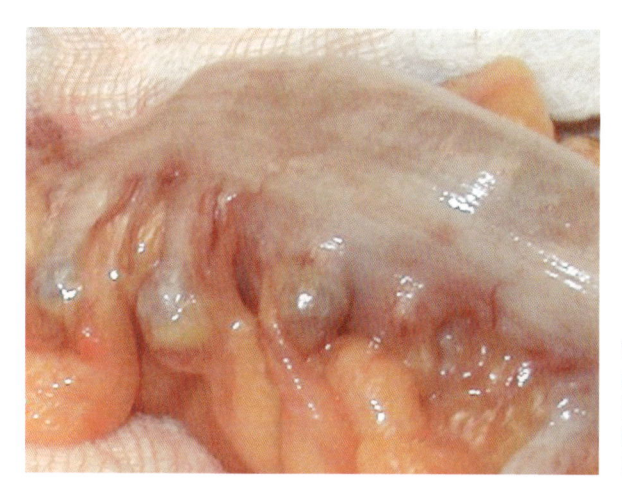

**Fig. 88  Diverticulosis of large intestine**
Peroperative picture.
Quiescent finding, large diverticula with long necks

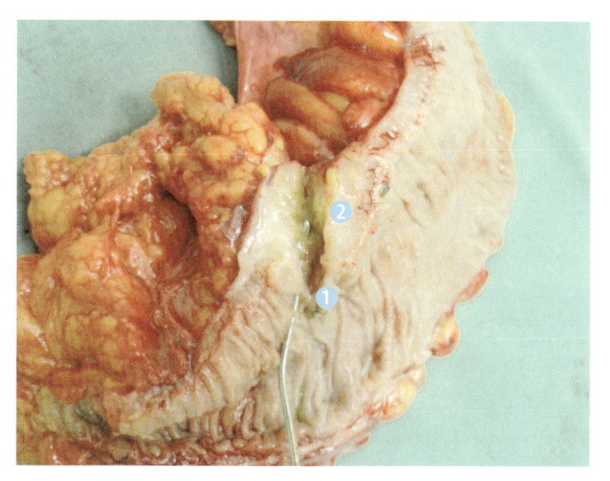

**Fig. 89  Fistula of diverticular origin**
Postoperative picture: probe inserted into fistula in the site of its internal orifice (1); postinflammatory fibrosis (2) in proximity of fistula

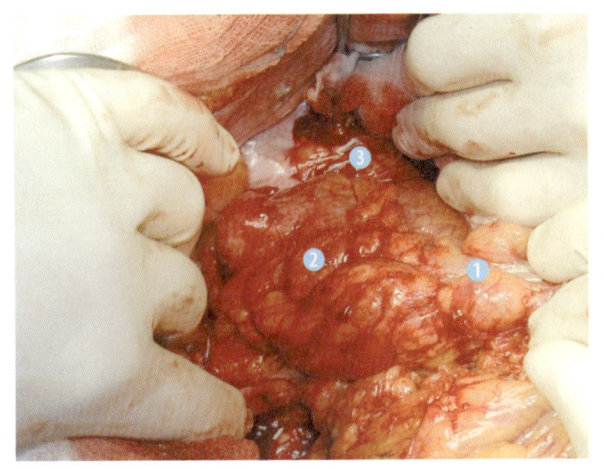

## SURGERY OF THE SMALL AND LARGE INTESTINES, RECTUM AND ANUS

**Fig. 90  Pericolic inflammatory mass in diverticulitis**
Peroperative picture:
1) Unaffected segment of descending colon
2) Infiltrate around sigmoid colon
3) Continuation of infiltrate into pelvis

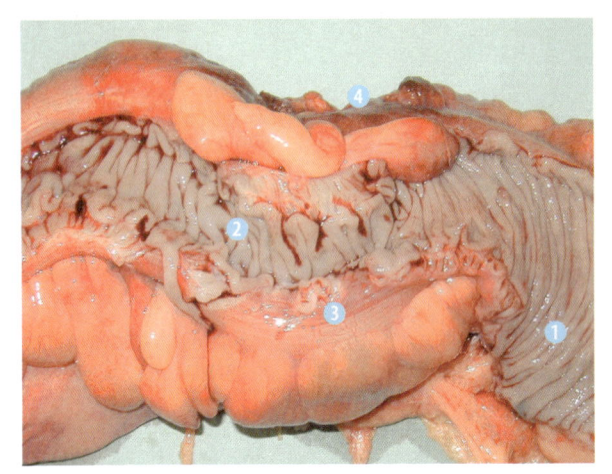

**Fig. 91  Stenosis of sigmoid colon in diverticulitis**
Postoperative picture:
1) Unaffected segment
2) Relative stenosis of lumen
3) Widened wall affected by inflammation and fibrosis
4) Intestinal hyperemia and inflammatory infiltration visible from outside

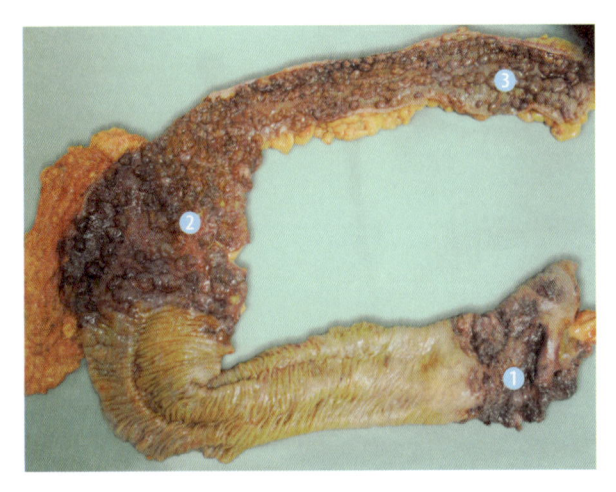

**Fig. 92a  Ulcerative colitis**
Resected tissue of large intestine with typical involvement
Postoperative picture:
1) Cecum
2) Transverse colon
3) Rectosigmoid colon

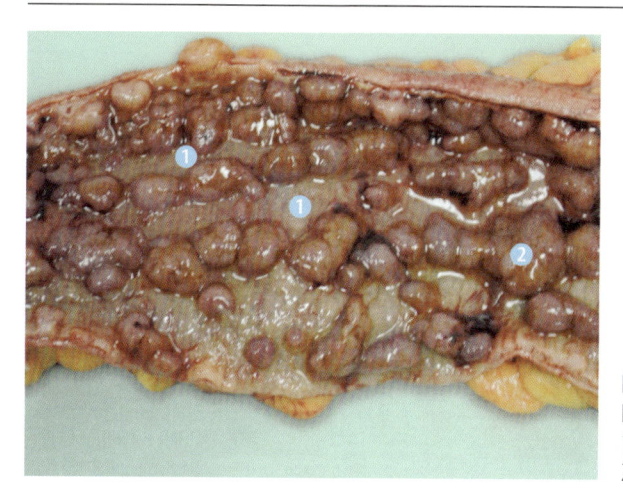

## SURGERY OF THE SMALL AND LARGE INTESTINES, RECTUM AND ANUS

**Fig. 92b  Ulcerative colitis**
Detail of resected tissue:
1) Typical longitudinal ulcerations
2) Hyperplastic polyps

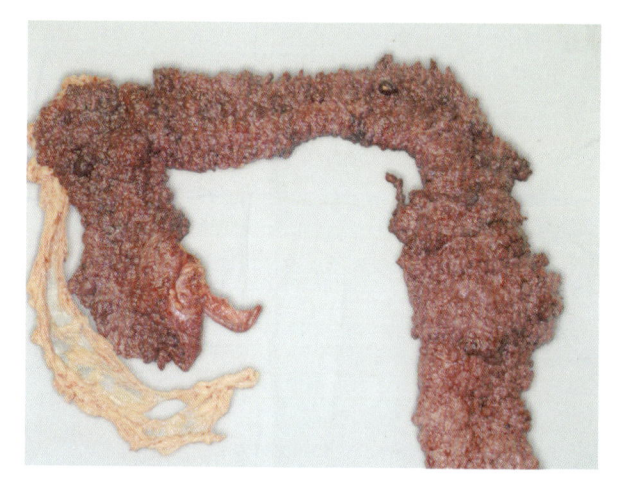

**Fig. 93a  Familiar adenomatous polyposis**
Resected tissue of large intestine
Postoperative picture:
Polyps do not leave any segment of mucosa unaffected

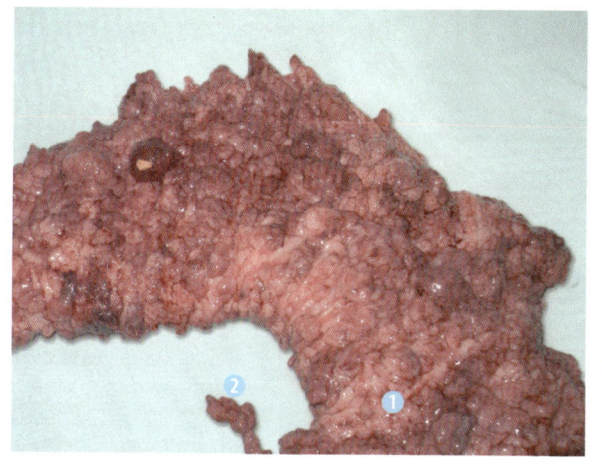

**Fig. 93b  Familiar adenomatous polyposis**
Detail of resected tissue:
1) Cecum filled with polyps
2) Appendix

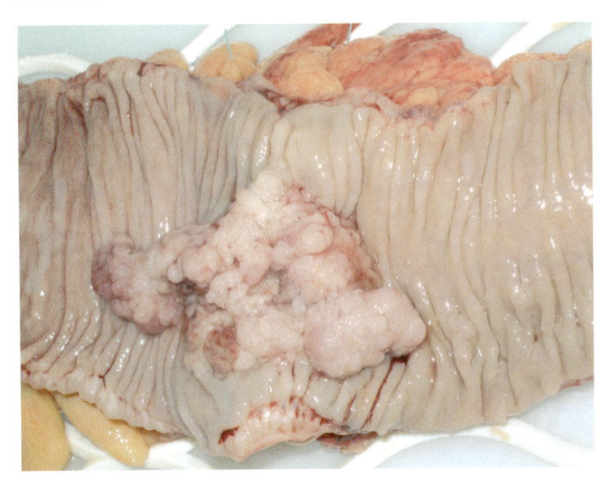

# SURGERY OF THE SMALL AND LARGE INTESTINES, RECTUM AND ANUS

**Fig. 94  Rectal villous adenoma**
Postoperative picture

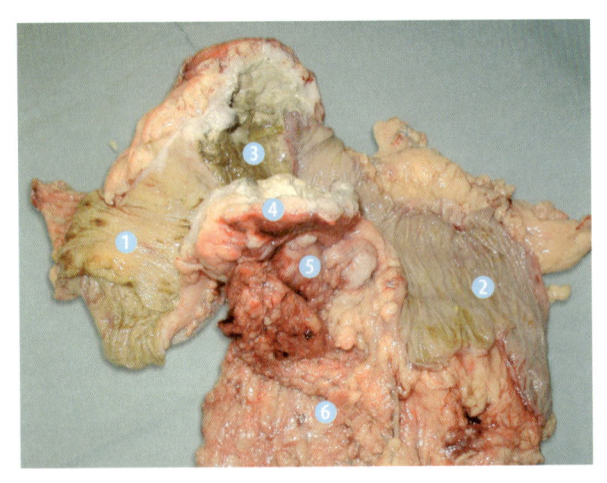

**Fig. 95  Carcinoma of colon splenic flexure**
Postoperative picture:
1) Transverse colon
2) Beginning of descending colon
3) Tumor with central necrosis
4) Tumorous and fibrous remodeling of intestinal wall
5) Enlarged paracolic lymph node
6) Greater omentum

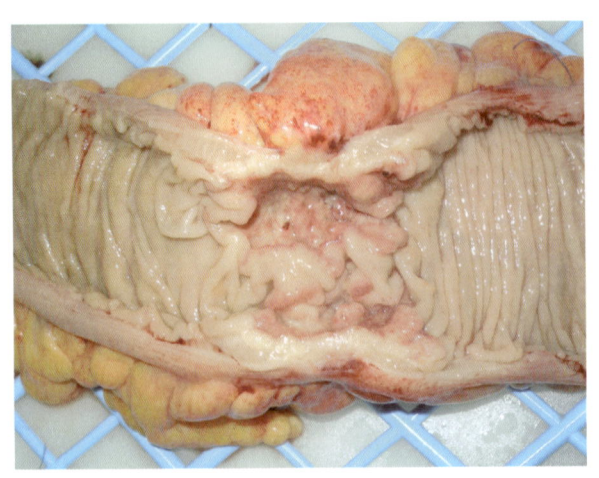

**Fig. 96  Carcinoma of sigmoid colon – scirrhus**
Postoperative picture – resected tissue with circular stenotic tumor

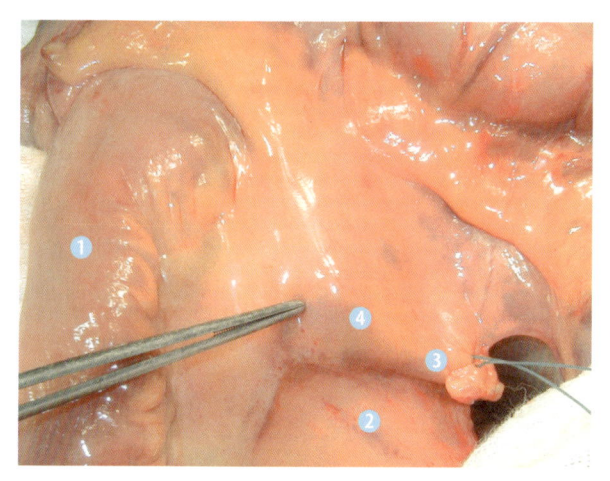

# SURGERY OF THE SMALL AND LARGE INTESTINES, RECTUM AND ANUS

**Fig. 97a  Lymph node involvement of mesentery**
Postoperative picture:
1) Ascending colon
2) Mesentery
3) Site of vessel disruption marked with ligation
4) Enlarged lymph node

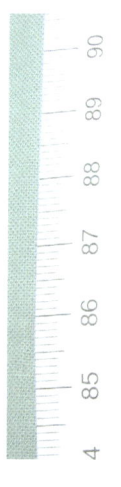

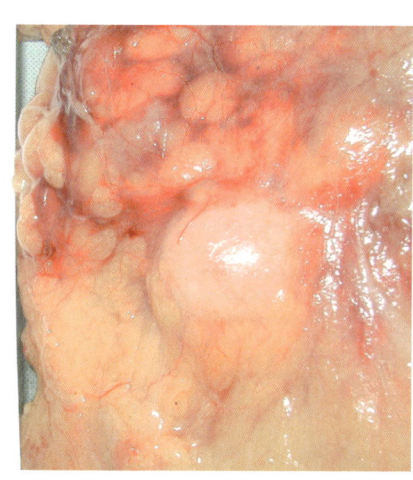

**Fig. 97b  Lymph node involvement of mesentery**
Detail:
Prominent enlarged lymph node of mesocolon

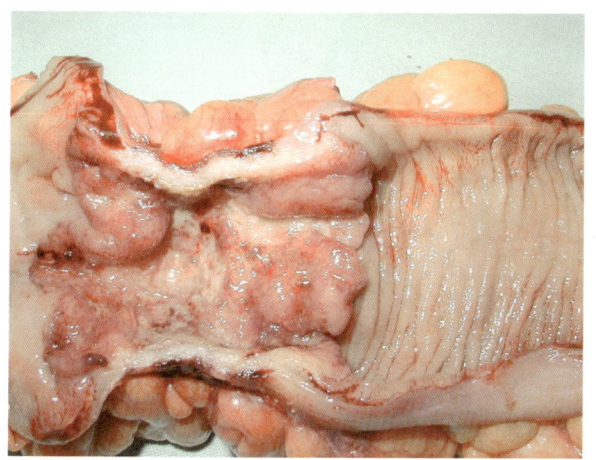

**Fig. 98  Exulcerated stenotic rectal tumor**
Postoperative picture, resected tissue

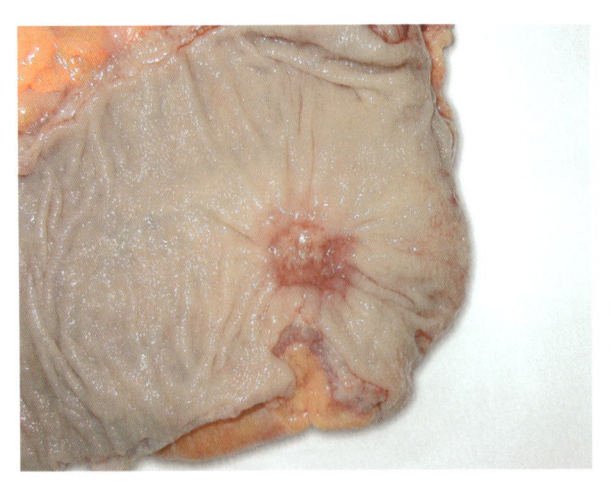

SURGERY OF THE SMALL AND LARGE INTESTINES, RECTUM AND ANUS

Fig. 99  Rectal carcinoma after neoadjuvant radiochemotherapy
Postoperative picture, resected tissue. Residue of original tumor that has regressed after treatment can be seen in the middle of the picture.

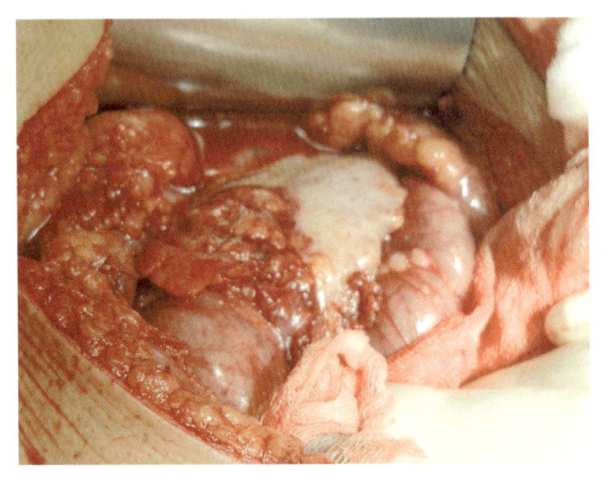

Fig. 100  Carcinosis of peritoneum in generalized colorectal carcinoma
Peroperative picture. All viscera are affected by tumor dissemination; confluent tumor infiltration of omentum can be seen in the middle of the picture.

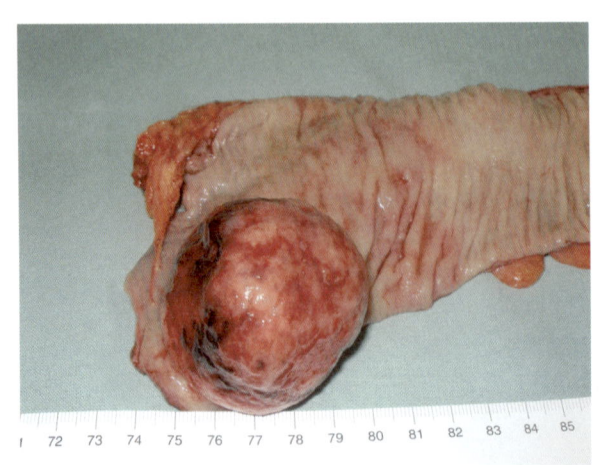

Fig. 101  Rectal lymphoma
Postoperative picture, resected tissue

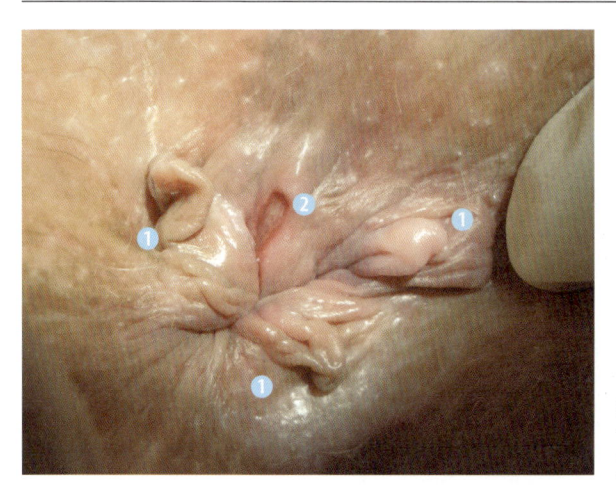

SURGERY OF THE SMALL AND LARGE INTESTINES, RECTUM AND ANUS

Fig. 102   Anal fissure
1) Skin plicae
2) Fissure

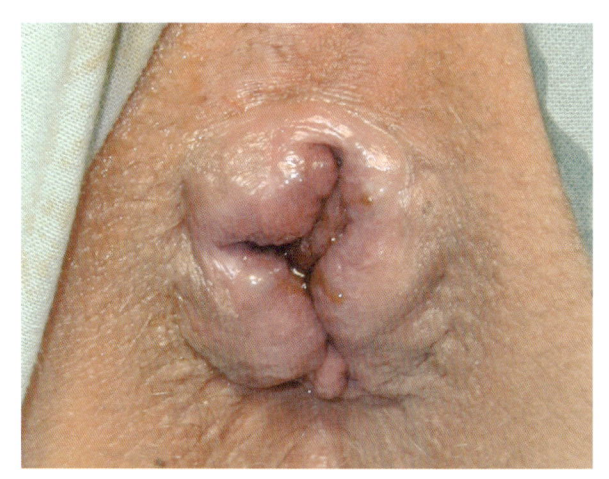

Fig. 103   Hemorrhoids
Large external hemorrhoids in typical localization, identical with internal hemorrhoids

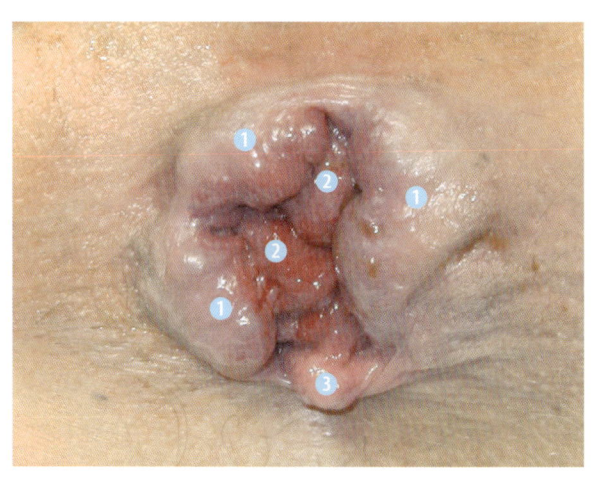

Fig. 104   Hemorrhoids
Besides large external hemorrhoids (1), internal hemorrhoids (2) can be also seen, one of them permanently prolapsing outside (3)

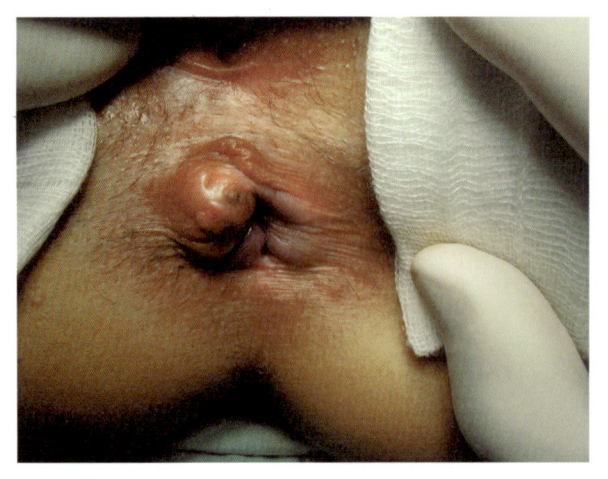

**SURGERY OF THE SMALL AND LARGE INTESTINES, RECTUM AND ANUS**

Fig. 105  Acute thrombosis of hemorrhoid

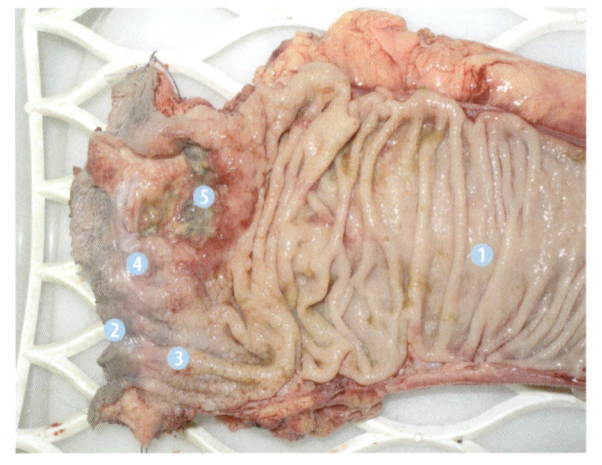

Fig. 106  Carcinoma of anal canal
Postoperative picture, resected tissue:
1) Rectal ampulla
2) Skin anal margin
3) Anal dentate line
4) Tumor
5) Central necrosis of the tumor

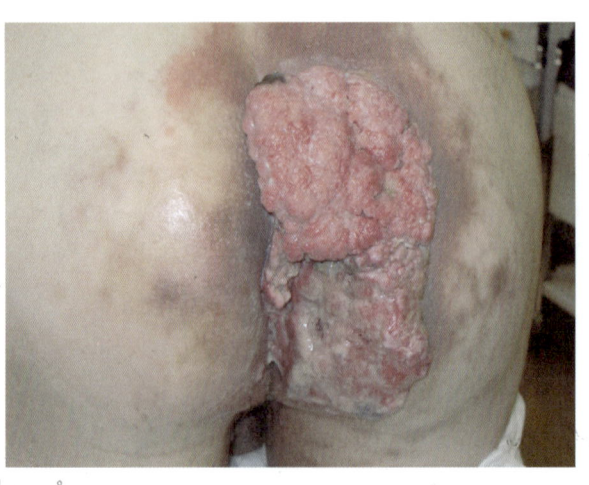

Fig. 107  Advanced anal carcinoma

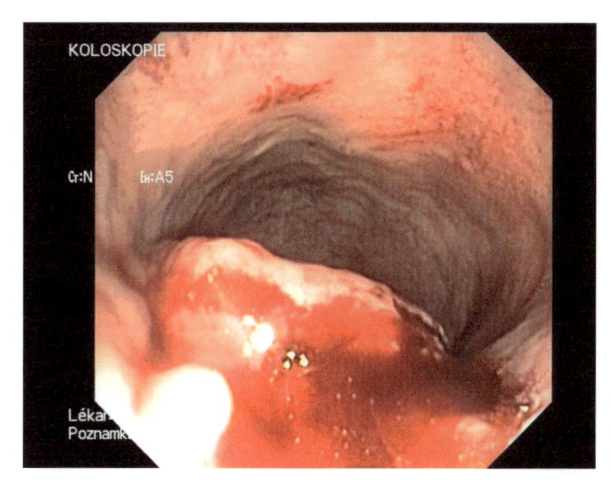

## SURGERY OF THE SMALL AND LARGE INTESTINES, RECTUM AND ANUS

Fig. 108 Tumor of descending colon
Endoscopy

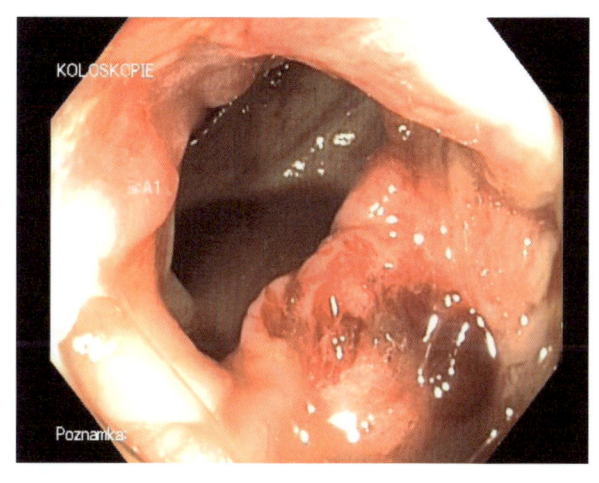

Fig. 109 Bleeding tumor of ascending colon
Endoscopy

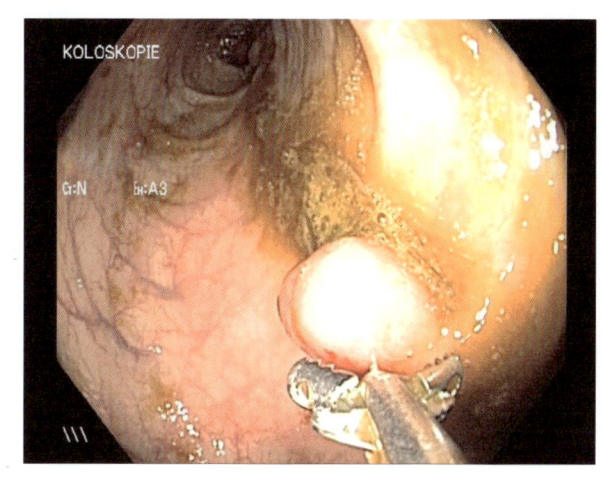

Fig. 110 Polyp of large intestine before starting biopsy
Endoscopy

LIVER SURGERY

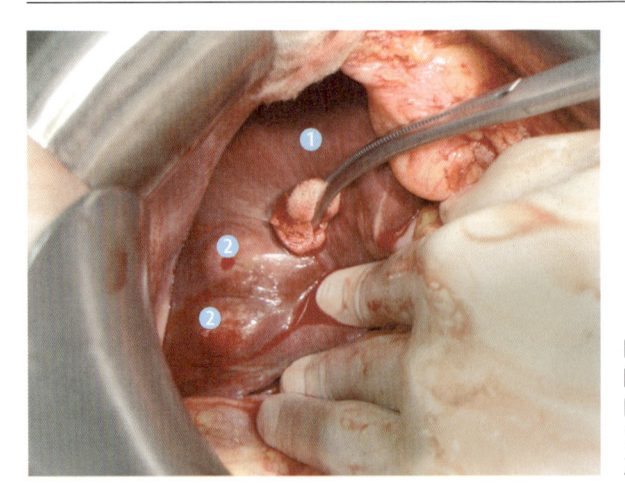

**Fig. 111 Tumor metastases in liver**
Peroperative picture:
1) Hepatic tissue
2) Metastasis

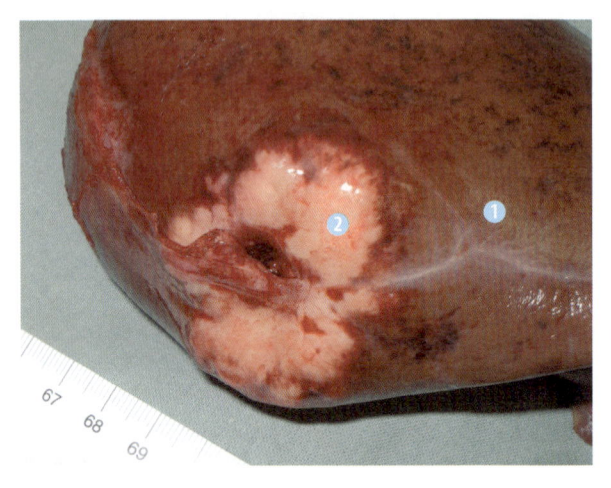

**Fig. 112 Tumor metastasis in liver – detail**
Resected hepatic tissue:
1) Hepatic tissue
2) Metastasis

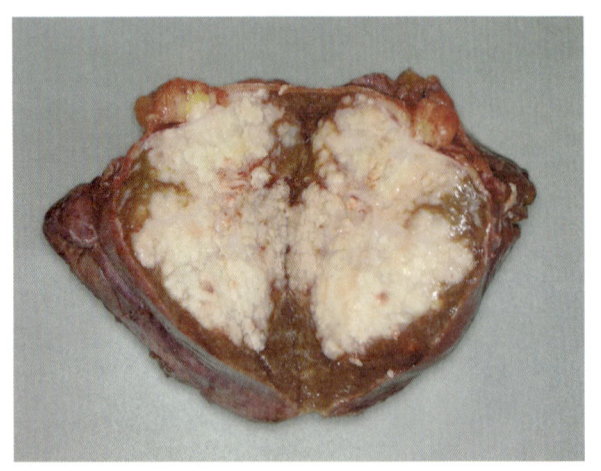

**Fig. 113 Metastasis of colorectal carcinoma into liver**
Resected hepatic tissue after bisegmentectomy (seg. V, VI)

LIVER SURGERY

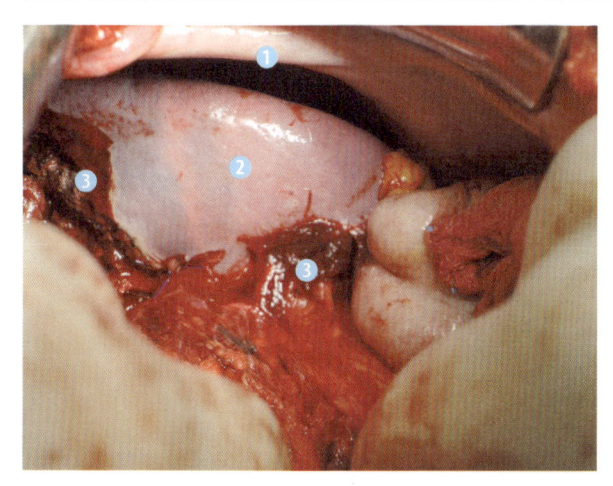

**Fig. 114 Liver injury after blunt abdominal trauma**
Laparotomy:
1) Costal margin
2) Uninjured part of the liver
3) Deep fissure of the liver

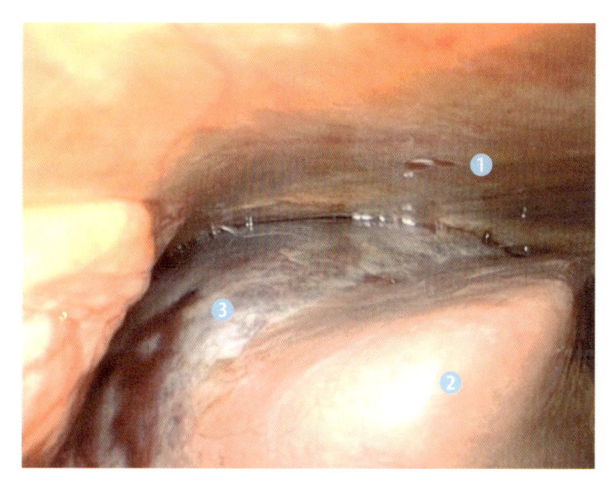

**Fig. 115 Subcapsular liver hematoma**
Laparoscopic picture:
1) Subphrenic region on the right side
2) Unaffected part of the liver
3) Visible subcapsular hematoma

GALLBLADDER AND EXTRAHEPATIC BILE DUCTS

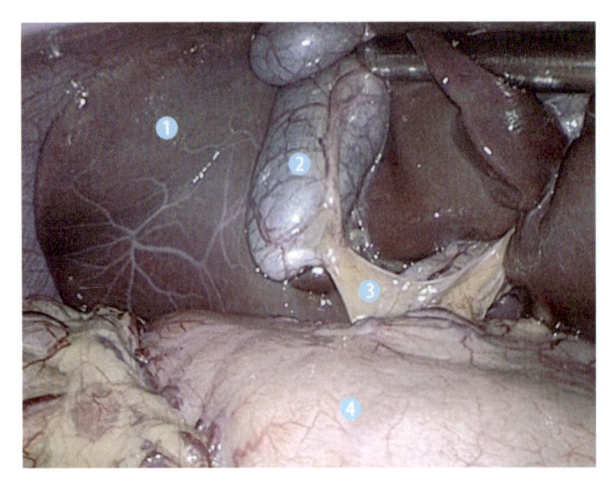

**Fig. 116 Gallbladder**
Laparoscopy:
1) Liver
2) Gallbladder (lifted up with a surgical instrument together with the liver)
3) Fat tissue around cystic duct and cystic artery
4) Anterior surface of stomach

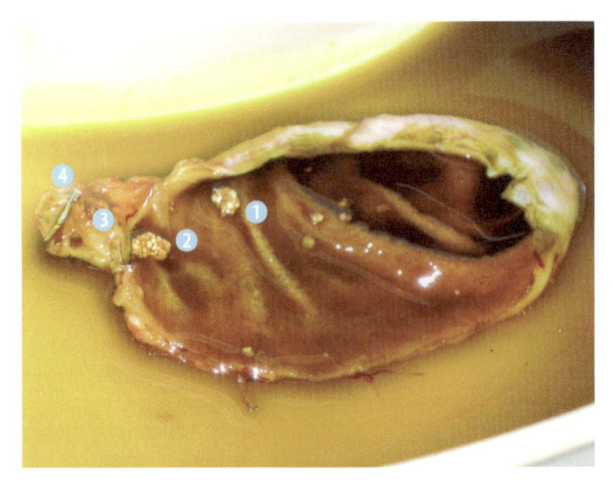

**Fig. 117 Gallbladder cut open after operation**
1) One of several stones of various size
2) Gallstone in gallbladder neck
3) Cystic duct
4) Closure with a clip

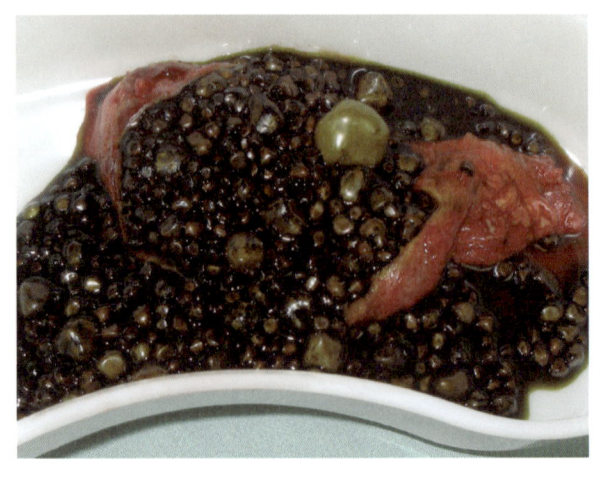

**Fig. 118 Gallbladder completely filled with small gallstones**

## GALLBLADDER AND EXTRAHEPATIC BILE DUCTS

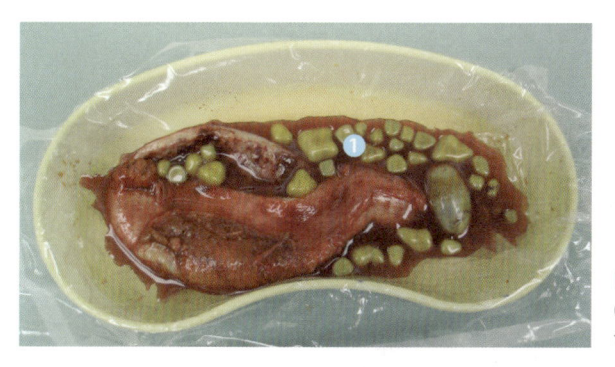

**Fig. 119  Gallbladder**
Gallstones of various size, some of them facet stones (1)

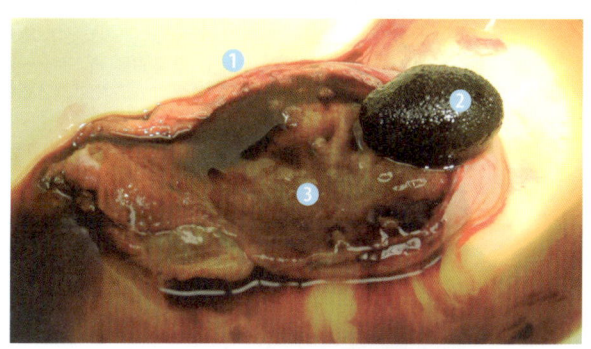

**Fig. 120  Phlegmonous calculous cholecystitis**
1) Gallbladder wall altered by inflammation
2) Large solitary stone
3) Gallbladder mucosa altered by inflammation

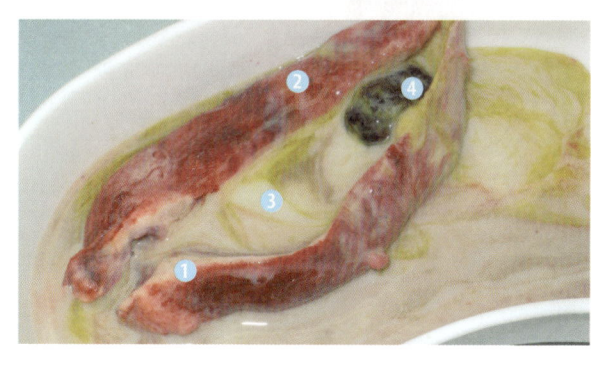

**Fig. 121  Gallbladder empyema**
Postoperative picture, gallbladder cut open:
1) Gallbladder wall thickened due to inflammation
2) Hyperemia of serosa
3) Pus evacuated from gallbladder into a bowl
4) Large solitary stone

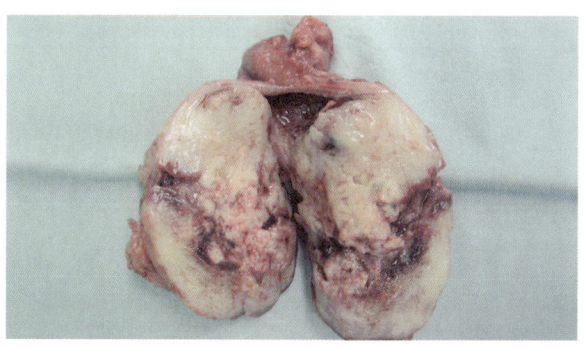

**Fig. 122  Tumor of gallbladder**
Cross-section — removed gallbladder is completely filled with tumorous masses

Chapter 11

## PANCREAS

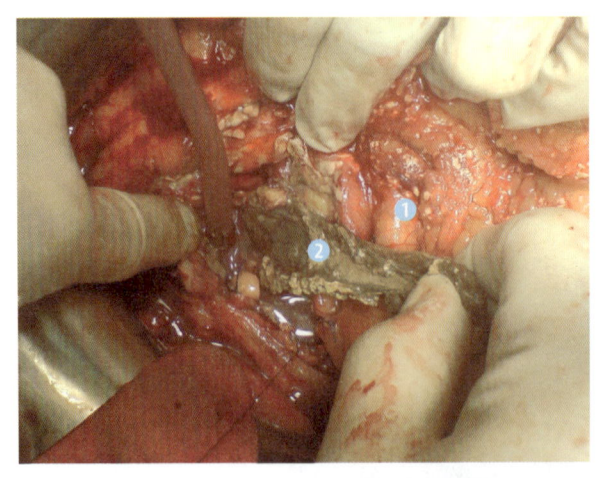

**Fig. 123 Acute necrotizing pancreatitis**
Peroperative picture – necrectomy:
1) Loop of small intestine – jejunum
2) Necrotic pancreatic tissue

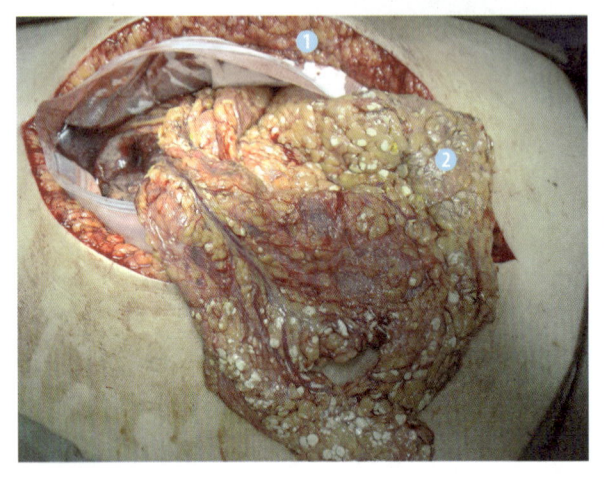

**Fig. 124 Acute pancreatitis**
Peroperative picture during repeated surgical session:
1) Laparostomy with plastic film and zipper for temporary abdominal closure
2) Greater omentum with well visible Balser's necroses (whitish foci)

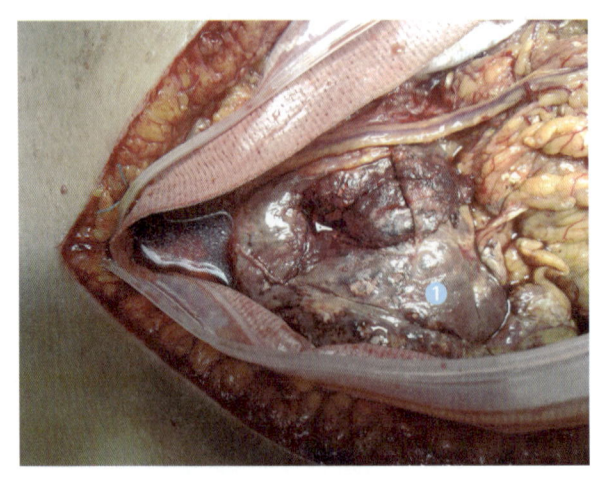

**Fig. 125 Acute pancreatitis**
Peroperative picture during repeated surgical session – detail:
1) Necroses in omental bursa

PANCREAS

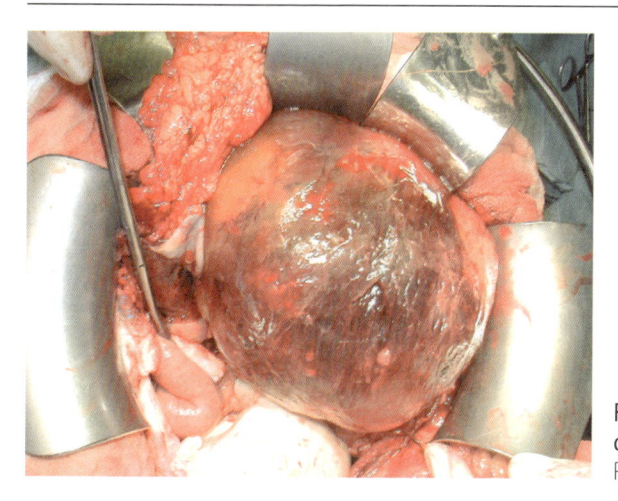

**Fig. 126 Mucinous pancreatic cystadenoma**
Peroperative picture

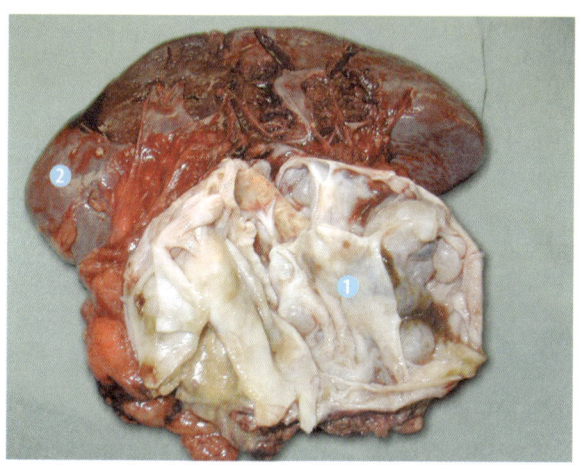

**Fig. 127 Mucinous pancreatic cystadenoma**
Postoperative picture – resected tissue:
1) Cystadenoma
2) Pancreatic tissue

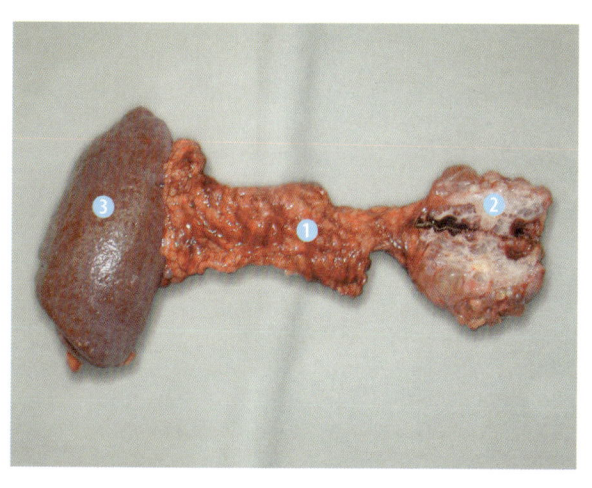

**Fig. 128 Serous pancreatic cystadenoma**
Postoperative picture of resected tissue:
1) Pancreas
2) Cystadenoma
3) Spleen

SPLEEN SURGERY

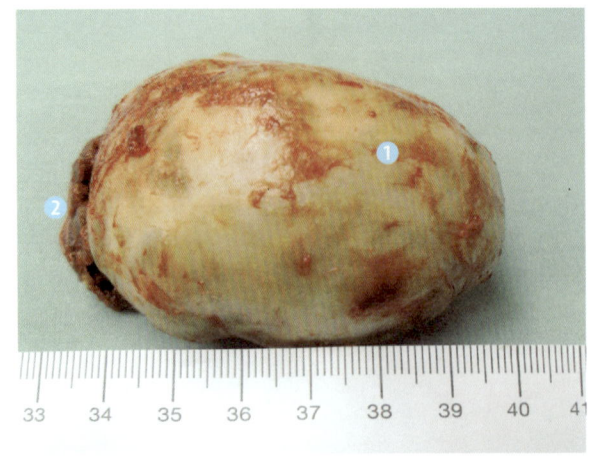

**Fig. 129  Splenic cyst**
Postoperative picture:
1) Cyst fills in a major part of the spleen
2) Residue of splenic tissue on the edge

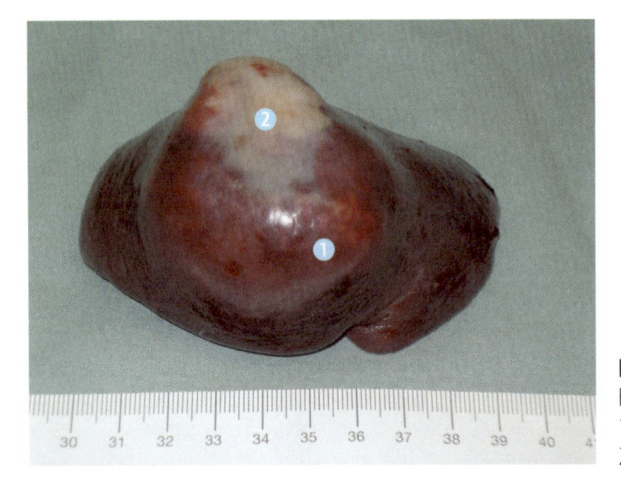

**Fig. 130  Splenic lymphoma**
Postoperative picture:
1) Intact splenic tissue
2) Focus of lymphoma

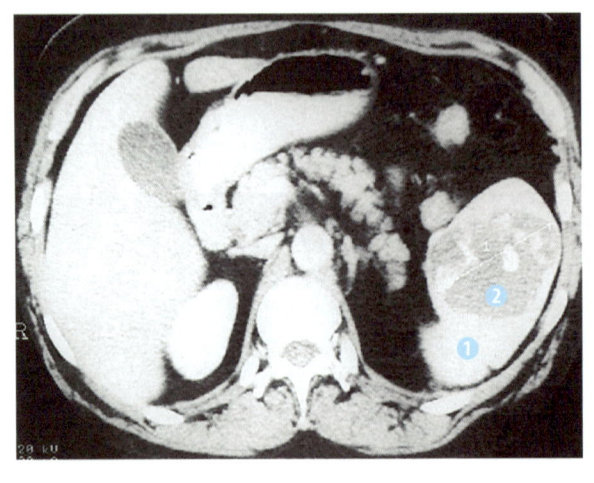

**Fig. 131  Cavernous structure in the spleen**
CT scan:
1) Preserved intact splenic parenchyma
2) Pathological focus in the spleen

SPLEEN SURGERY

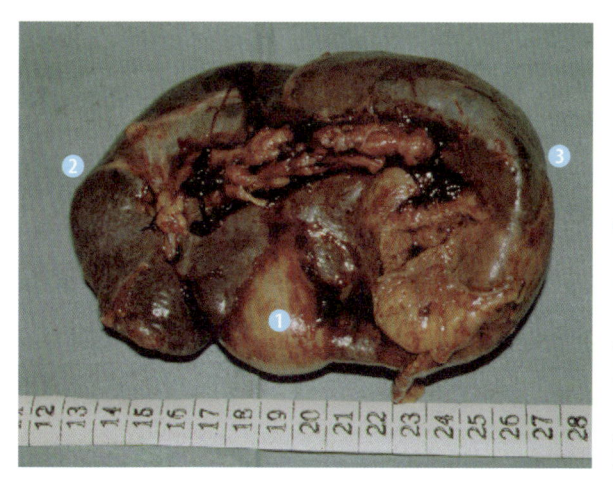

**Fig. 132 Spleen with cavernous structure**
Postoperative picture
(CT scan on the previous picture)
Focus cannot be observed from outside.
Anatomical orientation:
1) Hilum
2) Upper pole
3) Lower pole

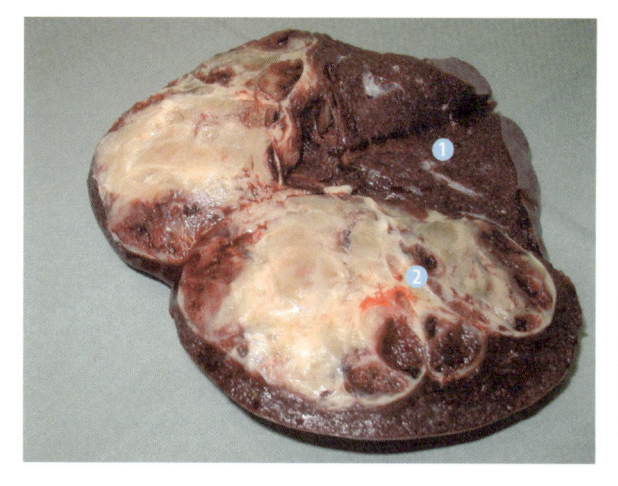

**Fig. 133 Cavernous hemangioma of the spleen**
Cross-section of removed spleen:
1) Residues of original tissue
2) Septa and necroses in hemangioma

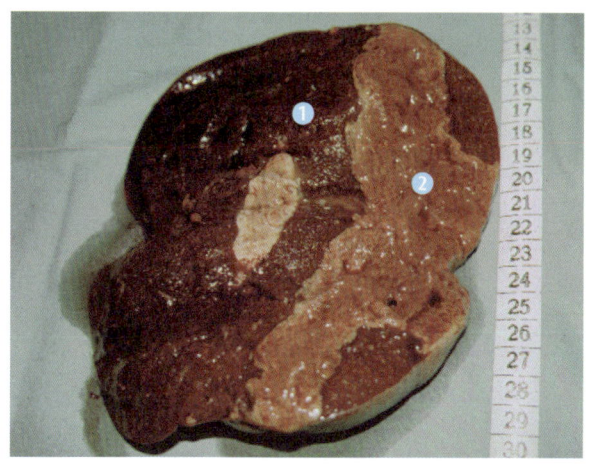

**Fig. 134 Splenic infarction**
Postoperative picture:
1) Intact parenchyma
2) Area of infarction

## ILEUS – INTESTINAL IMPASSABILITY

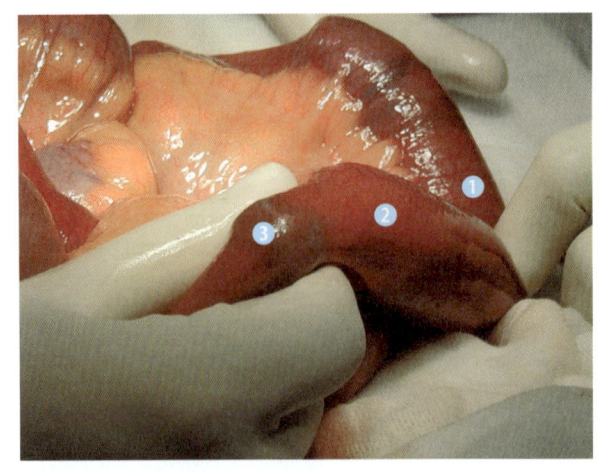

**Fig. 135   Biliary ileus**
Peroperative picture:
1) Hyperemic and edematous ileum
2) Dilatation of intestine
3) Gallstone

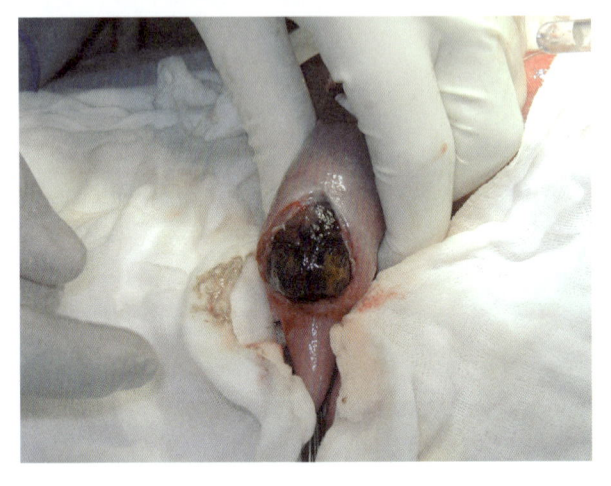

**Fig. 136   Biliary ileus**
Peroperative picture:
Enterotomy with gallstone

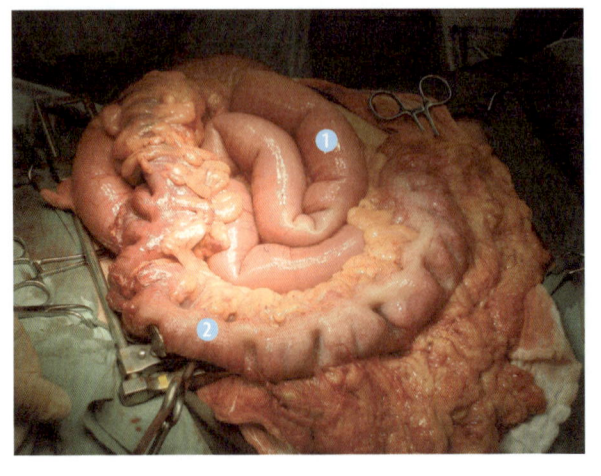

**Fig. 137   Obstructive ileus**
Peroperative picture:
1) Dilatation of small intestine loops
2) Dilatation of colon, hastration still visible

## ILEUS – INTESTINAL IMPASSABILITY

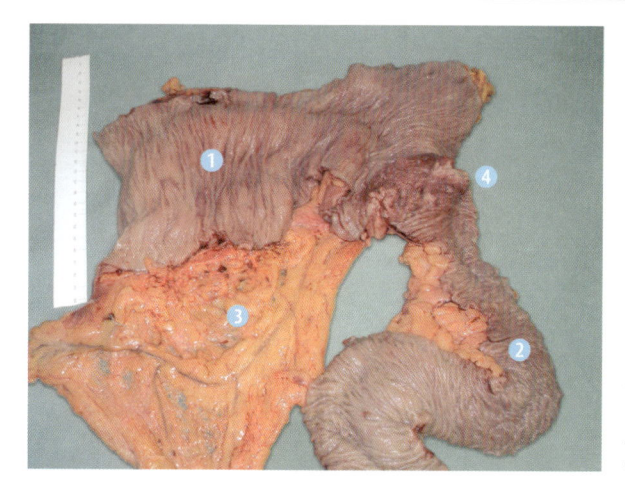

**Fig. 138 Obstructive ileus caused by tumor of descending colon**
Resected intestinal tissue:
1) Suprastenotic intestinal dilatation
2) Non-dilated intestine below the tumor
3) Part of greater omentum
4) Stenotic tumor

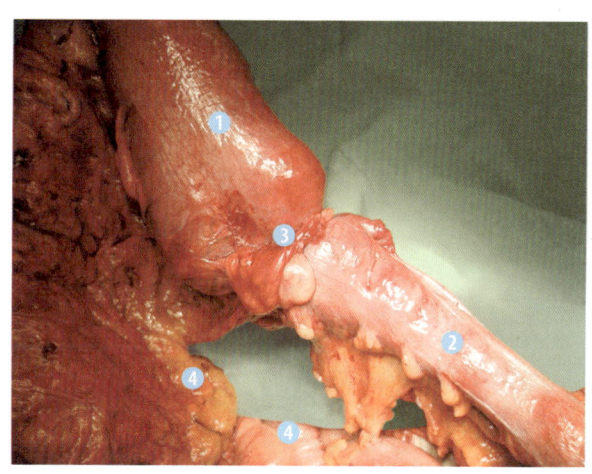

**Fig. 139 Restored intestinal continuity after resection – primary anastomosis**
1) Oral intestinal segment, evacuated and toned
2) Aboral non-dilated segment
3) End-to-end anastomosis
4) Defect between edges of mesocolon, before closing with suture

## PERITONITIS

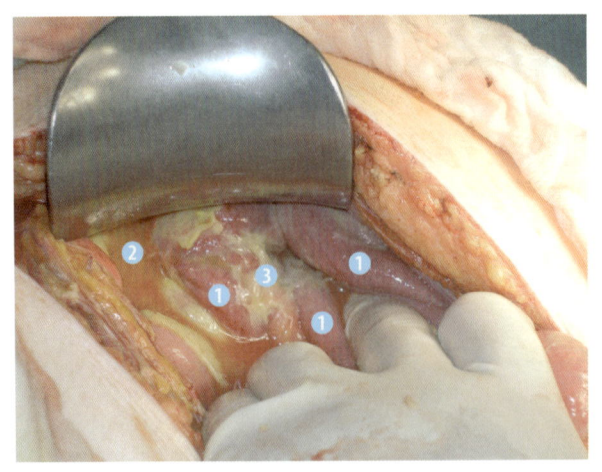

**Fig. 140 Purulent peritonitis due to intestinal perforation**
Peroperative picture, laparotomy, view to hypogastrium:
1) Small intestine
2) Purulent effusion
3) Fibrinous pseudomembranes

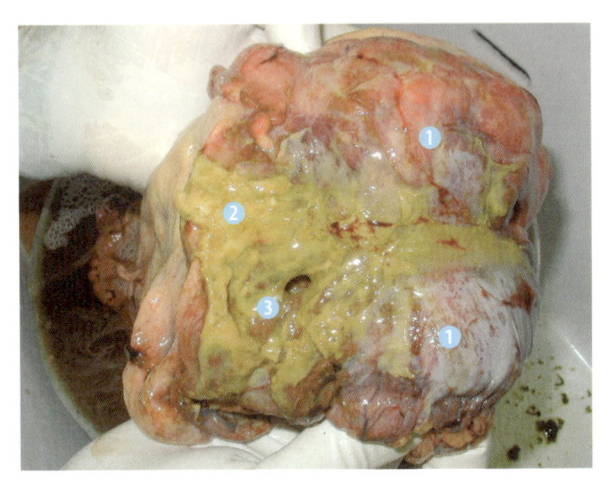

**Fig. 141 Perforation of small intestine**
Peroperative picture:
1) Convolute of loops of terminal ileum
2) Purulent fibrinous pseudomembranes
3) Perforation aperture

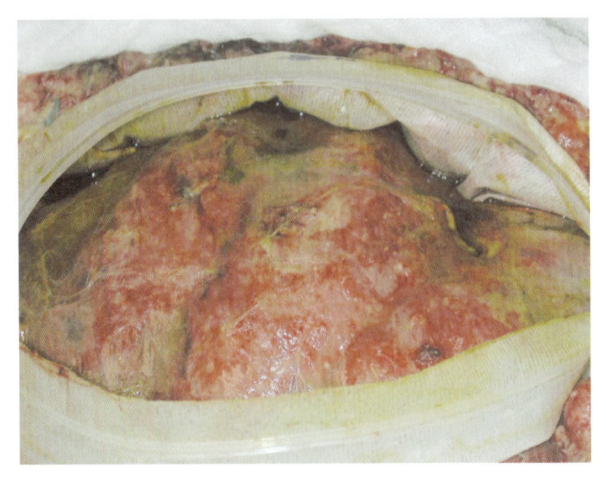

**Fig. 142 Stercoral peritonitis after multiple perforations of small intestine**
Picture of laparotomy with temporary closure with zipper. Convolute of loops of small intestine and effusion with intestinal content can be observed.

## PERITONITIS

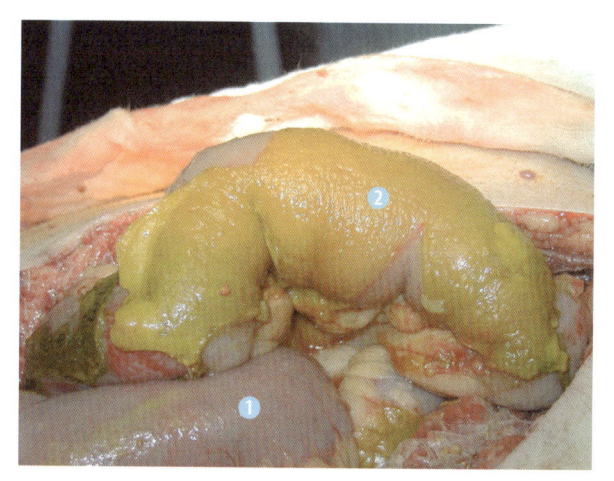

**Fig. 143 Fibrinous pseudomembranes in late phase of purulent peritonitis**
Laparotomy, peroperative picture:
1) Loop of small intestine
2) Loop of small intestine with adherent fibrinous pseudomembrane

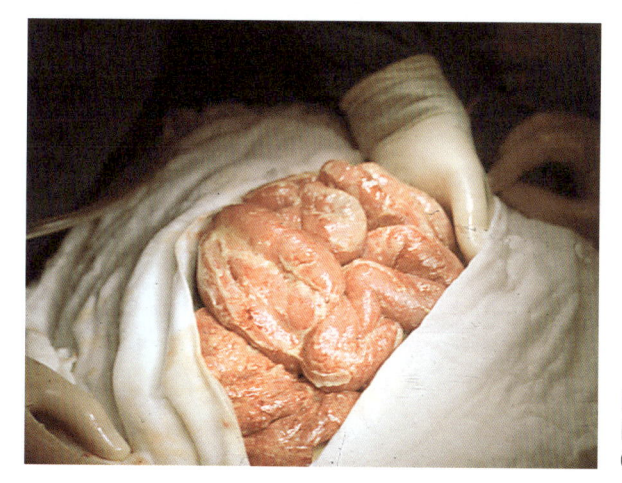

**Fig. 144 Plastic peritonitis**
Peroperative picture:
Convolute of loops of small intestine

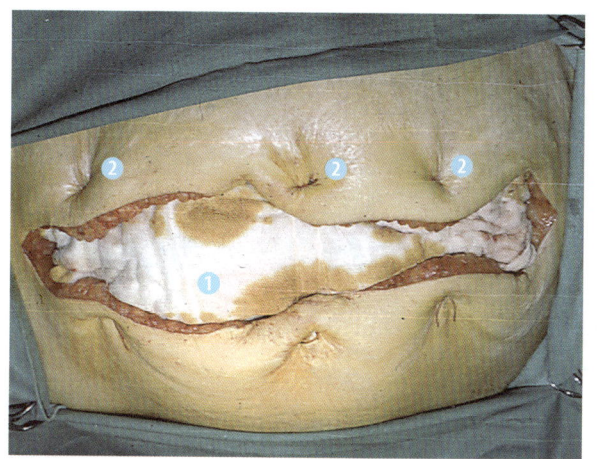

**Fig. 145 Laparostomy in peritonitis**
Temporary closure of laparotomic wound:
1) Viscera are covered with a drape
2) Retained stitches

## VASCULAR SURGERY

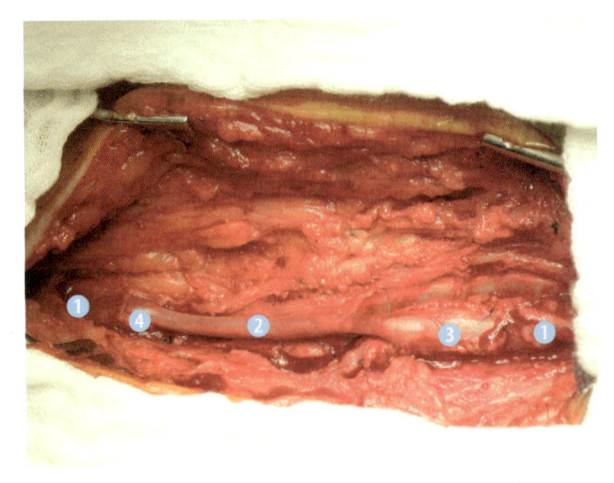

**Fig. 146  Interposition of venous graft from great saphenous vein to superficial femoral artery**
Peroperative picture:
1) Superficial femoral artery
2) Venous bypass
3) Proximal anastomosis
4) Distal anastomosis

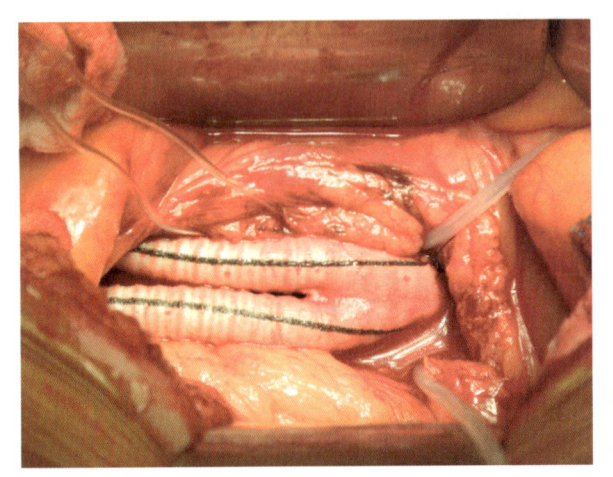

**Fig. 147  Proximal part of aortobifemoral bypass prosthesis**
Peroperative picture

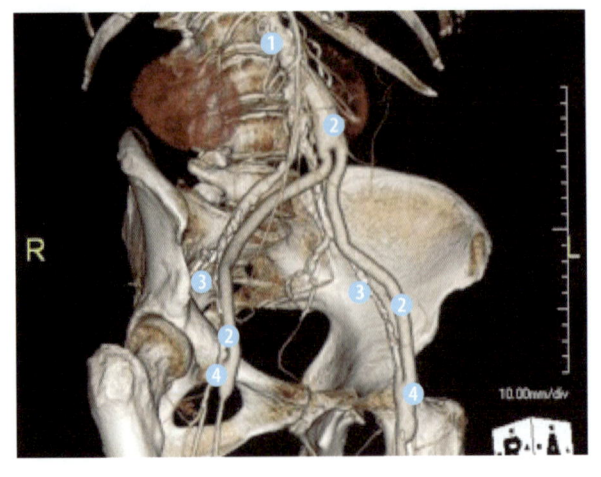

**Fig. 148  Aortobifemoral bypass**
CT angiography:
1) Abdominal aorta
2) Aortobifemoral bypass (prosthesis)
3) Affected pelvic bloodstream
4) Common femoral artery

VASCULAR SURGERY

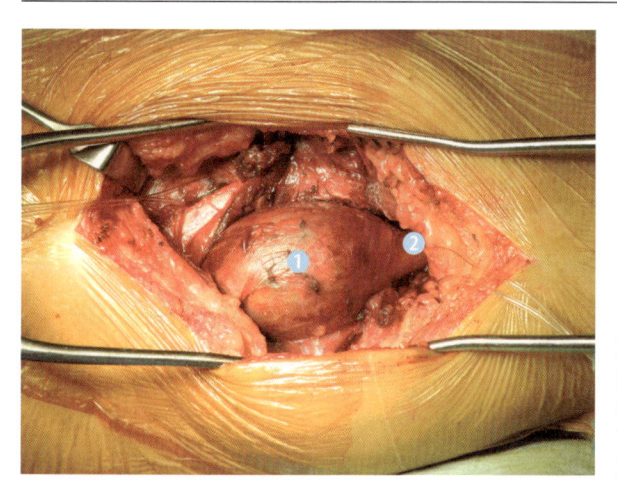

**Fig. 149  Aneurysm of popliteal artery**
Peroperative picture:
1) Aneurysm
2) Popliteal artery

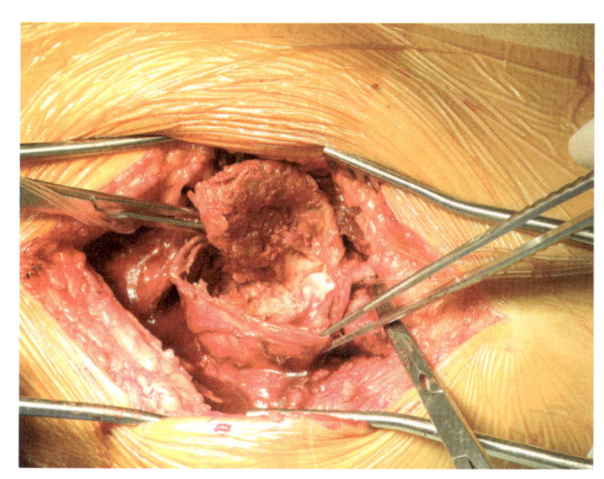

**Fig. 150  Open aneurysm of popliteal artery**
Peroperative picture:
Interior of the aneurysm filled in with atheromatous cell debris

CARDIAC SURGERY

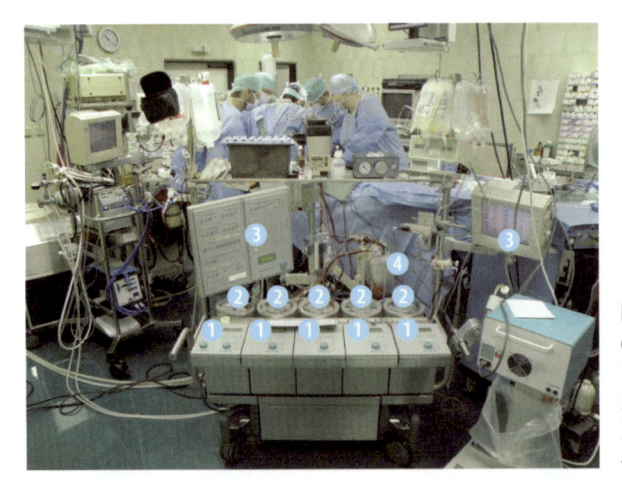

Fig. 151 Machine for extracorporeal circulation
1) Control panels
2) Rotating pumps
3) Monitors
4) Oxygenator and reservoir

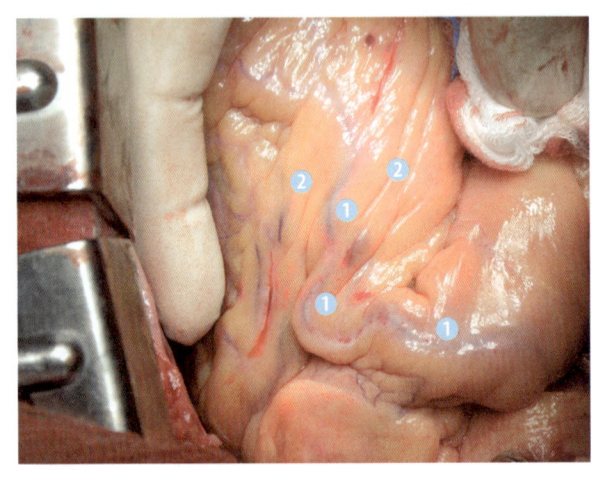

Fig. 152 Coronary artery
Peroperative picture:
1) Coronary artery
2) Epicardium

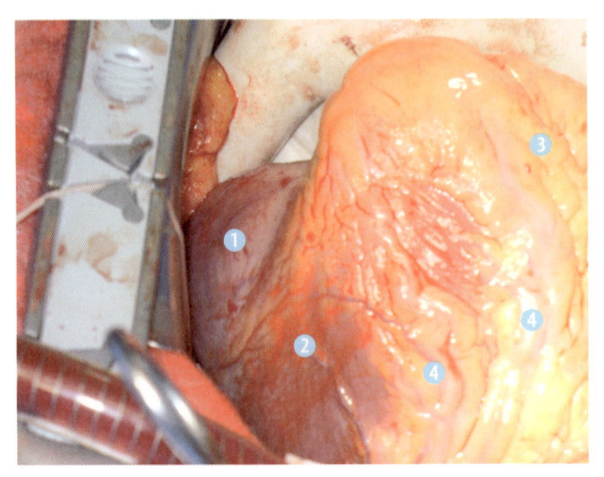

Fig. 153 Aneurysm of left ventricle
Peroperative picture:
1) Aneurysm of left ventricle
2) Myocardium of left ventricle
3) Epicardium
4) Coronary artery

CARDIAC SURGERY

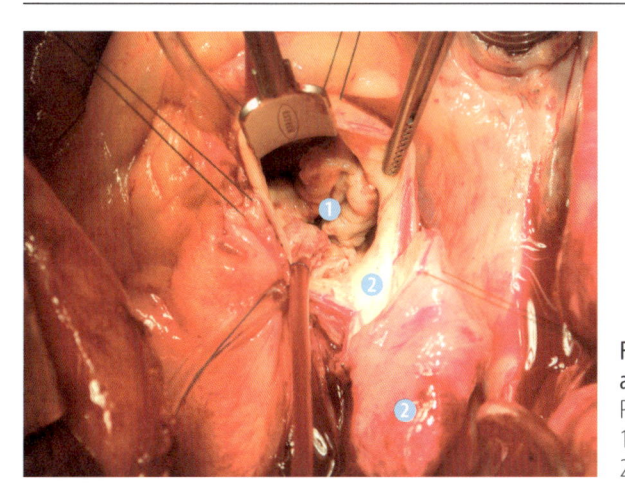

**Fig. 154  Calcificated bicuspid aortic valve**
Peroperative picture:
1) Calcificated bicuspid aortic valve
2) Ascending aorta

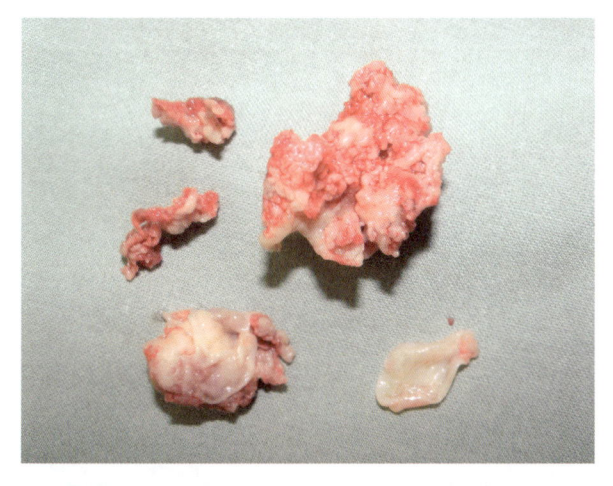

**Fig. 155  Excised calcificated aortic valve**

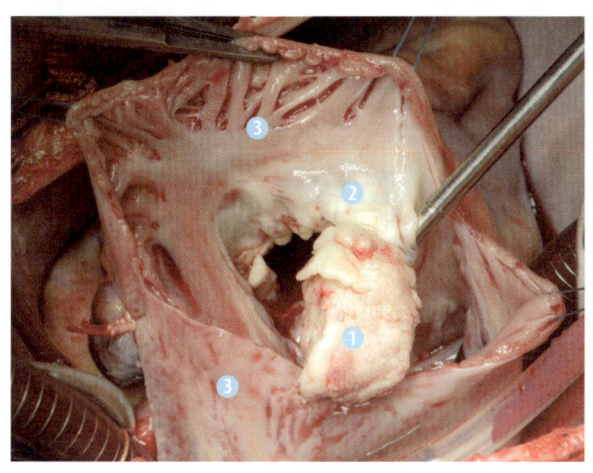

**Fig. 156  Infectious endocarditis**
Tricuspid valve. Vegetation.
Peroperative picture:
1) Vegetation
2) Anterior flap of tricuspid valve
3) Right atrium wall

CARDIAC SURGERY

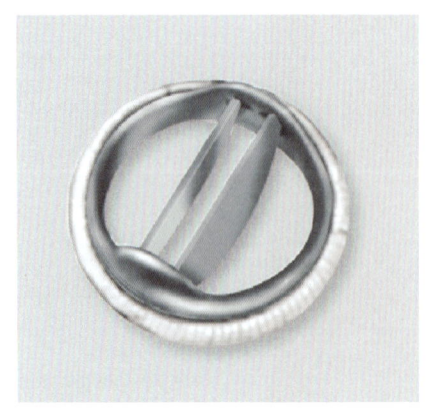

Fig. 157  Mechanical valve prosthesis

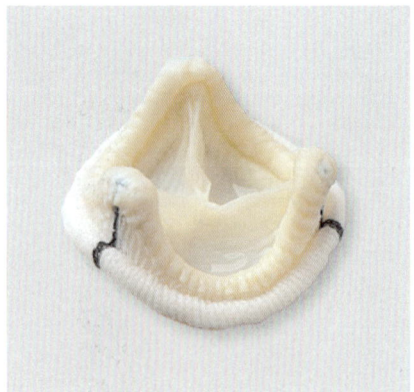

Fig. 158  Biological valve prosthesis

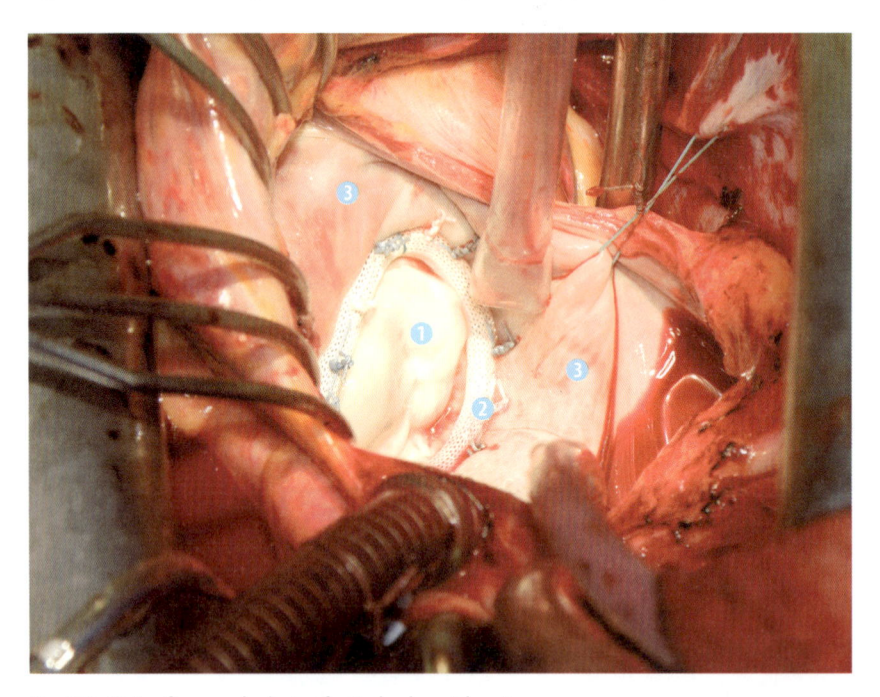

Fig. 159  State after annuloplasty of mitral valve with a ring
Peroperative picture:
1) Anterior flap of mitral valve
2) Ring
3) Left atrial wall

### CARDIAC SURGERY

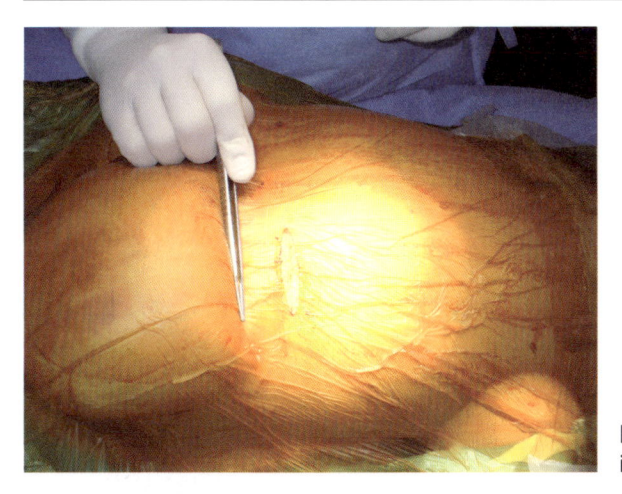

**Chapter 22**

Fig. 160 Skin incision for mini invasive surgery on mitral valve

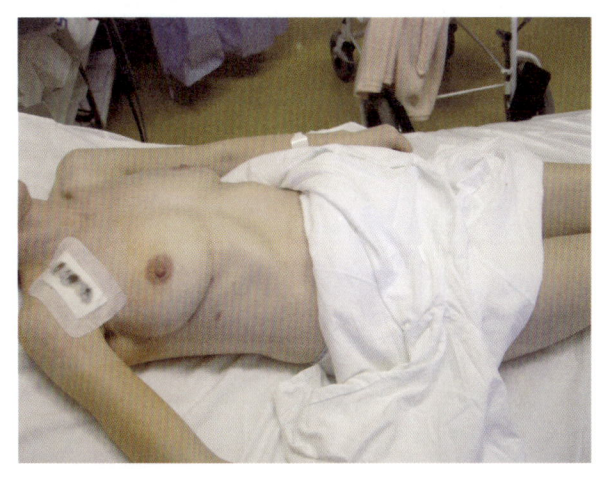

Fig. 161 Patient 11th day after mini invasive surgery

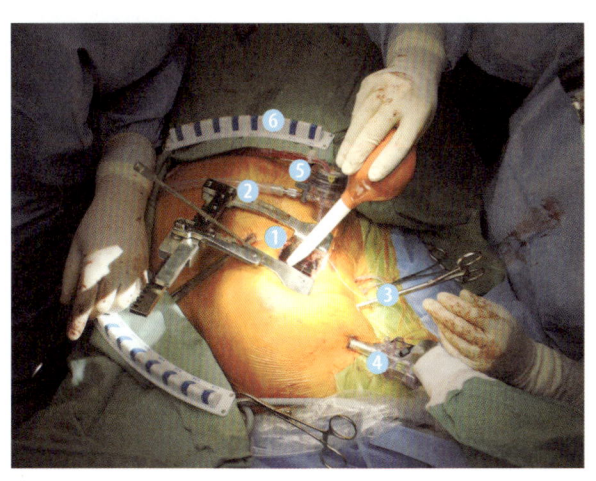

Fig. 162 Anterolateral thoracotomy for mini invasive (video-assisted) surgery on mitral valve
Peroperative picture:
1) Anterolateral thoracotomy in the 4th intercostal space
2) Retractor
3) Clamp on ascending aorta introduced through the 4th intercostal space
4) Optical system (camera + light) introduced via port in the 3rd intercostal space
5) Suction and insufflation of $CO_2$ via inserted port in the 5th intercostal space
6) Stitch holders

**CARDIAC SURGERY**

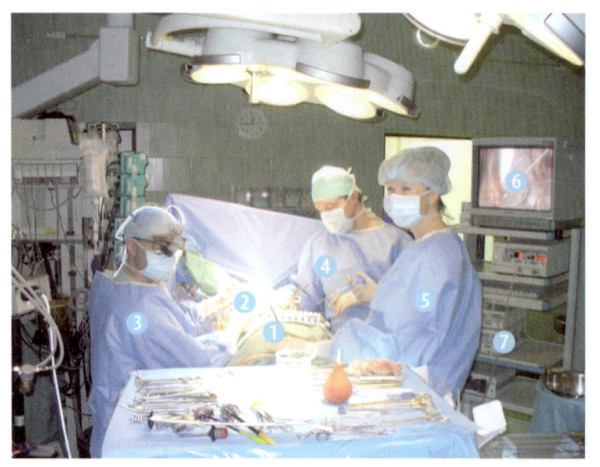

Fig. 163  Operating room layout during video-assisted operation
Peroperative picture:
1) Patient
2) Operative field
3) Operating surgeon
4) Assisting surgeon
5) Surgical technologist
6) Screen where the image from camera placed on the chest is transmitted
7) Source of light

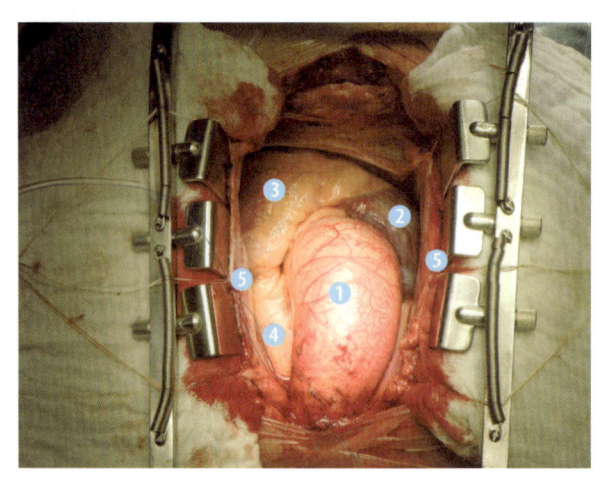

Fig. 164  Aneurysm of ascending aorta
Peroperative picture:
1) Ascending aorta (aneurysm)
2) Right atrium
3) Right ventricle
4) Pulmonary artery
5) Pericardium (open and fixed to distractor)

## CARDIAC SURGERY

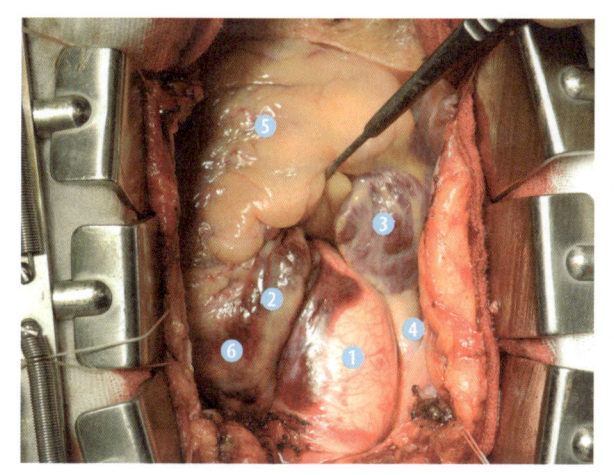

**Fig. 165 Acute aortic dissection**
Peroperative picture:
1) Ascending aorta with hemorrhaged wall
2) Hemorrhaged epicardium
3) Right atrium
4) Superior caval vein
5) Right ventricle
6) Pulmonary artery covered with hemorrhagic epicardium

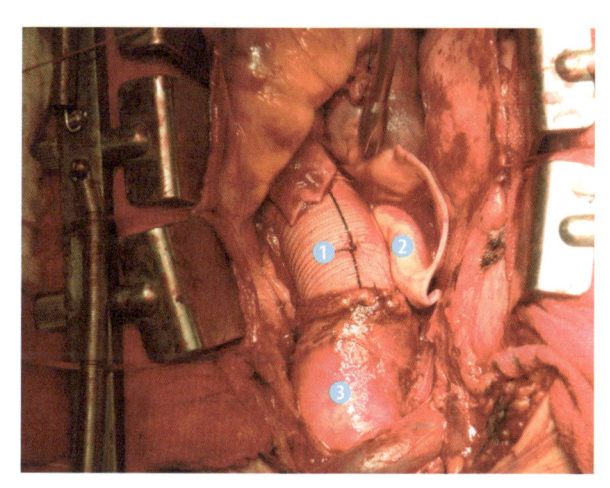

**Fig. 166 Replacement of ascending aorta with prosthesis**
Peroperative picture:
1) Prosthesis
2) Original wall of the aneurysm
3) Ascending aorta

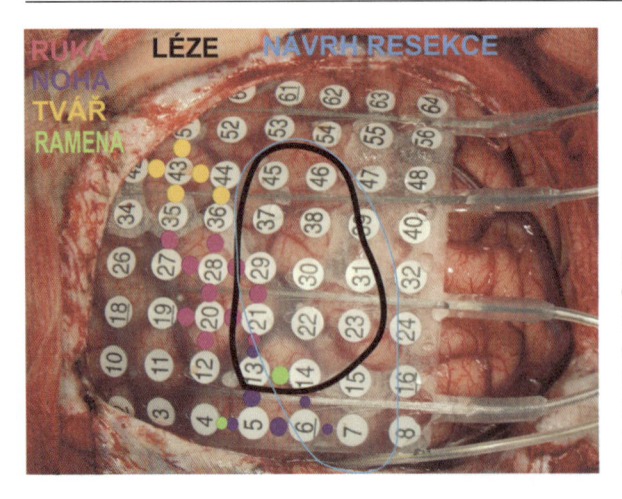

**Fig. 167 Epileptosurgical operation in precentral region**
Peroperative corticography employing subdural electrodes. Frame with 64 contact sites with marked results of stimulation, motor cortex and planned extent of resection

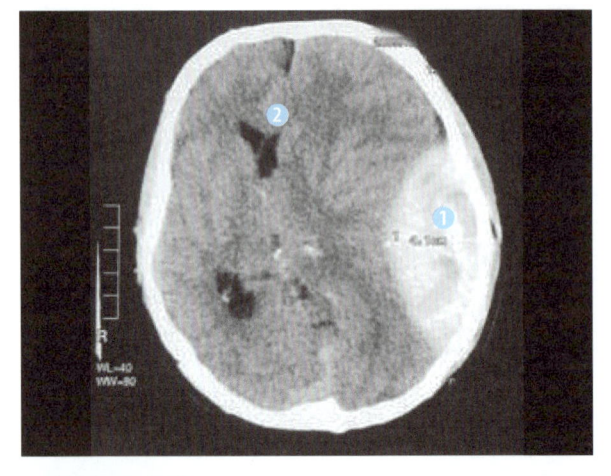

**Fig. 168a Epidural hematoma – frontotemporal region on the left side**
CT scan in axial plane:
1) Typical lenticular shape of coagulated hematoma
2) Dislocation of midline and ventricular system

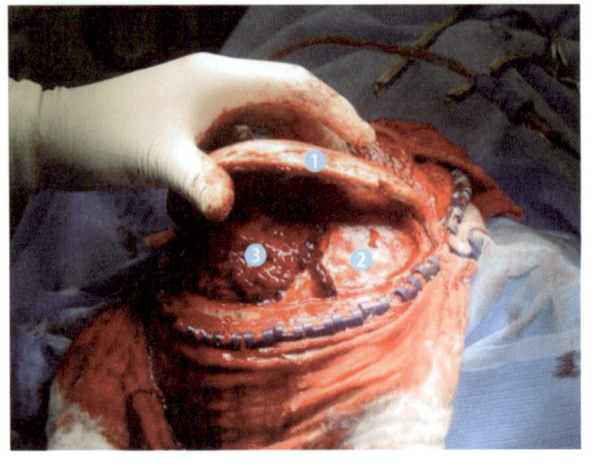

**Fig. 168b Epidural hematoma – frontotemporal region on the left side**
Peroperative picture, coagulated hematoma after removing bone flap:
1) Bone flap
2) Meninx
3) Hematoma

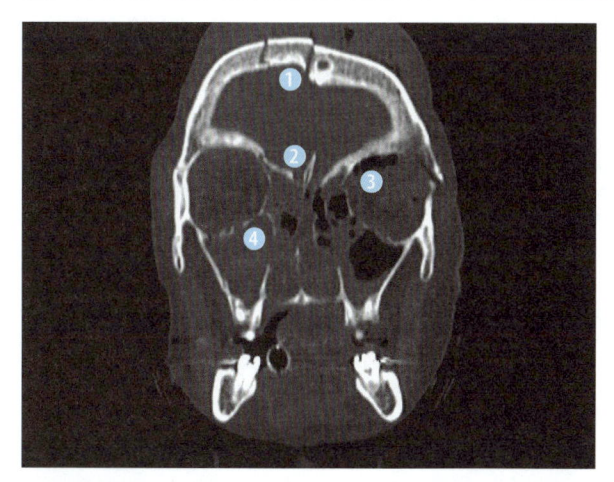

**Fig. 169 Frontobasal injury**
CT scan in coronal plane:
1) Fracture of frontal bone
2) Fracture of base of skull
3) Pneumo-orbit
4) Bleeding to paranasal sinuses

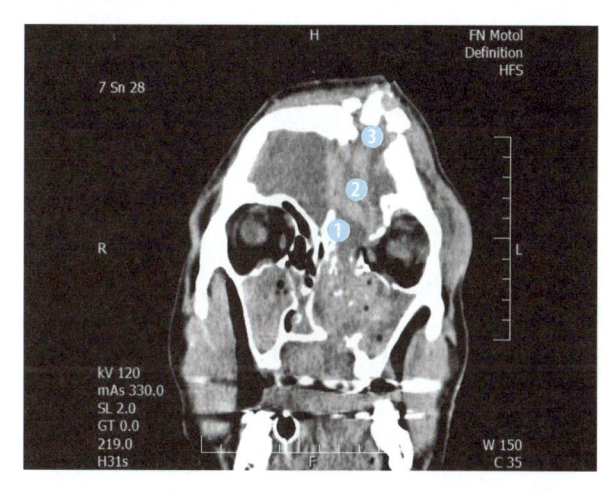

**Fig. 170a Gunshot injury of facial skeleton, base of anterior cranial fossa and frontal lobe**
CT scan, coronal plane:
1) Shot penetration through the base
2) Gunshot wound with devastation of frontal lobe
3) Exit wound on frontal convexity

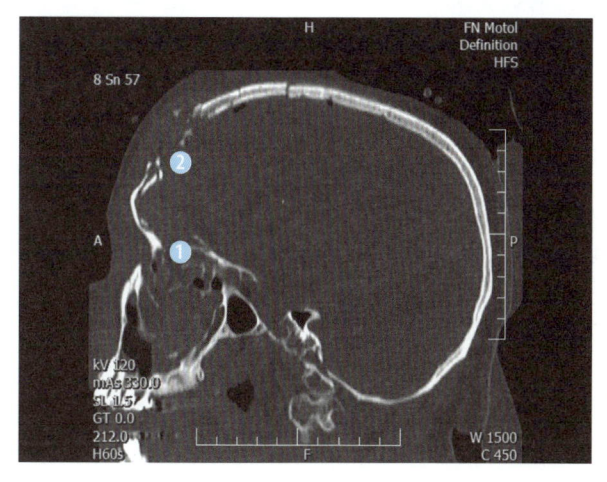

**Fig. 170b Gunshot injury of facial skeleton, base of anterior cranial fossa and frontal lobe**
CT scan, sagittal plane:
1) Shot penetration through the base
2) Exit wound on frontal convexity

NEUROSURGERY

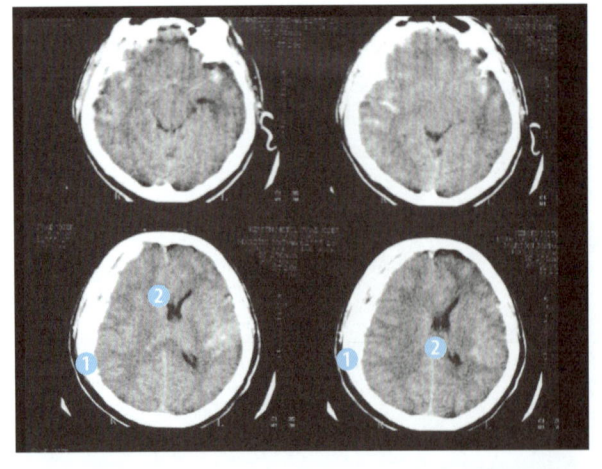

**Fig. 171 Acute subdural hematoma**
CT scan, axial plane:
1) Crescent hyperdense structure above hemisphere
2) Midline dislocation with compression of ventricular system

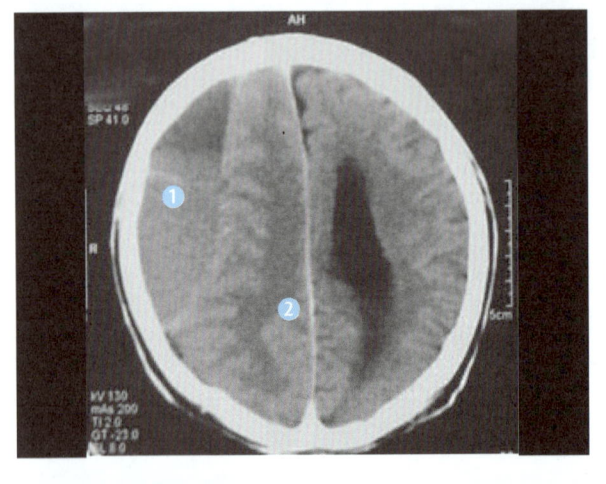

**Fig. 172 Subdural hematoma**
Chronic
CT scan, axial plane:
1) Hypodense structure above right hemisphere
2) Midline dislocation with disappeared ventricle

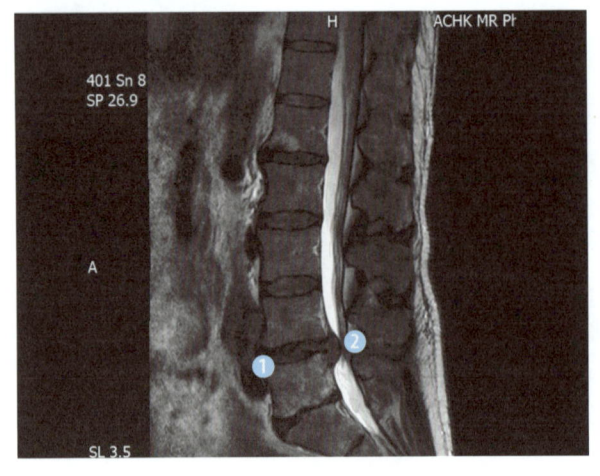

**Fig. 173 Spinal disc herniation**
In space L4-L5
MRI, sagittal plane:
1) Space L4-L5
2) Herniation with compression of dural sac

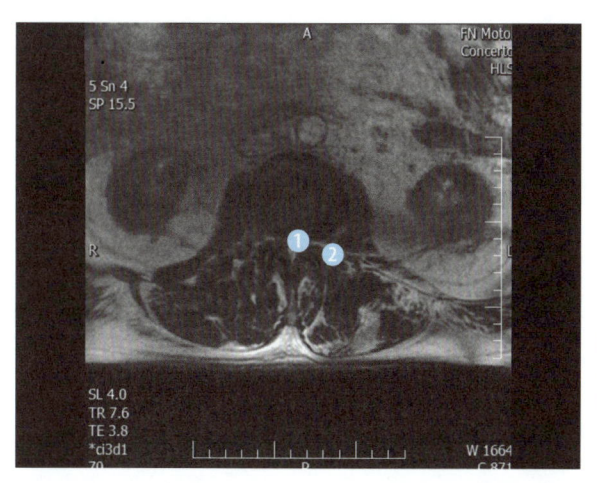

**Fig. 174 Stenosis of vertebral canal in degenerative disease**
MRI in axial plane:
1) Critical stenosis
2) Hypertrophic changes in bones

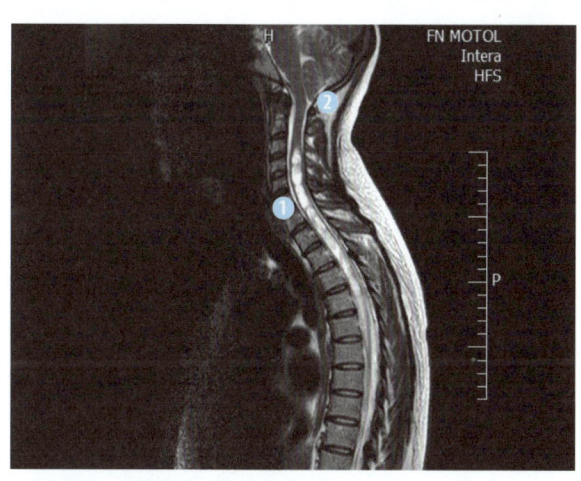

**Fig. 175 Extensive syringomyelic changes in Chiari malformation I**
MRI in sagittal plane, T2 sequence:
1) Syringomyelic cavities
2) Tonsillar descent

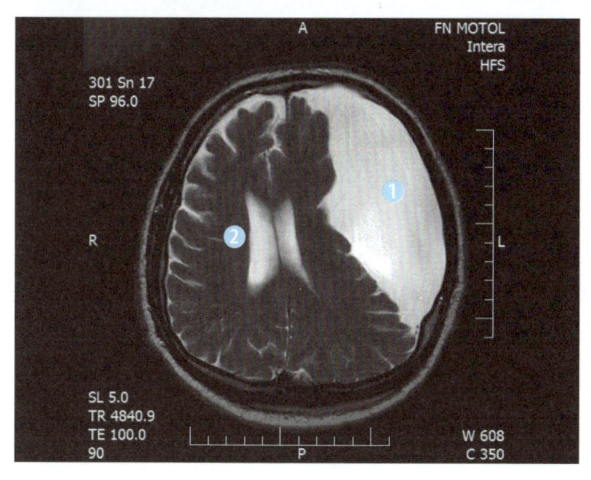

**Fig. 176 Arachnoid cyst with expansive behavior replacing major part of left hemisphere**
MRI:
T1 weighted image of coronal projection
1) Arachnoid cyst
2) Dislocation of ventricular system

NEUROSURGERY

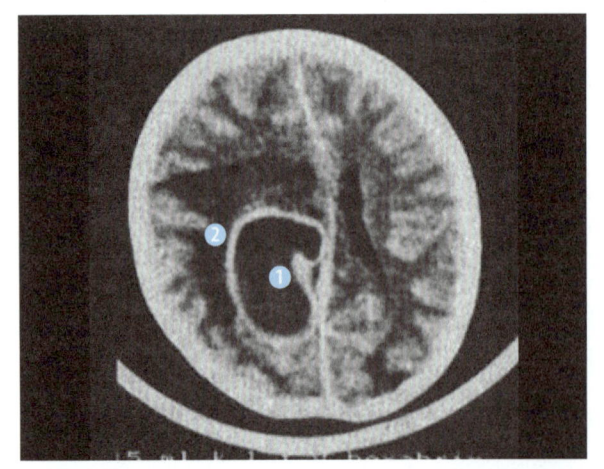

**Fig. 177 Cerebral abscess in right paramedian area with collateral edema and pressure on the midline**
Postcontrast CT scan, axial plane:
1) Abscess cavity
2) Marked hyperdense rim

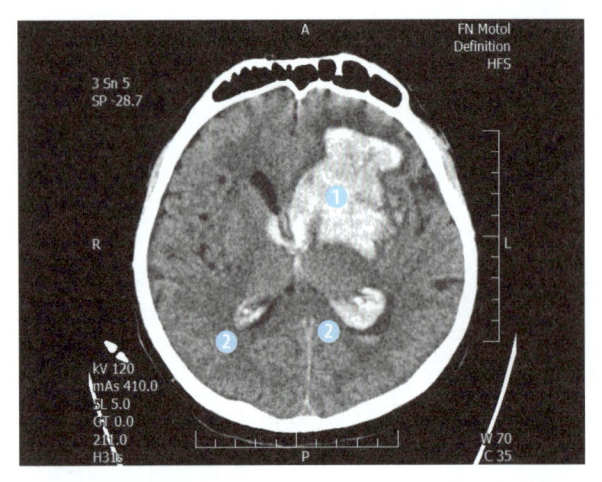

**Fig. 178 Intracerebral hypertonic hemorrhage on the left side penetrating into ventricular system**
CT scan in axial plane:
1) Intraparenchymatous hematoma
2) Hemorrhage in occipital horns of lateral ventricles

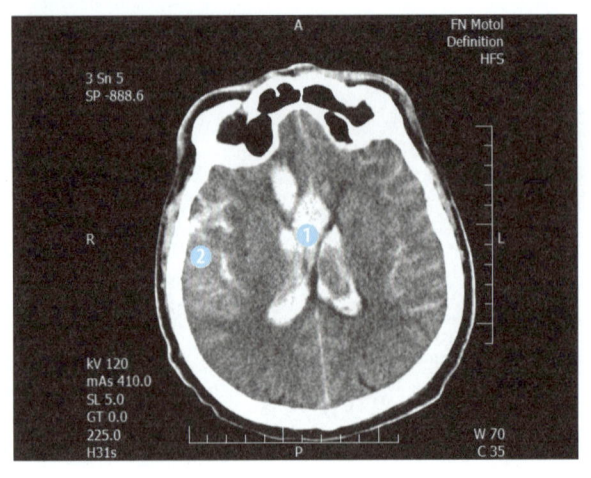

**Fig. 179 Subarachnoid hemorrhage due to rupture of aneurysm**
CT scan in axial plane:
1) Hemocephalus of the third ventricle and both lateral ventricles
2) Hemorrhage in subarachnoid space

NEUROSURGERY

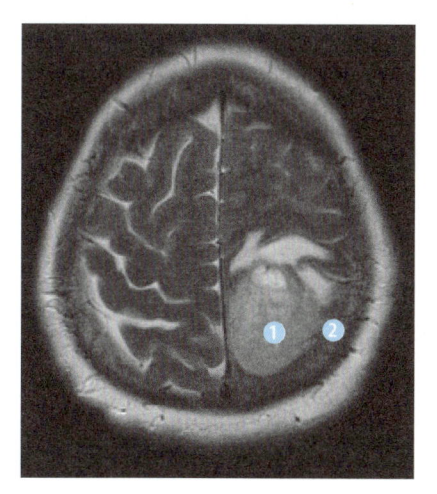

**Fig. 180a  Glioblastoma in left parieto-occipital area**
MRI: T2 weighted image in axial plane
1) Tumor
2) Edema

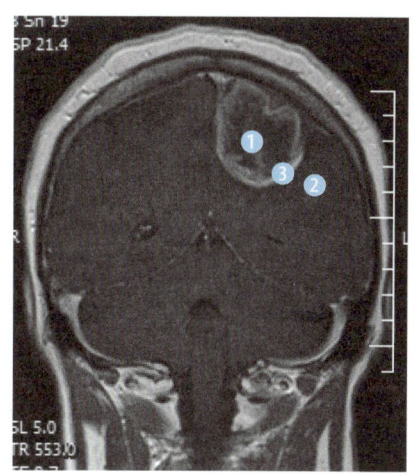

**Fig. 180b  Glioblastoma in left parieto-occipital area**
MRI: T1 weighted image in coronal plane, post-contrast enhancement of the tumor
1) Tumor
2) Edema
3) Post-contrast enhancement of the tumor

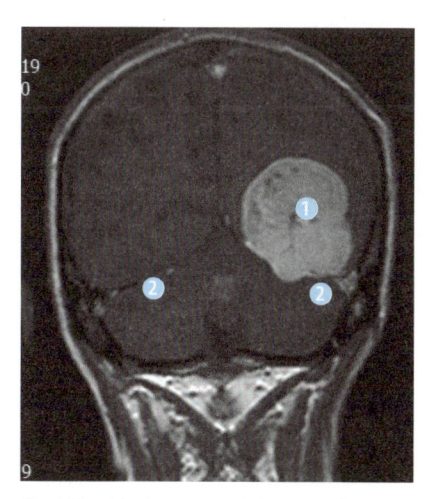

**Fig. 181a  Meningioma in left occipital area arising from tentorium**
MRI: T1weighted image with application of contrast agent – in coronal plane:
1) Tumor
2) Tentorium

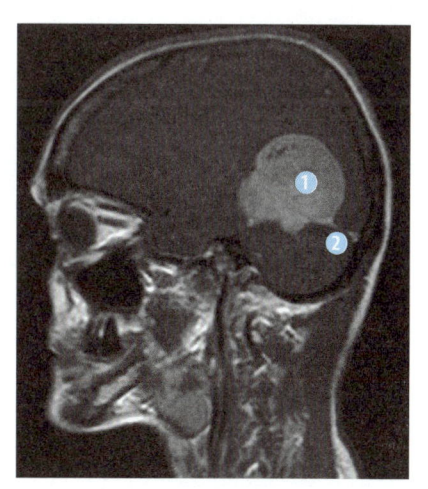

**Fig. 181b  Meningioma in left occipital area arising from tentorium**
MRI: T1weighted image with application of contrast agent – in sagittal plane:
1) Tumor
2) Tentorium

MODERN TECHNIQUES OF CUTTING

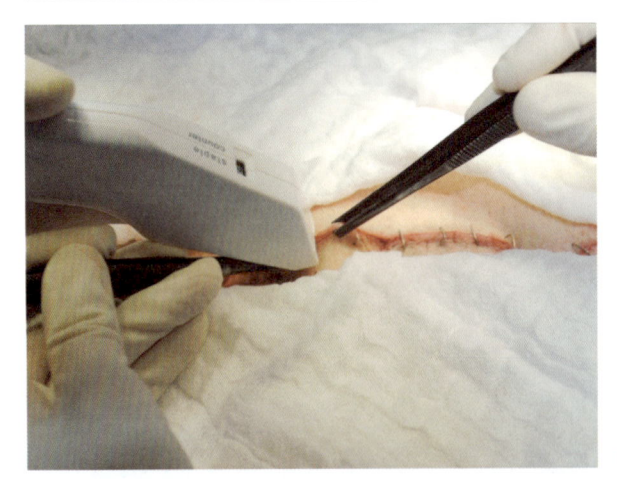

Fig. 182  Skin stapler

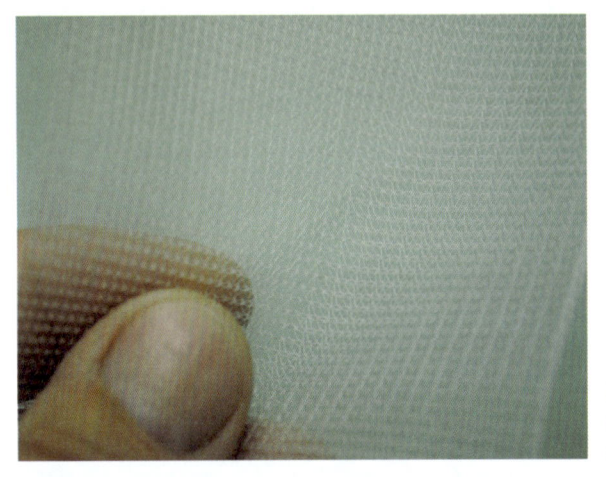

Fig. 183a  Surgical mesh for repair of hernias and abdominal wall defects

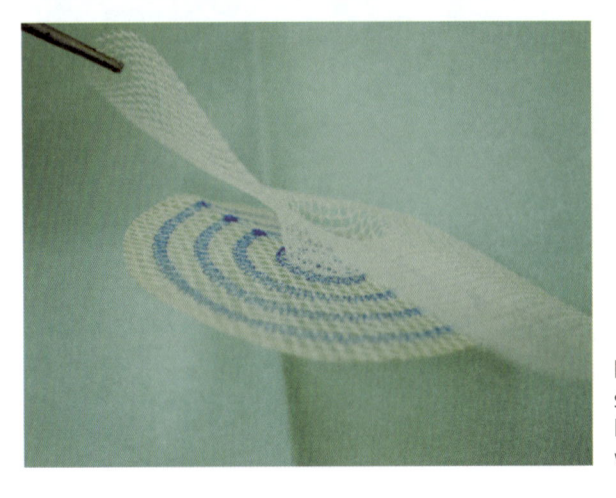

Fig. 183b  PHS (Prolene hernia system)
Implant for inguinal hernia repair, with retention in hernia

## MODERN TECHNIQUES OF CUTTING

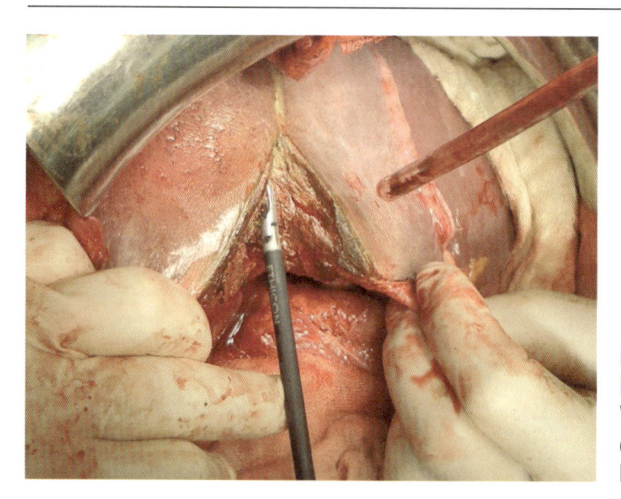

Chapter 24

**Fig. 184  Harmonic scalpel**
Peroperative picture:
Working end of the equipment, dissecting in resection line during liver resection

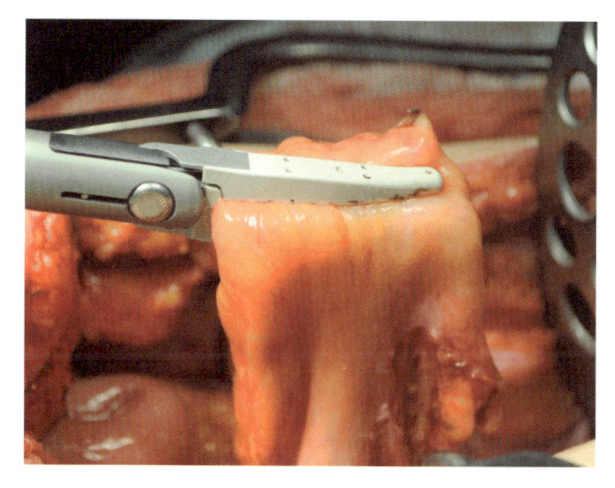

**Fig. 185  LigaSure™**
Peroperative picture:
Working end of the equipment

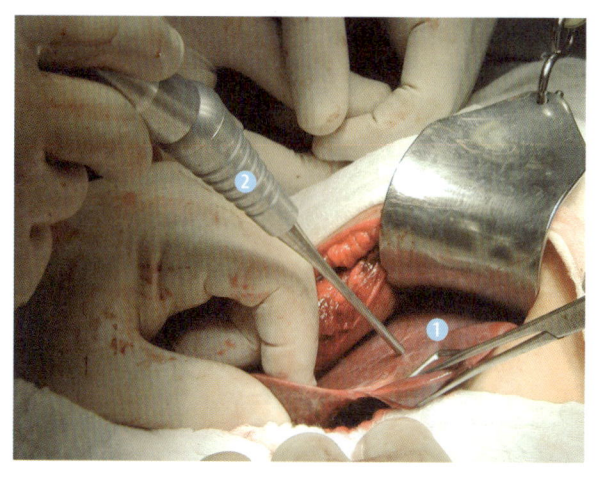

**Fig. 186  CUSA**
Peroperative picture, CUSA during liver resection:
1) Liver
2) Working end of the equipment

## MODERN TECHNIQUES OF CUTTING

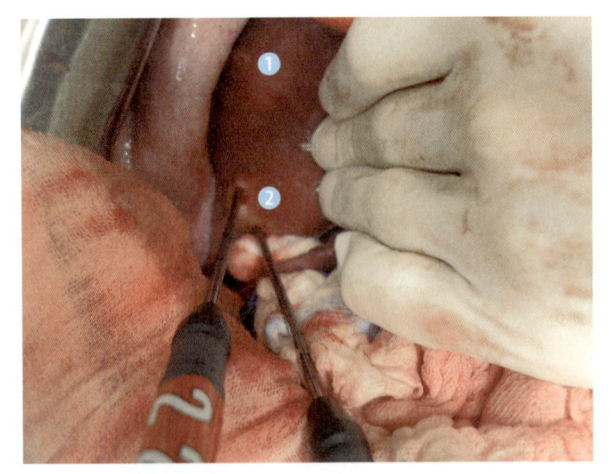

Fig. 187　Radiofrequency ablation (RFA) of liver metastases of colorectal carcinoma
Peroperative picture:
1) Liver
2) Metastasis with placed RFA probe

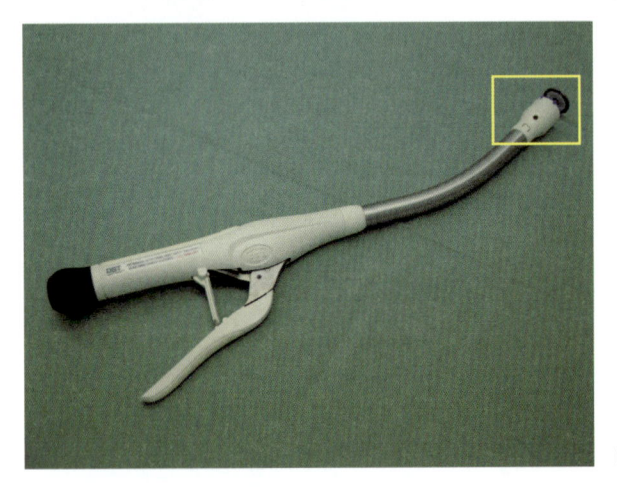

Fig. 188a　Endoluminal stapler

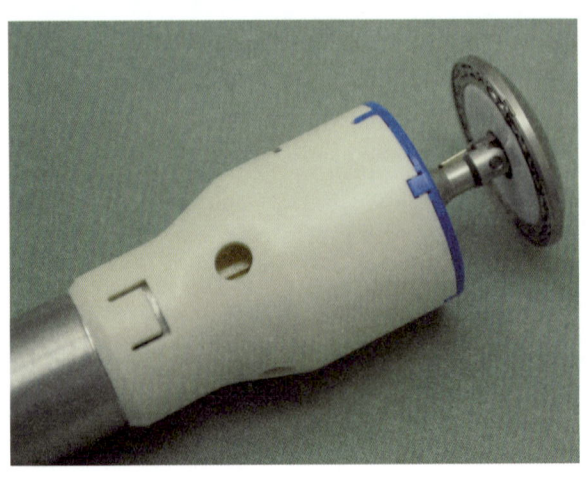

Fig. 188b　Working end
Detail of the previous picture

**MODERN TECHNIQUES OF CUTTING**

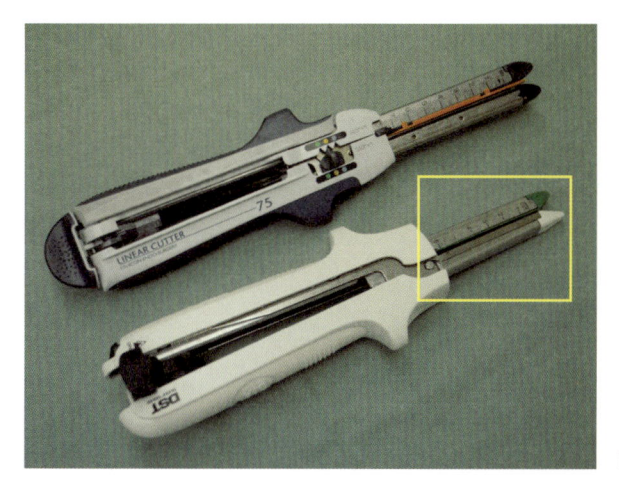

**Chapter 24**

Fig. 189a  Linear stapler

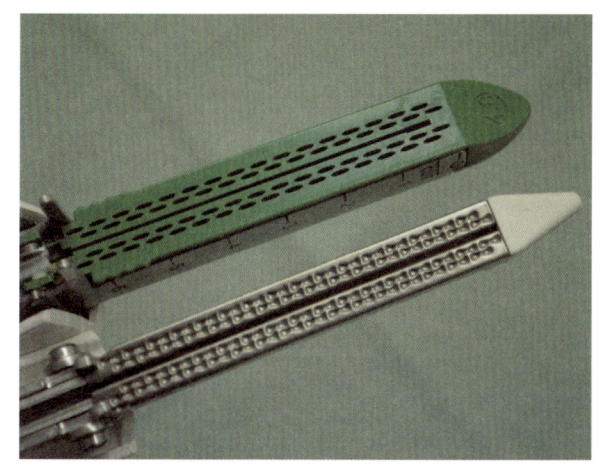

Fig. 189b  Detail of working part of the equipment

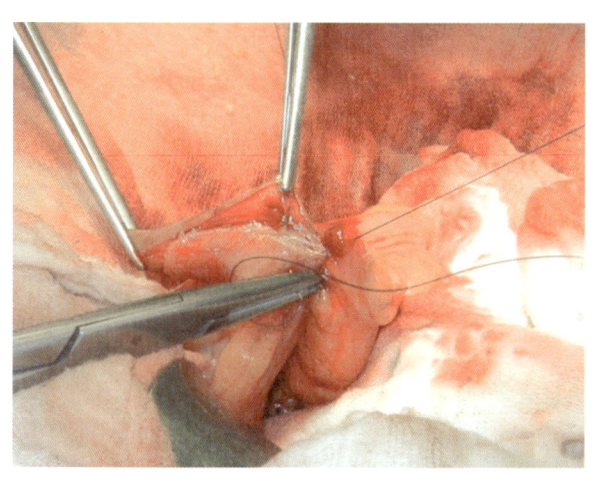

Fig. 190  Large intestine anastomosis
End-to-end, with continuous extramucosal circular completely absorbable monofilament atraumatic suture

## MODERN TECHNIQUES OF CUTTING

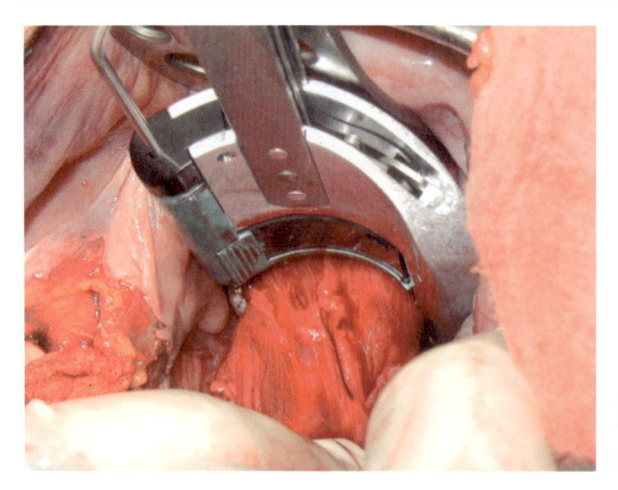

**Fig. 191a  Rectal resection**
Transection and closure of rectum with linear stapler

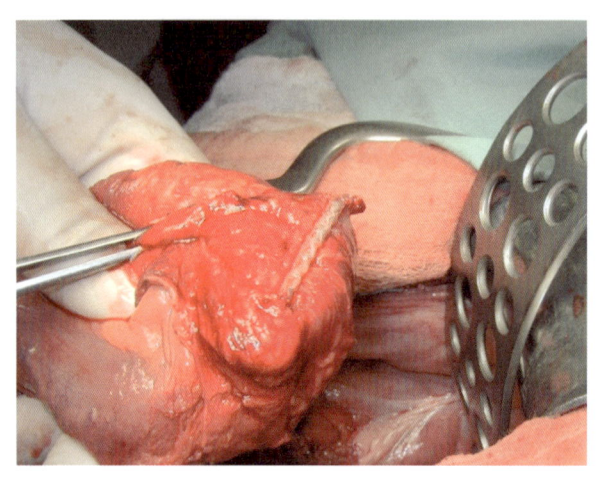

**Fig. 191b  Rectal resection**
Transection and closure of rectum. Final state

**MODERN TECHNIQUES OF CUTTING**

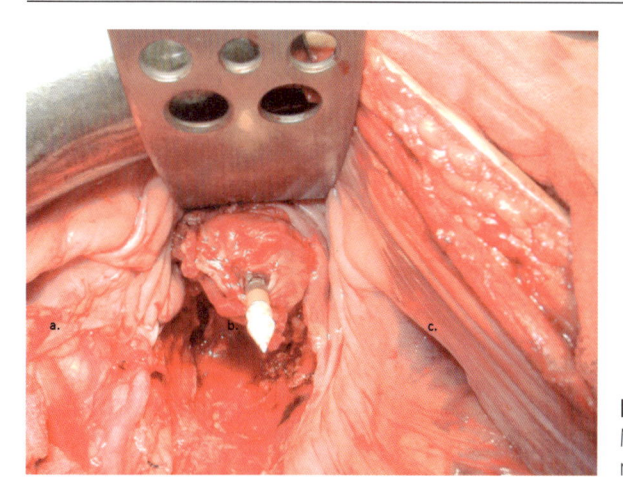

**Fig. 192a   EEA stapler**
Mechanical anastomosis after rectal resection, EEA stapler placed in rectum

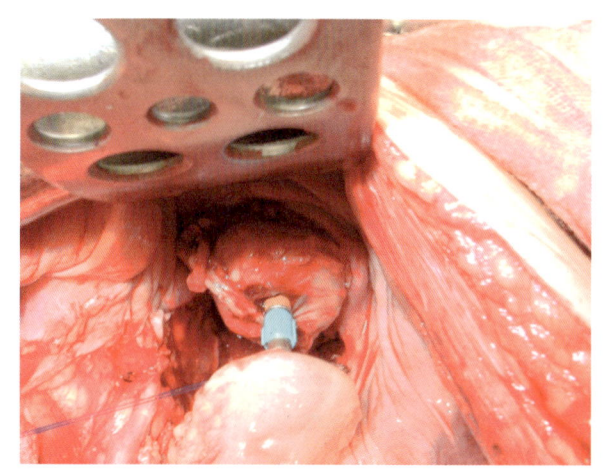

**Fig. 192b   EEA stapler**
Approximation of anastomosed intestinal segments

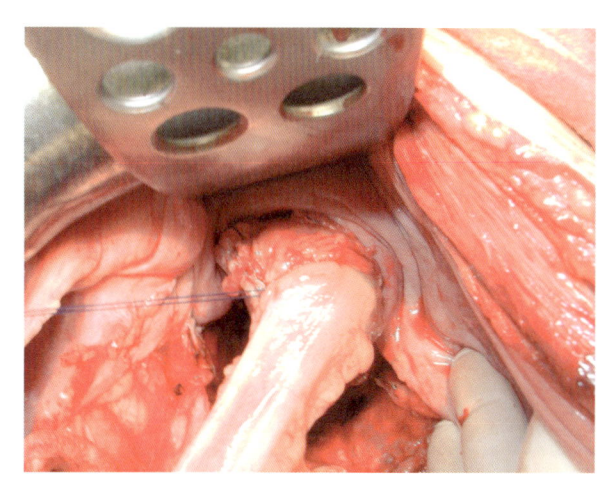

**Fig. 192c   EEA stapler**
Final state after creating colorectal stapler anastomosis

Chapter 24

561

MODERN TECHNIQUES OF CUTTING

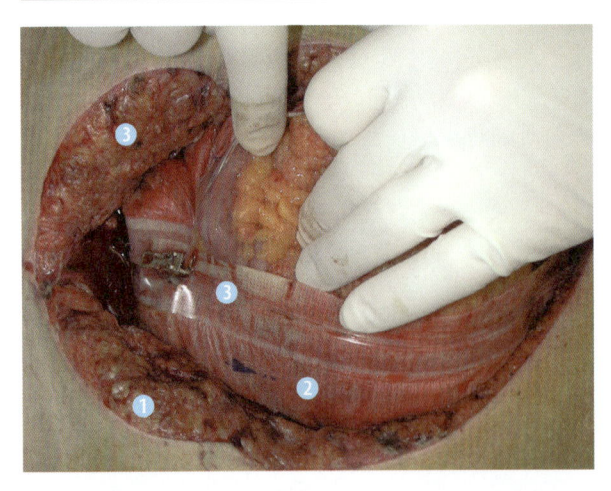

**Fig. 193a Laparostomic set for temporary closure of abdominal cavity**
1) Laparotomic edges
2) Membrane fixed to laparotomic edge
3) Zipper closure

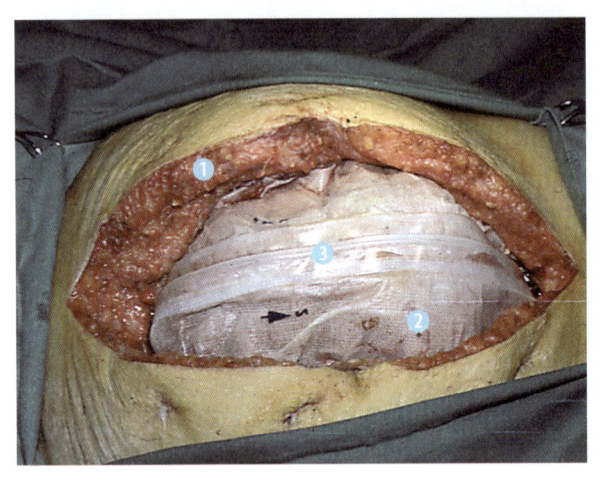

**Fig. 193b Laparostomic set for temporary closure of abdominal cavity**
After closing the zipper
1) Laparotomic edges
2) Membrane fixed to laparotomic edge
3) Zipper closure

MODERN TECHNIQUES OF CUTTING

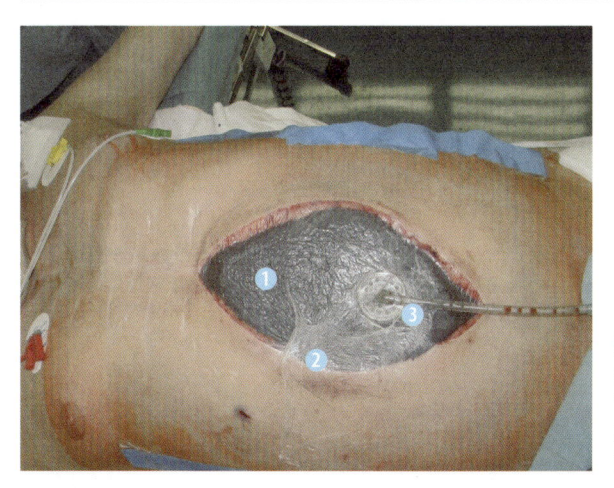

Fig. 194 VAC (Vacuum assisted closure)
1) Porous sponge
2) Covering membrane
3) Connector to vacuum pump

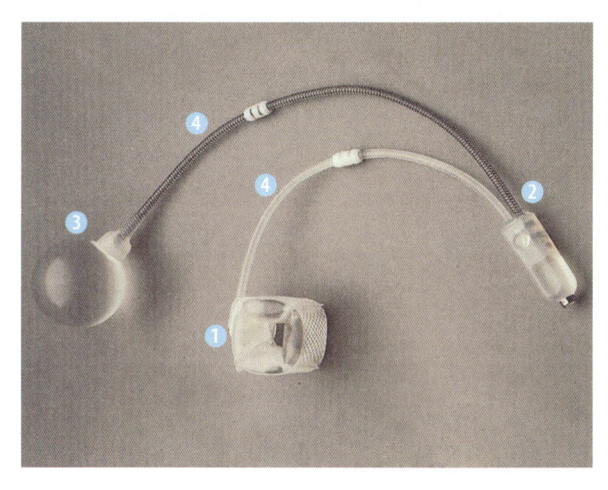

Fig. 195 ABS, Artificial bowel sphincter
1) Sphincter cuff
2) Control valve
3) Reservoir
4) Connecting tube

## INTENSIVE CARE IN SURGERY

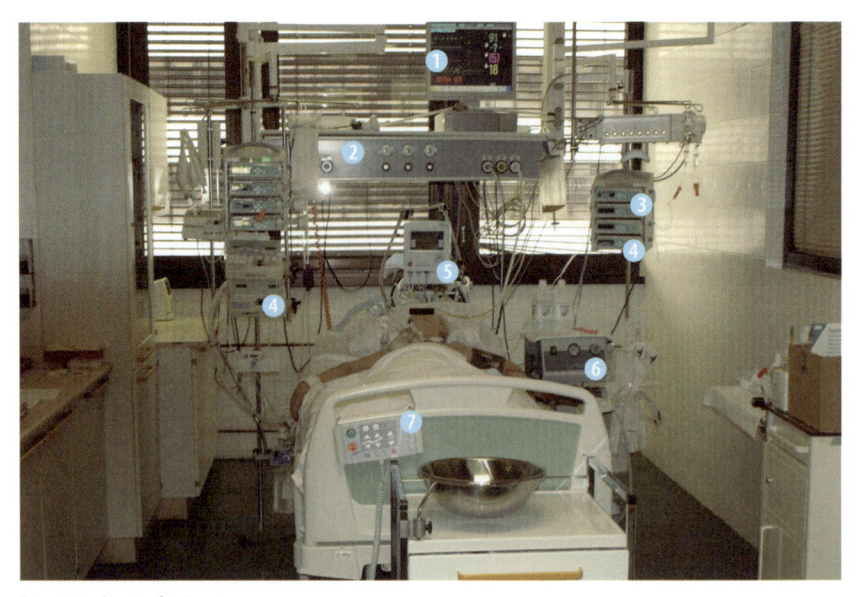

**Fig. 196 Surgical intensive care**
Example of a bed of intensive anesthesiological and resuscitative care:
1) Monitor of vital functions, 2) Central medical gas supply, 3) Linear perfusor, 4) Infusion pump, 5) Mechanical ventilator, 6) Suction unit, 7) Electric bed control

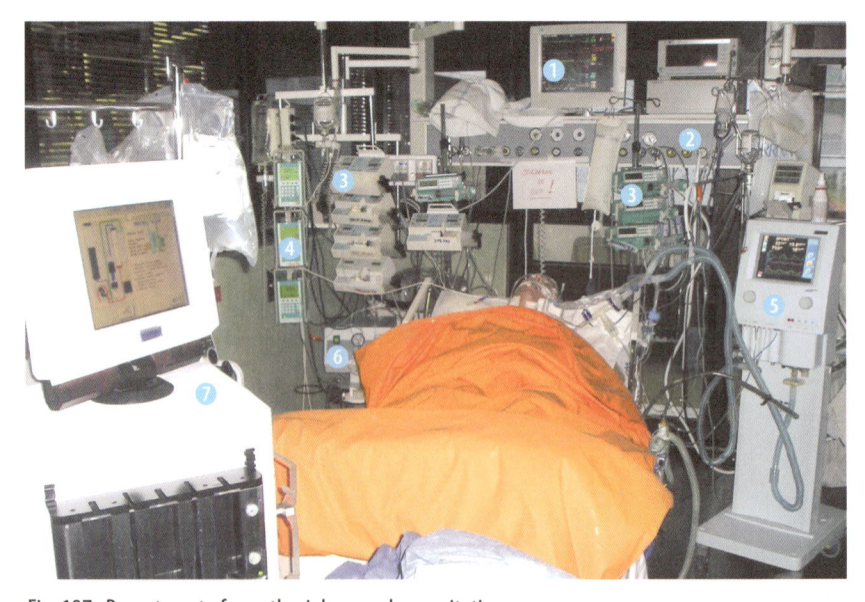

**Fig. 197 Department of anesthesiology and resuscitation**
1) Monitor of vital functions, 2) Central medical gas supply, 3) Linear perfusor, 4) Infusion pump, 5) Mechanical ventilator, 6) Suction unit, 7) Machine of extracorporeal elimination

MULTIMODAL ONCOLOGICAL TREATMENT

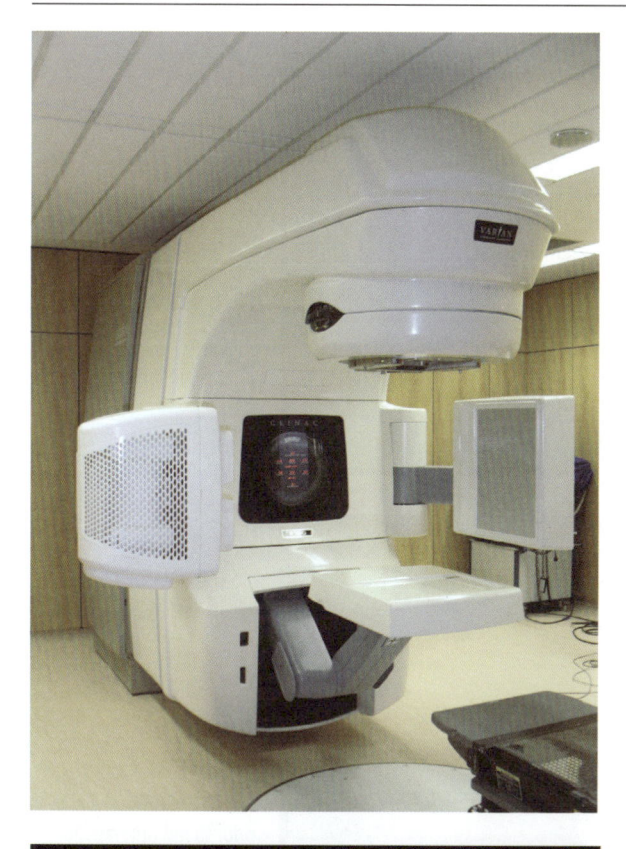

Chapter 33

Fig. 198 Linear accelerator – Clinac 2100C

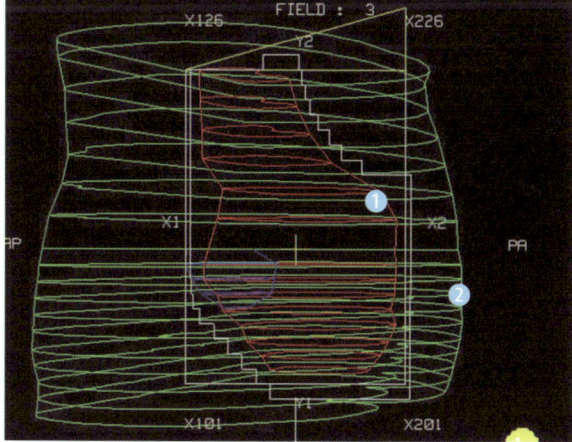

Fig. 199 Scheme of planning prior to radiotherapy for rectal tumor
1) Drawn planning target volume
2) Input field shaped by collimator

MULTIMODAL ONCOLOGICAL TREATMENT

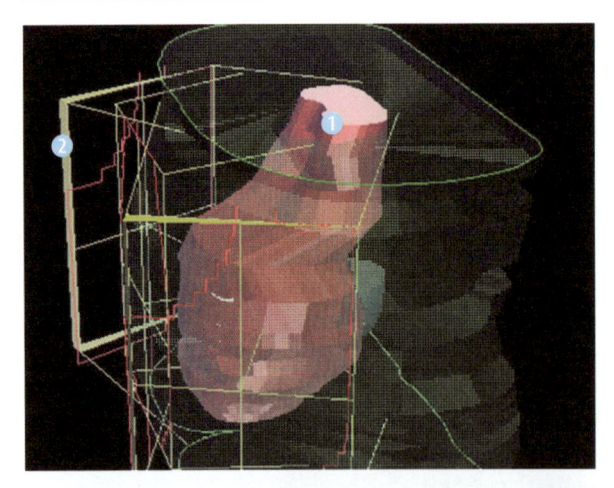

Fig. 200 Scheme of planning prior to radiotherapy for rectal tumor
1) 3D image of the total volume
2) Input radiation field

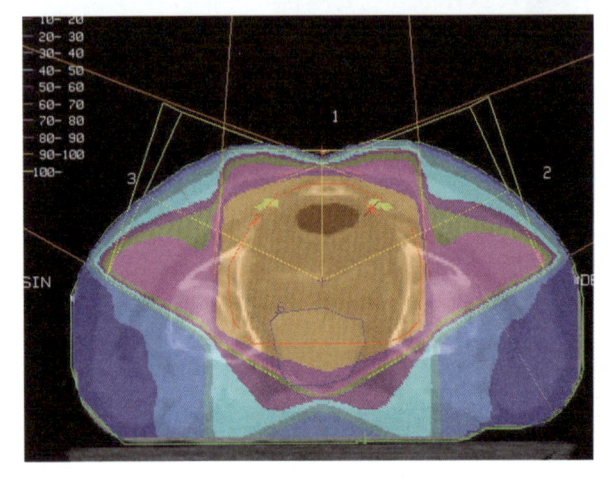

Fig. 201 Scheme of planning prior to radiotherapy for rectal tumor
CT section showing dose distribution in target volume and in adjacent healthy tissue

**AUTHORS**

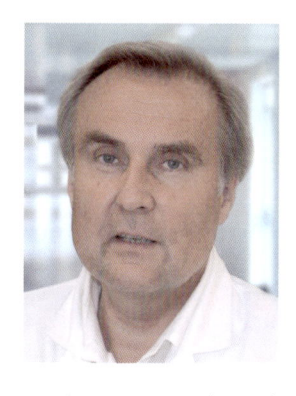

## Prof. Jiří Hoch, MD, PhD

The Head of the Department of Surgery, 2nd Faculty of Medicine, Charles University Prague and University Hospital Motol. As the leading surgeon of the 2nd Faculty of Medicine he authored Czech language Textbook of Surgery in 2001, with the second and third editions in 2003 and 2011, respectively. Among remarkable achievements, Professor Jiří Hoch authored another book entitled Acute Colon Surgery and co-authored several other books – Thyroid Gland Surgery, Gastrointestinal Bleeding, Sentinel Lymph-Node in Surgery of Solid Tumors, and The Blood Supply of the Large Intestine. He initiated publishing a Textbook of Traumatology in 2004 and several other books on surgery topics in Jessenius book series of Maxdorf Publishing, Prague.

In accordance with the department's needs, since the start of his professional career Jiří Hoch has been focusing his interest and efforts on *acute surgery, surgical oncology, coloproctology and surgical treatment of colorectal cancer*.

Professor Jiří Hoch is a member of the Board of the Czech Surgical Society / Czech Medical Association of J. E. Purkyně (CzMA JEP), the Chair of Coloproctology Section of the Czech Surgical Society, the Deputy Chair of the Society for Gastrointestinal Oncology, the national delegate in European Society for Coloproctology, member of several foreign societies and journal editorial boards, incl. editorial board of the journal European Surgery.

In 2007 Jiří Hoch commemorated legacy and tradition of Professor Bohuslav Niederle, MD (1907–2000) – the founder of the Motol Hospital Department of Surgery – in the book Niederle Reminescences published on the occasion of the 100th anniversary of Professor Niederle's birth.

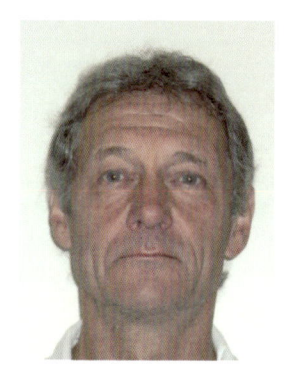

## Assoc. Prof. Jan Leffler, MD, PhD

The Deputy Head for Education, the Department of Surgery, 2nd Faculty of Medicine, Charles University Prague and University Hospital Motol. He has been engaged in pre- and postgradual education in surgery and gastroenterology since 1982, as a teacher and a member of examining comissions as well. Jan Leffler is the Vice-Dean of the 2nd Faculty of Medicine.

*Professional focus: intensive medicine, gastric and hepato-pancreato-biliary surgery*. From a long-term perspective Jan Leffler is devoted first of all to pancreatic surgery – acute pancreatitis, pancreatic cancer and cystic lesions of pancreas. He authored many papers on the topic both in Czech and foreign journals and also the book entitled Acute Pancreatitis – Where Are We Aiming? He co-authored all three editions of the Textbook of Surgery.

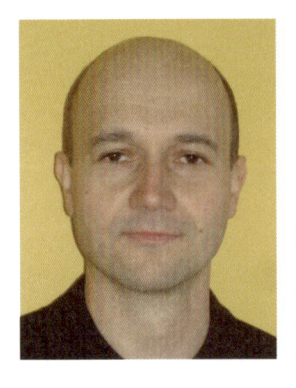

### Petr Bavor, MD

Assistant Professor, the Department of Surgery, 2nd Faculty of Medicine, Charles University Prague and University Hospital Motol. *Professional focus: endocrinology and intensive medicine.*

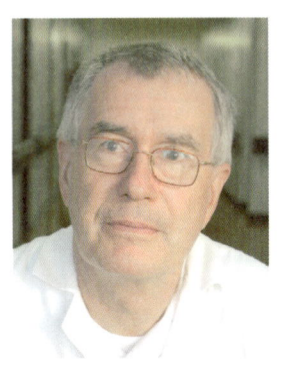

### Prof. Karel Cvachovec, MD, PhD, MBA

The Head of the Department of Anesthesiology and Resuscitation, 2nd Faculty of Medicine, Charles University Prague and University Hospital Motol. The President of the Committee of the Czech Society of Anesthesiology and Intensive Care Medicine. Member of the presidium of the Czech Medical Association of J. E. Purkyně (CzMA JEP), the honorary member of several foreign professional societies. *Professional focus: anesthesia in cardiovascular surgery, hemocoagulation in intensive care, care for critically ill patients, mechanical support of vital functions, health care economics and quality assessment.*

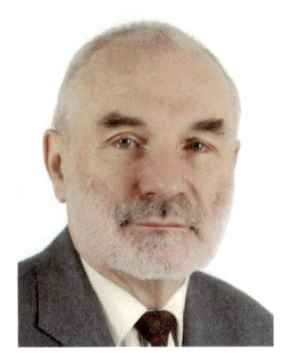

### Prof. Petr Goetz, MD, PhD

Former Head of the Institute of Biology and Medical Genetics, 2nd Faculty of Medicine, Charles University Prague and University Hospital Motol, former Vice-Dean of the faculty, the President of the Czech Society of Medical Genetics, member of the European Society of Medical Genetics, member of the board of the Union of Czech Physicians. *Professional focus: medical genetics, molecular medicine, oncogenetics.*

## AUTHORS

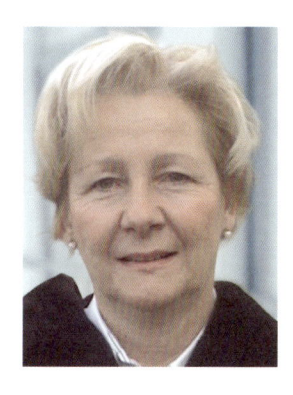

**Ivana Hochová, MD**

The Head of the Department of Clinical Hematology, University Hospital Motol. Member of the scientific committee of the Czech Myelodysplastic-Syndrome-Group of the Czech Society of Hematology. *Professional focus: hemato-oncology in adults.*

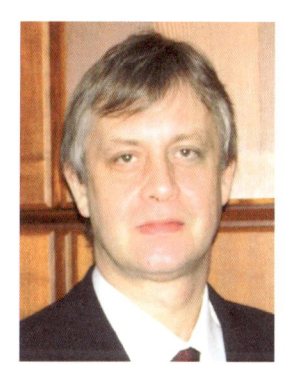

**Zbyněk Jech, MD**

Senior consultant, the Department of Surgery, 2$^{nd}$ Faculty of Medicine, Charles University Prague and University Hospital Motol. Member of the Czech Surgical Society and German Society of Surgery. *Professional focus: coloproctology, surgical oncology.*

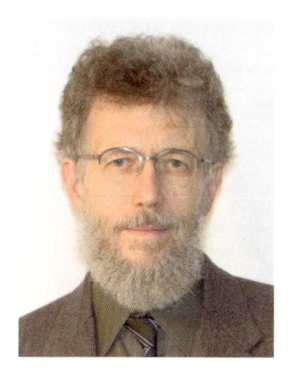

**Prof. Roman Kodet, MD, PhD**

The Head of the Institute of Pathology and Molecular Medicine, 2$^{nd}$ Faculty of Medicine and University Hospital Motol, the Vice-Dean of the faculty. Member of the Society for Pediatric Pathology and of several other professional societies. *Professional focus: oncopathology.*

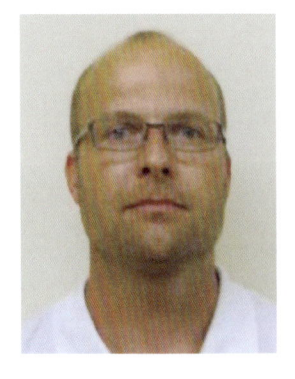

**Tomáš Krejčí, MD**

Assistant Professor, the Department of Surgery, 2nd Faculty of Medicine, Charles University Prague and University Hospital Motol. *Professional focus: surgical oncology, hepato-pancreato-biliary surgery.*

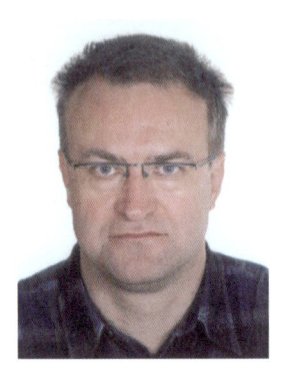

**Jiří Lisý, MD, PhD**

Assistant Professor and Deputy Head for Education, the Department of Imaging Methods, 2nd Faculty of Medicine, Charles University Prague and University Hospital Motol. Member of the Czech Society of Radiology, European Society of Radiology. *Professional focus: neuroradiology, head and neck imaging, abdominal diagnostics.*

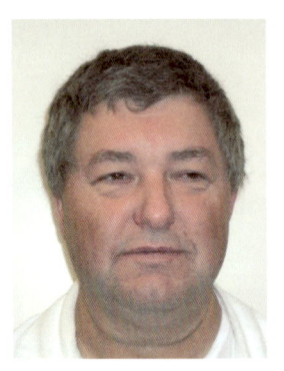

**Jan Neumann, MD, PhD**

The Head of the Intensive Care Unit, the Department of Surgery, 2nd Faculty of Medicine, Charles University Prague and University Hospital Motol. *Professional focus: intensive care in surgery, nutritional support.*

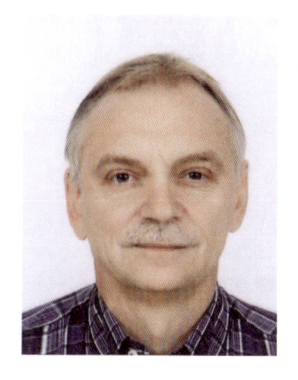

### Otakar Nyč, MD, PhD

The Head of the Institute of Medical Microbiology, 2nd Faculty of Medicine, Charles University Prague and University Hospital Motol. Member of the Committee of Antibiotic Politics of the Czech Medical Association of J. E. Purkyně, the Vice-President of the Central Co-ordination Group of the National Antibiotic Program of the Ministry of Health, member of the Committee of the Society for Medical Microbiology CzMA JEP, member of Working group for ATB Resistance Monitoring. *Professional focus: rational use of antibiotics.*

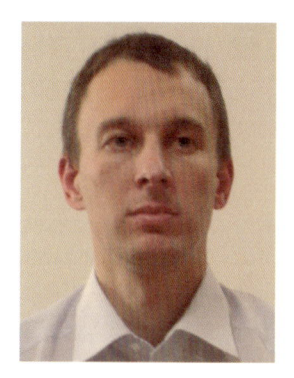

### Filip Pazdírek, MD

Assistant Professor, the Department of Surgery, 2nd Faculty of Medicine, Charles University Prague and University Hospital Motol. *Professional focus: gastrointestinal surgery, surgical endoscopy, intensive care.*

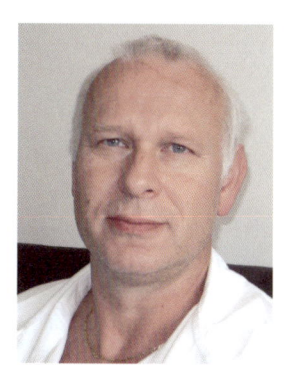

### Ronald Pospíšil, MD

The Head of the Department of Surgery, Regional Hospital Kladno. *Professional focus: thoracic surgery, surgical oncology.*

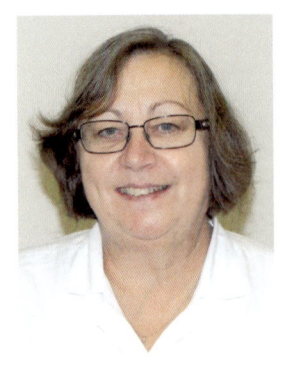

**Assoc. Prof. Jana Prausová, MD, PhD, MBA**

The Head of the Department of Radiotherapy and Oncology, University Hospital Motol. The Head of the Complex Oncology Centre, University Hospital Motol. Assoc. professor, Department of Pediatric Hematology and Oncology, 2nd Faculty of Medicine. *Professional focus: oncology, radiotherapy, management of breast and colorectal cancer.*

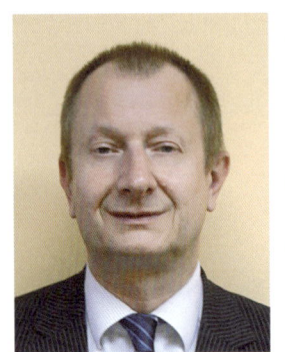

**Assoc. Prof. Miloslav Roček, MD, PhD, FCIRSE, EBIR**

The Head of the Department of Imaging Methods, 2nd Faculty of Medicine, Charles University Prague and University Hospital Motol. The President of the Committee of the Czech Society of Intervention Radiology, Section of Pediatric Radiology CzMA JEP, member of the Committee of the Czech Society for Vascular Access, Czech Society for Radiology and Czech Society of Angiology CzMA JEP and a member of SCIVR, CIRSE, ESCR. Member of the editorial board of European Journal of Vascular Medicine. *Professional focus: endovascular intervention.*

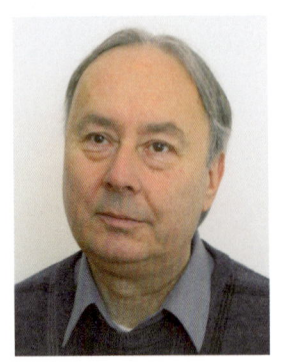

**Jan Schwarz, MD**

Assistant Professor, the Department of Surgery, 2nd Faculty of Medicine, Charles University Prague and University Hospital Motol. *Professional focus: gastrointestinal surgery, surgical endoscopy.*

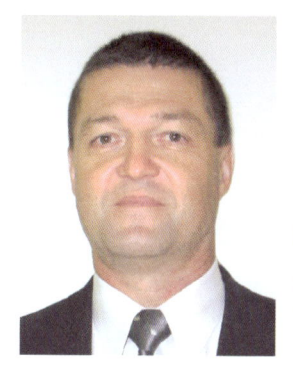

**Jiří Svoboda, MD**

The Head of the Department of Surgery, Regional Hospital Příbram. *Professional focus: miniinvasive surgery, abdominal and gastrointestinal surgery, advanced laparoscopy.*

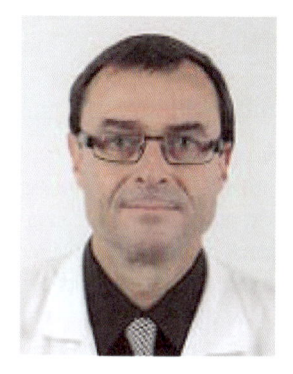

**Assoc. Prof. Marek Šetina, MD, PhD**

The Head of the Complex Cardiovascular Center, General University Hospital, Prague. Member of the Czech Society for Cardiovascular Surgery, Czech Society of Cardiology, European Association for Cardio-Thoracic Surgery, Society of Thoracic Surgerons, Mayo Alumni. Member of the editorial board of the journal Intervention and Acute Cardiology. *Professional focus: cardiac valves reconstruction, minimally invasive video thoracoscopy in cardiovascular surgery.*

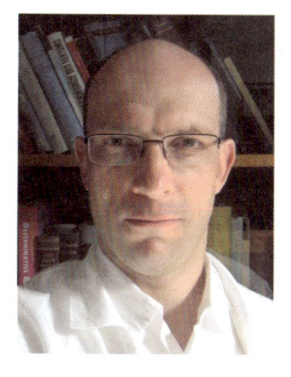

**Assoc. Prof. Jaromír Šimša, MD, PhD**

The Head of the Department of Surgery, 1st Faculty of Medicine and Thomayer Hospital, Prague. The Chair of the Section of Young Surgeons of the Czech Surgical Society CzMA JEP. *Professional focus: surgical oncology, detection of lymphatic system affection.*

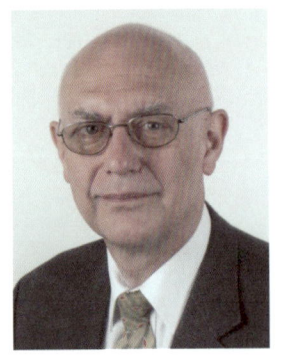

### Jaroslav Špatenka, MD, PhD

The Head of the Transplant Centre, University Hospital Motol. Member of several both Czech and foregin professional societies, member of the EATB Board (European Association of Tissue Banks), member of the Board of the Czech Transplant Society. *Professional focus: kidney transplant and HD access in children, banking, and use of cardiac valve alotransplants, transplant of chest organs.*

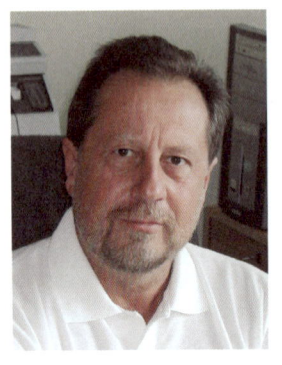

### Assoc. Prof. Michal Tichý, MD, PhD

The Head of the Department of Neurosurgery, University Hospital Motol. Member of several Czech professional societies, member of European asociation of Pediatric Neurosurgery, member of International Association of Pediatric Neurosurgery, member of the Committee for Pediatric Neurosurgery of the World Federation of Neurosurgery Societies. *Professional focus: neurooncology, congenital abnormalities of CNS, surgical treatment of epilepsy and spasticity.*

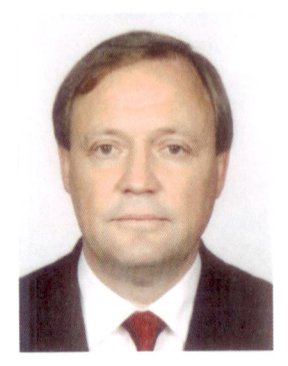

### Martin Wald, MD, PhD

Assistant Professor, the Department of Surgery, 2nd Faculty of Medicine, Charles University Prague and University Hospital Motol. Science secretary of the Czech Society for Lymphology. Member of the European and of the World Societies of Lymphology, German Society of Surgery, national delegate of European Journal of Lymphology and Related Problems. *Professional focus: mammology, diagnostics and surgical treatment of lymphedema.*

*By the time the third Czech editition of the Textbook of Surgery had been completed, all the authors were members of the University Hospital Motol staff.*

# INDEX

# INDEX

## A

abdominal aorta
– affections *284*
– aneurysm *284*
– – treatment *285*
– closure of the bifurcation *282, 285*
abdominal trauma *242*
– blunt *245*
abdominal wall *89*
– contusions *242*
– developmental defects *95*
– iatrogenic injuries *244*
– penetrating injuries *243*
abscess *36*
– brain *343*
– breast *64*
– perianal and periproctal *152, 153*
accessory breast *65*
acid-base homeostasis *399*
acute abdomen *127, 210*
– biochemical serum assessments *216*
– blood count *216*
– classification *211*
– diagnostics *212*
– differential diagnostics *218*
– endoscopy *217*
– imaging assessments *216*
– laparoscopy *217*
– non trauma based *211*
– per rectum examination *215*
– physical examination *214*
– pseudosurgical abdominal events *219*
– supplementary and auxiliary assessments *215*
– trauma based *211*
– urine assessment *216*
adenoma *32*
adhesions *137*
adjustable gastric band *394*
afferent loop syndrome *123*
achalasia *98*
– risk of tumor development *99*
achlorhydria *113*
alcohol *191*

alkaline reflux gastritis *123*
allograft
– arterial *267*
– venous *267*
allotransplantation *361*
analgesia *421*
– continuous epidural *429*
– patient controlled *429*
– postoperative *429*
analgosedation *421*
analysis of nucleic acids *448*
anastomosis *268*
– blockage *122*
anemia *109*
anesthesia *421*
– anesthetic plan *425*
– ASA classification *425*
– body temperature *427*
– caudal *422*
– consultation prior to the procedure *424*
– epidural *422*
– intravenous local *423*
– outpatient *428*
– peroperative provisions and administration *426*
– pharmaceuticals *423*
– postoperative *428*
– premedication *426*
– preoperative period *424*
– preparing the patient for surgery *426*
– selection *425*
– spinal *422*
– subarachnoid *422*
– techniques *421*
– wakes up *428*
anesthesiologist, collective cooperation *429*
aneurysm *275*
– aortic *317*
– false *276*
– of the left ventricle *308*
– thoracic *317*
angiology, invasive *265*
angioplasty *273*
antiaggregant therapy *416*

# INDEX

antibiotic prophylaxis  405, 411, 412
antibiotic therapy  405, 409
anticoagulation therapy  295
antithrombotic prophylaxis  413
anus  126, 150
- benign affections  154
- surgeries  157
- tumors  155
anusitis
- fissure  154
- prolapse  154
- sphincter incontinence  154
aortic arch branches  277
aortic coarctation  324
aortic dissection
- type A  319
- type B  319
aphonia  31
appendectomy, laparoscopic  260
appendix  138
- insufficiency of the stub  260
- perforated  140
arachnoid cysts  340, 341
argon-plasma coagulation  358
arrhythmias, surgical therapy  319
arteries
- arteria femoralis communis
- - acute closure  283
- arteria femoralis profunda, reconstruction  287
- arteria poplitea
- - acute closure  283
- - affection  289
- - aneurysm  290
- - injuries  275
- - renal  290
- - supplying intestines  291
- - supplying lower limbs  282
- - supplying the upper limbs  280
- - acute arterial closures  280
- - chronic affection  280
arteriotomy  276
arteriovenous fistula  276
arteriovenous malformation  346
artificial vascular replacements  267
ascendent aorta, injuries  323
ascites  183
atherosclerosis  290
atresia of the colon  140
atrial fibrillation  319
atrium septum defect  324

autograft  316
- arterial  267
- venous  266
autoimmune diseases, surgical therapy  30
autopsy  445
autotransplantation  361
axillary lymphadenectomy  71

# B

bacterial flora  126
bariatric surgery  392
Barrett's esophagus  101
basal impression  338
basal invagination  338
Bentall operation  318
bezoars  116
bile acids  126
bile duct  171
- cysts  176
- strictures  176
bile duct diseases  *see* gallbladder and bile duct diseases
biliary colic  172
biliary ileus  172
biliopancreatic diversion  394
biodegradable anastomotic rings  360
biological therapy  455
biopsy  447
biotin  126
bleeding
- from esophageal varices  252
- in the GIT  249
- in the subarachnoid space  346
- occult  130
- postoperative  31
- surgical patients  417
blood gases  399
blood pressure  181, 311, 397
blotting techniques  448
body mass index (BMI)  391
brain abscess  343
brain diseases, vascular  344
brain injuries  329
- commotion  330
- diffusion axonal  331
- primary  330
brain tumors  347
- brain-stem  354
- cerebellar  353

579

- craniopharyngioma *351*
- extradural *355*
- glial *348*
- hemispheral *348*
- hypophyseal adenomas *350*
- intradural *355*
- meningeomas *349*
- midline and intraventricular *349*
- pineal region *350*
- pontocerebellar angle *352*
- sellar region *350*
- visual tract *352*

Braun's entero-enteroanastomosis *121*
breast cancer
- complications of surgical therapy *74*
- examination of the sentinel lymph nodes *389*
- medical surveillance after therapy *76*
- prognosis *74*
- therapy *71*
- TNM classification *70*

breast conserving surgery *72*
breast disease
- classification *63*
- diagnosis
- - biopsy *69*
- - breast lump *66*
- - clinical examination *66*
- - cytology *69*
- - deformation *67*
- - discharge *68*
- - histopathological and immunohistochemical assessment *69*
- - imaging methods *68*
- - laboratory assessments *69*
- - medical history *65*
- - pain *67*
- - reddening and edema *67*

breast incisions *71*
breast lump *66*
breast reconstruction *77*
bronchiectasis *53*
Brunner's glands *108*
buess surgical rectoscope *360*
bypass
- aortobifemoral *286*
- aortocoronary *301*
- femoropopliteal *287, 290*

# C

CA 19-9 *130, 149, 189, 200*
calcium serum levels *24*
Calot's triangle *259*
capnography *398*
capnometry *398*
carbuncle *20*
carcinoid syndrome *136*
carcinoma *see also* tumor
- anaplastic *27*
- follicular *27*
- medullar *27*
- papillary *27*

cardiac failure *304*
cardiac rupture with tamponade *322*
cardiac surgery *298*
- history and present days *298*
- mini-invasive procedures *320*
- preoperative examinations *301*
- surgical approaches *302*

cardioplegic solution *300*
Caroli's syndrome *167*
carpal tunnel syndrome *338*
caudal syndrome *336*
C-cells producing calcitonin *443*
cells
- G cells *108*
- chief *107*
- mucous *108*
- parietal *107*

central venous catheters *471*
cerebrovascular accident *277*
cervical ribs *34*
cervico-cranial anomalies *338*
circulatory instability *235*
circumscriptive myxedema *26*
cirrhosis *260*
clinical-pathological correlation *456*
clinical-pathological seminars *446*
CNS, infectious disease *342*
coagulation set *258*
colitis
- ischemic *145*
- ulcerative *143*

collection of organs *364*
colon
- mesenchymal tumors *146*
- perfusion disorder *145*

colonoscopy *254*
coma *27*
compartment syndrome *273*

# INDEX

comprehensive decongestive therapy *76*
compressive neck syndromes *34*
computed tomography (CT) *69*
congenital anorectal malformations *151*
congenital heart defects *323*
consciousness, monitoring *399*
constriction syndromes *338*
coronary artery disease *302*
– clinical symptoms *304*
– coronary bypass *305*
– – off-pump technique *307*
– diagnostics
– – CT angiography *304*
– – selective coronarography *304*
– therapy *304*
cranial osteomyelitis *344*
craniocerebral injuries *328*
craniopharyngioma *351*
C-reactive protein *189*
cricopharyngeal dysfunction *96*
Crohn's disease *132*
– complications *133*
– large intestine *143*
– prognosis *135*
– therapy *134*
crural circulation *283*
– affection *290*
CT assessment *109*
curttage/excisioen of the tissue *447*
cystic hygroma colli *20*

## D

Dandy-Walker complex *338*
deep venous circulation of the thigh and crus
– affection *294*
– chronic closures *294*
– phlebothrombosis *294*
degenerative spinal disorders *335*
Department of Anesthesiology and Resuscitation *396*
desmoid *95*
devascularization procedures *118*
diabetes mellitus *393*
digestion *126*
disseminated intravascular coagulopathy *418*
diverticula *254 see also* esophagus, diverticula
diverticulitis *141*

diverticulosis *141*
double bypass *305*
drainage *42*
– of the pancreatic area *194*
ductography, in breast disease diagnosis *68*
dumping syndrome *123*
duodenotomy *116*
dysphagia *103*

## E

ECG curve *397*
ecchymosis *329*
efferent loop syndrome *122*
EGFR receptor in tumor cells *455*
electrosurgical (electrocoagulation) units *358*
embolectomy *272*
embolism *271*, *277*
– in superior mesenteric artery *157*
– treatment *272*
embolization *470*
emulsifying fats *171*
en bloc resection of the lymph nodes *27*
endocrine orbitopathy *26*
endoscopes, flexible *255*
endoscopic procedures
– hemostasis *109*, *184*, *250*, *251*
– injuries *245*
– papillotomy *174*
– retrograde cholangiopancreatography *193*, *466*
– sonography *109*
endostapler *263*
energy requirement in critically patients *403*
epidural abscess *343*
epilepsy
– surgical therapy *356*
– – anteromedial temporal resections *356*
– – extratemporal resection *357*
– – stimulation of the nervus vagus *357*
epileptosurgical procedures *356*
esophageal injury, perforation *99*
esophageal spasm *96*
esophageal varices, bleeding *183*
– nonsurgical treatment *184*
– prophylaxis of relapses *186*
– surgical treatments *185*
esophagogastroduodenoscopy *109*

esophagus *61*
– adenocarcinoma *103*
– achalasias *98*
– bleeding *100*
– burns *100*
– diverticula *97*
– – epiphrenic *97*
– – pulsion *97*
– – traction *97*
– – Zenker's *97*
– motility disorders *96*
– squamous cell carcinoma *103*
– tumors *102*
– – actinotherapy *105*
– – chemotherapy *105*
– – radical surgery *104*
exenteration of the axilla *73*
extracorporeal circulation, machine *300*

## F

familial adenomatous polyposis *146*, *440*
fast-track concept *402*
fat necrosis of the breast *64*
fever *26*, *235*
fibrocystic mastopathy *64*
fibromatosis *95*
fistulae *153*
fistulectomy *153*
fistulotomy *153*
flow cytometry *448*
fluidothorax *see* pleural effusion
Fogarty catheter *272*
folic acid *126*
fractionation *434*
frozen tissue *451*
functional hepatic circulation *181*
fundoplication, according to Nissen-Rossetti *102*
furuncles *20*

## G

gallbladder *171*
gallbladder and bile duct diseases *172*
– basic surgical *177*
– clinical findings *173*
– imaging methods *174*
– laboratory assessments *173*
– prognosis *179*
– treatment *175*
– tumorous *176*
Gardner's syndrome *146*
gas and stool stoppage *213*
gastrectomy
– subtotal *115*, *121*
– total *114*, *121*
gastric evacuation disorders *199*
gastric resection *112*, *118*
– Roux-en-Y anastomosis *120*
– type I *119*
– type II *119*
gastric tumors *113*
– classification according to Laurint *113*
– TNM classification *114*
gastritis *109*
– diffuse antral *110*
– focal atrophic *110*
– chronic *113*
– chronic diffuse *110*
gastroduodenal surgeries
– complications *122*
– local *116*
gastroduodenal ulcer disease
– complications *112*
– surgical therapy *111*
gastroduodenum, examinations *109*
gastroenteroanastomoses *118*
gastrostomy, according to Witzel *118*
gastrotomy *116*, *117*
G cells *108*
generalized inflammatory response *191*
giarrhea *213*
GIT hemorrhage *249*
– aorto-enteral fistula *253*
– lower *254*
– pharmacotherapy *252*
– therapy *250*
– tumors *253*, *254*
– upper *251*
– urgent endoscopy *250*
GIT passage disorders *212*
GIT surgeries, using a thoracic approach *61*
Glasgow coma scale *330*
goiters
– diffuse *25*
– endemic *24*
– eufunctional *24*
– nodular *28*
– surgical therapy *28*
goiter size stages (WHO) *23*

# INDEX

Graser's diverticula *131*
gynecomasty *65*

## H

H2-receptor blockers *111*
harmonic (ultrasound) scalpel *358*
heart contusion *322*
heart injuries *321*
– blunt injuries *321*
– penetrating *322*
heart transplantation *321*
Helicobacter pylori *109*
hematemesis *109*, *213*, *249*
hematochesis *109*, *249*
hematoma
– epidural *331*
– intracerebral *345*
– subdural *332*
hemicolectomy *263*
hemodialysis *296*
hemodynamically stable *246*
hemorrhage, subarachnoid *346*
hemorrhagic shock *249*
hemorrhoids *254*
– external *152*
– internal *151*
hemothorax *46*, *59*
heparin *280*, *300*, *415*
– low-molecular-weight *415*, *470*
hepatic insufficiency *417*
hepaticojejunoanastomosis according to Roux *176*
hereditary breast and ovarian cancer syndrome *441*, *442*
hereditary non-polyposis colorectal cancer *147*, *439*
hernias *89*
– accreted *91*
– acquired *90*
– classification *89*
– clinical aspects *90*
– complications *90*
– congenital *90*
– diaphragmatic *105*
– external, internal *89*
– femoral *92*
– foramen of winslow *94*
– incarceration *90*
– – Richter's *90*
– – W-shaped Maydl's *90*

– inflammations *94*
– inguinal *92*
– – laparoscopic solution *261*
– in scars *94*
– internal *94*
– irreponible *90*
– mixed *106*
– paraesophageal *105*
– perivesical *94*
– reponible *90*
– scrotal *92*
– sliding *90*
– sliding hiatal *105*
– therapy *91*
– Treitz's *94*
– tumors *94*
– umbilical *93*
– ventral *94*
hiccups *see* singultus
Hippocratic elastic ligature *154*
Hirschsprung's disease *140*
histopathological examination *446*
hoarseness *31*
homograft *316*
hydrocephalus *341*
hydrothorax *43*
hypercalcemia *33*
hyperparathyrosis *32*
– primary *32*
– secondary *33*
– tertiary *34*
hyperperistalsis *196*
hyperplasia *32*
hyperthyroidism *23*, *25*
hypothyroidism *23*

## Ch

Chagas disease *98*
Charcot's triad *173*
Chiari malformation *339*
cholecystectomy *175*
– conventional *177*
– laparoscopic *178*, *258*
cholecystolithiasis *172*, *258*
choledocholithiasis *172*
choledocholithotomy *259*
cholelithiasis *175*, *191*
chronic arterial closures *274*
chylothorax *46*

## I

icterus (jaundice) *163*, *201*
idiopathic esophageal dilatation *98*
idiopathic proctocolitis *143*
ileofemoral thrombosis *293*
ileus *220*, *222*
- classification *220*
- colonoscopy *227*
- diagnostics *224*
- examination *225*
- functional *221*
- imaging methods *225*
- laboratory assessments *227*
- large intestinal *222*
- obstruction *220*
- paralytic *221*
- spastic *221*
- state *149*
- symptomatology *223*
- therapy
- – conservative *228*
- – surgical *228*
- vascular *221*
immunohistochemical methods *448*
immunoprophylaxis *419*
immunosuppression *387*
infection *405*
- content of pathological cavities *408*
- foreign material *408*
- microbiological diagnostics *407*
- nosocomial *406*
- post-splenectomy *419*
- primary sterile body fluids *408*
- skin and soft tissues *407*
- splenectomy *419*
- surgical site infection *405*
- – diagnostics *407*
- – risk factors *407*
- wounds and defects *407*
inflammations *20*, *63*
inflammatory gallbladder disease *175*
inguinal hernioplasty, laparoscopic *261*
injuries
- blunt *276*
- deceleration *276*
- of the posterior wall of the artery *275*
- of the soft skull covers *328*
- to soft tissues of the thoracic wall *59*
- trocar *257*
insertion of an intragastric balloon *393*

insulinomas *203*
insulin secretion *187*
intensive care *395*
intervertebral disk *336*
intestinal content *126*
intestinal diseases
- diagnosis
- – angiography *129*
- – CT assessment *129*
- – defecography *129*
- – endoscopy *129*
- – laboratory methods *130*
- – magnetic resonance imaging *130*
- – physical examination *128*
- – radiography *128*
- – ultrasound examination *129*
- symptoms *127*
intestinal obstruction *142*, *149*
- postoperational *221*
- prognosis *230*
- therapy *227*
intestinal vascular events *157*
intestinal vascular supply *125*
intestine *see* large/small intestine
intestines *157*
intra-abdominal abscesses *240*
intracranial hypertension *330*
intrathoracic procedures *278*
irigography *128*
irrigation and suction systems *258*
ischemic problems in the upper limbs *277*

## K

Klatskin tumors *177*

## L

laparoscopic colorectal procedures *262*
large intestine *125*
- congenital anomalies *140*
- Crohn's disease *143*
- diverticular disease *141*
- tumors *145*, *147*
- – complication *149*
- – palliative procedures *149*
- – therapy *149*
- – TNM classification *148*
large vein affections *291*
large vessel affections

INDEX

– central (intrathoracal) *277*
– peripheral *278*
large vessel injuries *275*
lavage of the abdominal *175*
leiomyosarcoma *79*
lentigo maligna *83*
Lerich syndrome *285*
LigaSureTM *359*
liposarcoma *79*
liver disease *163, 373*
– abscess *167*
– basic laboratory assessments *165*
– benign *166*
– cell adenoma *168*
– CT assessment *166*
– cystadenoma *167*
– cysts *166*
– focal nodular hyperplasia *168*
– hemangioma *168*
– hepatocellular carcinoma *169*
– Child-Pugh classification *165*
– cholangiogenic carcinoma *169*
– cholangiolithiasis *167*
– imaging methods *165*
– malignoma *169*
– metastases *169*
– parasitary cysts *167*
– ultrasonography *165*
liver injuries *245*
– complications *248*
– diagnostics *245*
– symptoms *245*
– therapy *246, 247*
liver, surgical anatomy *164*
liver transplantation *186*
lobectomy, total *30*
lumbar spine disease *336*
lumen of the vessel *318*
lungs
– anatomical notes *47*
– examination methods *48*
– inflammatory diseases *52*
– types of surgical operations *53*
lung tuberculosis *53*
lymphadenopathy *20*
lymphatic system
– insufficiency *see* lymphedema
– intestinal *125*
lymph drainage *76*
lymphedema *67, 74, 76, 389*
lymph nodes *19*

lymphotropic patent blue *389*
Lynch syndrome *439*

## M

magnetic resonance mammography (MRM) *69*
malabsorptive operations *394*
malignant fibrous histiocytoma *79*
malignant tumors, surgical therapy *28*
Mallory-Weiss syndrome *253*
mammary dysplasia *64*
mammary gland *63, 461*
mammography *68, 461*
mastectomy
– breast reconstruction *77*
– halsted radical *72*
– modified radical *72*
mastitis *63*
mastopathy *64*
maximally sparing surgery *see* mini-invasive (minimal access) surgery
Meckel's diverticulum *131*
mediastinal flutter *41*
mediastinitis *262*
– acute *54, 99*
mediastinum
– anatomical notes *54*
– mediastinal emphysema *56*
– mediastinal tumors, Diviš classification *55*
medullary thyroid carcinoma
– correlation genotype-phenotype *444*
– gene nature *444*
meduloblastoma *354*
megacolon *141*
mechanical cardiac supports *321*
melanoblastoma *156*
melanoma *83*
– acral lentiginous *85*
– adjuvant therapy *88*
– causes *85*
– Clark classification *84*
– classification *83*
– diagnostics
– – ABCDE rule *86*
– – examination of regional lymph nodes *86*
– – minor symptoms *87*

- examination of the sentinel lymph nodes *389*
- follow-up examinations *88*
- lymphadenectomy *87*
- metastases extirpation *88*
- nodular *84*
- prognosis *88*
- radical surgical excision *87*
- risk factors *85*
- staging *83*
- superficial spreading *83*
- therapy *87*
- TNM classification *83, 85*

melena *109, 249*
Ménétrier's disease *116*
meningeomas *349*
Merkel cells carcinoma *390*
mesocolon *125*
metabolic syndrome *393*
meteorism *195*
mini-invasive (minimal access) surgery *256*
- disadvantage *257*
- instrumentation *258*
- insufflated gas *257*
- robotic systems *258*

minimally invasive direct coronary artery bypass *307*
molecular diagnostics at the gene level *446*
monitoring *427*
- acid-base homeostasis *399*
- blood gases *399*
- cardiovascular system *397*
- consciousness *399*
- measurement of diuresis *399*
- postoperative *396*
- respiratory rate *398*
- respiratory system *397*
- volume of drained fluids *399*

monoanesthesia *421*
mRNA expression *446*
mucosectomy *109*
Muir-Torre syndrome *439*
multi-organ harvesting *365*
- explantation *369*
- perfusion *368*
- preparation *367, 368*
- techniques *367*

multiple endocrine neoplasia
- preventive follow-up *443*
- type 1 (MEN 1) *442*
- type 2 (MEN 2) *443*

multiple organ dysfunction syndrome *233*
muscle relaxation *424*
myocardial contusion *322*
myocardial infarction
- mechanical complications *307*
myocardial necrosis *304*
myonephropatic-metabolic syndrome *274*

# N

natural orifice transluminal endoscopic surgery *264*
nausea *108, 212*
neck cysts *19*
Neisseria meningitidis *419*
nephrolithiasis *32*
nerve blocks *423*
neurological disorders after surgical therapy of breast cancer *75*
neuromuscular disorder *98*
neurosurgery *328*
neutropenia, surgical treatment *416*
Nissen-Rossetti fundoplication *262*
nutrition *400*
- enteral *400, 401*
- parenteral *402*
- perioperative *404*
- screening *400*

# O

obesity
- classification *391*
- treatment *392*

obstruction icterus *172*
occult bleeding *130*
odynophagia *103*
oliguria *235*
omphalitis *94*
omphaloenteric duct, persistent *95*
oncological treatment, multimodal *431*
- ablative therapy *435*
- biological targeted therapy *436*
- hormonal therapy *435*
- chemotherapy *433, 434*
- medical team *432*
- prognostic and predictive factors *432*

# INDEX

- radiotherapy *434*
- surgical treatment *432*

OPSI syndrome *208*

optochiasmatic-hypothalamic gliomas *352*

organ collection *362*
- cold ischemia *363, 369*
- warm ischemia *362, 368*

organ donation *365*
- cadaveric donors *366*
- living donor *366*
- marginal donors *387*

organ preservation *363*

organ transplantation *see* transplantation

osteochondrosis in the cervical area *337*

osteomyelitis of the ribs and sternum *37*

ostium secundum type defect *324*

otorrhea *329*

## P

pain
- colicky *223*
- in the epigastrium *188, 195, 199, 201*
- in the muscles *274*
- lumbar spine *337*
- of the anterior wall *235*
- peritoneal *235*
- somatic *212*
- spinal *335*
- visceral *212*

pancreatic disease
- clinical findings *188*
- cystic processes *199*
- imaging methods
- – angiography *190*
- – contrast spiral CT *189*
- – endoscopic retrograde cholangiopancreatography *190*
- – functional tests *190*
- – magnetic resonance *190*
- – percutaneous transhepatic cholangiography *190*
- – ultrasonography *189*
- laboratory assessments *189*
- symptoms *188*
- tumors *200*
- – examination methods *201*
- – palliative surgery *204*
- – therapy *203*
- – TNM classification *202*

pancreatitis
- acute *191, 193*
- chronic *195, 196*
- resection procedures *198*

pangastritis *110*

parathormone *32*

parathyroid glands *31*

parenchymatous organs, contusions *242*

paresis of the laryngeal recurrent nerve *31*

pathology *445*
- bioptic *446*
- bioptic examination after surgical procedures *450*
- collaboration with a surgeon in lymph node examination *452*
- cutting of samples *452*
- detection of diagnostically and prognostically significant molecules *454*
- examination of resected tissue after neoadjuvant therapy *453*
- examinations after organ transplantations *454*
- generalization of optimum practice *455*
- perioperative bioptic examination *448*
- photo documentation *452*
- preoperative examination *447*

pectoral muscles atrophy *75*

pelvic arteries, acute closure *282*

pelvic circulation, affection *286*

pelvic vein affections *293*

pepsin precursors *107*

peptic ulcer, Forrest classification *251*

percutaneous cholecystotomy *466*

percutaneous transhepatic cholangiography *466*

percutaneous transluminar angioplasty (PTA) *470*

perianal hidradenitis *154*

periappendicular abscess *139*

pericolic abscesses *142*

pericolic infiltrate *141, 142*

perioperative bioptic service *449*

peripheral nerve injuries *334*

peritoneum *232*

peritonitis *142*

- after irradiation (plastic) *234*
- biliary *172*
- classification *233*
- clinical symptoms *234*
- CT assessment *237*
- definition *231*
- diagnostics *236*
- diffuse biliary *260*
- indications for surgical treatment *237*
- laboratory findings *236*
- microbiological examination *234*
- native abdominal radiography *236*
- pathophysiology *232*
- primary *233*
- prognosis *241*
- secondary *233*
- tertiary *234*
- therapy
- – complications *240*
- – lavage of the abdominal cavity *239*
- – surgical *238*
- thoracic scan *236*
- tuberculous *234*
- ultrasonography *236*
peroperational cholangiography *259*
Peutz-Jeghers syndrome *146*
phlegmones *20*
plasty
- anterior *93*
- of the papilla *179*
- posterior *93*
- total extraperitoneal *93*
- transabdominal preperitoneal *93*
platybasia *338*
plenies sign *214*, *235*
pleura *39*
- effusion *43*
- malignant mesothelioma *46*
pleural tumors
- benign *46*
- malignant *46*
- TNM classification *46*
pneumothorax
- iatrogenic *41*
- open *41*, *42*
- secondary *41*
- spontaneous *40*
- tension *41*, *42*
polypectomy *109*

polyps *113*, *254*
- hamartomatous *146*
- hyperplastic *146*
- inflammatory *146*
- neoplastic *145*
polytetrafluorethylen *268*
portal hypertension *181*
- clinical findings *182*
- complications *182*, *183*
- pathophysiology *182*
- postsinusoidal *182*
- resinusoidal *181*
- sinusoidal *181*
- symptoms *182*
- transjugular intrahepatic portosystemic shunt (TIPS) *472*
portal vein thrombosis *419*
positron emission tomography (PET) *69*
postcholecystectomy syndrome *180*
postmastectomy pain syndrome *75*
postradiation brachial plexitis *75*
preservation by continuous perfusion *387*
pressure overload *309*
proctalgia fugax *154*
proton-pump inhibitors *111*
pruritus ani *154*
pseudocysts *199*
pseudosurgical abdominal events *219*
pulmonary abscess *53*
pulmonary contusion *60*
pulmonary embolism *413*
pulse oximetry *398*
puncture-lavage of the abdominal cavity *193*
pyloroplasty *116*
pyothorax *44*

## Q

Quick test
- in aortic replacement *315*
- in the mitral replacement *315*

## R

radiodiagnostics
- abdominal trauma *469*
- abdominal wall *463*
- appendicitis *464*
- esophagus *463*

- gallbladder  *466*
- gastroduodenum  *463*
- chest traumas  *460*
- chest wall  *458*
- ileus  *468*
- large intestine  *465*
- liver  *465, 466*
- lungs  *459*
- lung tumors  *460*
- lymph nodes  *457*
- mammary glands  *462*
- mammography  *461*
- mediastinum  *461*
- pancreatic tumors  *467*
- pancreatitis  *467*
- pleura  *459*
- salivary glands  *457*
- small intestine  *464*
- soft tissues  *463*
- spleen  *468*
- thyroid gland  *457*

radioiodine  *26*
radiology, interventional  *469*
- arterial  *470*
- transplanted organs  *472*
- venous  *471*
ras gene  *455*
rectum  *126, 150*
- surgeries  *157*
- tumors  *155*
reflux disease (esophagitis)  *100, 102, 262*
rejection  *384*
- immune reaction  *454*
reperfusion syndrome  *274*
retractors  *360*
rhinorrhea  *329*
rib fractures  *58, 59*
rings for reconstructions of the mitral or tricuspid valve  *316*
rotation disorders  *140*
Roux-en-Y anastomosis  *120, 121, 394*

## S

Santorini's duct  *187*
scalene syndrome  *34*
Scopinaro operation  *394*
self-expanding metal stent  *466*
sentinel lymph node  *86, 388*
- dissection  *73*
- examination  *87, 390*
- possibilities of detection  *389*
sepsis  *234*
- pathophysiology  *232*
septum defect
- atrioventricular  *325*
- ventricular  *325*
serosa  *125*
shunts  *296, 297*
- selective portosystemic  *185*
- ventriculoperitoneal  *342*
Schloffer tumor  *95*
single incision laparoscopic surgery  *264*
singultus (hiccups)  *213*
skull fractures  *328*
small intestine  *124*
- adhesions  *137*
- carcinoid  *136*
- congenital anomalies  *130*
- ileus  *222*
- tumors  *135, 136*
soft tissue tumors
- definitive resection  *80*
- diagnostics  *79*
- en bloc resection  *82*
- histological classification and specification  *82*
- chemotherapy  *82*
- incidence  *79*
- localization  *79*
- magnetic resonance imaging  *80*
- palliative purposes  *82*
- radiation therapy  *82*
- surgical treatment  *79*
- symptoms  *79*
- ultrasound examination  *80*
somnolence  *27*
specialized/surgical ICU  *395*
spine and spinal cord injuries  *333*
- classification  *334*
spleen
- anatomy  *205*
- function and physiology  *205*
- injury  *206*
- malformations  *206*
- surgery  *206*
splenectomy  *208, 419*
splenomegaly  *209*
spondylolisthesis  *337*

Staphylococcus aureus *406*
steal syndromes *277*
stenosis of the spinal canal *336*
stent graft *318*
sternal fractures *59*
stomach *107*
- inflammations *109*
strangulation *213, 221*
stridor *31*
stripping (removal) *295*
subdural empyema *343*
submucous resection *109*
subtotal resection of the thyroid gland (STE) *30*
superficial femoral artery, affection *287*
superior thoracic aperture syndrome *35*
surgery
- anesthesiology and resuscitation *420*
- bariatric *391*
- cardiac surgery *298*
- diaphragm *96*
- duodenal *107*
- esophagus *96*
- gastric *107*
- hematological issues *413*
- imaging methods *457*
- infection *405*
- intensive care *395*
- liver *163*
- mammary gland *63*
- mini-invasive *255*
- neck *19*
- neurosurgery *328*
- pancreas *187*
- small and large intestine *124*
- spleen *205*
- thoracic *35*
- vascular *265*
surgical site infections *405*
suture *116*
- surgical *118*

# T

tachycardia *26, 235*
tachypnea *235*
tension free plasty *91*
tetany *31*
tetralogy of Fallot *326*
thoracic drainage *42*
thoracic empyema *see* pyothorax

thoracic outlet syndrome *34, 281*
thoracic traumas *57*
- complications *61*
thoracic wall
- anatomical notes *35*
- benign skeletal tumors *38*
- benign tumors of soft tissues *37*
- diseases *35*
- infections *36*
- malignant primary skeletal tumors *38*
- malignant secondary skeletal tumors *39*
- malignant tumors of soft tissues *38*
- phlegmona *36*
- surgeries *39*
thoracophrenolaparotomy *61*
thoracoscopy *263*
three-artery system RIA, RC and ACD *304*
thrombocytopenia *416, 417*
thrombocytosis *419*
thrombolysis *272, 470*
thrombophlebitis, superficial *295*
thromboprophylaxis *414*
thyroid disorders
- assessment *23*
- complications of surgeries *31*
- CT examination *23*
- fine needle aspiration biopsy *24*
- indirect laryngoscopy *24*
- laboratory parameters *24*
- scintigraphy *23*
- sonography *23*
- SPECT/CT *24*
- surgical therapy *28*
- – partial procedures *30*
- – surgical procedure *30*
- symptoms *21*
thyroidectomia fere totalis *30*
thyroidectomy, total *27, 30*
thyroid gland *21, 29*
- malignant tumors *27*
thyroid inflammations *28*
thyroiditis
- acute *28*
- De Quervain subacute *28*
- Hashimoto's chronic *28*
- Riedel's fibrotizing chronic *28*
thyrostatics *26*
thyrotoxic crisis *26*
thyrotoxicosis *25*

# INDEX

– autoimmune  *25*
– autonomous  *25*, *26*
– immunogenic  *25*
thyroxine  *24*
tissue adhesives and hemostatics  *359*
TNM classification
– breast cancer  *70*
– esophagus tumors  *103*
– gallbladder tumors  *177*
– gastric tumors  *114*
– large intestine tumors  *148*
– lung tumors  *50*
– melanoma  *84*
– pancreatic tumors  *202*
– pleural tumors  *46*
– thyroid gland tumors  *27*
total extraperitoneal approach  *261*
transabdominal preperitoneal
    approach  *261*
transduodenal papillosphincterotomy  *179*
transitory ischemic attack  *277*
transjugular intrahepatic portosystemic
    stent shunting (TIPSS)  *184*
transparietal punctures, injuries  *245*
transplantation
– complications  *384*
– future  *386*
– heart  *375*
– – orthotopic  *376*
– immunosuppression  *384*
– intestinal  *384*
– kidney  *372*
– – contraindications  *371*
– – from a living donor  *373*
– – preemptive  *373*
– liver  *373*
– – contraindications  *374*
– – child recipients  *375*
– – orthotopic  *185*
– lung  *380*
– – contraindication  *381*
– – single  *382*
– multi-organ  *384*
– pancreas  *382*
transplant centers  *363*
transplantology
– history  *361*
– in today's medicine  *362*
transposition of the great arteries  *326*
triiodothyronine  *24*
trocars – ports  *258*

Trypanosoma cruzi  *98*
TSH  *24*
tumor  *20* see also carcinoma
– anus  *155*
– brain  *347*
– breast  *71*
– cardiac  *319*
– cystic  *200*
– duodenal  *115*
– esophagus  *102*
– gallbladder and extrahepatic
    pathway  *176*
– gastric  *113*
– large intestine  *145*
– lung  *49*
– malignant melanoma  *83*
– mediastinal  *55*
– pancreas  *200*
– periampullary  *203*
– pleural  *46*
– rectum  *155*
– soft tissue  *38*, *78*
– thoracic wall  *38*
– thyroid gland  *27*
tumor genetics  *437*
tumor markers  *130*
Turcot's syndrome  *146*

## U

ulcer  *110*
– duodenal  *111*
– gastric  *111*
– peptic  *131*
– therapy  *111*
ulnar sulcus syndrome  *338*
ultrasound dissector  *359*
units of intermediary care  *395*
upper dyspeptic syndrome  *108*
upper endoscopy  *114*
urachus, persistent  *95*

## V

vacuum assisted closure  *360*
vagotomy  *112*
– selective  *122*
– superselective (proximal)  *122*
– truncal  *121*
valves
– aortic

– – congenital stenosis *327*
– – insufficiency *309*
– – stenosis *308*
– – surgical therapy *310*
– biological *315*
– mechanical *315*
– mitral
– – insufficiency *312*
– – stenosis *311*
– – surgical therapy *313*
– pulmonary, isolated stenosis *327*
– tricuspid *314*
– – treatment *314*
valvular defects *308*
valvular replacements *315*
valvular surgery *302*
varices
– esophageal *100*, *183*, *252*
– spider and small *295*
– trunk *295*
– veins *265*, *295*
vascular accident
– hemorrhagic *345*
– ischemic *344*
vascular approaches for hemodialysis *296*
vascular connection *267*
vascular prostheses *267*, *318*
vascular replacement and sutures *266*
– basic methods *269*
– bypass (bridging) *269*
– endarterectomy *270*
– kinking *271*
– plastic *269*
– re-implantation *271*
– replacement *269*
– shortening *271*

vena cava filter *471*
vena cava inferior, closure *292*
vena cava superior, closure *292*
venous graft *305*
venous pressure, central *397*
venous thromboembolism, postoperative *413*
Veres security needle *259*
vestibular schwannoma *352*
video-assisted surgery, in cardiosurgery *320*
video-assisted technique *263*
video-thoracoscopic procedures, in the thoracic cavity *263*
visceral arteries *290*
vitamin K *126*
volvulus of the stomach *115*
vomiting *108*, *212*

# W

waiting lists for individual organs *365*
warfarin therapy
– before an urgent operation *415*
– preoperative management *414*
Wirsung's duct *187*
Wobenzym *76*

# X

xenotransplantation *361*, *387*

# Y

Y-Roux resection *176*